HANDBOOK OF
Mentalizing

in Mental Health Practice

SECOND EDITION

HANDBOOK OF
Mentalizing
in Mental Health Practice

SECOND EDITION

Edited by

Anthony Bateman, M.A., FRCPsych

Peter Fonagy, Ph.D., FBA, FMedSci, FAcSS

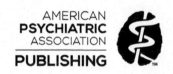

AMERICAN
PSYCHIATRIC
ASSOCIATION
PUBLISHING

American Psychiatric Association Publishing
800 Maine Avenue SW
Suite 900
Washington, DC 20024-2812
www.appi.org

Library of Congress Cataloging-in-Publication Data
Names: Bateman, Anthony, editor. | Fonagy, Peter, 1952– editor. | American
  Psychiatric Association Publishing, issuing body.
Title: Handbook of mentalizing in mental health practice / edited by Anthony
  Bateman, Peter Fonagy.
Description: Second edition. | Washington, DC : American Psychiatric
  Association Publishing, [2019] | Includes bibliographical references and
  index.
Identifiers: LCCN 2019004494 (print) | LCCN 2019005158 (ebook) | ISBN
  9781615372508 (ebook) | ISBN 9781615371402 (alk. paper)
Subjects: | MESH: Psychotherapy—methods | Mentalization
Classification: LCC RC480.5 (ebook) | LCC RC480.5 (print) | NLM WM 420 | DDC
  616.89/14—dc23
LC record available at https://lccn.loc.gov/2019004494

British Library Cataloguing in Publication Data
A CIP record is available from the British Library.

This book is dedicated to Professor George Gergely,
a clinician developmentalist,
in gratitude for inspiring all of us
who work within the mentalizing frame.

Contents

Part I
Principles

1 Introduction 3
Peter Fonagy, Ph.D., FBA, FMedSci, FAcSS
Anthony Bateman, M.A., FRCPsych

2 Contemporary Neuroscientific Research 21
Martin Debbané, Ph.D.
Tobias Nolte, M.D., M.Sc.

3 Assessment of Mentalizing 37
Patrick Luyten, Ph.D.
Saskia Malcorps, M.Sc.
Peter Fonagy, Ph.D., FBA, FMedSci, FAcSS
Karin Ensink, Ph.D., M.A. [Clin. Psych.]

4 Mentalizing, Resilience, and Epistemic Trust 63
Peter Fonagy, Ph.D., FBA, FMedSci, FAcSS
Elizabeth Allison, D.Phil.
Chloe Campbell, Ph.D.

5 Mentalizing and Trauma 79
Patrick Luyten, Ph.D.
Peter Fonagy, Ph.D., FBA, FMedSci, FAcSS

Part II
Clinical Practice

Part III
Specific Applications

CONTRIBUTORS

Elizabeth Allison, D.Phil.
Research Department of Clinical, Educational and Health Psychology, University College London

Nina Arefjord, Cand.Psychol.
Specialist in Clinical Psychology. The Bergen Clinics Foundation, Norway

Eia Asen, M.D.
Consultant Psychiatrist, Anna Freud National Centre for Children and Families, London

Dawn Bales, Ph.D.
MBT Specialism Lead, Viersprong Institute for Studies on Personality Disorders

Anthony Bateman, M.A., FRCPsych
Visiting Professor, University College London; Affiliate Professor in Psychotherapy, Copenhagen University; Consultant to Anna Freud National Centre for Children and Families, London

Dickon Bevington, M.A., M.B.B.S., MRCPsych, PGCert
Medical Director, Anna Freud National Centre for Children and Families, London; Consultant in Child and Adolescent Psychiatry, Cambridgeshire and Peterborough NHS Foundation Trust, Cambridge, United Kingdom

Efrain Bleiberg, M.D.
Professor, Menninger Department of Psychiatry and Behavioral Sciences, Baylor College of Medicine, Houston, Texas

Chloe Campbell, Ph.D.
Research Department of Clinical, Educational and Health Psychology, University College London

Martin Debbané, Ph.D.
Associate Professor, Faculty of Psychology and Educational Sciences, University of Geneva; Department of Psychiatry, University of Geneva School of Medicine, Switzerland; Research Department of Clinical, Educational and Health Psychology, University College London

Karin Ensink, Ph.D., M.A. [Clin Psych]
Professor, École de Psychologie, Université Laval, Québec, Canada

Sebastian Euler, M.D.
Head of Department for Consultation, Liaison and Emergency Psychiatry and Senior
Researcher, University Hospital Zürich, Switzerland

Peter Fonagy, Ph.D., FBA, FMedSci, FAcSS
Professor of Contemporary Psychoanalysis and Developmental Science, University
College London; Chief Executive, Anna Freud National Centre for Children and Families, London

Peter Fuggle, Ph.D.
Clinical Director, Anna Freud National Centre for Children and Families, London

Thorsten-Christian Gablonski, Dipl.-Psych.
Research Assistant, Institute for Psychosocial Prevention, Heidelberg University,
Germany, and Institute for Psychology, Alpen-Adria-Universität Klagenfurt, Austria

Sune Bo Hansen, Cand.Psych.Aut., Ph.D.
Psychiatric Research Unit, Region Zealand, Slagelse, Denmark

Dominik Havsteen-Franklin, Ph.D.
Professor, Department of Arts and Humanities, Brunel University London, United
Kingdom

Mickey Kongerslev, M.Sc., Ph.D.
Head of the Centre of Excellence for Personality Disorder, Psychiatric Research Unit,
Region Zealand; Adjunct Associate Professor, Department of Psychology, University
of Southern Denmark, Slagelse, Denmark

Alessandra Lemma, M.A., M.Phil., D.Clin.Psych.
Professor, Anna Freud National Centre for Children and Families; Visiting Professor,
University College London

Karin Lindqvist, M.Sc.
Clinical Psychologist, The Erica Foundation, Stockholm, Sweden

Kari Lossius, Cand.Psychol.
Specialist in Clinical Psychology, The Bergen Clinics Foundation, Norway

Patrick Luyten, Ph.D.
Professor, Faculty of Psychology and Educational Sciences, KU Leuven; Research Department of Clinical, Educational and Health Psychology, University College London

Norka Malberg, Psy.D., LPC, Ed.M., M.S.
Assistant Clinical Professor, Yale Child Study Center, New Haven, Connecticut

Saskia Malcorps, M.Sc.
Faculty of Psychology and Educational Sciences, KU Leuven, Belgium

Nick Midgley, Ph.D.
Co-Director, Child Attachment and Psychological Therapies Research Unit (ChAPTRe),
Anna Freud National Centre for Children and Families/University College London

Katharina Morken, Cand.Psychol., Ph.D.
Specialist in Clinical Psychology. The Bergen Clinics Foundation, Norway

Anna Motz, B.A., C.Foren.Psychol., DipClinPsych
Consultant Clinical and Forensic Psychologist, Family Assessment and Safeguarding Service, Oxford, England

Nicole Muller, M.Sc.
Children and Youth Psychotherapist and Family Therapist, CAMHS De Jutters, The Hague, The Netherlands

Tobias Nolte, M.D., M.Sc.
Clinical Research Associate, The Wellcome Centre for Human Neuroimaging, University College London, and Anna Freud National Centre for Children and Families, London

Sheila Redfern, Ph.D.
Consultant Clinical Psychologist and Head of Specialist Clinical Services: Trauma and Maltreatment (STAMS), Anna Freud National Centre for Children and Families, London

Paul Robinson, M.D., FRCP, FRCPsych
Principal Teaching Fellow, Division of Medicine, University College London

Trudie Rossouw, M.B.Ch.B., F.F.Psych., MRCPsych, M.D. (Res)
Consultant Child and Adolescent Psychiatrist, The Priory Hospital North London, United Kingdom

Ellen Safier, M.S.W., LCSW
Clinical Assistant Professor, Menninger Department of Psychiatry and Behavioral Sciences, Baylor College of Medicine, Houston, Texas

Carla Sharp, Ph.D.
Professor and Director of Clinical Training, Department of Psychology, University of Houston, Texas

Sebastian Simonsen, Ph.D.
Senior Researcher and Clinical Psychologist, Psykoterapeutisk Center Stolpegård, Denmark

Finn Skårderud, M.D., Ph.D.
Psychiatrist, Institutt for Mentalisering, Oslo, Norway

Mary Target, M.Sc., Ph.D.
Professor, Research Department of Clinical, Educational and Health Psychology, University College London

Svenja Taubner, Prof. Dr. Phil.
Director, Institute for Psychosocial Prevention, Heidelberg University, Germany

Brandon Unruh, M.D.
Instructor in Psychiatry, McLean Hospital, Harvard Medical School, Belmont, Massachusetts

Jessica Yakeley, M.B. B.Chir., MRCP, FRCPsych
Consultant Psychiatrist in Forensic Psychotherapy; Director of the Portman Clinic and Director of Medical Education, Tavistock & Portman NHS Foundation Trust, London

Disclosures of Interest

The following contributors to this textbook have indicated a financial interest in or other affiliation with a commercial supporter, manufacturer of a commercial product, and/or provider of a commercial service as listed below:

Anthony Bateman, M.A., FRCPsych   receives honoraria for MBT training and for lectures on related topics, and receives royalties from books including books on mentalizing.

Dickon Bevington, M.A., M.B.B.S., MRCPsych, PGCert   receives royalties from a book published on AMBIT (*Adaptive Mentalization-Based Integrative Treatment: A Guide for Teams to Develop Systems of Care*, by Bevington D, Fuggle P, Cracknell L, and Fonagy P, Oxford University Press, 2017) and is employed by the Anna Freud National Centre for Children and Families, from which charitable organization AMBIT trainings are delivered, though without direct financial benefit to the author who is in a salaried post.

Peter Fonagy, Ph.D., FBA, FMedSci, FAcSS   is Chief Executive of the Anna Freud National Centre for Children and Families, London, UK, which benefits from short courses and training programs it provides in relation to a range of mentalization-based treatments; he holds research grants on mentalizing-related research at University College London, which bring research income to the university.

Patrick Luyten, Ph.D.   has been involved in the development, evaluation, training, and dissemination of mentalization-based treatments.

Brandon Unruh, M.D.   receives royalty payments from Springer Publishing for a book on borderline personality disorder.

The following contributors stated that they had no competing interests during the year preceding manuscript submission:

Elizabeth Allison, D.Phil.; Nina Arefjord, Cand.Psychol.; Eia Asen, M.D.; Dawn Bales, Ph.D.; Efrain Bleiberg, M.D.; Chloe Campbell, Ph.D.; Martin Debbané, Ph.D.; Karin Ensink, Ph.D., M.A. [Clin Psych]; Sebastian Euler, M.D.; Peter Fuggle, Ph.D.; Thorsten-Christian Gablonski, Dipl.-Psych.; Sune Bo Hansen, Cand.Psych.Aut., Ph.D.; Dominik Havsteen-Franklin, Ph.D.; Mickey Kongerslev, M.Sc., Ph.D.; Alessandra Lemma, M.A., M.Phil., D.Clin.Psych.; Karin Lindqvist, M.Sc.; Kari Lossius, Cand.Psychol.; Norka Malberg, Psy.D., LPC, Ed.M., M.S.; Saskia Malcorps, M.Sc.; Nick Midgley, Ph.D.; Katharina Morken, Cand.Psychol., Ph.D.; Anna Motz, B.A., C.Foren.Psychol., DipClinPsych; Nicole Muller, M.Sc.; Tobias Nolte, M.D., M.Sc.; Sheila Redfern, Ph.D.; Paul Robinson, M.D., FRCP, FRCPsych; Trudie Rossouw, M.B.Ch.B., F.F.Psych., MRCPsych, M.D. (Res); Ellen Safier, M.S.W., LCSW; Carla Sharp, Ph.D.; Sebastian Simonsen, Ph.D.; Finn Skårderud, M.D., Ph.D.; Mary Target, M.Sc., Ph.D.; Svenja Taubner, Prof. Dr. Phil.; Jessica Yakeley, M.B. B.Chir., MRCP, FRCPsych

PREFACE

The aim of the first edition of this book was to summarize how the concept of mentalizing and its application in clinical work were influencing and changing mental health practice. Much has happened over the 7 years since the first edition was published in terms of our understanding of mentalizing and its use in clinical practice. This inevitably means that this book bears only a limited resemblance to the previous edition, even though its aim is the same: to summarize the current state of clinical and research work on mentalization-based approaches in mental health practice. All the chapters have been rewritten, the book has been reorganized, and many new authors have contributed to it. For the editors, this is of course highly gratifying. These changes reflect a vibrant field undergoing significant development along a number of dimensions that are important for mental health. First, the range of mental disorders for which the mentalization-based treatment (MBT) approach has been found to be helpful has substantially increased and now includes psychosis. Yet there is further to go, with only limited research to date in learning disability and autistic spectrum disorder, for example. Alongside this expansion, there has been an increase in the range of contexts within which the approach has been shown to be of value. Beyond its origins in partial hospitalization (i.e., day hospitals in Europe), MBT as a guiding framework has been found to be useful in outpatient and community settings, and in the broader context of children, adolescents, couples, and families, and the social contexts where we find them, such as schools and even prisons.

Perhaps more important than the extension of clinical reach and intervention domains is the generalizability of the framework to an understanding of the social context of mental health. The model advanced in this book goes beyond an understanding of the development of mentalizing and its vicissitudes and aims to provide an understanding of the role of mentalizing in a range of social processes. These encompass relationships between parents and children, the experience of childhood adversity, the nature of learning nested in interpersonal communication, and, most ambitiously, an understanding of the emergence and maintenance of mental disorder. In case this is mistaken for hubris, neither the editors nor any of the authors of these chapters suggest that mentalizing provides an adequate account of such a massive range of issues. However, we do feel that mentalizing is so central to the human condition that for it to have no role in such key social processes is improbable.

The ambition of this book is therefore threefold. First, to be useful to practitioners, regardless of their model of practice, to enable them to take a mentalizing perspective to whatever their objective may be in relation to their work. Second, to outline some coherent and tried-and-tested approaches to the treatment of some common and generally hard-to-treat conditions for which MBT may provide a genuine, effective alternative. Third, and present in all the chapters without exception, to outline a conceptual frame that may help focus all our minds on this all-important facet of our uniquely human existence—that of imagining ourselves and others as behaving in line with beliefs and feelings, and the thoughts and wishes they generate. It is this facet that may be critical to maintaining a stance to one another that is based on a capacity to imagine that others think, feel, and suffer just as we do.

The extensive application of mentalizing and its influence in clinical services is remarkable and bears some explanation. First, mentalizing is a transdiagnostic concept and so is applicable to a range of mental health conditions. This is illustrated by a series of chapters on different conditions, including trauma (Chapter 5), personality disorders (Chapters 19–21), eating disorders (Chapter 22), depression (Chapter 23), substance use disorder (Chapter 24), and psychosis (Chapter 25). Second, focusing on mentalizing helps people consider how teams, systems, and services interact to facilitate or undermine interventions and the delivery of services; a nonmentalizing team and system has a negative impact on clinical care by creating an environment that impedes the implementation of reliable and responsive pathways to care and the realization of skillful treatment. So, in this book, we consider mentalizing and teams (Chapter 13) and mentalizing and wider systems (Chapter 14). Third, there is increasing empirical research on the developmental origins of mentalizing and how a focus on mentalizing can improve outcomes for patients. All the chapters in this book outline some of the research related to the topic under discussion. This aims to persuade clinicians to integrate mentalizing into their clinical practice, using many of the techniques described to enhance mentalizing (see Chapters 6–8, for example). How a focus on mentalizing increases resilience to adversity, perhaps protecting individuals from relapse, and improves therapeutic outcomes is discussed in Chapters 4 and 10, respectively. Finally, its position as a well-developed component of the literature on neurobiology and higher-order cognition (see Chapter 2) and its central place in research on child and adolescent development (see Chapters 15–18) mean that mentalizing benefits from a number of different strands of research, ranging from neurobiology through child development to adult psychopathology. We hope that this second edition of *Handbook of Mentalizing in Mental Health Practice* captures all these strands and brings them together in a coherent manner. We have tried to reduce repetition between chapters, but it is likely that we have missed some examples, for which we apologize. At least our worry can be mollified by the knowledge that repetition is a driver of learning.

All concepts related to higher-order cognition, such as mentalizing, refer to information-processing mechanisms that do not rely on a static, fixed set of specialized brain regions and fixed neuroanatomical connections. Higher-order cognition is thought to operate by optimizing neural resources and creating routes between processing systems. Normally, neural networks are believed to manifest collective behaviors, which become apparent in second- or higher-order parameters coming to govern contextual information-processing modes. The core distinguishing feature of these hypothetical constructs is that they relate to brain structure as a hierarchy of layers of abstraction and assume a top-down influence on lower orders of this neural pyramid.

All the above concepts assume that a process, something like self-awareness, can dynamically control local biophysical and biochemical parameters to facilitate access to particular processing units, which have physical locations, and simplify the control of the complex device that is the brain, functioning as an information-processing system. In this type of conceptualization, we assume that the brain functions as some kind of interpreter of code and that mentalizing occurs in a kind of virtual workspace. In their chapter on the neurobiology of mentalizing (Chapter 2), Debbané and Nolte go beyond these elaborations of the neuroscience of mentalizing and review cognitive, developmental, and affective neuroscience findings, as well as exciting new findings based on the computational approach to neuroscience. New neuroscientific paths are charted in their chapter that will enrich our conceptualization of the self, draw us closer to a physical account of selfhood, and allow us to explore embodied aspects of mentalizing.

From an evolutionary point of view, mentalizing may indeed provide a degree of resilience in the face of potential structural damage to the neural architecture by rearranging processes within the brain and assuring "business as usual" notwithstanding adverse conditions. Thinking about actions in terms of thoughts and feelings, using knowledge of these mental states to master life challenges by responding to psychological challenges effectively on the basis of psychological knowledge, or designating them as "just thoughts" that do not need to be acted on—or, by contrast, that need to be seriously and maturely considered (for the purpose of reflection, as in reflective functioning)—all serve the purpose of creating a higher-order process above cognition (including cognition regarding emotions). Being able to measure this higher-order process of mentalizing has been the subject of controversy and some research since the previous edition of this book. In Chapter 3, which discusses assessment, Luyten and colleagues suggest that mentalizing is an important clinical construct both across different individuals and in different settings and times within an individual. They set out the measurement approaches and techniques currently available to assess this variability.

The importance of mentalizing as a pathway to resilience is discussed in Chapter 4. Fonagy and colleagues use an understanding of imagination as a key component of the mentalizing process in their account of how mentalizing can protect from mental disorder by enhancing understanding of a stressful social context. At the same time, they draw attention to the vulnerability that imagination creates when it is unbridled.

The key to mitigating the long-term effects of personal trauma in childhood and later life is resilience of the individual and family in the face of adversity. A temporary loss of mentalizing is particularly likely to be encountered in individuals whose emotion regulation is poor and who have experienced early adversity. In Chapter 5, Luyten and Fonagy discuss the complex relationship between trauma, mentalizing, and the ubiquitous outcome of early adversity, namely, mental disorder. The very definition of trauma in childhood entails an understanding of mentalizing and the child's isolation from other minds. When adversity is experienced without the benefit of social referencing, long-term sequelae can readily arise. The availability of other minds—which helps to ensure individuals' capacity to envision mental states in themselves and others—serves as a moderator (as outlined in Chapter 4): this capacity generates resilience. The impact of trauma, which is in part mediated by disruption of the attachment system, serves to render mentalizing less robust. Failure to mentalize effectively—in particular, relying on the mode of thinking that we describe as *psychic equivalence* (see Chapter 1)—makes the memory of trauma at times indistinguishable from present reality. In the extreme, this cascade from mentalizing to ineffective mentalizing can generate posttraumatic stress disorder (PTSD). At a more moderate level, it causes a distrust in social relationships and a withdrawal from a social-cognitive process on which all humans depend if we are to adjust and reference our understanding of our own states of mind through interpersonal interactions. The disruption of this flow of knowledge and personal calibration generates a vulnerability and "rigidity" that perhaps all mental disorders share. Improving mentalizing through improving social connections should thus be an important element of trauma-focused treatment. As such, Chapter 5 points to a specific model of understanding the benefit of all psychological therapies in terms of reestablishing the flow of social communication rooted in mentalizing. Trauma disrupts the capacity to represent subjective experience; failure of mentalizing results in internal experience being given the same status as physical reality. This generates the problems commonly encountered in PTSD, namely, reexperiencing, cognitive avoidance, and emotion dysregulation (arousal). This formulation implies that addressing mentalizing problems more specifically in PTSD may improve outcomes.

MBT as a clinical approach originated in individual therapy but has grown substantially beyond its original focus of supporting individuals with a diagnosis of borderline personality disorder (BPD), as this book demonstrates. In Chapter 6, Bateman and colleagues provide a detailed picture of techniques that can be used in individual therapy or other adaptations that promote mentalizing in people with personality disorder, based around findings from measures of fidelity that suggested that some techniques were not implemented skillfully—or even at all— by clinicians.

As the theoretical focus of MBT has increasingly moved beyond the dyadic to the social domain, the importance of mentalizing in the context of group therapy has come to the foreground. Bateman and colleagues have updated the MBT approach to groups, and in Chapter 7, they discuss how the group approach has evolved from its original role as an adjunct to individual therapy, to a core and often separate therapeutic approach used with adolescents and other special groups.

Family therapy represents a logical elaboration of the MBT model, particularly when it comes to offering treatment to children and addressing the problems that couples in conflict face. Asen and Midgley, in Chapter 8, attempt to reconcile the well-established systemic approach and the tried-and-tested techniques it entails with the model of mentalizing around which this book is organized. The authors join together the explicit family model of MBT with applications in which selected systemic techniques are co-opted into MBT to help deal with family interactions dominated by pre-mentalizing modes. Chapter 9, by Bleiberg and Safier, similarly uses old and new side by side to facilitate interventions with couples in conflict. Their clinical presentations beautifully illustrate how addressing issues of partners who chronically mis-imagine each other's mental states may be efficiently addressed using techniques simply focused on enhancing mentalizing.

In Chapter 10, Fonagy and colleagues present an ambitious reformulation of the psychological mechanisms underpinning not just MBT but perhaps many other talking therapies, couching their speculation in the framework of *epistemic trust*. They suggest that for an individual, the experience of feeling his or her personal narrative in some of its complexity being understood by someone else enhances epistemic trust, which opens the individual's mind to the possibility of change through learning. In this process, the accurate perception of how the individual is perceived is a vital component, which is powerfully enhanced through the strengthening of mentalizing capacity.

Chapter 11 describes a new departure for MBT. The previous edition of this book had little or no coverage of expressive therapies such as music or art therapy. Havsteen-Franklin, an art therapist, describes work that has undoubtedly enriched the field, whereby those practicing interventions rooted in expression through a range of artistic modalities can be seen to focus their clients on a deepening of their experience of mental states through the use of metaphor. The exploration of nuances of emotional experience and the emergence of a language for what is internal and private in the context of intersubjective sharing is at the core of mentalizing. Perhaps the most important contribution of this initial summary of arts-based forms of mentalizing intervention is that mentalizing can be a shared language for what has been traditionally a fragmented field.

It is unlikely to have been a historical accident that MBT was developed in the context of partial hospitalization or day hospitals. This "transitional" stage provided us, the editors of this book, with an opportunity to organize a single set of core principles applicable to what was—and remains—a multifaceted treatment process, which, without a common anchor point such as mentalizing, all too often lacks coherence. In Chapter 12, Bales illustrates how the elements of provision of partial hospitalization for individuals with severe personality disorder can be brought into a single frame using MBT principles. The chapter describes how cognitive-behavioral therapy, writing groups, art therapy, family therapy, and other approaches can be joined together in a coherent program using the shared aim of creating a mentalizing environment, supported by coordinated therapeutic work, which is itself embedded through *intervision*—that is, staff "practicing what they preach" and generating a mentalizing team environment.

Just as mentalizing is the lingua franca of interpersonal interaction and social collaboration, so mentalization-based treatments have the capacity to provide a common framework for professionals who are working collaboratively in principle, but in practice often operate in professional and service silos. The mentalization-based approach has in many ways found a real home in guiding collaboration between members of a treatment team—and between teams—working with those who have the least resources and greatest need. In Chapter 13, Bevington and Fuggle present a revolutionary approach for helping teams working with "hard-to-reach" young people and families, who tend to use an unusually large proportion of resources. The work described goes beyond the interface with clients, and focuses on working with teams and their beliefs, emotions, wishes, and desires, including the ever-present risk of professional shame and the reality of emotional exhaustion. Beyond this, MBT principles can address the inevitable "dis-integration" that arises between agencies when tackling this challenging clinical population, and counteract the tendency for individuals and teams to shut down, insist on familiar ways of working, and become closed to learning new approaches.

The interface between social groups and individual mentalizing capacity is directly addressed by Asen and colleagues in Chapter 14. Building on the social model of mentalizing described in detail in Chapter 10, Chapter 14 turns the relationship of social and mentalizing processes on its head, exploring the extent to which social symptoms can be seen as a product of varying degrees of mentalizing that characterize the function of social systems. The chapter tackles the social systems at the heart of human culture, including schools and the justice system, and culture itself.

It is paradoxical that a developmentally rooted model such as MBT up until recently has said little about addressing mental health problems in children. This gap is now addressed by Midgley and colleagues in Chapter 15, who provide an innovative mentalizing model that addresses the needs of children whose problems with mentalizing manifest as emotional and behavioral challenges. The authors present a focused, short-term program of intervention, which, while rooted in psychodynamic principles, draws on features from a number of evidence-based approaches and extends the transdiagnostic approach adopted by MBT to a developmental group (age 5–12 years) in which mental health problems can represent the largest proportion of disease burden.

The intellectual roots of the mentalizing model lie in the developmental process. Mentalizing emerges in the context of family and other early social interactions. Given our assumption that variability in mentalizing is at least in part accounted for by variability in the quality of childhood experience, it is axiomatic that our approach should be able to contribute to the highly influential clinical literature on parenting. Parenting interventions are part of both prevention and treatment, and form part of most guidelines for pediatric mental and physical health. Parents are laden with an enormous social responsibility in Western culture in relation to the well-being of the next generation. Can the mentalizing approach make a genuine contribution to relieving this burden? Redfern's chapter on the Reflective Parenting model (Chapter 16) outlines the specific focus that attunement-oriented interventions can adopt in relation to mentalizing, which includes direct intervention with the caregiver. Developing cognitive and intuitive awareness in relation to the child's internal states and enhancing the parents' awareness of their own mentalizing in relation to their interactions with the child create an advantageous context for learning mentalizing. The chapter is practical in its focus and makes an important specific contribution to the caregiver–child relationship in the context of looked-after children, foster carers, and adoptive parents, where the challenge to mentalizing is acute.

Young people with emerging personality disorder have been a focus of mentalization-based therapies since the initial development of this approach to clinical practice. In Chapter 17, Sharp and Rossouw offer comprehensive and up-to-date information on the clinical roots of BPD in adolescence, and place this in the context of the developmental task of adolescence—the establishment of a coherent and integrated sense of self. Sharp is the originator of the concept of *hypermentalizing*—a tendency to elaborate models of internal states in the absence of relevant evidence—and has highlighted the particular association of hypermentalizing with emerging BPD in adolescence. The empirical evidence gathered to support the notion that emerging difficulties in adolescence that are consistent with the diagnosis of BPD are rooted in failures of mentalizing is compelling. The therapeutic approach described by the authors is clearly laid out and comprehensively illustrated with material drawn from the authors' practice.

A major, and frequently challenging, developmental task for adolescents is understanding their own experiences and the way these interact with the thoughts and feelings of others, particularly peers. A comprehensive chapter by Taubner and colleagues (Chapter 18) focuses on behavioral problems that can emerge when this process goes wrong—that is, when mentalizing is impaired or absent. The authors review the current understanding of the etiology of conduct disorder and place mentalizing in the context of complex multifactorial models. They outline the mentalizing approach to conduct problems, currently undergoing a treatment trial, which has many features that overlap with the classical MBT approach. The mentalizing approach they describe also offers innovative features specifically designed to tackle the challenges of engaging these young people in a therapeutic relationship and the particular problems that arise in the course of treatment, such as angry outbursts associated with interpersonal hypersensitivity.

The first clinical application of MBT was in relation to BPD. In fact, many of the conceptualizations and techniques that represent the common thread running through this volume have their origin in these early developments. Beyond the now reasonably well-known model of BPD, seen through the eyes of an MBT practitioner, Chapter 19, by Bateman and colleagues, presents an overview of the challenges presented by individuals with the diagnosis of BPD, and how these may be better tackled with appropriate understanding of the nature of the mentalizing deficits this diagnosis entails. There is much more in relation to this model in Chapters 4, 10, and 17, because of the fundamental role of this diagnosis as paradigmatic in the MBT model.

Chapters 20 and 21 outline recent extensions of the MBT model. Chapter 20, by Bateman and colleagues, was written in the midst of an ongoing randomized controlled trial of MBT for antisocial personality disorder (ASPD), which was initiated following promising outcomes from two pilot studies. The conceptual framework extends the notions of violence outlined briefly in Chapter 18 (focusing on conduct disorder) but integrates the clinical model with the new emerging model of psychopathology, in which the social context has increasing prominence. The intervention is group-based, and perhaps this chapter should be read alongside Chapter 7.

An exciting new contribution to this volume is the extension of the MBT model to avoidant and narcissistic personality disorders, described in Chapter 21 by Simonsen and Euler. The model adapted to the core pathology of individuals with these diagnoses is of course highly relevant to aspects of the presentation in BPD and ASPD, in which both grandiosity and avoidance may commonly be part of the clinical picture. It is helpful that the chapter also builds on both the conceptual model presented in Chapters 1 and 3 and throughout the book in terms of the dimensions of mentalizing, and identifies mentalizing clinical tools (described in more detail in other clinical chapters) that must be modified when treating patients with avoidant and narcissistic personality disorders.

Few clinicians would argue against the suggestion that a marked indicator of a pathological focus on eating is a deficit in mentalizing. In Chapter 22, Robinson and Skårderud explore the vicious cycle that can underpin eating disorders, whereby excessive concern with the physical world—in this case, with bodily appearance—can trigger anomalous eating patterns that in turn may generate characteristic nonmentalizing mental function (confusing belief with reality and experiencing subjective states as almost meaningless). In turn, these patterns may generate characteristic nonmentalizing mental function (i.e., confusing belief with reality and experiencing subjective states as almost meaningless), which then exacerbates the abnormal eating patterns, generating changes in brain function that further undermine the capacity for higher-order cognition. Whether the root of this process lies in early attachment problems is doubtful, but the disruption to current attachment relationships is un-equivocal. As we see attachment and the social network mediated by attachment re-lationships as critical in maintaining mentalizing, a relational approach aimed at improving mentalizing and engagement with family members, friends, and the wider community is likely to be beneficial to these individuals. The chapter proposes a range of therapeutic techniques that have been shown to be helpful in empirical and clinical work.

Interestingly, notwithstanding the affective background of the diagnostic condi-tions where mentalization-based therapeutic techniques emerged, depression has only recently become a specific focus of MBT. In Chapter 23, Luyten and colleagues provide a model for understanding the most common mental disorder within a men-talizing framework. They review evidence on the relationship between mood and mentalizing and bring in attachment history to help clarify the strong associations ob-served. They suggest that even in the context of brief therapeutic interventions for mild to moderate depression, disruptions of mentalizing are common, and that ad-dressing these disruptions enhances the extent to which patients can benefit from dy-namic interpersonal therapy. In this way, this chapter pioneers an entirely new but highly relevant context for the relevance of mentalizing to psychological therapies. Given the intense focus on emotions in most psychological interventions and the "in-verted U" that characterizes the relationship of arousal and mentalizing, it is axiom-atic that in the course of any therapy there will be failures of mentalizing when the patient is no longer in a position to process and benefit from the therapist's interven-tions. The techniques for helping recover mentalizing when it is lost therefore are po-tentially pertinent to all diagnoses and all treatment models.

A rich literature links personality disorders (particularly ASPD and BPD) to sub-stance use disorder. Arefjord and colleagues suggest, in Chapter 24, that substance use disorder may be seen as a way for individuals whose mentalizing is not robust to achieve a degree of stability in emotion regulation, self-cohesion, and continuity of in-terpersonal relationships. Unbalanced mentalizing is seen here as a vulnerability fac-tor because emotional experiences that are inadequately balanced by cognition are more intense and are thought to lead to almost catastrophic subjective experiences that demand to be addressed immediately. The would-be "pause button" of mental-izing is simply not present. This rationale for a mentalization-based approach to sub-stance use disorder is strong, but whether MBT is of sufficient potency to combat the urgency of emotional experiences associated with addiction realistically remains to be seen.

The current frontier of MBT is perhaps in the domain of management of psychotic conditions. In Chapter 25, Debbané and Bateman provide a model of how mentaliz-ing failure can generate psychotic states. The evidence for the social determinants of psychosis has only recently begun to be integrated, but the fact that attachment re-lates to expressions of psychosis from its earliest manifestations to its full expression, and its course and outcome, opens the door for a mentalizing account. The chapter strengthens the case by outlining potential neurobiological pathways that may be in-volved, which implicate mentalizing. From this evidence, the authors advance a com-pelling clinical model, in which a mentalizing-informed approach is adopted in the management of psychosis along its developmental continuum.

ACKNOWLEDGMENTS

It is impossible to thank all the people who have supported us in their different ways in the development of this book. Many people have given their time and expertise freely, commenting on our manuscript and making suggestions for improvement. For this, we thank them, and we hope that we can return their generosity. We are especially grateful to the team at University College London. A work of this complexity and length would have been impossible to produce without them. All the authors in this volume are aware that they had to get their chapters past Clare Farrar, whose critical faculties are second to none. She picked up inconsistencies, poor sentences, incomprehensible passages, and sloppy writing immediately, yet always made helpful suggestions for improvement; she recognized when the mentalizing framework was contradictory across chapters and asked for clarification; she kept a careful mental record of the main points of each chapter and suggested cross-links between chapters. Without her detailed editorial work, this book would not have the clarity and consistency we hope it now has. We are deeply grateful to her for her hard work and unfailing support. We would also like to thank Chloe Campbell and Liz Allison, who, with patience and quiet determination, also tried to keep us on task and contributed to many of the chapters of the book in different ways. Thank you.

Finally, we would like to acknowledge our intellectual indebtedness to a person who has not authored any of the chapters in this book yet whose name appears in almost every chapter. Professor George Gergely's contributions continue to identify ways in which the close experimental study of early social development can illuminate clinical work across a wide range of mental health settings and contexts, and this has been the case since the earliest phase of our work. We wish to express our gratitude and appreciation for his leadership by dedicating this second edition of the book to him.

Anthony Bateman, M.A., FRCPsych

Peter Fonagy, Ph.D., FBA, FMedSci, FAcSS

ACKNOWLEDGMENTS

PART I

Principles

CHAPTER 1

INTRODUCTION

Peter Fonagy, Ph.D., FBA, FMedSci, FAcSS
Anthony Bateman, M.A., FRCPsych

Mentalizing describes a particular facet of the human imagination: an individual's awareness of mental states in himself or herself and in other people, particularly in explaining their actions. It involves perceiving and interpreting the feelings, thoughts, beliefs, and wishes that explain what people do. This entails an awareness of someone else's circumstances, his or her prior patterns of behavior, and the experiences to which the individual has been exposed.

The idea that mentalizing is an act of imagination implies that any act of mentalizing is by its very nature uncertain; internal states are opaque, changeable, and quite often difficult to pin down, even in the individual's own mind. This means that any attempt to make sense of mental states is vulnerable to error or inaccuracy. Mentalizing is something people do most of the time, normally without giving it much conscious thought, and for all their efforts it is also something people quite often get somewhat wrong. Usually, this involves minor mismatches and adjustments as individuals correct themselves or update their understanding of what might be going on in response to feedback they receive.

The emphasis on imagination and the inherent lack of certainty in relation to mental states points to one of the ideas underpinning the mentalizing clinical approach: the *inquisitive stance.* The inquisitive stance is a style of interaction characterized by an expectation that an individual's mind may be influenced, surprised, changed, and enlightened by learning about another's mind. But this emphasis on the imagination, and on the intrapersonal and interpersonal uncertainty this entails, has also taken on a new role in our thinking about mental disorder and the social mind. As explored in more detail in Chapter 4 ("Mentalizing, Resilience, and Epistemic Trust") and Chapter 10 ("Therapeutic Models"), we suggest that the human imagination is both what

3

generates human social complexity and cultural creativity and what leaves individuals vulnerable to psychological disorder and psychic distress. Mentalizing is positioned within this as the interpersonal "workhorse" of the social imagination: it is the aspect of social cognition that enables individuals to make sense of the behavior of themselves and others, making cooperative and adaptive interaction possible.

The role of mentalizing as the imaginative linchpin between individuals' more abstract cognitive processes and their everyday interpersonal interactions is what makes it so therapeutically significant as the first place to approach a mind that feels lost or wildly out of kilter with other minds. The closeness of mentalization-based treatment (MBT) to art therapy (see Chapter 11, "Creative Arts Therapies") underscores the inherently creative nature of mentalizing. Forging a link with another mind is a creative process, as great artists self-evidently demonstrate by generating connections to millions of unique individual experiences.

DEVELOPMENTAL ORIGINS OF MENTALIZING AND THE IMPACT OF ADVERSITY

The potential to mentalize is partially a traitlike capacity: everyone is born with the capability to mentalize and with innate variations in strengths and natural competence, but the development of this constitutional capacity is scaffolded and modulated by the early social environment. We have used the development of language as an analogue of understanding this process: verbal competence has a genetic component, but the nature of an individual's command of language derives from the particular language spoken, and the way it is spoken, by those around the individual in his or her early environment (Neuman et al. 2011). The development of robust and balanced mentalizing depends on whether the young child's own mental states are adequately understood by caring, attentive, nonthreatening adults (Fonagy and Luyten 2016). Of particular importance is the child's experience of *marked mirroring* of their emotional reactions by an adult; this is the process by which the adult represents the child's affect in a manner that conveys recognition and understanding of the child's state at the same time as communicating a sense of coping with, rather than merely reflecting back, the child's affect (Fonagy et al. 2002; Gergely and Watson 1996). The experience of adequate mirroring interactions helps the child develop second-order representations of his or her own subjective experiences. This in turn positively influences the emergence of affect regulation and self-control (including attentional mechanisms and effortful control), as the development of the capacity to reflect on mental states provides the tools for these regulative processes. The therapeutic application of the recognition of the family's importance in the development and maintenance of mentalizing is discussed in Chapter 8, "Working With Families." Later in life, exposure to a wider environment (e.g., peers, teachers, friends) that fosters a focus on internal mental states is thought to broaden and strengthen the development of mentalizing (Fonagy and Luyten 2016), as explored in Chapter 14, "Social Systems: Beyond the Microcosm of the Individual and Family."

Developmental research has enabled tracking of the emergence of mentalizing skills across infancy and childhood. A key developmental milestone is measured by the *false-belief task*—a classic example being the "Smarties test," in which a child is shown a tube of Smarties (a type of sugar-coated chocolate confectionery popular in the United Kingdom) and then shown that the tube contains not Smarties, but pencils. When a third person—who has not been shown the real contents of the Smarties tube—enters the room, the child is asked what the third person will think is in the tube. By the age of 4 or 5, most children will reply that the third person will assume that it contains Smarties (this and similar tests are summarized in a meta-analysis by Wellman et al. [2001]). These children, who have developed a "theory of mind," understand that the other person has a different understanding of the situation from their own. This is an example of *explicit* mentalizing, which most younger children will be unable to perform. However, there is evidence that much younger children can show *implicit* mentalizing capacity. This was derived from a study of babies as young as 7 months, in which the baby is shown a simple video animation of a cartoon character that is present on-screen to see a ball entering a box. When the character walks off-screen (and therefore cannot see what is happening), the baby is shown the ball moving out of the box and falling out of sight, so that when the character returns the character has a false belief about the ball being in the box and the watching baby has a true belief that the ball has gone elsewhere. It is this condition, in which the baby is considering what the character (differently) believes about the ball's whereabouts, that holds the baby's attention for longest (Kovács et al. 2010). The presence of mechanisms for implicit, automatic computations about others' beliefs at such an early stage of development might suggest that they constitute a core, human-specific "social sense" and a cognitive precondition for elaborate social functioning (Kovács et al. 2010).

A sense of self and emotional agency emerges through mentalizing, initially via marked mirroring exchanges with the primary caregiver (Gergely and Watson 1996). Later, in mentalizing interactions, the caregiver puts the child's (and the caregiver's own) emotions into spoken words. Through these mentalizing narratives, the relationships surrounding and scaffolding the child's emotional world are demonstrated to the child (Fonagy and Target 1996). The ability of the caregiver to mentalize the infant well enough to mirror in this way is one of the benefits of being exposed to sensitive parenting. The caregiver is able to recognize the psychological complexity and emotional agency of the child; he or she can interpret the child's signals and respond to them appropriately, tolerating the child's expression of a wide range of emotions and adapting to them in a manner that is proportionate and unobtrusive (at least, enough of the time for this to be consistently felt by the child) (Target and Fonagy 1996). Securely attached infants therefore benefit from not just the physical but also the psychological proximity and availability of their caregiver(s). In normal circumstances, secure attachment and mentalizing develop hand in hand (Fonagy et al. 2008). Infants who are more securely attached tend to develop better mentalizing capacities in childhood; for example, they are more adept at inferring beliefs and more empathic in relating to their peers (de Rosnay and Harris 2002). Again, this seems commonsensical: by virtue of being mentalized, children become better mentalizers and, through a virtuous cycle, become more sensitive to and better able to appreciate the experience of being mentalized. This in turn enables them to become better mentalizers, and so on (Fonagy and Target 2007a).

Conversely, consistent or serious failures in the process of marked mirroring by early attachment figures lead to impairments in the capacity to reflect on the self and others, as they lead to unmentalized self-experiences—also called "alien-self" experiences—which do not validate the individual's experience and thus are felt as alien to the self (Fonagy and Target 2000). Such failures are to an extent part of the fabric of everyday life: as mentioned at the beginning of the chapter, no one can ever be certain about the accuracy of his or her ideas about another person's mind, and some misattunement in marked mirroring is to some extent an inevitable experience, and thus all persons have unmentalized mental states. However, in various forms of psychopathology—most paradigmatically, in the case of borderline personality disorder (BPD), and most often as the result of a combination of biological vulnerability and environmental circumstances—these alien-self experiences are so pronounced that they dominate the individual's subjectivity. This leads to a constant pressure to externalize these unmentalized self-experiences, which may be expressed in, for instance, the tendency to dominate the mind of others and/or various types of self-harming behavior (Fonagy and Luyten 2016).

Research has shown that, in contrast to the previously held view that full cognitive development has been achieved by early adolescence, the brain continues to undergo significant neurobiological change throughout adolescence, with particular implications for social cognition (Blakemore 2012; Blakemore and Mills 2014; Crone and Dahl 2012; Dumontheil et al. 2010; Váša et al. 2018). More research is needed into the developmental neurobiology of mentalizing, but there are suggestions that "while brain regions involved in social perception develop early in life, the fine-tuning or functional specialization of other regions of the social brain network may continue during adolescence" (Moor et al. 2012, p. 50). This is reflected in Moor et al.'s (2012) finding of slightly poorer performance in the Reading the Mind in the Eyes Test by 14- to 16-year-olds compared with adults. A growing body of literature on the ongoing development of the social brain across adolescence has led to the suggestion that this period should be regarded as a window of heightened developmental sensitivity in relation to social cognition (Blakemore and Mills 2014). In terms of clinical implications, this research suggests that adolescents with a predisposed weakness in their capacity for mentalizing (whether for genetic or environmental reasons, or an interaction between the two) may be particularly vulnerable when faced with the considerable developmental challenges of this life stage. Sharp and colleagues (Kalpakci et al. 2016; Sharp et al. 2016) have developed the concept of *hypermentalizing* to capture a particular mentalizing profile associated with emerging BPD in adolescence—an inclination to develop non-evidence-based and often elaborate presuppositions of internal states, as discussed more fully in Chapter 17, "Borderline Personality Pathology in Adolescence." We consider the notion of hypermentalizing as a distinguishing feature of emergent BPD to be particularly resonant in the context of recent thinking about the role of social imagination in psychopathology. We speculate that the overimaginative sensitivity that is characteristic of a hypermentalizing state in adolescence is an indication of developmental challenges in aligning the individual's social imagination adaptively in the context of the environmental and neurobiological flux of this period. The individual's experience of an overwhelming alien self, which is associated with violent behaviors toward others or toward himself or herself in the form of self-harm—particularly at moments of interpersonal stress or distress—is a further characteristic of the mentalizing difficulties associated with emerging disorder in adolescence.

DEVELOPMENT OF MENTALIZING IN THE CONTEXT OF EARLY ADVERSITY

The relationship between adversity—in particular, trauma in the context of attachment relationships—and mental disorder is discussed in Chapter 5, "Mentalizing and Trauma." To summarize the position as articulated there, we propose that the process by which trauma may cascade into psychopathology in some individuals works through mechanisms of adaptive response to the social environment, often in interaction with constitutional tendencies. We suggest that adverse experiences in the context of attachment relationships are potentially so significant because it is via these relationships that the child's first experiences of being mentalized take place, in the first instance, in infancy, often through the experience of embodied mentalizing (Fonagy and Target 2007b; Fotopoulou and Tsakiris 2017; see also Chapter 2, "Contemporary Neuroscientific Research"). Indeed, the caregiver's capacities to mentalize the infant and to provide contingent, appropriate emotionally regulatory touch have been shown to have a direct relationship with each other (Crucianelli et al. 2018; see also Shai and Belsky 2017). In instances of abuse, neglect, or maltreatment, the impact of this nonalignment of the child's needs with the reality of what he or she is experiencing constitutes a powerful signal to the child that the social environment is not one in which others' minds are sufficiently reliable or invested in his or her well-being. Mentalizing antedates the development of language, and maternal understanding of the child's mental state is experienced and communicated bodily, or at least paralinguistically, long before the appearance of the first word.

MULTIDIMENSIONAL NATURE OF MENTALIZING

Although we have so far tended to talk about mentalizing as a single entity or aptitude, neuroscientists have identified four different components, or *dimensions*, to mentalizing (Lieberman 2007), which reflect different social-cognitive processes:

1. Automatic versus controlled mentalizing.
2. Self versus other mentalizing.
3. Internal versus external mentalizing.
4. Cognitive versus affective mentalizing.

The neuroscience of the mentalizing dimensions is explained in Chapter 2, and their assessment and measurement are outlined in Chapter 3, "Assessment of Mentalizing." It is also helpful to distinguish the dimensions during clinical assessment of mentalizing (see Chapter 3), and they have significant clinical applications (e.g., see Chapter 19, "Borderline Personality Disorder").

To mentalize effectively requires the individual not only to be able to maintain a balance across these dimensions of social cognition but also to apply them appropriately according to context (Fonagy and Luyten 2009). In an adult with personality disorder, for example, consistently imbalanced mentalizing on at least one of these four dimensions would be evident. From this perspective, different types of psychopathology can be distinguished on the basis of different combinations of impairments along the four dimensions (which we refer to as different *mentalizing profiles*).

Automatic Versus Controlled Mentalizing

The most fundamental dimension to mentalizing is the spectrum between *automatic* (or *implicit*) and *controlled* (or *explicit*) mentalizing. Controlled mentalizing reflects a serial and relatively slow process, which is typically verbal and demands reflection, attention, awareness, intention, and effort. The opposite pole of this dimension, automatic mentalizing, involves much faster processing, tends to be reflexive, and requires little or no attention, intention, awareness, or effort. Several neuroscience researchers (Carver et al. 2017; Crespi et al. 2016; Jung 2014) have proposed models that juxtapose the pragmatic deductive mindset (at its extreme typified in autism) with a divergent thinking style of individuals who are more likely to display common mental disorders. Freud (1923/1961) was one of the first to point to a dichotomy between cognitive and experiential modes of functioning (Epstein 1994). Indeed, we can delineate a dichotomy between a reflexive, basic, responsive-to-emotion mode and a reflective, deliberative mental function (Carver et al. 2017). A large family of neuroscience-informed theories (e.g., Evans and Stanovich 2013; Kahneman 2011; Rothbart et al. 2003; Toates 2006) implicitly or explicitly envision this kind of dichotomy. In these theories a deliberative reflective system is opposed to the reflexive mode characterized by relative simplicity and responsiveness to affect (Metcalfe and Mischel 1999; Strack and Deutsch 2004).

In day-to-day life and ordinary social interaction, mentalizing tends to be automatic because most straightforward exchanges do not require more attention. Particularly in a secure attachment environment, when things are running smoothly on an interpersonal level, more deliberate or controlled mentalizing is not called for; in fact, the use of such a mentalizing style might hinder such interactions, making them feel unduly weighty or uncomfortably overwrought (hypermentalized). Both common-sense experience and neuroscience tell us that individuals relax controlled mentalizing and are less watchful of social intentions in a secure attachment environment; a parent playing with a child or close old friends reminiscing will conduct their exchanges along automatic, intuitive processes. However, when necessary, someone with normative mentalizing abilities will be able to switch to controlled mentalizing if the situation demands it. For example, when a child starts to cry during play, the parent will respond by explicitly asking about what has upset the child, or the person in conversation may detect a change in their friend's tone and mood and wonder whether the conversation has stumbled upon a difficult memory or association. In other words, well-functioning mentalizing involves the ability to switch flexibly and responsively from automatic to controlled mentalizing.

Mentalizing difficulties arise when an individual relies exclusively on automatic assumptions about the mental states of the self or others, which tend to be oversimplistic, or when the situation makes it difficult for the individual to apply his or her automatic assumptions appropriately. In fact, it could be that any psychotherapeutic intervention in essence involves challenging such automatic, distorted assumptions and requires the patient to make these assumptions conscious and attempt to reflect on them, in partnership with the clinician. In other words, any effective treatment is, at that level, about getting the patient to mentalize; we will return to this point later in this chapter.

Most experts agree that two systems for mentalizing arise from different neurocognitive mechanisms, both of which are specialized for thinking about and interpreting mental states (Apperly 2011). The *automatic* system develops early and tracks mental states in a fast and efficient way, while the *explicit* system develops later, operates more slowly, and makes greater demands on executive functions (working memory and inhibitory control). Explicit mentalizing allows an individual to explain and predict behavior and has a role in social regulation (McGeer 2007). In general, our impression is that the primary function of the "slow-reflective-conscious-explicit" system is to facilitate social interaction rather than to drive or motivate individual behavior. The making explicit (or "spelling out") of implicit assumptions helps in the coordination of social interactions that require shared awareness, which social collaboration demands (Fonagy and Allison 2016). However, it is the balance of automatic and controlled mentalizing that is critical for effective functioning. Explicit reflection cannot feel real unless it is contextualized by an intuitive awareness of the mental states that are being reflected on.

Stress and arousal, especially in an attachment context, bring automatic mentalizing to the fore and inhibit the neural systems that are associated with controlled mentalizing (Nolte et al. 2013). This has important implications for clinical work: any intervention that calls for reflection, by asking for clarification or elaboration on a thought, is by its very nature asking the patient to engage in controlled mentalizing. Many patients may perform relatively well (in terms of mentalizing) under low-stress conditions. However, under higher levels of stress, when automatic mentalizing naturally kicks in, the patient may find it much more difficult to activate the processes that underpin controlled mentalizing, and so will find it harder to understand and reflect on what might be happening.

Self Versus Other Mentalizing

This mentalizing dimension involves the individual's capacity to mentalize his or her own state—the *self* (including the individual's own physical experiences)—or the state of *others*. The two are closely connected, and an imbalance signals vulnerability in mentalizing both others and the self. Individuals with mentalizing difficulties are likely to preferentially focus on one end of the spectrum, although they may be impaired at both.

It is a central tenet of our attachment-based approach that a sense of self and the capacity to mentalize develop in the context of attachment relationships. The child observes, mirrors, and then internalizes his or her attachment figure's ability to represent and reflect mental states. Hence, the self and others, and the capacity to reflect on the self and others, are inevitably closely intertwined. In line with these assumptions, neuroimaging studies suggest that individuals' capacity to mentalize about others is closely related to their ability to reflect on themselves because the two capacities rely on common neural substrates (Lieberman 2007). Therefore, it is not surprising that disorders that are characterized by severe impairments in feelings of self-identity—most notably, psychosis and BPD—are also characterized by severe deficits in the ability to reflect about others' mental states.

However, this should not be taken to mean that individuals with an impaired capacity to mentalize themselves will always show similar impairments in the ability to mentalize others. Some individuals may have fewer universal impairments in mentalizing in relation to the self and others and have stronger skills at one or other end of this dimension. For example, individuals with antisocial personality disorder can often be surprisingly skilled in "reading the mind" of others, but typically lack any real understanding of their own inner world (see Chapter 20, "Antisocial Personality Disorder in Community and Prison Settings").

Still, following the neuroimaging literature, we can identify two distinct neural networks used in self-knowing and knowing others (Lieberman 2007; Northoff and Huang 2017; Northoff et al. 2011).

- The first of these is a *shared representation* system, in which empathic processing relies on shared representations of others' mental states. This represents a kind of "visceral recognition" that occurs while experiencing and observing others experiencing states of mind, which operates through a mirror-neuron motor-simulation mechanism (Lombardo et al. 2010).
- The second is the *mental state attribution* system, which relies more on symbolic and abstract processing (Ripoll et al. 2013).

In line with our expectation of the way the dimensions of mentalizing function, these two systems may be mutually inhibitory (Bardi et al. 2017; Brass et al. 2009), in that the neural regions most often recruited in the inhibition of imitative behavior are those involved in explicit mental-state attributions.

Internal Versus External Mentalizing

Mentalizing can involve making inferences on the basis of the *external* indicators of a person's mental states (e.g., facial expressions) or figuring out someone's *internal* experience from what an individual knows about the person and the situation the person is in. This dimension does not just refer to a process of focusing on the externally visible manifestations versus the internal mental state of others; it also includes the individual thinking about himself or herself and his or her own internal and external states. From the perspective of clinical assessment, the internal–external distinction is particularly significant in helping clinicians understand why some patients appear to be seriously impaired in their capacity to "read the mind" of others, yet they may be hypersensitive to facial expressions or bodily posture, giving the impression of being astute about others' states of mind. Individuals who have poor access to and great uncertainty about their subjective experience may come to a conclusion about what they are feeling from observing their own behavior as well as the reactions of others: for instance, their legs feel restless; therefore, they must be feeling anxious. The external focus can make a person extremely vulnerable to the observable behavior of others. The absence of confident knowledge about the internal world creates a thirst for clues from others' reactions, even when these are not directed at the individual. Seeing someone else anxiously fidget can stimulate an internal state of unease and worry to a greater extent than it might normally do if mentalizing was not imbalanced in favor of the external.

Mentalizing difficulties may become apparent only when the balance of internal and external cues used to establish the mental states of others is considered. For example, BPD patients often tend to hypermentalize emotions in others—including the clinician treating them. This is because they pay more attention to external indicators of mental states and their initial ideas are left unchecked by controlled/reflective mentalizing (which might limit the possibilities for attributing thoughts and feelings). For example, if the clinician leans back and opens his or her mouth even slightly, the patient may believe that this was a yawn indicating that the clinician is bored with him or her. If the clinician frowns, perhaps pensively, the patient may interpret this as looking angry or disgusted with him or her. There has been considerable research on BPD patients' hypersensitivity to facial cues; their performance in the Reading the Mind in the Eyes Test can be better than normal, creating an impression in clinicians that their patients are better-than-average mind-readers (sometimes called the *borderline empathy paradox*; Dinsdale and Crespi 2013). A focus on external features, in the absence of reflective mentalizing, makes an individual highly vulnerable in social contexts, because it generates the kind of interpersonal hypersensitivity well described by Gunderson and Lyons-Ruth (2008). In MBT, mentalizing interventions often need to start by examining the patient's interpretations of a person based on external cues and then consider possible plausible scenarios about what that person's internal states of mind may be, encouraging the patient to take into account the subtleties and complexities of people's internal worlds (Flasbeck et al. 2017).

Cognitive Versus Affective Mentalizing

Intense emotion appears to be incompatible with serious reflection on mental states. This point hardly needs to be made, but, as with much that is obvious, neuroimaging studies have provided biological confirmation. For example, emotional activation has been shown to limit people's ability to "broaden and build" in the face of stress—that is, to open up (broaden) their minds to new possibilities and to build on their personal resources that facilitate resilience and well-being (Fredrickson 2001). In a functional magnetic resonance imaging study of 30 healthy women, it was found that during a provocative confrontation, high emotional reactivity to threat suppressed recruitment of the mentalizing network (Beyer et al. 2014).

Cognitive mentalizing involves the ability to name, recognize, and reason about mental states (in oneself or others), whereas *affective* mentalizing involves the ability to understand the *feeling* of such states (again, in oneself or others), which is necessary for any genuine experience of empathy or sense of self. Some individuals give undue weight to either cognitive or affective mentalizing. Studies have suggested that BPD patients have a deficit of cognitive empathy (Harari et al. 2010; Ritter et al. 2011), which is coupled with heightened sensitivity toward any kind of emotional cue (Lynch et al. 2006). This suggests that these patients may have an emotional processing advantage, perhaps linked to a combination of amygdala overactivation and orbitofrontal cortex and prefrontal cortex regulatory deficits (Domes et al. 2009).

CONTEXT- AND RELATIONSHIP-SPECIFIC NATURE OF MENTALIZING

Mentalizing, then, is made up of different dimensions. Everyone is likely to be more or less skilled at some of these dimensions, or to have a tendency to veer toward one pole of a dimension, but individuals with personality pathology tend to have pronounced impairments along some of the dimensions, resulting in an imbalance in mentalizing and occasionally outright mentalizing failures. In this section we discuss the situations that are more likely to trigger mentalizing failures or difficulties. As well as being multidimensional, mentalizing changes over time, and particular situations and stimuli are more likely to lead to mentalizing difficulties. For instance, BPD patients may be able to perform mentalizing tasks relatively well in experimental settings, but when they become emotionally aroused (e.g., in a difficult interpersonal situation), they may show considerable confusion, as they become dominated by automatic assumptions about other people's internal states and find it challenging to reflect on and moderate these assumptions. In other words, when in a state of emotional arousal, they typically lose the ability for controlled mentalizing and are likely to struggle to imagine a rational scenario that might explain the states of mind of others. This is discussed further in Chapter 3, which gives an overview of how individual differences in relation to attachment histories can result in observable differences in mentalizing capacities as a response to arousal.

Heightened psychological arousal tends to cause the capacity for controlled mentalizing to become increasingly difficult to access, and automatic and nonreflective mentalizing starts to dominate. Up to a point this is a normal fight/flight response to stress, which has the advantage of allowing an immediate response to danger. However, in situations of social interpersonal stress, more complex, cognitive, reflective functioning may be more helpful, and an inability to use these more controlled and conscious skills can lead to real difficulties in dealing with other people. Given a certain amount of emotional arousal, it becomes hard to focus on someone else's point of view. When people are emotional, not only does it become much harder or even impossible for them to concern themselves with the other person's perspective; they can also be quick to make assumptions on the basis of flimsy observations. Individuals can become convinced that their point of view is the only valid one and ignore everything they know about the other person except what is relevant to support their point of view. Therefore, the degree to which an individual finds himself or herself affected by interpersonal stress may make a critical difference in his or her mentalizing skills across life experiences. It seems likely that the threshold for switching to an automatic (fight/flight) style of mentalizing will be lower in people who have been exposed to stress or trauma in early life. There may also be a genetic influence on the ease with which people are likely to switch to this automatic, uncontrolled mentalizing mode.

There is also some evidence that activation of the attachment system is linked to the deactivation of mentalizing. Imaging studies (e.g., Nolte et al. 2013) have shown that the brain areas normally associated with maternal and romantic attachments appear to suppress activity in brain regions associated with different aspects of cognitive control, including those associated with making social judgments and mentalizing. Anything that stimulates the attachment system (beyond stress-induced arousal), therefore, seems to bring with it a general loss of mentalizing capacity. A traumatic experience will arouse the attachment system, and attachment trauma may do so chronically. Hyperactivation of the attachment system in people with a history of trauma may account for the dramatic loss of mentalizing capacity experienced by some individuals in emotional situations that trigger their attachment-seeking instincts. Attachment trauma probably hyperactivates the attachment system because the person to whom the child needs to turn in a state of anxiety (their attachment figure, usually a parent) is the very person causing the fear in the first place (see Chapter 5). The quick-fire triggering of the attachment system in BPD may be a result of past trauma, and it shows itself in the tendency of BPD patients both to move to positions of intimacy with undue haste and to be vulnerable to the temporary loss of mentalizing in interpersonally intense situations.

Such moments of mentalizing failure are significant because they make it difficult for someone to relate to others in the context of an attachment relationship. When mentalizing fails in this way, there tends to be a reemergence of nonmentalizing modes of behavior, which can lead to powerful complications and profound disturbances in relationships. We will discuss these nonmentalizing modes next.

IMBALANCES IN MENTALIZING: PREMENTALIZING MODES

When mentalizing becomes disrupted (as typically happens in individuals with BPD, particularly in contexts of high arousal), individuals often fall back on prementalizing ways of thinking, which have parallels with the ways in which young children behave before they have developed full mentalizing capacities.

While the dimensions of mentalizing can reflect anomalies in terms of mechanisms, on the whole, that is not what the clinician sees. The whole-person perspective that clinicians are obliged to take must address the phenomenology or subjectivity of their patients; their experience is not that of a single brain mechanism out of kilter with the rest, but of a whole system functioning suboptimally. What the patient and the mentalizing clinician see is a product of a malfunctioning mentalizing system, driven by imbalances in the dimensions of mentalizing. We have grouped the outcomes of these malfunctions under three typical modes of nonmentalizing subjectivity for the purpose of clinical experience. The modes are termed *psychic equivalence mode*, *teleological mode*, and *pretend mode*. These nonmentalizing modes are important for the clinician to recognize and understand, as they tend to emerge in the consulting room and refer to aspects of the patient's experience. It is important to address them because they can cause considerable interpersonal difficulties and result in destructive behaviors.

In the **psychic equivalence mode**, thoughts and feelings become "too real" to a point where it is extremely difficult for the individual to entertain possible alternative perspectives. When mentalizing gives way to psychic equivalence, what is thought is experienced as being real and true, leading to what clinicians describe as "concreteness of thought" in their patients. There is a suspension of doubt, and the individual increasingly believes that his or her own perspective is the only one possible. Psychic equivalence is normal in a child of around 20 months who has not yet developed full mentalizing skills. Young children, and patients with BPD who are in this mode, describe an overriding sense of certainty about their subjective experience, whether this is that *"There is a monster under the bed"* or *"This medication is harming me."* Such a state of mind can be extremely frightening, adding a powerful sense of drama and risk to life experiences. The sometimes exaggerated reactions of patients are justified by the seriousness and "realness" with which they can experience their own and others' thoughts and feelings. The vividness and bizarreness of subjective experience can appear as quasi-psychotic symptoms and are also evident in the physically compelling memories associated with posttraumatic stress disorder.

In the **teleological mode**, states of mind are recognized and believed only if their outcomes are physically observable. Hence, the individual can recognize the existence and potential importance of states of mind, but this recognition is limited to very concrete situations. For example, affection is perceived to be true only if it is accompanied by physical contact such as a touch or caress. A patient who experiences mentalizing failure and falls into the teleological mode may express this by acting out, carrying out dramatic or inappropriate actions or behaviors in order to generate outcomes from others whose claims of subjective states (e.g., of being concerned about the patient) are not credible to the patient. The teleological mode appears in patients who are imbalanced toward the external pole of the internal–external mentalizing dimension—they are heavily biased toward understanding how people (and they themselves) behave and what their intentions may be in terms of what they physically do.

In the **pretend mode**, thoughts and feelings become disconnected from reality. In more extreme cases, this may lead to feelings of derealization and dissociation. A prementalizing young child creates mental models and pretend worlds, which the child can maintain only as long as these are completely separate from the real world (e.g., as long as an adult does not interrupt the game or spoil it by "getting it wrong"). Similarly, patients in pretend mode can discuss experiences without contextualizing them in any kind of physical or material reality, as if they were creating a pretend world. The patient may hypermentalize (see Chapter 17) or *pseudomentalize*, a state in which they may say much about states of mind but with little true meaning or connection to reality. Attempting psychotherapy with patients who are in this mode can lead to lengthy discussions of internal experience that has no link to genuine experience. A patient who shows considerable cognitive understanding of mentalizing states but little affective understanding may often hypermentalize. This state can often be difficult to distinguish from genuine mentalizing, but it tends to involve excessively lengthy narratives, devoid of a real affective core or of any connection to reality. On first impressions, hypermentalizing can lead clinicians to believe that they are working with an individual with extraordinary mentalizing capacities, but after a little while they discover that they are unable to resonate with the feelings underlying their patient's mentalizing efforts. In addition, because in pretend mode there are no real feelings or emotional experiences providing the individual with constraints, the individual may misuse his or her cognitive capacity in self-serving ways (e.g., to get others to care for or feel compassion toward him or her, or to control or coerce others).

The nonmentalizing modes are generated by imbalances within the dimensions of mentalizing. Psychic equivalence is inevitable if emotion (affect) dominates cognition. Teleological mode follows from an exclusive focus on external features to the neglect of the internal. Pretend mode and hypermentalizing are unavoidable if reflective, explicit, controlled mentalizing is not well established. The normal predominance of nonmentalizing in the early years of life can be predicted from what is known about the developmental unfolding of mentalizing capacities. For example, as affect-focused mental-state thinking antedates more cognitive mentalizing (Harris et al. 2016), psychic equivalence (and the anxieties that accompany it) will almost inevitably be part of the life of a child age 3–5 years.

The three prementalizing modes are particularly important to identify in patients, as they are often accompanied by a pressure to externalize unmentalized aspects of the self (alien self parts, discussed earlier in this chapter). This may be demonstrated in attempts to dominate the mind of others, self-harm, or other types of behavior that in the teleological mode are expected to relieve tension and arousal, a feature typical of BPD.

OSTENSIVE CUES AND EPISTEMIC TRUST

We have sought to establish distortions in the development of the capacity for balanced mentalizing as a further implication, beyond attachment itself, of traumatic or atypical caregiving experiences, often in interaction with a biological predisposition. No sooner have we made a place for mentalizing alongside attachment than we are seeking to make space for another social-cognitive process that may be implicated in mental disorders. We arrive at this position by considering the question *Why do we mentalize*?

Mentalizing may be helpful in all kinds of ways, but we argue that its predominant function is to enable everyone to navigate their social environment (Fonagy and Allison 2016) and to make community life easier. Human consciousness more generally depends on and is shaped by social experience, and that which is conscious is confirmed by the social context: thoughts and feelings are recognized through other people's reactions, thoughts, and feelings. At a certain point in human evolution, the capacity for social interaction was harnessed for the communication of knowledge. Once individuals are capable of producing abstract conceptual tools, they can create a belief independent of physical value, something of potentially enormous benefit; it makes far greater technological advancement and social complexity possible. Higher-order social cognition allows humans to establish an agreed social reality, which can take the form of reasoning, law, and morality; this agreement of social reality is dependent on explicit mentalizing (Heyes and Frith 2014). However, there is also a danger inherent in creating something with no physical reality, and that is the risk of individuals becoming unmoored in their own social imagination, unable to align their social imagination with the wider environment in a way that can provide them with access to the comfort, perspective, cooperation, and shared knowledge that arise from being accurately in touch with other minds. The risk of psychopathology is thus an inescapable flipside to the evolution of social imaginative thinking, and the reason why mental health disorders have not been selected out of the population (and, in fact, appear to affect up to four-fifths of people at some point in their life; see Schaefer et al. 2017) is that the social imaginative capabilities, which drive the capacity for mental disorder, are also so advantageous.

We suggest that by disrupting mentalizing, traumatic or atypical attachments undermine progress toward another fundamental social-cognitive developmental achievement and compromise the ability to access other minds in a way that supports the alignment of the social imagination: the ability to read cues that stimulate epistemic trust. *Epistemic trust* is defined as openness to the reception of social knowledge that is regarded as personally relevant and of generalizable significance. Epistemic trust enables everyone to receive the social knowledge that allows them to navigate the social environment, maximizing the benefits that can be obtained from working cooperatively with others, and letting them access other minds to help them use the social imagination in a benign and constructive manner. These social-cognitive processes (attachment, mentalizing, and epistemic trust) all use the same relational pipeline (attachment relationships) for different functions. They are not the same thing—attachment is much older, in evolutionary terms, and exists across many species—but they are heuristically connected because of the way humans have evolved to care for infants and young children.

This thinking on the role of epistemic trust builds on the ground-breaking work of the Hungarian psychologists Gergely and Csibra about the evolutionary importance of human infants' capacity to learn from their primary caregivers. According to their theory, human beings have evolved to both teach and learn new and relevant cultural information, and to do this they have evolved particular sensitivity to forms of communication that indicate opportunities for this kind of learning. As part of this process of communication, a caregiver signals to a child that what he or she is conveying to the child is relevant and can be considered useful and valid cultural knowledge. These signals have been termed *ostensive cues*. Human infants have been shown to be attuned to paying particular attention to these cues (Csibra and Gergely 2011). Ostensive cues from the caregiver include eye contact, turn-taking contingent reactivity, and the use of a special vocal tone (so-called "motherese"), all of which appear to trigger a special mode of learning in the infant. We believe that this happens because the ostensive cues indicate to the infant that the caregiver recognizes him or her as an individual, and as a thinking and feeling (i.e., mentalizing) "agent." In brief, sensitive responding to the child's needs fosters not just a general confidence that he or she matters as a person, but also serves to open the child's mind more generally to receive new information as relevant and to alter his or her beliefs and modify future behavior accordingly.

Ostensive cues thus trigger epistemic trust: they show that what the caregiver is trying to convey is relevant and significant and should be remembered. A securely attached child is more likely to treat his or her caregiver as a reliable source of knowledge, and this inclination to trust is likely to generalize to other people in a position to teach them. By contrast, individuals whose social experiences have led them to a state of chronic epistemic mistrust, in which (perhaps because they are hypermentalizing) they imagine the motives of the communicator to be malign, will appear to be resistant to new information. They might come across as rigid and stubborn, or even deliberately uncooperative, because they treat new knowledge from communicators as suspicious, spurious, or irrelevant, and will not internalize it (i.e., they will not modify their internal mental structures to accommodate it). Their epistemic trust has been undermined by their previous experiences, and as a consequence an evolutionarily prepared channel for the acquisition of personally relevant information is partially blocked. We suspect that it is less likely to be the frank brutality of physical abuse that undermines epistemic trust (although, of course, it can do just that), and that genetic predisposition, in combination with neglect, emotional abuse, and/or attachment trauma (see Chapter 5), will play a larger role in rendering an individual excessively vulnerable to distrusting information from others.

Access to social knowledge from others is essential in working out how to manage the interpersonal environment. At times, all people experience some uncertainty in relation to their beliefs and intuitions and look for input and reassurance from others.

This is more likely to be the case for an individual whose disrupted mentalizing has rendered his or her sense of social understanding fragile. Yet, even though such an individual's need for confirmation may be more intense than normal and anxiously sought, the content of any reassuring communications may be rejected, their meanings confused or even misinterpreted as having hostile intent, leaving the individual in a state of chronic uncertainty yet without access to satisfying or meaningful resolution. A person whose channels for learning about the social world have been obstructed—for example, one whose social experiences with caregivers during childhood have caused a breakdown in epistemic trust—is stuck in a general state of uncertainty and permanent *epistemic vigilance*. An individual with a history of trauma has little reason to trust others and will reject information that is inconsistent with his or her existing beliefs. Rejecting social information in this way will create an apparent rigidity or reluctance to change. This rigidity is underpinned by epistemic mistrust and a state that may be characterized as "hearing but not listening."

Clinicians may end up describing these individuals as "hard to reach," yet these individuals are simply showing what may be a reasonable adaptation to a social environment where information from most attachment figures is "tagged" as likely to be misleading. Notwithstanding the behavior of a parent or a partner as faultlessly supportive and invariably acting in the patient's interest, or a clinician who consistently offers valuable and accurate advice, the patient apparently takes no notice, ignores the evidence of cooperativeness and support, and continues to feel abandoned, betrayed, and unsupported. It is as if these patients are blind to the evidence presented to them, because it runs contrary to their beliefs. According to this perspective, the destruction of trust in social knowledge is a key mechanism in pathological personality development.

SOCIAL AND CULTURAL CONTEXT OF MENTALIZING

As discussed in the preface to this book, the mentalizing approach to mental health has come a long way. Its applications have been extended to inform the treatment of several different mental health disorders, such as psychosis (Chapter 25), depression (Chapter 23), and eating disorders (Chapter 22), as well as personality disorders (Chapters 19, 20, and 21). The model has been developed for use in a range of settings and modalities, such as parenting (Chapters 15 and 16), couples and family therapy (Chapters 8 and 9), art therapy (Chapter 11), and services designed to help some of the most vulnerable and traditionally considered "hard to reach" individuals (Chapter 13). This extension of the clinical range of mentalizing-related work is particularly valuable to us as our theoretical framework has developed to place ever greater emphasis on systems and the wider cultural context of mentalizing (see Chapter 14).

More recently, the human capacity for individuals to imagine themselves in relation to their surrounding social environment and culture in a way that is attuned with an interpersonally shared and agreed-on social reality as being key to mental health has been suggested (see Chapter 4). It is on the basis of the reasonable congruence of an individual's imaginations and narratives with other people's imaginations and narratives about who he or she is that individuals are able to develop a tolerable and workable sense of self and to communicate with others in a cooperative and meaningful way. One implication of this is that the way individuals mentalize is crucial to their being able to perform the social communicative tasks that underpin the creation of a coherent sense of self and adaptive relationships. If individuals' social imagination—of which mentalizing is one component—is not sufficiently aligned with social reality, they are vulnerable to thinking about their own or others' minds in ways that are inaccurate or maladaptively diffuse. There is a further implication to this emphasis on the cultural context, which lies beyond a focus on the individual's social imagination going awry. Several questions follow: How can clinicians hope to support the mentalizing of individuals in a social environment that does not reasonably contribute to the maintenance of balanced mentalizing? What if the social environment does not support the alignment of the individual's social imagination, whether through lack of access to other minds (in a hostile or highly isolated and fragmented social world) or through the cognitive distortions that may underpin cultural functioning (in a social environment in which pretend mode prevails)? We hope and believe that it is this wider social context of mentalizing, and our human collective responsibility to support it, that will be at the core of mentalizing endeavors in the future.

REFERENCES

Apperly IA: Mindreaders: The Cognitive Basis of "Theory of Mind." Hove, UK, Psychology Press, 2011

Bardi L, Six P, Brass M: Repetitive TMS of the temporo-parietal junction disrupts participant's expectations in a spontaneous Theory of Mind task. Soc Cogn Affect Neurosci 12(11):1775–1782, 2017 28981914

Beyer F, Münte TF, Erdmann C, et al: Emotional reactivity to threat modulates activity in mentalizing network during aggression. Soc Cogn Affect Neurosci 9(10):1552–1560, 2014 23986265

Blakemore SJ: Development of the social brain in adolescence. J R Soc Med 105(3):111–116, 2012 22434810

Blakemore SJ, Mills KL: Is adolescence a sensitive period for sociocultural processing? Annu Rev Psychol 65:187–207, 2014 24016274

Brass M, Ruby P, Spengler S: Inhibition of imitative behaviour and social cognition. Philos Trans R Soc Lond B Biol Sci 364(1528):2359–2367, 2009 19620107

Carver CS, Johnson SL, Timpano KR: Toward a functional view of the p factor in psychopathology. Clin Psychol Sci 5(5):880–889, 2017 29057170

Crespi B, Leach E, Dinsdale N, et al: Imagination in human social cognition, autism, and psychotic-affective conditions. Cognition 150:181–199, 2016 26896903

Crone EA, Dahl RE: Understanding adolescence as a period of social-affective engagement and goal flexibility. Nat Rev Neurosci 13(9):636–650, 2012 22903221

Crucianelli L, Wheatley L, Filippetti ML, et al: The mindedness of maternal touch: An investigation of maternal mind-mindedness and mother-infant touch interactions. Dev Cogn Neurosci pii:S1878–9293(17)30084–1, 2018 29402735 [Epub ahead of print]

Csibra G, Gergely G: Natural pedagogy as evolutionary adaptation. Philos Trans R Soc Lond B Biol Sci 366(1567):1149–1157, 2011 21357237

de Rosnay M, Harris PL: Individual differences in children's understanding of emotion: the roles of attachment and language. Attach Hum Dev 4(1):39–54, 2002 12065029

Dinsdale N, Crespi BJ: The borderline empathy paradox: evidence and conceptual models for empathic enhancements in borderline personality disorder. J Pers Disord 27(2):172–195, 2013 23514182

Domes G, Schulze L, Herpertz SC: Emotion recognition in borderline personality disorder—a review of the literature. J Pers Disord 23(1):6–19, 2009 19267658

Dumontheil I, Apperly IA, Blakemore SJ: Online usage of theory of mind continues to develop in late adolescence. Dev Sci 13(2):331–338, 2010 20136929

Epstein S: Integration of the cognitive and the psychodynamic unconscious. Am Psychol 49(8):709–724, 1994 8092614

Evans JS, Stanovich KE: Dual-process theories of higher cognition: advancing the debate. Perspect Psychol Sci 8(3):223–241, 2013 26172965

Flasbeck V, Enzi B, Brüne M: Altered empathy for psychological and physical pain in borderline personality disorder. J Pers Disord 31(5):689–708, 2017 28072040

Fonagy P, Allison E: Psychic reality and the nature of consciousness. Int J Psychoanal 97(1):5–24, 2016 26602060

Fonagy P, Luyten P: A developmental, mentalization-based approach to the understanding and treatment of borderline personality disorder. Dev Psychopathol 21(4):1355–1381, 2009 19825272

Fonagy P, Luyten P: A multilevel perspective on the development of borderline personality disorder, in Developmental Psychopathology Vol 3: Maladaptation and Psychopathology, 3rd Edition. Edited by Cicchetti D. New York, Wiley, 2016, pp 726–792

Fonagy P, Target M: Playing with reality: I. Theory of mind and the normal development of psychic reality. Int J Psychoanal 77(Pt 2):217–233, 1996 8771375

Fonagy P, Target M: Playing with reality: III. The persistence of dual psychic reality in borderline patients. Int J Psychoanal 81(Pt 5):853–873, 2000 11109573

Fonagy P, Target M: Playing with reality: IV. A theory of external reality rooted in intersubjectivity. Int J Psychoanal 88(Pt 4):917–937, 2007a 17681900

Fonagy P, Target M: The rooting of the mind in the body: new links between attachment theory and psychoanalytic thought. J Am Psychoanal Assoc 55(2):411–456, 2007b 17601099

Fonagy P, Gergely G, Jurist E, et al: Affect Regulation, Mentalization, and the Development of the Self. New York, Other Press, 2002

Fonagy P, Gergely G, Target M: Psychoanalytic constructs and attachment theory and research, in Handbook of Attachment: Theory, Research, and Clinical Applications, 2nd Edition. Edited by Cassidy J, Shaver PR. New York, Guilford, 2008, pp 783–810

Fotopoulou A, Tsakiris M: Mentalizing homeostasis: The social origins of interoceptive inference. Neuro-psychoanalysis 19:3–28, 2017

Fredrickson BL: The role of positive emotions in positive psychology. The broaden-and-build theory of positive emotions. Am Psychol 56(3):218–226, 2001 11315248

Freud S: The ego and the id (1923), in The Standard Edition of the Complete Psychological Works of Sigmund Freud. Edited by Strachey J. London, Hogarth Press, 1961, pp 1–59

Gergely G, Watson JS: The social biofeedback theory of parental affect-mirroring: the development of emotional self-awareness and self-control in infancy. Int J Psychoanal 77(Pt 6):1181–1212, 1996 9119582

Gunderson JG, Lyons-Ruth K: BPD's interpersonal hypersensitivity phenotype: a gene-environment-developmental model. J Pers Disord 22(1):22–41, 2008 18312121

Harari H, Shamay-Tsoory SG, Ravid M, et al: Double dissociation between cognitive and affective empathy in borderline personality disorder. Psychiatry Res 175(3):277–279, 2010 20045198

Harris PL, de Rosnay M, Pons F: Language and children's understanding of mental states. Curr Dir Psychol Sci 14:69–73, 2016

Heyes CM, Frith CD: The cultural evolution of mind reading. Science 344(6190):1243091, 2014 24948740

Jung RE: Evolution, creativity, intelligence, and madness: "Here Be Dragons." Front Psychol 5:784, 2014 25101040

Kahneman D: Thinking, Fast and Slow. New York, Farrar, Straus, & Giroux, 2011

Kalpakci A, Vanwoerden S, Elhai JD, et al: The independent contributions of emotion dysregulation and hypermentalization to the "double dissociation" of affective and cognitive empathy in female adolescent inpatients with BPD. J Pers Disord 30(2):242–260, 2016 25905730

Kovács AM, Téglás E, Endress AD: The social sense: susceptibility to others' beliefs in human infants and adults. Science 330(6012):1830–1834, 2010 21205671

Lieberman MD: Social cognitive neuroscience: a review of core processes. Annu Rev Psychol 58:259–289, 2007 17002553

Lombardo MV, Chakrabarti B, Bullmore ET, et al; MRC AIMS Consortium: Shared neural circuits for mentalizing about the self and others. J Cogn Neurosci 22(7):1623–1635, 2010 19580380

Lynch TR, Rosenthal MZ, Kosson DS, et al: Heightened sensitivity to facial expressions of emotion in borderline personality disorder. Emotion 6(4):647–655, 2006 17144755

McGeer V: The regulative dimension of folk psychology, in Folk Psychology Re-Assessed. Edited by Hutto D, Ratcliffe MM. Dordrecht, Netherlands, Springer, 2007, pp 137–156

Metcalfe J, Mischel W: A hot/cool-system analysis of delay of gratification: dynamics of willpower. Psychol Rev 106(1):3–19, 1999 10197361

Moor BG, Macks ZA, Güroglu B, et al: Neurodevelopmental changes of reading the mind in the eyes. Soc Cogn Affect Neurosci 7(1):44–52, 2012 21515640

Neuman SB, Newman EH, Dwyer J: Educational effects of a vocabulary intervention on preschoolers' word knowledge and conceptual development: a cluster-randomized trial. Read Res Q 46:249–272, 2011

Nolte T, Bolling DZ, Hudac CM, et al: Brain mechanisms underlying the impact of attachment-related stress on social cognition. Front Hum Neurosci 7:816, 2013 24348364

Northoff G, Huang Z: How do the brain's time and space mediate consciousness and its different dimensions? Temporo-spatial theory of consciousness (TTC). Neurosci Biobehav Rev 80:630–645, 2017 28760626

Northoff G, Qin P, Feinberg TE: Brain imaging of the self—conceptual, anatomical and methodological issues. Conscious Cogn 20(1):52–63, 2011 20932778

Ripoll LH, Snyder R, Steele H, et al: The neurobiology of empathy in borderline personality disorder. Curr Psychiatry Rep 15(3):344, 2013 23389774

Ritter K, Dziobek I, Preissler S, et al: Lack of empathy in patients with narcissistic personality disorder. Psychiatry Res 187(1–2):241–247, 2011 21055831

Rothbart MK, Ellis LK, Rueda MR, et al: Developing mechanisms of temperamental effortful control. J Pers 71(6):1113–1143, 2003 14633060

Schaefer JD, Caspi A, Belsky DW, et al: Enduring mental health: prevalence and prediction. J Abnorm Psychol 126(2):212–224, 2017 27929304

Shai D, Belsky J: Parental embodied mentalizing: how the nonverbal dance between parents and infants predicts children's socio-emotional functioning. Attach Hum Dev 19(2):191–219, 2017 27852170

Sharp C, Venta A, Vanwoerden S, et al: First empirical evaluation of the link between attachment, social cognition and borderline features in adolescents. Compr Psychiatry 64:4–11, 2016 26298843

Strack F, Deutsch R: Reflective and impulsive determinants of social behavior. Pers Soc Psychol Rev 8(3):220–247, 2004 15454347

Target M, Fonagy P: Playing with reality: II. The development of psychic reality from a theoretical perspective. Int J Psychoanal 77(Pt 3):459–479, 1996 8818764

Toates F: A model of the hierarchy of behaviour, cognition, and consciousness. Conscious Cogn 15(1):75–118, 2006 15996485

Váša F, Seidlitz J, Romero-Garcia R, et al; NSPN consortium: Adolescent tuning of association cortex in human structural brain networks. Cereb Cortex 28(1):281–294, 2018 29088339

Wellman HM, Cross D, Watson J: Meta-analysis of theory-of-mind development: the truth about false belief. Child Dev 72(3):655–684, 2001 11405571

CHAPTER 2

Contemporary Neuroscientific Research

Martin Debbané, Ph.D.
Tobias Nolte, M.D., M.Sc.

As clinicians, we often ask how much neuroscience can meaningfully add to the art of clinical intervention and psychotherapy. Yet, when we consider how neuroscientific research has influenced the mentalization-based approach to psychotherapy—that is, mentalization-based treatment (MBT)—it becomes difficult to ignore some essential contributions. For example, the importance of early attachment relationships in the development of social cognition represents a key building block of MBT's conceptual edifice. Work on the neurobiology of attachment (Carter and Porges 2013) and the epigenetic effects of attachment trauma (Meaney 2010) provide the mechanistic evidence required to more broadly legitimize research into early attachment dynamics and to pursue therapeutic avenues targeting attachment representations and social learning from close relationships. Building on work from attachment theory and affective neuroscience, the MBT approach adopted a biobehavioral switch model (Arnsten et al. 1999; Mayes 2000), to the point of integrating it into clinical work and training (Bateman and Fonagy 2016) (see Chapter 6, "Individual Therapy Techniques"). Indeed, in vivo, the arousal-mediated switching between controlled and automatic mentalizing constitutes a key indicator in the frame-by-frame monitoring of a therapeutic session. The switch model quickly became a favorite clinical tool for therapists in reading the therapeutic process, enabling them to detect temporary breakdowns in mentalizing and to select the most appropriate therapeutic action along an arousal-sensitive spectrum of interventions, from supportive validation to mentalizing the relationship (Bateman and Fonagy 2004, 2006).

In 2009, responding to external critique around issues of concept definition and boundaries, Fonagy and Luyten (2009) put forward an integrative operationalization of mentalizing, specifying eight interrelated systems (i.e., automatic, controlled, internal, external, cognitive, affective, self, and other); the choice of these systems derives directly from cognitive neuroscience studies using magnetic resonance imaging to investigate neural function, and more specifically from the field of social cognitive neuroscience (Lieberman 2007). Today, clinical decisions in the consulting room are often made on the basis of the so-called mentalizing dimensions (see Chapter 1, "Introduction"), which guide the MBT practitioner's selection of clinical interventions (see Chapter 6). Although these dimensions have not yielded new therapeutic techniques per se, they usefully organize some of the thinking that takes place in clinicians' minds as they work through the complexity of their clinical encounters.

In this chapter we will briefly summarize how neuroscience contributes to the understanding of attachment and the mentalizing dimensions, as proposed elsewhere (Fonagy and Luyten 2009; Luyten and Fonagy 2015). Following this summary, we will present some of the latest advances in the neuroscience of mentalizing, which come from the field of cognitive, developmental, and affective neuroscience, and more recently from the computational approach to neuroscience. These recent developments will then lead us to consider how neuroscientific research enriches the understanding of key concepts such as selfhood, embodied mentalizing, and communication under conditions of epistemic trust. Finally, we will consider the mechanisms underlying general psychopathology within an MBT framework.

NEUROSCIENTIFIC BUILDING BLOCKS OF MBT

In the past 30 years, emotions have become a legitimate object of study in neuroscience (Sander and Scherer 2009), and this has greatly facilitated the integration of neurobiological and neuroimaging research findings into clinical concepts and therapeutic approaches. MBT is a treatment that focuses on affect, as lived within the intrapersonal as well as the intersubjective realms of experience. As such, contemporary neuroscience related to affect and its regulation, both within early attachment relationships and during development, is relevant to the understanding of mentalizing phenomena in the consulting room.

Attachment and Parenting

As informed by research that spans from anthropology to basic neuroscience, we know that the specific survival needs of the immature mammalian brain lead the infant to seek proximity to an attachment figure who provides both caregiving and co-regulation of affect. Within emerging attachment bonds, the infant's affiliative motivation and the parents' caregiving are sustained at the neurobiological level by cross-talk between the dopaminergic and oxytocinergic systems in the brain (Ebert and Brüne 2018). Through processes of contingent interactions (i.e., biobehavioral synchrony; see Feldman 2017), early experiences shape the social brain as a "situated" dialectic organ—that is to say, as being primarily influenced by and oriented toward the social environment of the individual's developmental niche. In the interplay between striatal regions, subcortical regions (amygdala and hypothalamus), and a network of neocortical areas (anterior cingulate, medial prefrontal, and orbitofrontal cortices), a sense of relatedness and reciprocity can be studied from the behavioral down to the neurobiological levels of investigation.

The basic neural machinery that develops in the sensitive period of mother–infant attachment (Feldman 2017) is repurposed and modified, sometimes substantially, through later relationships because of the brain's potential for plasticity. Good-enough caregiving experiences are imbued with a sense of regularity, trust, and communicative means that enable the infant to learn from the wider social group under conditions of epistemic trust (see Chapter 4, "Mentalizing, Resilience, and Epistemic Trust").

There is also growing evidence that such provision for a child's early needs, and the formation of attachment bonds, are facilitated by well-defined processes in the parental brain (see, e.g., Kim et al. 2016; Rutherford et al. 2015). Again, neuromodulators play a critical role in gating and coordinating the corticolimbic networks that interact to support parents' brain responses to their infants. These include circuitry for arousal and salience, which motivate parental reward and guide instrumental as well as reflective capacities. Together, these afford the parental brain and mind the sustained sensitivity required to detect and respond to infant cues. Thus, within attachment relationships, this complex interplay between biology, behavior, and representation gives rise to the parents' conceiving of their babies as essentially intentional beings with a propensity to find their mind (or self) in the mind of mentalizing caregivers (see Chapter 15, "Children").

Stress and Arousal

A central tenet of the MBT framework pertains to the influence affective arousal exerts on mentalizing. In other words, MBT centers on the question of how balanced mentalizing can be maintained or recovered if it is temporarily compromised as a result of an activated attachment system (Nolte et al. 2013). The therapeutic framework has integrated the switch model of Arnsten et al. (1999) and Mayes (2000) as a pivotal tool in how information about mental states of self and others is processed and emotions are modulated. Simply put, optimal arousal works in favor of good mentalizing, whereas suboptimal arousal (too low or too high for the individual's threshold) perturbs it. This principle is simple only on the surface; the variations of affective arousal within a therapeutic exchange can be subtle but sometimes quite fierce, swift, and generally difficult to predict. The clinical presentation of dysregulated arousal may differ according to the patient's dominant psychopathology (e.g., the different presentations of emotional dysregulation patterns in borderline, antisocial, and schizotypal personality disorders); in a similar vein, the triggers that modify and gate arousal variations are idiosyncratic to each patient. The biobehavioral switch model on which the MBT framework draws stipulates that an arousal-dependent switch occurs between mainly prefrontally mediated slow, controlled, and reflective modes of processing and posterior/subcortically mediated rapid, automatic, and reflexive modes of processing. Threat stimuli and distress, but also motivational arousal (e.g., sexual, appetitive), whether externally or internally generated, will adaptively shut down slow, serial processing mediated by the prefrontal cortex and its projections, in favor of the fight/flight/freeze or seeking and lust biobehavioral systems. One of the hallmarks of any psychopathological state is its ability to alter the affective switch point, which, in turn, affects the robustness of prefrontal functioning as well as the delay in down-regulating an overactivation of the affective system.

Neuroimaging studies have demonstrated that attachment-related interpersonal stress can lead to partial deactivation of the neural circuitry underpinning social cognition (e.g., Debbané et al. 2017; Nolte et al. 2013; Vrticka et al. 2014), thereby compromising the stress-buffering effect of mentalizing (see Chapter 17, "Borderline Personality Pathology in Adolescence" and Chapter 19, "Borderline Personality Disorder"). From a neurobiological standpoint, arousal within significant relationships implicates neuropeptides such as opioids, oxytocin, and vasopressin, and is further modulated by the stress regulation of the hypothalamic-pituitary-adrenal (HPA) axis. There is now increasing evidence that attachment security serves a protective function by promoting resilience to the impact of stress, mainly via anxiolytic and trust-enhancing effects, mediated primarily by oxytocin (Feldman et al. 2007; Heinrichs and Domes 2008; Powers et al. 2006). Moreover, studies investigating stress responsivity in both humans and animals have demonstrated that secure attachment leads to an "adaptive hypoactivity" of the HPA axis (Gunnar and Quevedo 2007). Conversely, stress and interpersonal hypervigilance impact HPA axis functioning, in the sense of chronic wear and tear. This posits that the initially regulatory and anticipatory functions of the HPA axis can also confer vulnerability to psychopathology (Lupien et al. 2009; Schulkin 2011). The core emotional regions of the brain (the frontolimbic circuit) are the primary and central mediators of stress load via the HPA axis and represent the main interface between changes in the environment and the individual's (mentalized) accommodation to it.

From Neural Circuits to Mentalizing Dimensions

The controlled-to-automatic switch provoked by increased arousal does not constitute the sole domain of influence that affect may have on mentalizing. Fonagy and Luyten (2009) have very usefully described four key mentalizing dimensions that, communicating via hypothetical underlying neural circuits, balance the mentalizing activity: 1) automatic–controlled; 2) internal–external; 3) self–other; and 4) cognitive–affective (see Table 2–1 for a full description of these dimensions).

The term *dimensions* has introduced some confusion regarding the relationship between the resulting eight polarities of mentalizing processes, especially given the fact that they are preferentially presented as pairs (as above). It is important to remember that each polarity represents a putative system and that all systems are interrelated and neutrally embedded in structural-functional brain dynamics. In certain situations, particularly when computing resources are scarce (as in situations of high arousal), the activity of each system competes with that of other systems. Cooperation/competition relationships are more likely to arise between automatic and/or controlled processing, involving content that can be more or less internal (e.g., thoughts, feelings) or external (e.g., perceptions, body postures), based on the perspective of self and/or other, focusing on cognitive and/or affective features. Therefore, while pairings describe oppositions in neural processing that have been described in the literature, it is important to remember that all systems relate to each other in the brain.

Furthermore, the validity of the pairings proposed by a number of studies constitutes only one of many ways in which "information processing" can be divided. Recent work on cognitive systems and information processing proposes a layered, hierarchical approach to information processing, which may also inform our field of work (Rudrauf et al. 2017). While this approach is still too new to be formalized into the MBT model, it should be kept in mind that the dimensional configuration is a clinically useful way to conceptualize the processes of the minds of patients, and even the

TABLE 2–1.	Polarities, features, and proposed neural circuits of mentalizing dimensions	
Polarity	**Features**	**Neural circuits**
Automatic	Unconscious, parallel, fast processing of social information that is reflexive and requires little effort, focused attention, or intention; therefore, prone to bias and distortions, particularly in complex interpersonal interactions (i.e., when arousal is high).	Amygdala Basal ganglia Ventromedial prefrontal cortex (VMPFC) Lateral temporal cortex (LTC) Dorsal anterior cingulate cortex (dACC)
Controlled	Conscious, verbal, and reflective processing of social information that requires the capacity to reflect consciously and deliberately on and make accurate attributions about the emotions, thoughts, and intentions of self and others. Relies heavily on effortful control and language.	Lateral prefrontal cortex (LPFC) Medial prefrontal cortex (MPFC) Lateral parietal cortex (LPAC) Medial parietal cortex (MPAC) Medial temporal lobe (MTL) Rostral anterior cingulate cortex (rACC)
Internal	Understanding one's own mind and that of others through a direct focus on the mental interiors of both the self and others.	Medial frontoparietal network (more controlled)
External	Understanding one's own mind and that of others based on external features (e.g., facial expressions, posture, prosody).	Lateral frontotemporoparietal network (more automatic)
Self–Other	Shared networks underpin the capacity to mentalize about the self and others.	Shared representation system (more automatic) vs. mental state attribution system (more controlled)
Cognitive–Affective	Mentalizing may focus on more cognitive features (more controlled), such as belief–desire reasoning and perspective taking vs. more affective features (more automatic), including affective empathy and mentalized affectivity (the feeling and thinking-about-the-feeling).	Cognitive mentalizing involves several areas in the prefrontal cortex; affectively oriented mentalizing seems to be particularly related to the VMPFC.

minds of therapists. However, it does not represent the only way to conceptualize mentalizing processes. As we will explain below, computational approaches may provide a promising avenue to complement and enrich current ways of thinking about mentalizing.

What appears crucial to most neuroscientific approaches to mentalizing is that the neural dynamics involved, in concert, enable the mind to

- Distinguish reality from psychological interior and fantasy.
- Sustain the emergence of an embodied self that can experience effective agentive properties.
- Experience interactions as meaningful.
- Engage in perspective taking and, more generally, imaginative thinking.

COMPUTATIONAL APPROACH TO NEUROSCIENCE: IMPLICATIONS FOR MBT

Basic Principles in Computational Neuroscience

As explained earlier in this chapter, it is our view that experience-dependent reorganization of the brain's structure-function relationships affords individuals with the potential for lifelong adaptation. Resilience, from that viewpoint, is governed by higher-order cognition (HOC), which comprises a variety of psychological mechanisms, such as perspective taking, metacognition, executive function, attention, memory, general intelligence, and self-awareness. In the brain, this translates into HOC as the overarching process of rerouting structural and functional connections between ensembles of neuron populations or networks (see, e.g., Fonagy and Bateman 2016; Rudrauf 2014). Thereby, new routes for information processing between regions are created (e.g., after structural damage resulting from a neurological event). The resulting optimized neural architecture seeks to compensate for the compromised structure by generating an alternative set of brain connections to sustain functional resilience in the face of partial organ failure.

Mentalizing in a broader (i.e., HOC) sense is a prime candidate in order to dynamically preserve or recover adaptive functioning, which supports psychological resilience and robustness in the face of challenges impacting the brain. When both neural integrity and the integrity of the felt self are under threat (e.g., during childhood adversity, illness, prolonged distress in maladaptive relationships, dissociative symptoms, or traumatic experiences), HOC acts as a compensatory cognitive reserve (Stern 2009) to rearrange computations in the brain to ensure "business as usual" (Fonagy and Bateman 2016). Heuristically speaking, the human capacity for imaginative activity may constitute one of the crucial mechanisms enabling abstraction, separation of thoughts from feelings, perspective taking, and reappraisal, which are key to flexible and resilient thinking abilities (see Chapter 4).

One of the most promising approaches to studying these phenomena in a principled empirical way is computational neuroscience and computational psychiatry, with an emphasis on psychopathology. Computational psychiatry is a nascent discipline at the intersection of computational neuroscience, psychology, and psychiatry. It holds the promise to get closer to "carving nature at its joints" and to provide insight into the key mechanisms underpinning mental functioning and psychopathology. Computational psychiatry offers the advantage of investigating the associations between brain function, the interplay with the environment the brain is trying to model or act on, and psychiatric symptoms via formulized computational processes (Friston et al. 2014; Montague et al. 2012; Stephan and Mathys 2014).

Active inference, as one of the main principles driving this new approach, posits that the brain performs so-called Bayesian inference processes. In the heuristics of this framework, the brain is viewed as not just a passive filter of input, but rather a "statistical organ that generates hypotheses or fantasies that are tested against sensory evidence" (Friston et al. 2014, p. 148). This notion is of particular importance, as navigating the social world requires constant modeling of other people, as well as approximating what intentional states might underpin their behaviors or one's own, so as to generate coherent self-with-other experiences.

Recognizing discrepancies between an individual's own assumptions (his or her prior beliefs about the causes of what is perceived) and reality generates "surprise" or "unbound energy." Such a mismatch then leads to a neural alert, the so-called *prediction error signals*, which in turn incline the system to update the relevant working hypotheses as the individual accumulates more and new evidence or information. Through preexisting mental structures, the individual's generative models of self and other are also afforded greater or lesser precision via top-down neuromodulatory gain control mechanisms. These prescribe how prone the revisions of the individual's beliefs are to rigidity—or indeed flexibility. Here, a parallel may be drawn to the notion of *learning from experience* (see Chapter 1).

The main contention of computational neuroscience is that neural functioning shapes sensory input into experience according to Bayesian probabilistic calculus. As captured by Holmes and Slade (2018, p. 151), in healthy minds, "discrepancies between prediction and input are: (a) identified, via 'tolerating uncertainty,' (b) explored, by *action* aimed at reducing uncertainty, (c) leading, finally, to cognitive restructuring and updating of 'prior' probabilities." A mentalizing therapist helps patients to bear the inevitable uncertainty intrinsic to knowledge about mental states; the therapist further models affect regulation, stimulates reflection, and scaffolds the exploration of alternative perspectives so that the process of thinking and imagining can be rekindled, constantly reshaped, and updated through experience.

From a developmental perspective, the generation of meaning in infancy may be examined in the biobehavioral synchronies (and asynchronies) with caregivers and the physical environment, the pressures to regulate allostatic challenges (both continuous life stressors and particular traumatic events), and the reappraisal (i.e., mentalizing) of caregiving experiences, all from the point of view of Bayesian principles. In typically developing infants, the accompanying basic generative models or beliefs undergo constant revision and refinement. In other words, "a baby's brain is in the game of minimizing surprise, while acting epistemically to reduce expected surprise (i.e., uncertainty)," about the novel events it is constantly encountering (Friston 2017, p. 43). The baby, adjusting to a specific developmental niche, can be understood as "conforming to one imperative; namely, to maximize the evidence for its own existence" (Friston 2017, p. 43), captured by the notion of a self-evidencing brain that strives to make sense of what is going on inside and around him or her. In a computational neuroscience framework, mental ill health (ranging from normal to psychopathology) can be understood in terms of atypical developmental patterns underpinning computational aspects of such inference.

Modeling the computations that sustain ongoing experience-dependent adaptation in life may generate empirical tools that can inform the existing mentalizing framework to better conceptualize the processes that contribute to health and to psychopathology. Significant conceptual contributions from this approach bear relevance for a deepened understanding of how aspects of mentalizing are indeed implemented neurally. These concepts go beyond identifying which network of brain areas is involved when a particular process is being called into action; rather, they seek to uncover the algorithms underlying how neural populations perform their computations. For instance, these new approaches are concerned with the inference of self and other representations (Moutoussis et al. 2014), interoception and homeostasis of the self when engaged with the outside world (Gu et al. 2013; Seth 2013), and compulsivity (Hauser et al. 2016), and may yield a kind of deep cognitive phenotyping (Hula et al. 2015; Xiang et al. 2012). These conceptual contributions can be complemented further by tangible examples and applications focused on, for instance, social learning (Diaconescu et al. 2017), the therapeutic process (Moutoussis et al. 2017), and theory of mind in two-party interactions (Hula et al. 2018). In this sense, the computational neuroscience framework affords the possibility of learning not only from therapeutic experience but also from neuroscientific modeling, such as virtual reality settings or simulated interpersonal processes, thereby increasing the potential for research on mentalizing in health and psychopathology.

A paradigmatic example of such experimental tasks serves to illustrate recent developments in research. A recent study by Hula et al. (2018) characterized the establishment, breakdown, and repair of trust signals in a two-party economic exchange task, the canonical Trust Game. This game evolves iteratively over 10 rounds of an interaction between two players. The *recursive modeling* required—that is, the making sense of what is going on—captures the individual's own social signals sent to the other, and the individual's thinking about his or her partner, as well as the potential representation of the self in the counterpart. Critically, the model should include the individual's updating of the beliefs underlying these interpersonal theory of mind assumptions, along the lines of: "*If I behave in this particular way, my partner may respond contingently; he's coming into the interaction with a set of expectations from previous experiences and adjusting his style of playing in the light of new exchanges just made with me (and the same holding true for myself).*" Additional parameters that can be modeled and traced across the interaction include the horizon for future-action planning as a temporal aspect of mentalizing, an index of guilt or inequality aversion, and the propensity for irritation that precipitates and responds to ruptures in cooperation. At this stage it remains an empirical question for future research to establish the value and validity of these markers—for instance, in clustering patient groups along new continua of interpersonal problems. These markers certainly represent a new avenue for research and perhaps will assist in predicting differential responses to treatment. In addition, the artificial intelligence revolution will inevitably have an impact on the field of MBT by challenging traditional views of understanding mental ill health.

Embodied Mentalizing and the Development of the Self

At this juncture readers may ponder how the cross-talk between computational neuroscience and the clinical MBT framework is currently taking place. A number of publications have employed the term *embodied mentalizing* as a key construct offering the opportunity to bridge the neuroscientific and clinical levels of analysis (Debbané et al. 2016; Fonagy and Campbell 2017; Fotopoulou and Tsakiris 2017; Luyten et al. 2012; Shai and Belsky 2011). Luyten et al. (2012, p. 125) define embodied mentalizing as "the capacity to see the body as the seat of emotions, wishes and feelings and the capacity to reflect on one's own bodily experiences and sensations and their relationships to intentional mental states in the self and others." Embodied mentalizing involves "the processes needed to *detect*, *identify* and *regulate* signals coming from one's body to harness them with one's mind" (Debbané et al. 2016, p. 12). As Fotopoulou and Tsakiris (2017) hypothesize, these psychological depictions of embodied mentalizing could be amenable to the field of computational neuroscience, albeit with an operationalized notion that seeks to capture its computational rather than clinical essence:

> We define "embodied mentalization" here as the inferential brain process by which primary sensorimotor and multisensory signals are progressively integrated and schematized to form multiple, predictive models of our embodied states in given environments. These models are not understood as static body representations in the brain (e.g., "body schema" vs. "body image") but rather as "hypothetical" (probabilistic, inferential), dynamic and generative processes (they are constantly updated against received error signals). (p. 8)

Common to these depictions of embodiment in mentalizing is the dynamic, integrative nature of a kind of mentalizing founded upon the signals coming from the body: mentalizing is the process of melding sensations, affects, and thoughts into novel dispositions, which will themselves be employed as raw material in subsequent mentalizing processes. Critically, this process is initiated within the very first infant–caregiver interactions and pursued throughout development.

The increased attention paid to embodied mentalizing is in line with early insights from the field of psychoanalytic psychosomatics, namely that mentalizing represents a suite of processes responsible for the regulation and transformation of physiological activation through higher-order psychological processes (Lecours and Bouchard 1997; Marty 1991). In infancy, it is the HOCs coming from the parents' minds, through their caregiving gestures, that assume most of this regulation, or indeed, metabolization. As Shai and Belsky (2011) point out, parental embodied mentalizing is initially nonverbal and implicit. That is to say that infants *find their mind in their caregivers' arms*. The concepts of holding, handling, and presenting (Winnicott 1960) can be revisited as types of embodied engagements whereby caregivers employ their body to communicate their mentalizing of the infant's internal states (Fonagy and Campbell 2017). Critically, these embodied engagements present a model of the infant from the caregiver's perspective, which at the neuroscientific level assists the infant to integrate the primary sensory and multisensory signals (Fotopoulou and Tsakiris 2017), and on which predictive models will spatially, affectively, and cognitively orient the infant to explore the environment. Furthermore, the infant's nascent generative (probabilistic inferential) models will be dynamically updated in relation to so-called "error signals"—that is, through attention to novelty.

These neuroscientific considerations have important implications concerning how, from the mentalization-based framework, the development of the self is conceptualized (Fonagy et al. 2002). Typically, such a perspective stresses the importance of contingent and marked mirroring in the establishment of a continuity of selfhood. This critical observation is echoed in computational neuroscience: if the brain is designed to elaborate hierarchical generative models of the world, then the infant brain will fundamentally seek to differentiate self versus nonself causes of sensations. As Friston (2017, p. 44) suggests: "It follows that the first job of structure learning is to distinguish between the causes of sensations that can be attributed to self and those that cannot. If we assume that the fundamental self versus nonself distinction is an imperative for subsequent (hierarchical) elaboration of a model…this is the first structural inference an infant has to accomplish." Friston (2017) underlines how infants are "self-evidencing," thereby producing sensations (e.g., through body movements, communicative signals) that provide the material on which the internal–external and self–nonself distinctions can be forged. The self-evidencing baby does not live in a relational vacuum: the caregiver's response to the baby's behaviors will contribute to the increasingly sharpened self–other distinction. A developmental and potentially clinically relevant issue arises when feedback from the environment is fuzzy: this could be the result of unmarked mirroring (Fonagy et al. 2002), or of atypical neurodevelopment, which leaves the infant's brain vulnerable to deficits in decoding social feedback signals (Jones and Klin 2013). In other words, the self-evidencing baby critically requires predictable input from the caregiver to integrate self–other boundaries. When this input is missing or incomprehensible, or when it is conveyed in a highly affective and "unmarked" fashion, it carries the opposite effect—that of blurring the self–other boundary, which can sustain the development of maladaptive, disorganized internal working models, as attachment research has shown. Future research will need to elucidate how hierarchical inferential models put forward by computational neuroscience relate to internal working models examined in attachment research. We can already see how computational neuroscience provides new methodology for the examination of development of the self in the baby (e.g., see Cittern et al. 2018) and throughout ontogeny.

The Nature of Psychopathology: The "p" Factor and the Brain

From the preceding section, we can appreciate how the concept of embodied mentalizing generates interest not only in the brain bases of psychopathology but also in the multisensory nature of signals that require integration to sustain adaptive development. This leads us to reflect on the nature of the coming-into-being of a stable and continuous self, and opens the possibility for finer-grained studies of the earliest manifestations of developmental psychopathology, such as autism spectrum disorder, which critically implicates atypical multisensory integration (Iarocci and McDonald 2006) and often disturbed evolution of agency and the sense of self. These future neuroscientific studies may also pave the way to a more complex mechanistic understanding of the development of the self in contexts of early trauma and abuse and, more specifically, the new methodologies established could assist in further exploring the emergence of disorganized attachment.

More generally, clinicians may reflect on how advances in neuroscience more broadly, and computational neuroscience in particular, may afford learning opportunities concerning the nature of psychopathology. Findings have demonstrated that some individuals are more prone to persistent and severe psychopathology, as captured by a general vulnerability index, referred to as the *p (psychopathology) factor* (Caspi et al. 2014) (see Chapter 4). Additional promising models of psychopathology, such as the network approach to mental disorders (Borsboom and Cramer 2013), which does not assume latent psychopathological factors but examines the nature of the interactions between symptoms and their underlying psychopathological processes in the dynamics of mental illness and health, can lend themselves to neuroscientific investigations. In line with both these contemporary accounts, computational neuroscience may shed light on both environmental and constitutional contributions to this general vulnerability or propensity to persistent psychopathology. Furthermore, computational neuroscience can help identify key computational processes and brain–behavior interactions of compromised functioning (e.g., suboptimal recruitment of HOCs). With evidence emerging that casts the p factor as being strongly associated with high levels of childhood maltreatment and low mentalizing capacity (Gibbon et al. 2018), the neural underpinnings of mental-state processing will illuminate transdiagnostic brain–behavior relationships that will help to understand why certain symptoms cluster together.

With regard to psychopathology, such computational models can be informative for identifying where a single patient is located along a continuum of problems (Stephan et al. 2017), as well as identifying endophenotypes of higher-order mental processing that cut across traditional diagnoses. Most importantly, these new approaches may shed light on aspects of brain structure-function relationships underpinning resilience processes (Kalisch et al. 2015), possibly facilitated by epistemic trust in others and the resulting broaden-and-build process in relation to social support and learning from other mentalizing minds (Fonagy et al. 2015). Critically, computational neuroscience may assist in furthering knowledge of the following: 1) the three therapeutic communication systems (see Chapter 4); 2) how insights gained in the consulting room are generalized in the social world of the patient; and 3) how the "inferential organ" of the patient is made more receptive to external influence and more amenable to being updated on the basis of interpersonal and social experience.

CONCLUSION

Our aim in this chapter was to convey how neuroscience research and MBT as a treatment approach are involved in a fertile exchange that can mutually benefit research and clinical practice. Neuroscience has proven vital in identifying some putative mechanistic (and now probabilistic) models that enrich the mentalization-based framework. Distinguishing the different poles of feeling and thinking about self and others provided a clinically useful and neuroscientifically grounded model to capture the phenomenology of what patients bring to the consulting room. We conjecture that the next period of neuroscientific effort will get at the "how"; it will address the complex dynamics sustaining the integration of sensory, affective, perceptual, and cognitive processes underlying individuals' capacity to makes sense of and to learn from their experiences, inner world, and behaviors.

Future research into the neurobiology of social cognition could address the following areas in order to inform the development of new therapies and the shaping and evaluation of care pathways:

1. *Dynamic aspects* of mentalizing, which take into account contextual and relationship-specific features.
2. *Ecological validity* of research paradigms that approximate to real-life experiences, including the impact of affective arousal and other emotional states.
3. *Longitudinal research* assessing the neurobiology of mentalizing from a lifetime perspective, starting with its origins in infancy, and incorporating what developmental psychopathology has contributed (e.g., equifinality and multifinality, differential susceptibility, twin studies to discern genetic and environmental factors as well as their coupling).

4. Employment of insights gained from these future neuroscientific endeavors in psychotherapy outcome studies that will critically contribute to increased knowledge about the *mechanisms of change* in psychotherapy

Moreover, to facilitate a mechanistic understanding of psychopathology, future advances might focus on the complex interplay between mentalizing as a core capacity of human communication and its role in fostering resilience in the context of adversity. This approach could shed further light on the protective role of social cognitive capacities via their contribution to structural-functional plasticity in the developing and adjusting brain.

A better mechanistic understanding of how canonical microcircuits of the mentalizing neural network in the brain orchestrate and update beliefs about relational experiences (including those schemata that are recruited without a person's awareness) can identify computational building blocks of self–other inference. Furthermore, a new generation of neuroimaging techniques ("hyperscanning" of interacting brains and noninvasive optically pumped magnetoencephalography that allow the registration of brain signals during movement and engagement with others in the environment [Montague et al. 2002]), as well as the accompanying methodological developments, may generate new insights into how two or more mentalizing brains influence one another (e.g., Bolis and Schilbach 2017). Entraining flexible thinking (balanced mentalizing) and thereby openness to psychological knowledge through epistemic trust results in learning from a social environment that is experienced as benign and offering support. Thus, a final extension to such between-brain processes and their neural machinery (with parent–infant or therapist–patient as paradigmatic dyads) will most probably include the investigation of how broader social networks and the wider social environment are represented and experienced.

In conclusion, it appears that neuroscience, much like the clinical approach to mentalizing, is returning to a focus on "the body," through research on embodiment and nonverbal communication. After a strong effort to delineate the cognitive and representational systems that sustain mentalizing, the bodily sources of communication and learning via ostensive signaling are stimulating rejuvenated interest, which is complemented by the development of novel methodological tools. Computational neuroscience, mathematical simulation, and the like are candidate contributors that may fail or succeed to inform the updating of mentalizing models in clinical practice.

REFERENCES

Arnsten AF, Mathew R, Ubriani R, et al: Alpha-1 noradrenergic receptor stimulation impairs prefrontal cortical cognitive function. Biol Psychiatry 45(1):26–31, 1999 9894572

Bateman A, Fonagy P: Psychotherapy for Borderline Personality Disorder: Mentalization-Based Treatment. Oxford, UK, Oxford University Press, 2004

Bateman A, Fonagy P: Mentalization-Based Treatment for Borderline Personality Disorder: A Practical Guide. Oxford, UK, Oxford University Press, 2006

Bateman A, Fonagy P: Mentalization-Based Treatment for Personality Disorders: A Practical Guide. Oxford, UK, Oxford University Press, 2016

Bolis D, Schilbach L: Beyond one Bayesian brain: Modeling intra- and inter-personal processes during social interaction: Commentary on "Mentalizing homeostasis: The social origins of interoceptive inference" by Fotopoulou and Tsakiris. Neuro-psychoanalysis 19:35–38, 2017

Borsboom D, Cramer AO: Network analysis: an integrative approach to the structure of psychopathology. Annu Rev Clin Psychol 9:91–121, 2013 23537483

Carter CS, Porges SW: The biochemistry of love: an oxytocin hypothesis. EMBO Rep 14(1):12–16, 2013 23184088

Caspi A, Houts RM, Belsky DW, et al: The p factor: One general psychopathology factor in the structure of psychiatric disorders? Clin Psychol Sci 2(2):119–137, 2014 25360393

Cittern D, Nolte T, Friston K, et al: Intrinsic and extrinsic motivators of attachment under active inference. PLoS One 13(4):e0193955, 2018 29621266

Debbané M, Salaminios G, Luyten P, et al: Attachment, neurobiology, and mentalizing along the psychosis continuum. Front Hum Neurosci 10:406, 2016 27597820

Debbané M, Badoud D, Sander D, et al: Brain activity underlying negative self- and other-perception in adolescents: the role of attachment-derived self-representations. Cogn Affect Behav Neurosci 17(3):554–576, 2017 28168598

Diaconescu AO, Mathys C, Weber LAE, et al: Hierarchical prediction errors in midbrain and septum during social learning. Soc Cogn Affect Neurosci 12(4):618–634, 2017 28119508

Ebert A, Brüne M: Oxytocin and social cognition. Curr Top Behav Neurosci 35:375–388, 2018 29019100

Feldman R: The neurobiology of human attachments. Trends Cogn Sci 21(2):80–99, 2017 28041836

Feldman R, Weller A, Zagoory-Sharon O, et al: Evidence for a neuroendocrinological foundation of human affiliation: plasma oxytocin levels across pregnancy and the postpartum period predict mother-infant bonding. Psychol Sci 18(11):965–970, 2007 17958710

Fonagy P, Bateman AW: Adversity, attachment, and mentalizing. Compr Psychiatry 64:59–66, 2016 26654293

Fonagy P, Campbell C: What touch can communicate: Commentary on "Mentalizing homeostasis: the social origins of interoceptive inference" by Fotopoulou and Tsakiris. Neuro-psychoanalysis 19:39–42, 2017

Fonagy P, Luyten P: A developmental, mentalization-based approach to the understanding and treatment of borderline personality disorder. Dev Psychopathol 21(4):1355–1381, 2009 19825272

Fonagy P, Gergely G, Jurist EL, et al: Affect Regulation, Mentalization, and the Development of the Self. New York, Other Press, 2002

Fonagy P, Luyten P, Allison E: Epistemic petrification and the restoration of epistemic trust: a new conceptualization of borderline personality disorder and its psychosocial treatment. J Pers Disord 29(5):575–609, 2015 26393477

Fotopoulou A, Tsakiris M: Mentalizing homeostasis: the social origins of interoceptive inference. Neuro-psychoanalysis 19:3–28, 2017

Friston KJ: Self-evidencing babies: Commentary on "Mentalizing homeostasis: The social origins of interoceptive inference" by Fotopoulou and Tsakiris. Neuro-psychoanalysis 19:43–47, 2017

Friston KJ, Stephan KE, Montague R, et al: Computational psychiatry: the brain as a phantastic organ. Lancet Psychiatry 1(2):148–158, 2014 26360579

Gibbon L, Nolte T, Fonagy P: Modelling Axis I and personality disorder symptomatology and its associations with childhood trauma and mentalizing. University College London, 2018

Gu X, Hof PR, Friston KJ, et al: Anterior insular cortex and emotional awareness. J Comp Neurol 521(15):3371–3388, 2013 23749500

Gunnar M, Quevedo K: The neurobiology of stress and development. Annu Rev Psychol 58:145–173, 2007 16903808

Hauser TU, Fiore VG, Moutoussis M, et al: Computational psychiatry of ADHD: neural gain impairments across Marrian levels of analysis. Trends Neurosci 39(2):63–73, 2016 26787097

Heinrichs M, Domes G: Neuropeptides and social behaviour: effects of oxytocin and vasopressin in humans. Prog Brain Res 170:337–350, 2008 18655894

Holmes J, Slade A: Attachment in Therapeutic Practice. London, Sage, 2018

Hula A, Montague PR, Dayan P: Monte Carlo planning method estimates planning horizons during interactive social exchange. PLOS Comput Biol 11(6):e1004254, 2015 26053429

Hula A, Vilares I, Dayan P, et al: A model of risk and mental state shifts during social interaction. PLOS Comput Biol 14(2):e1005935, 2018 29447153

Iarocci G, McDonald J: Sensory integration and the perceptual experience of persons with autism. J Autism Dev Disord 36(1):77–90, 2006 16395537

Jones W, Klin A: Attention to eyes is present but in decline in 2–6-month-old infants later diagnosed with autism. Nature 504(7480):427–431, 2013 24196715

Kalisch R, Müller MB, Tüscher O: A conceptual framework for the neurobiological study of resilience. Behav Brain Sci 38:e92, 2015 25158686

Kim P, Strathearn L, Swain JE: The maternal brain and its plasticity in humans. Horm Behav 77:113–123, 2016 26268151

Lecours S, Bouchard MA: Dimensions of mentalisation: outlining levels of psychic transformation. Int J Psychoanal 78(Pt 5):855–875, 1997 9459091

Lieberman MD: Social cognitive neuroscience: a review of core processes. Annu Rev Psychol 58:259–289, 2007 17002553

Lupien SJ, McEwen BS, Gunnar MR, et al: Effects of stress throughout the lifespan on the brain, behaviour and cognition. Nat Rev Neurosci 10(6):434–445, 2009 19401723

Luyten P, Fonagy P: The neurobiology of mentalizing. Pers Disord 6(4):366–379, 2015 26436580

Luyten P, van Houdenhove B, Lemma A, et al: A mentalization-based approach to the understanding and treatment of functional somatic disorders. Psychoanal Psychother 26:121–140, 2012

Marty P: Mentalisation et Psychosomatique. Paris, Empêcheurs de Penser en Rond, 1991

Mayes LC: A developmental perspective on the regulation of arousal states. Semin Perinatol 24(4):267–279, 2000 10975433

Meaney MJ: Epigenetics and the biological definition of gene x environment interactions. Child Dev 81(1):41–79, 2010 20331654

Montague PR, Berns GS, Cohen JD, et al: Hyperscanning: simultaneous fMRI during linked social interactions. Neuroimage 16(4):1159–1164, 2002 12202103

Montague PR, Dolan RJ, Friston KJ, et al: Computational psychiatry. Trends Cogn Sci 16(1):72–80, 2012 22177032

Moutoussis M, Fearon P, El-Deredy W, et al: Bayesian inferences about the self (and others): a review. Conscious Cogn 25:67–76, 2014 24583455

Moutoussis M, Shahar N, Hauser TU, et al: Computation in psychotherapy, or how computational psychiatry can aid learning-based psychological therapies. Computational Psychiatry 2:50–73, 2017

Nolte T, Bolling DZ, Hudac CM, et al: Brain mechanisms underlying the impact of attachment-related stress on social cognition. Front Hum Neurosci 7:816, 2013 24348364

Powers SI, Pietromonaco PR, Gunlicks M, et al: Dating couples' attachment styles and patterns of cortisol reactivity and recovery in response to a relationship conflict. J Pers Soc Psychol 90(4):613–628, 2006 16649858

Rudrauf D: Structure-function relationships behind the phenomenon of cognitive resilience in neurology: insights for neuroscience and medicine. Adv Neurosci (Hindawi) 2014:1–28, 2014

Rudrauf D, Bennequin D, Granic I, et al: A mathematical model of embodied consciousness. J Theor Biol 428:106–131, 2017 28554611

Rutherford HJ, Wallace NS, Laurent HK, et al: Emotion regulation in parenthood. Dev Rev 36:1–14, 2015 26085709

Sander D, Scherer KR: The Oxford Companion to Emotion and the Affective Sciences. Oxford, UK, Oxford University Press, 2009

Schulkin J: Social allostasis: anticipatory regulation of the internal milieu. Front Evol Neurosci 2:111, 2011 21369352

Seth AK: Interoceptive inference, emotion, and the embodied self. Trends Cogn Sci 17(11):565–573, 2013 24126130

Shai D, Belsky J: When words just won't do: introducing parental embodied mentalizing. Child Dev Perspect 5:173–180, 2011

Stephan KE, Mathys C: Computational approaches to psychiatry. Curr Opin Neurobiol 25:85–92, 2014 24709605

Stephan KE, Schlagenhauf F, Huys QJM, et al: Computational neuroimaging strategies for single patient predictions. Neuroimage 145(Pt B):180–199, 2017 27346545

Stern Y: Cognitive reserve. Neuropsychologia 47(10):2015–2028, 2009 19467352

Vrticka P, Sander D, Anderson B, et al: Social feedback processing from early to late adolescence: influence of sex, age, and attachment style. Brain Behav 4(5):703–720, 2014 25328847

Winnicott DW: The theory of the parent-infant relationship. Int J Psychoanal 41:585–595, 1960 13785877

Xiang T, Ray D, Lohrenz T, et al: Computational phenotyping of two-person interactions reveals differential neural response to depth-of-thought. PLOS Comput Biol 8(12):e1002841, 2012 23300423

CHAPTER 3

ASSESSMENT OF MENTALIZING

Patrick Luyten, Ph.D.

Saskia Malcorps, M.Sc.

Peter Fonagy, Ph.D., FBA, FMedSci, FAcSS

Karin Ensink, Ph.D., M.A. [Clin. Psych.]

In clinical practice and research it is sometimes helpful to consider mentalizing as a unitary construct (*"This patient has severe impairments in mentalizing"*), but in most cases more detailed assessment and monitoring of a patient's mentalizing capacities with respect to the different dimensions underlying mentalizing are indicated. Different types of psychopathology are characteristically associated with specific imbalances between the dimensions of mentalizing; that is, there may be impairments in one dimension but not the others (Allen et al. 2008; Luyten and Fonagy 2015). Hence, detailed assessment of a patient's mentalizing capacities along each dimension yields important diagnostic information that can also be used to tailor a specific treatment approach. For instance, although the programs of mentalization-based treatment (MBT) for patients with borderline personality disorder (BPD) and for those with antisocial personality disorder (ASPD) share many features, they also have a number of important differences that are related to the specific types of mentalizing impairments that differentiate patients with the two disorders (discussed later in this chapter; see also Chapter 20, "Antisocial Personality Disorder in Community and Prison Settings"). As effective treatment should lead to a decrease in dissociations between mentalizing capacities and thus to a more balanced and flexible use of the different dimensions of mentalizing, it is important for therapists to be able to tailor treatment to these specific dissociations or imbalances. Hence, the formulation of a so-called *mentalizing profile*—that is, a profile detailing the individual's mentalizing skills with respect to each of the dimensions of mentalizing (Luyten et al. 2012)—is particularly helpful in adapting treatment to the patient's needs. This profile also informs therapists about the types of relationships and associated mentalizing impairments that are likely to develop, serving as the first *transference tracers*—that is, similarities between the way the patient relates to other people in his or her life and to the treating clinician (Bateman and Fonagy 2016).

Mentalizing is typically also heavily dependent on context—in particular, attachment contexts (Luyten et al. 2012). With increasing arousal (often linked to specific types of relationships or interactions), effective mentalizing becomes increasingly difficult (Luyten and Fonagy 2015). This response is in keeping with the biobehavioral switch model of the relationship between stress and automatic and controlled mentalizing (Figure 3–1). It is therefore imperative to explore the extent to which the patient's mentalizing capacities are context- and relationship-specific. Individual differences in the use of primary and secondary attachment strategies are key in understanding the dynamic relationship between arousal or stress and mentalizing. Thus, the assessment of mentalizing also requires detailed attention to the attachment history of the individual. This assessment will also yield important information concerning broader contextual factors that together with the individual's attachment history, may have influenced his or her capacity for epistemic trust (i.e., the capacity to trust others as a source of knowledge about the social world and to consider this knowledge as personally relevant and generalizable to the self; see Chapter 4, "Mentalizing, Resilience, and Epistemic Trust") and, thus, mentalizing (Fonagy et al. 2015).

In this chapter we first discuss the dimensions underlying mentalizing and how they form the basis for a detailed assessment of mentalizing along the different dimensions. Second, we provide an overview of the role of arousal in relation to attachment history and mentalizing, pointing to important individual differences in mentalizing capacities. We end this chapter by providing detailed guidelines concerning the assessment of mentalizing in routine clinical practice and for research purposes.

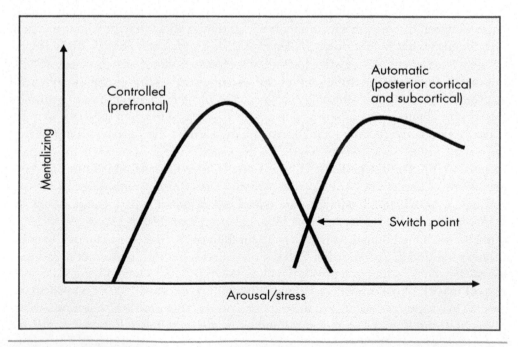

FIGURE 3–1. Biobehavioral switch model of the relationship between stress and controlled versus automatic mentalizing.

DIMENSIONS OF MENTALIZING AND MENTALIZING PROFILES

As described in Chapter 1 ("Introduction"), mentalizing is underpinned by four dimensions, each with its own relatively distinct neural circuits: 1) automatic–controlled, 2) internal–external, 3) self–other, and 4) cognitive–affective (Fonagy and Luyten 2009; Luyten et al. 2012). Mentalizing thus is an umbrella concept. This has two important implications for assessment. First, although mentalizing is sometimes conceptualized as a unitary concept, mentalizing is in fact all about the *balance* between the four dimensions underlying mentalizing, and about potential *imbalances* between the two poles of each dimension. Patients with BPD features, for instance, are typically overly sensitive to the emotional states of others at the expense of reflective awareness of their own states of mind. They are also easily overwhelmed by the affective states of both themselves and others, often have little capacity for cognitive control, and are typically highly attuned to external features (e.g., facial expressions, posture), which leads them to jump to conclusions about internal mental states, resulting in erroneous and overly negative assumptions about what others think and feel about them. Effective mentalizing thus involves a balance between the various systems that are involved in the individual's thinking and feeling about himself or herself and others. As an illustrative example, Figure 3–2 represents prototypical mentalizing profiles of patients with BPD, ASPD, and narcissistic personality disorder (NPD).

A second implication of this multidimensional view is that mentalizing is an overarching concept or construct that encompasses related constructs such as empathy, mindfulness, and theory of mind (ToM). The different dimensions underlying mentalizing are again helpful in this context. Empathy and ToM, for instance, involve mentalizing with regard to others, whereas mindfulness involves mentalizing about the self and concerns basic physical and emotional sensations and experiences in particular. In terms of the cognitive–affective dimension, most theory and research on empathy and mindfulness have focused on the affective processes involved in each, whereas research on ToM has typically focused on cognitive features involved in mentalizing with regard to others (e.g., belief-desire reasoning), although more recent formulations pay more attention to affective features involved in ToM. This also means that assessment methods that have been developed in research on these related constructs can be used as proxy measures of different features or components of mentalizing, as explained in more detail later in this chapter.

MENTALIZING, AROUSAL, AND INDIVIDUAL DIFFERENCES IN ATTACHMENT

Arousal typically impedes effective mentalizing. Under increasing arousal, there is a switch from controlled mentalizing—that is, conscious, reflective, and verbal consideration of mental states of the self and others—to more automatic mentalizing, which is marked by fast and nonreflective processing of (social) information (Arnsten 1998; Mayes 2006) (see Figure 3–1). From an evolutionary perspective, this switch has a clear survival value (Lieberman 2007; Mayes 2006). In response to stress, the fight/flight response is best subserved by the swift processing of social information. In the complex interpersonal world, however, such automatic processing of social information has

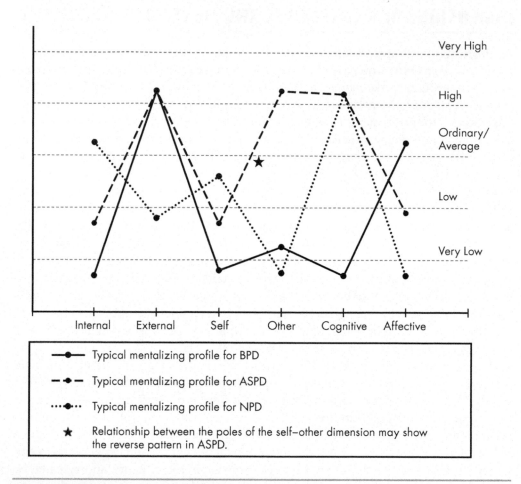

FIGURE 3–2.   Prototypical mentalizing profiles for borderline, narcissistic, and antisocial personality disorder.

ASPD=antisocial personality disorder; BPD=borderline personality disorder; NPD=narcissistic personality disorder.

many disadvantages, particularly in individuals who are characterized by a low threshold for such a switch.

The biobehavioral switch model depicted in Figure 3–1 proposes that individual differences in the use and strength of attachment hyperactivation and deactivation strategies in response to stress determine three key parameters in this switch from controlled to automatic mentalizing. These parameters are as follows: 1) the threshold (intercept) at which the switch happens, 2) the strength of the relationship between stress and the activation of controlled versus automatic mentalizing (the slope), and 3) the time to recovery from stress (i.e., return to controlled mentalizing).

Secure attachment has been related to the capacity to retain high levels of mentalizing even in high arousal contexts, and to recover mentalizing relatively rapidly after it has been temporarily lost (Table 3–1). The combination of security of attachment and high levels of mentalizing is also typically related to "broaden and build" (Fredrickson 2001) cycles that reinforce feelings of secure attachment, personal agency, and mentalizing ("build"), and are associated with a genuine interest in and openness to others and new social information and contexts ("broaden") (Mikulincer and Shaver 2007). Genuine mentalizing thus also fosters the capacity for epistemic trust and *salutogenesis*, the capacity to benefit from positive features in the environment. Our newest formulations link these features (effective mentalizing leading to genuine interest in the mind of others and epistemic trust in knowledge that others transfer) to resilience in the face of adversity (Fonagy et al. 2017a, 2017b; see also Chapter 4). Indeed, individuals with these features typically seek out others in times of need ("relationship recruiting") and have the capacity to let others "recalibrate" their mind in adaptive ways.

TABLE 3–1.   Attachment strategies, arousal, and mentalizing

Attachment strategy	Threshold for switch	Strength of automatic response	Recovery of controlled mentalizing
Secure	High	Moderate	Fast
Hyperactivating	Low: hyperresponsivity	Strong	Slow
Deactivating	Relatively high: hyporesponsive, but failure under increasing stress	Weak, but moderate to strong under increasing stress	Relatively fast
Disorganized	Incoherent: hyperresponsive, but often frantic attempts to downregulate	Strong	Slow

Individuals who primarily rely on *attachment hyperactivating strategies* (typical for anxiously attached individuals, such as those with a preoccupied attachment style) also tend to seek out others in times of distress, yet they typically have the underlying belief that others will not be there for them or will eventually reject or abandon them. This leads to often desperate efforts to find support and relief, as expressed in demanding and claiming behaviors. Attachment hyperactivating strategies have been associated with a low threshold for deactivation of brain areas involved in controlled mentalizing, and thus individuals with these features tend to have a low threshold for switching to automatic mentalizing (see Table 3–1) (Luyten and Fonagy 2015). Moreover, they tend to be highly sensitive to signs of rejection and abandonment, have an increased time to recovery of mentalizing after it has been lost, and experience severe lapses in mentalizing.

Attachment deactivating strategies, which are typically observed in avoidant individuals (e.g., those with fearful-avoidant and dismissive attachment), are characterized by the denial of attachment needs, and often strong assertions of their own autonomy, independence, and strength when faced with stress. These individuals are often able to keep controlled mentalizing "online" (i.e., active and engaged) for longer and tend to recover quickly from lapses in mentalizing (Vrticka et al. 2008; see Table 3–1), which may lead clinicians to erroneously attribute genuine mentalizing capacities to these individuals. However, mentalizing in these individuals is best described as *pseudomentalizing*; particularly in high arousal contexts, their mentalizing tends to become overly cognitive, without any affective basis. This imbalance in the cognitive–affective dimension explains the pretend-mode character of many of their narratives (see Chapter 1): they do not genuinely reflect on what they and/or others *feel* in a given situation, but relate often complex narratives about what happened to them that at first sight seem understandable but lack any affective grounding in reality. This type of pseudomentalizing is often observed in patients with NPD features or in those with functional somatic disorders.

Furthermore, as arousal increases, attachment deactivating strategies typically break down, resulting in the resurgence of defended-against feelings of insecurity and negative self-representations (Mikulincer et al. 2004). It is therefore imperative to increase the level of arousal to challenge these deactivating strategies when attempting to assess mentalizing in these individuals. This is typically done, for example, when administering the Adult Attachment Interview (e.g., Fonagy et al. 1996; Levinson and Fonagy 2004), which includes demand questions related to affectively highly charged issues such as separation and loss.

Studies have also shown that individuals who primarily rely on attachment deactivating strategies tend to show a dissociation between subjective and biological stress (e.g., blood pressure, skin conductance) (Dozier and Kobak 1992; Luyten et al. 2013). In terms of assessment, paying attention to so-called somatic markers of emotion (Abbass 2015), such as sweating, hand-clenching, or dizziness, is therefore important. Somatic markers of emotion in the absence of any conscious awareness of emotion in these individuals reveal important discrepancies between an apparently composed and coherent narrative that seems to be indicative of genuine mentalizing, and the pretend-mode quality of such narratives. Similarly, individuals who rely on attachment deactivating strategies often appear too calm for the situation (e.g., when relating a history of abuse or neglect without showing any signs of distress) or attribute obvious signs of distress to external factors (e.g., "*I feel suddenly dizzy, but this is because I haven't had breakfast this morning*") or cannot explain what is happening to them ("*I have no idea what is happening to me now, have never experienced this before, this must be coincidence*")—responses that are indicative of pretend mode and/or teleological functioning. Finally, when probed for examples illustrating general statements about attachment relationships, these individuals often cannot provide them, or they provide examples demonstrating exactly the opposite. For instance, a patient emphatically argued that he had always had a good relationship with his son. When asked for an example, he recounted how he and his son would frequently get into a fight about the son's lack of interest in school.

Finally, individuals with *disorganized attachment* tend to use both attachment hyperactivating and deactivating strategies when confronted with stress, often switching between the two strategies. This typically confuses the clinician, as the patient tends to switch from marked hypomentalizing to hypermentalizing, often in a matter of seconds (Bateman and Fonagy 2004) (see Table 3–1).

Secondary attachment strategies limit broaden-and-build cycles and inhibit behavioral systems implicated in resilience, such as exploration and affiliation (Insel and Young 2001; Mikulincer and Shaver 2007; Neumann 2008). Hence, these strategies limit epistemic trust and salutogenesis, and manifest themselves in epistemic credulity, epistemic hypervigilance, epistemic freezing, or epistemic petrification, or as any combination of these (see Chapter 4).

In fact, the loss of effective mentalizing associated with secondary attachment strategies leads to the reemergence of more automatic, prementalistic modes of experiencing the subjective reality of both the self and others—that is, *psychic equivalence, pretend mode,* and *teleological mode* (Bateman and Fonagy 2016). These nonmentalizing modes also are often associated with a tendency to externalize nonmentalized experiences (i.e., alien-self experiences), particularly in individuals with a marked history of trauma (see Chapter 5, "Mentalizing and Trauma"). Table 3–2 provides examples of the impact of the pressure of alien-self experiences on mentalizing that can be seen as special cases of hypomentalizing and hypermentalizing.

TABLE 3–2. **Consequences of the pressure to externalize alien-self parts for mentalizing**

Examples	Markers
Intrusive pseudomentalizing	The person "knows" what others are feeling or thinking; this is experienced by others as intrusive.
Destructively inaccurate mentalizing	Mental states are induced either explicitly or implicitly in others (e.g., ranging from simple emotional states such as guilt or shame to complex mental states such as victim–perpetrator states).
Disavowal of mentalizing	The person refuses to reflect on mental states.

UNSTRUCTURED CLINICAL ASSESSMENT OF MENTALIZING

The views outlined in this chapter have a number of important implications for the assessment of mentalizing in clinical practice. First, the following are required: 1) a systematic exploration of mentalizing in different arousal contexts and 2) the use of active probing and challenging. Particularly in individuals who rely on attachment deactivating strategies, "testing the limits" is required to assess mentalizing capacities. Gross imbalances in mentalizing capacities across different contexts or relationships are particularly important to note, as are impairments in mentalizing that are related to specific contexts or attachment relationships (e.g., when the individual is talking about his or her partner, or about partner relationships more generally).

Second, the assessment of mentalizing in the context of a new attachment relationship with an assessor needs to be explored. Does the patient show an awareness of the mental states of the assessor? For instance, the patient who relates a history of abuse might appropriately warn the assessor that what he or she is about to tell is shocking, or, by contrast, might relate such a history without any attention to the impact this might have on the assessor. Some patients might even assume that the assessor or therapist "knows" everything the patient knows (i.e., assuming that all knowledge is shared knowledge); this assumption is typical of many patients with BPD features. For instance, the patient comes into the therapist's office and immediately starts complaining about a person at work, but without explaining who that person is or what has happened; or the patient begins to tell a very detailed story about how "Jessica" played such an important role when she was a child and teenager, but without explaining who Jessica is. Similarly, is the patient interested in the mind of the assessor (*"What do you think?"*), and is he or she open to (novel) perspectives offered by the assessor? Finally, is the patient able to allow the assessor to co-regulate stress and arousal during the assessment interview, particularly "when the going gets tough"? Does this lead to a recovery of effective mentalizing or does mentalizing spiral out of control when the assessor attempts to validate or normalize the patient's experience?

Finally, assessment of mentalizing involves close attention to individual differences in the use of secondary attachment strategies, and the extent to which these differ depending on the type of attachment relationship.

A comprehensive assessment of mentalizing should be based on two to three sessions with the patient. The first session could start with a detailed review of the patient's attachment history, moving from past to current attachment relationships, and exploring to what extent the patient sees any links between his or her attachment history and presenting problems. As noted earlier, explicit probing using so-called demand questions is typically called for. Examples of such questions include *"Do you know why your parents/partner acted as they did?" "Do you think what happened to you as a child is related to the way you are as an adult?" "How has your relationship with your parents changed since childhood?" "In what ways have you changed since childhood?" "How did you feel when your parents seemed to prefer your sister over you?"* and *"Do you think your upbringing is related in any way to your problems now?"*

The second session could focus on areas that were not (or insufficiently) explored during the first interview and could also explore the patient's mentalizing skills with regard to his or her presenting symptoms. For instance, does the patient see any relationship between his or her tendency to self-harm and what is happening to him or her in terms of mental states? Does such probing lead to a loss of mentalizing (*"Why do you ask questions like that? I can't see the point"*), and how extensive are these losses of mentalizing? Is the patient able to recover mentalizing when the assessor moves on to another topic? Patients might be completely overwhelmed by such probing and might defensively begin to try to dominate the mind of the assessor (*"Why are you asking such questions? Do you think it is all my fault then? Do you know what you are suggesting, as if I have anything to do with what is happening to me?"*), or may engage in excessive mentalizing in an attempt to find some meaningful connection between his or her life history and presenting problems (e.g., in patients with obsessive–compulsive or somatoform disorders), often using "canned language."

In cases where a third assessment session is indicated, the assessor might want to revisit certain features of the patient's life history and gauge the patient's response to the assessor's first attempt to meaningfully link the patient's life history to presenting problems.

From the information gathered through these initial assessment interviews, assessors should ideally consider the following steps in arriving at a comprehensive assessment of mentalizing.

1. Make an assessment of the patient's *overall mentalizing* capacities. The assessor should first consider the overall level of mentalizing of the patient (see Boxes 3–1 and 3–2), in a manner similar to the scoring of the Reflective Functioning Scale on the Adult Attachment Interview (Table 3–3).

TABLE 3–3.   Reflective Functioning Scale

Score	Description	Level
9	**Full or exceptional:** Interviewee's answers show exceptional sophistication; are surprising, quite complex, or elaborate; and consistently manifest reasoning in a causal way using mental states.	Moderate to high reflective functioning
7	**Marked:** Numerous statements indicating full reflective functioning, which show awareness of the nature of mental states and explicit attempts at teasing out mental states underlying behavior.	
5	**Definite or ordinary:** Interviewee shows several instances of reflective functioning, even if prompted by the interviewer rather than emerging spontaneously from the interviewee.	
3	**Questionable or low:** Some evidence of consideration of mental states throughout the interview, albeit at a fairly rudimentary level.	Negative to limited reflective functioning
1	**Absent but not repudiated:** Reflective functioning is totally or almost totally absent.	
−1	**Negative:** Interviewee systematically resists taking a reflective stance throughout the interview.	

2. The assessment of overall mentalizing capacities should be followed by the drawing of a *mentalizing profile* (see Figure 3–2), by plotting an individual's mentalizing capacities first for each of the different dimensions separately and then making a consideration of the compensatory and/or mutually reinforcing relationships between the various dimensions and poles. Notes should be made concerning 1) discrepancies in mentalizing both within and among the dimensions (see Boxes 3–3 to 3–6), and 2) how context and specific (types of) relationships may be responsible for such discrepancies. Hence, the assessment of mentalizing includes actively probing the patient's capacity for controlled mentalizing and looking for when there is a switch to more automatic, biased mentalizing; for mentalizing based on internal as well as external features of the self and others; for the patient's own internal states and those of others; and for the integration of cognition and affect in mentalizing. Assessors should actively increase the arousal in the session (within reason) to "test the limits" of the patient's capacity for controlled mentalizing. For instance, the assessor should ask questions that actively probe for mentalizing, such as "*What do you feel now? You just seemed to shiver when you were talking about your boss; what does that mean*"? (externally based/self) and "*When he looked at you like that, what did you think he thought about you?*" (externally based/other). Contrary moves are often useful in this context to shift the perspective from self to other or vice versa: "*You have been talking now about yourself, but how do you think he feels about the whole situation?*" Contrary moves may also be particularly useful to uncover potential discrepancies in mentalizing, as in patients who are unable to switch from their own perspective to that of others, or who revert to pseudomentalizing, as in patients who seem to invent a "just-so" story on the spot, often to

BOX 3-1. **What does good mentalizing look like?**

- Security of mental exploration and openness to discovery; internal freedom and interest in exploring even painful memories and experiences.

- Acknowledgment of the opaqueness and tentativeness of mental states.

- Genuine interest in the mental states of the self and others, and their relation.

- Adaptive flexibility in switching from automatic to controlled mentalizing.

- Acknowledgment of the changeability of mental states, including awareness of the developmental perspective (i.e., that the individual's own attachment history influences current ways of relating to self and others).

- Integration of cognitive and affective features of self and others ("embodied mentalizing").

- Sense of realistic predictability and controllability of mental states.

- Ability to regulate distress in relation to others.

- Relaxed and flexible, not "stuck" in one point of view.

- Can be playful, with humor that engages rather than hurting or distancing.

- Can solve problems by "give and take" between own and others' perspectives.

- Describes his or her own experience, rather than defining other people's experience or intentions.

- Conveys "ownership" of his or her behavior rather than a sense that it "happens" to him or her.

- Open to and curious about other people's perspectives, and expects to have his or her own views extended by those of others.

Relational strengths
- Curiosity.
- Safe uncertainty.
- Contemplation and reflection.
- Perspective taking (including the recognition that others may have different thoughts, feelings, and opinions).
- Forgiveness.
- Impact awareness.
- Nonparanoid attitude.

Perception of own mental functioning
- Developmental perspective.
- Realistic skepticism.
- Internal conflict awareness.
- Self-inquisitive stance.
- Awareness of the impact of affect.
- Acknowledgment of unconscious and preconscious functioning.
- Belief in changeability.

BOX 3–1. What does good mentalizing look like? *(continued)*

Self-representation

- Rich internal life.
- Autobiographical continuity.
- Advanced explanatory and listening skills.

General values and attitudes

- Tentativeness.
- Humility (moderation).
- Playfulness and humor.
- Flexibility.
- "Give and take."
- Responsibility and accountability.

BOX 3–2. What does bad mentalizing look like?

- Dominance of unreflective, naive, distorted, automatic assumptions.
- Unjustified certainty about internal mental states of self and/or others.
- Rigid adherence to own perspective or excessively flexible in changing perspectives.
- Overly focused on external or internal features of self and other, or complete neglect of one or both ("mind-blindness").
- Inability to consider both self and other perspectives.
- Emphasis on either cognitive or affective aspects of mentalizing (i.e., overly analytical versus being overwhelmed by states of mind of self and/or others).
- Excessively sparse or overdetailed mentalizing.
- Focus on external factors (e.g., government, school, colleagues, neighbors).
- Focus on "empty," purely behavioral personality descriptors (e.g., "tired," "lazy") or diagnoses.
- Lack of interest in mental states, or defensive attempts to avoid mentalizing by becoming aggressive or manipulative, using denial, changing the subject, or otherwise being noncooperative (e.g., *"I don't know"*).

please the assessor. We have often noticed that assessors fail to increase the arousal level in the session (e.g., by the use of demand questions and contrary moves); this leads to erroneous conclusions concerning the mentalizing capacities of their patients, ones that either overestimate or underestimate these capacities.

3. Assessing each of the dimensions of mentalizing also leads to a consideration of the different *parameters of the biobehavioral switch model* of mentalizing discussed earlier: a) the activation gradient of mentalizing (i.e., the proclivity of the individual to mentalize); b) the switch point between controlled and automatic mentalizing; and c) the time to recovery of controlled mentalizing (see Figure 3–1 and Box 3–6). The influence of the use of attachment hyperactivating and deactivating strategies on these

BOX 3–3.   **Internally and externally focused mentalizing**

- Awareness of internal and external features of self and others, and the relationship between the two.

- Sensitivity to external and internal features of self and others.

- Ability to perceive and to self-correct initial impressions based on external features and to let others correct these impressions (e.g., *"My first thought seeing his face was that he couldn't be trusted, but I immediately realized that I was prejudiced"; "Something in the way he talked bothered me, but I quickly realized that this was because he reminded me of someone I once had a serious disagreement with"*).

BOX 3–4.   **Mentalizing with regard to self and others**

- Presence of egocentrism (i.e., to see others in terms of self versus degree of control or inhibition of own perspective).

- Liability to emotional contagion (self–other diffusion with regard to mental states) versus defensive separation from mental states of others.

- Response to contrary moves, particularly flexibility to move between self and other perspectives.

- Ability to integrate embodied knowledge with more reflective knowledge of self and others.

BOX 3–5.   **Cognitive and affective mentalizing**

- Tendency to see "mind-reading" as an intellectual, rational game.

- Tendency for either cognitive or affective hypermentalizing (pseudomentalizing).

- Tendency to become overwhelmed by affect when thinking about states of mind.

- Ability for *mentalized affectivity* and *embodied mentalizing* (i.e., to integrate cognitive knowledge and affective knowledge of the self and others).

parameters should be assessed, and, again, the assessor should carefully register whether these parameters differ across specific attachment relationships.

4. A detailed assessment of mentalizing capacities also entails an assessment of what happens when effective mentalizing breaks down. That is, what are the "preferred" *nonmentalizing modes* that become active in the patient, and to what extent do they lead to a pressure to externalize nonmentalized states of mind (see Box 3–7)? It is important to note in this context that the nonmentalizing modes are not mutually exclusive. Psychic equivalence often involves teleological thinking (*"He has never liked me, I know for sure because he never answers any of my calls; next time I'll do the same when he rings me"*). Nonmentalizing modes may be associated with a relatively mild tendency to externalize nonmentalized (i.e., alien-self) experiences. For instance, patients who have a tendency to revert to the teleological mode may try to achieve some control over unmentalized experiences by means of action (e.g., exercising or working excessively) and/or attributing distress purely to objective causes (e.g., a virus or working conditions). In more extreme cases, there may be a constant pressure to externalize alien-self experiences that might lead to

BOX 3–6.   Automatic and controlled mentalizing in specific contexts and relationships

- Are there global impairments in mentalizing (e.g., marked automatic mentalizing based on distorted assumptions about the self and others) or more partial difficulties?

- Are there marked discrepancies between mentalizing in nonstressful versus stressful conditions, or are mentalizing levels approximately equally high or low in both conditions?

- What is the optimal stress level for adequate mentalizing?

- Are there differences related to self–other and context, particularly attachment relationships (e.g., gross imbalances between mentalizing about self and others or between different attachment figures)?

- How extensive is failure of mentalizing under stress?

- What is the time to recovery (e.g., relatively quick versus slow)?

- Is there the ability to self-correct and be corrected by others, even under high stress levels?

- Is there a sense of sufficient and realistic security in the relationship to the assessor or therapist (e.g., patients may feel very stressed and/or be constantly on their guard, or alternatively may show an unrealistic sense of security, as if they have known the therapist for years)?

- Are there specific attachment relationships or contexts that lead to impairments in mentalizing?

BOX 3–7.   Nonmentalizing and pseudomentalizing modes

- Pretend mode (i.e., reasoning about mental states but without any real connection to reality).

- Psychic equivalence mode (i.e., concrete understanding)—for example, *"You do not love me because you didn't call me"*; *"I know you are in love with me, because you smiled at me."*

- Teleological mode (i.e., internal states of mind are reduced to observable behavior)— for example, *"The only time I feel loved is when you are near me."*

- Pseudomentalizing: mostly self-serving, improbable, and inaccurate.

  - Intrusive: the individual "knows what others think."

  - Overactive (hypermentalizing): excessively detailed, decoupled from (affective) reality.

  - Destructively inaccurate: denial of others' internal states and replacing them with the individual's own construction—for example, *"You want to destroy me, I'm sure. Don't deny it. There's no way you can ever deny this."*

a tendency to self-harm or harm others, or to attempt to dominate, control, and/ or manipulate the mind of others either unconsciously (as, for instance, in many patients with BPD) or consciously (as in patients with ASPD).

5. In an assessment of mentalizing, examples of online (i.e., immediate) mentalizing in the session—and particularly the extent to which the individual shows evidence of the self-correcting function of mentalizing and is able to use the assessor's presence and interventions to co-regulate arousal and recover from mentalizing lapses—are

important. These typically provide a more reliable and valid estimate of mentalizing than do examples of more offline (i.e., retrospective) mentalizing, particularly in patients with high levels of attachment-deactivating strategies.

6. Finally, the assessor should determine to what extent mentalizing impairments are linked to problems with epistemic trust and salutogenesis. To what extent have mentalizing impairments led to a disorder in social communication—that is, an inability to benefit from input from the environment—and in the patient's capacity to recalibrate his or her mind in relation to others? Again, evidence of such recalibration and genuine interest in the mind of the assessor should be seen as a positive indication with potentially important consequences for prognosis and treatment response.

STRUCTURED ASSESSMENT OF MENTALIZING

More structured assessment of mentalizing (e.g., for research purposes) might be thought of in similar ways as the clinical assessment of mentalizing. Numerous measures have been developed that tap into an individual's overall mentalizing capacities or more specific areas of mentalizing problems. These measures, which are summarized in Table 3–4, include the Reflective Functioning Scale (Fonagy et al. 1998), a broad measure of mentalizing that is scored on the Adult Attachment Interview (Hesse 2008) or similar interviews, such as the Child Attachment Interview (Shmueli-Goetz et al. 2008; Target et al. 2003), the Object Relations Inventory (Diamond et al. 1991), or transcripts of psychotherapy sessions (Karlsson and Kermott 2006; Szecsödy 2008). The Reflective Functioning Scale has also been used to assess mentalizing with regard to specific issues or symptoms, such as anxiety symptoms (Rudden et al. 2006, 2009), depressive themes (Taubner et al. 2011), trauma (Berthelot et al. 2015), and specific attachment figures or relationships (Diamond et al. 2003).

More recently, the Reflective Functioning Questionnaire has been developed as a broad self-report measure specifically designed to assess severe impairments in mentalizing, as are typically observed in individuals with BPD (Fonagy et al. 2016; Ha et al. 2013). Levy et al. (2005) have reported preliminary evidence for a clinician-rated multidimensional Reflective Functioning Scale, and several other efforts to develop general measures of mentalizing are currently under way.

Other measures focus on relationship-specific mentalizing, such as a modification of the Reflective Functioning Scale to be scored on the Parent Development Interview (Slade 2005; Slade et al. 2007) or on the Working Model of the Child Interview (Schechter et al. 2005). The work of Elizabeth Meins and colleagues (Meins et al. 2012), who developed a maternal mind-mindedness scale, also deserves a prominent place in this context. This scale taps into a caregiver's online mentalizing with regard to his or her child and can be scored on different types of narrative material (Meins and Fernyhough 2015). The Parental Reflective Functioning Questionnaire (Luyten et al. 2017) assesses various dimensions of parental mentalizing. Various experimental tasks can be used to assess general or relationship-specific mentalizing in children and adolescents (Sharp and Fonagy 2008).

There is also a broad range of well-validated measures available to assess different dimensions of mentalizing in young people as well as in adults. Table 3–4 provides some examples to assist researchers (and clinicians) in selecting measures that tap into

TABLE 3–4.   Measures assessing the dimensions of mentalizing

	Self–Other		Cognitive–Affective		Internal–External		Automatic–Controlled	
	Self	Other	Cognitive	Affective	Internal	External	Automatic	Controlled
Questionnaires								
Beliefs about Emotions Scale (Rimes and Chalder 2010)	X	(X)	X	X	X			X
Toronto Alexithymia Questionnaire (Bagby et al. 1994)	X		X	X	X			X
Kentucky Inventory of Mindfulness—Describe and Act With Awareness subscales (Baer et al. 2004)	X		X	X	X		(X)	X
Mindful Attention Awareness Scale (Brown and Ryan 2003)	X		X	X	X		(X)	X
Levels of Emotional Awareness Scale (Lane et al. 1990)	X	X	X	X	X			X
Psychological Mindedness Scale (Shill and Lumley 2002)	X	X	X	X	X			X
Interpersonal Reactivity Index—Perspective Taking subscale (Davis 1983)		X	X	X	X			X
Empathy Quotient (Lawrence et al. 2004)	X	X	X	X	X		(X)	X
Mayer-Salovey-Caruso Emotional Intelligence Test (Salovey and Grewal 2005)	X	X	X	X	X	X	(X)	X
Reflective Functioning Questionnaire (Fonagy et al. 2016)	X	X	X	X	X	(X)		X
Parental Reflective Functioning Questionnaire (Luyten et al. 2017)	X	X	X	X	X	(X)		X
Mentalizing Stories for Adolescents (Vrouva and Fonagy 2009)		X	X	X	X	(X)		X
Basic Empathy Scale (Jolliffe and Farrington 2006)	X	X	X	X	X			X
Difficulties in Emotion Regulation Scale—Lack of Emotional Clarity/Awareness subscales (Gratz and Roemer 2004)	X		X	X	X			X
Mentalization Scale (Dimitrijevic et al. 2018)	X	X	X	X	X			X
Mentalization Questionnaire (Hausberg et al. 2012)	X	X	X	X	X	(X)	(X)	X

TABLE 3–4.　Measures assessing the dimensions of mentalizing (*continued*)

	Self–Other		Cognitive–Affective		Internal–External		Automatic–Controlled	
	Self	Other	Cognitive	Affective	Internal	External	Automatic	Controlled
Questionnaires (*continued*)								
Mentalized Affectivity Scale (Greenberg et al. 2017)	X		X	X	X			X
Reflective Functioning Questionnaire for Youths (Ha et al. 2013)	X	X	X	X	X	(X)		X
Reflective Functioning Questionnaire for Children (Ensink et al. 2018a)	X	X	X	X	X	(X)		X
Interviews/narrative coding systems								
Adult Attachment Interview—Reflective Functioning Scale (Fonagy et al. 1998)	X	X	X	X	X	(X)	(X)	X
Parent Development Interview–Reflective Functioning Scale (Slade et al. 2004)	X	X	X	X	X	(X)	(X)	X
Working Model of the Child Interview—Reflective Functioning Scale (Grienemberger et al. 2005)	X	X	X	X	X	(X)	(X)	X
Pregnancy Interview–Maternal Reflective Functioning Scale (Slade and Patterson 2005)	X	X	X	X	X	X	(X)	X
Panic Specific Reflective Functioning Interview—Panic Specific Reflective Functioning Scale (Rudden et al. 2006)	X	(X)	X	X	X	(X)	(X)	X
Brief Reflective Functioning Interview—Reflective Functioning Scale (Rudden et al. 2005; Rutimann and Meehan 2012)	X	X	X	X	X	(X)	(X)	X
Toronto Structured Interview for Alexithymia (Bagby et al. 2006)	X		X	X	X		(X)	X
Mental States Measure and Grille de l'élaboration verbale de l'affect (Bouchard et al. 2008)	X	X	X	X	X	(X)	(X)	X
Metacognition Assessment Scale (Carcione et al. 2007)	X	X	X	X	X		(X)	X

TABLE 3–4. **Measures assessing the dimensions of mentalizing** *(continued)*

	Self–Other		Cognitive–Affective		Internal–External		Automatic–Controlled	
	Self	Other	Cognitive	Affective	Internal	External	Automatic	Controlled
Interviews/narrative coding systems *(continued)*								
Intentionality Scale (Hill et al. 2007)	X	X	X	X	X	(X)	(X)	X
Internal State Lexicon (Beeghly and Cicchetti 1994)	X	X	X	X	X	(X)	(X)	X
Reflective Functioning Rating Scale (Meehan et al. 2009)	X	X	X	X	X	(X)	(X)	X
Theory of Mind Assessment Scale (Bosco et al. 2009)	X	X	X	X	X	(X)		X
Mini Parental Reflective Functioning Interview (Ensink et al. 2018a, 2018b)	X	X	X	X	X	(X)	(X)	X
Child Attachment Interview—Child and Adolescent Reflective Functioning Scale (Ensink et al. 2016a)	X	X	X	X	X	(X)	(X)	X
Trauma Reflective Functioning Scale (Ensink et al. 2014a)	X	X	X	X	X	(X)	(X)	X
Experimental/observational tasks								
Reading the Mind in the Eyes Test (Baron-Cohen et al. 2001)		X	X	X	X	X		X
Reading the Mind in the Voice Test (Golan et al. 2007)		X	X	X		X		X
Reading the Mind in Films Task (Golan et al. 2008)		X	X	X		X		X
International Affective Picture System (Lang et al. 2008)		X	X	X	X	X		X
NimStim Set of Facial Expressions (Tottenham et al. 2009)		X	X	X		X		X
Face morphs (Bailey et al. 2008)	X	X	X	X		X	(X)	X
Dynamic body expressions (Pichon et al. 2009)		X	X	X		X	(X)	X
Electromyography of facial mimicry (Sonnby-Borgström and Jönsson 2004)	(X)	X	(X)	X		X	X	
Affect labeling (Lieberman et al. 2007)		X	X	X		X		X
Movie for the Assessment of Social Cognition (Dziobek et al. 2006)		X	X	X	X	X	(X)	X
Trust Task (King-Casas et al. 2008)	(X)	X	X	X	X			X

TABLE 3–4. Measures assessing the dimensions of mentalizing *(continued)*

	Self–Other		Cognitive–Affective		Internal–External		Automatic–Controlled	
	Self	Other	Cognitive	Affective	Internal	External	Automatic	Controlled
Experimental/observational tasks *(continued)*								
Interoceptive sensitivity (Barrett et al. 2004)	X		X	X	X			X
Empathy for pain in others (Hein and Singer 2008)	(X)	X	X	X		X	X	X
Manipulating body consciousness (Brass et al. 2007; Lenggenhager et al. 2007)	X	X	X	X	X	X	X	X
Test battery for perception and recognition of facial emotion expressions (Wilhelm et al. 2014)	X	X	X	X	X	X	(X)	X
Animated Theory of Mind Inventory for Children (Beaumont and Sofronoff 2008)	X	X	X	X	X	X	(X)	X
Maternal mind-mindedness (Meins and Fernyhough 2015)	X	X	X	X	X	(X)	(X)	X
Maternal mind-mindedness (on free play mother–child interaction; Meins et al. 2012)	X	X	X	X	X	(X)	(X)	X
Maternal Accuracy Paradigm (Sharp et al. 2006)	X	X	X	X	X	(X)	(X)	X
Strange Stories Task (Happé 1994; White et al. 2009)	X	X	X	X	X			X
False belief picture sequencing task (Baron-Cohen et al. 1986; Langdon and Coltheart 1999; Langdon et al. 1997)	X	X	X		X			X
Cartoon-based assessment of mentalizing skills (Brüne et al. 2016; Ghiassi et al. 2010)	X	X	X	X	X	(X)		X
Faux Pas Test (Baron-Cohen et al. 1999)	X	X	X	X	X	(X)		X
Affect Task for Children (Ensink et al. 2014b)	X	X	X	X	X	(X)		X
Affective Knowledge Test (Denham 1986)		X	X	X	X	(X)	X	X
Mentalizing about the Self—Interview for Preschoolers (Laurent et al. 2018b)	X		X	X	X	X		X

TABLE 3–4. Measures assessing the dimensions of mentalizing *(continued)*

	Self–Other		Cognitive–Affective		Internal–External		Automatic–Controlled	
	Self	Other	Cognitive	Affective	Internal	External	Automatic	Controlled
Performance-based measures								
Thematic Apperception Test (Murray 1943)	(X)	X	X	X	X	X	(X)	X
Projective Imagination Test (Blackshaw et al. 2001)	(X)	X	X	X	X	X	(X)	X
Children's Play Therapy Instrument (Kernberg et al. 1998)	X	X	X	X	X	X	X	X
Mirror Paradigm (Ensink et al. 2016b)	X		X	X	X	X	X	X
Squiggle Paradigm (Ensink et al. 2017)	X	X	X	X	X	X	X	X
Therapist Mental Activity Scale (Ensink et al. 2013)	X	X	X	X	X	X	X	X

Note. X indicates that the measure captures the relevant pole or dimension of mentalizing; (X) indicates that the measure assesses certain features of the relevant pole or dimension of mentalizing but mainly captures other poles or dimensions of mentalizing.

the mentalizing impairments that are typical of specific patient populations. For instance, researchers interested in patients with functional somatic problems may want to select measures that tap into basic (embodied) mentalizing, rather than assuming that these patients are characterized by severe impairments in mentalizing about others. Similarly, researchers of ASPD might want to include measures in their research protocol that tap into cognitive and affective features of mentalizing about self and others.

A range of clinical research measures for assessing mentalizing in therapists and parents, children and adolescents, and mentalizing regarding trauma have been developed by Ensink and colleagues. To assess mentalizing in clinicians, Ensink et al. validated the Therapist Mental Activity Scale and used it to assess the effectiveness of training programs geared to develop therapists' mentalizing about complex patients (Ensink et al. 2013). The Mini Parental Reflective Functioning Interview was validated to assess parental reflective functioning about infants and children in pediatric practice and predicts parenting behavior and infant attachment (Ensink et al. 2018b). In addition, the Squiggle Paradigm facilitates assessment of parents' reflective stance while engaging their children in a collaborative task and interpreting their communication, and is potentially useful for planning interventions with parents (Ensink et al. 2017). Furthermore, in the context of working with patients with histories of trauma, the Trauma Reflective Functioning Scale (Ensink et al. 2014a) facilitates assessment of reflective functioning regarding trauma, which has been shown to be associated with couple adjustment and infant attachment.

Instruments have also been developed to assess mentalizing in young children and adolescents. The Child and Adolescent Reflective Functioning Scale (Ensink et al. 2016c) has been developed to assess mentalizing regarding self and others in children ages 8–12, which has been shown to be associated with trauma, child psychopathology, dissociation, physiological regulation, and parental reflective functioning (Ensink et al. 2016a). A questionnaire version, the Reflective Functioning Questionnaire for Children (Ensink et al. 2018a), was adapted to complement the Reflective Functioning Questionnaire for Youths (Ha et al. 2013). In addition, mentalizing about the embodied self can be assessed with the Mirror Paradigm (Ensink et al. 2016b) to identify child and adolescent mentalizing difficulties in this area associated with distress, psychopathology, and trauma. Other measures of specific dimensions of mentalizing have been validated, including the Affect Task for Children (Ensink et al. 2014b) and Strange Stories Task (Happé 1994). For preschoolers, the POKO video-based assessment, as well as puppet interviews, has been adapted to assess emerging mentalizing (Ensink and Achim 2016; Laurent et al. 2018a, 2018b). Furthermore, mentalizing in pretend play can be assessed with the Children's Play Therapy Instrument, and this has been shown to predict child reflective functioning (Tessier et al. 2016). In parallel, mentalizing techniques used in play therapy can be assessed using the schema elaborated by Muñoz Specht et al. (2016).

Importantly, tasks that have been developed within social neuroscience approaches are increasingly allowing researchers to disentangle different dimensions of mentalizing. Contemporary imaging methods are steadily improving, providing better opportunities to assess more implicit, automatic mentalizing, particularly as most measures of mentalizing developed so far require conscious (and thus explicit and controlled) mentalizing as well as considerable cognitive abilities. Indeed, most of the measures listed in Table 3–4 require the individual to have some sort of cognitive reflection, control, and modulation of response. For instance, in completing the Reading the Mind in the Eyes Test (Baron-Cohen et al. 2001), which purportedly captures emotion recognition, participants are required to integrate their cognitive and affective knowledge about emotions. This is also the case for measures that have been explicitly developed to distinguish between aspects of cognitive and affective mentalizing, such as Baron-Cohen and Wheelwright's (2004) measure of cognitive versus affective empathy, and measures of cognitive and affective alexithymia (Bermond and Vorst 1998). Some experimental tasks enable a better distinction between cognition and affect in mentalizing (and the integration between the two) (Shamay-Tsoory et al. 2009), but more work is needed to improve their ecological validity.

Similarly, there is a growing number of mentalizing tasks that involve online, "hot" mentalizing as opposed to more offline, "cold" self-report measures. The former methods will undoubtedly play a more prominent role in future research, particularly as these measures may be more ecologically valid in capturing mentalizing as it typically unfolds in real-life situations.

Hence, a rather daunting task awaits the field, not only to meet the urgent need for well-validated, more sophisticated measures of the different facets of mentalizing, but also to facilitate the application of these measures in routine clinical practice. We hope that this chapter will inform and guide such efforts.

CONCLUSION

The comprehensive assessment of mentalizing involves an assessment of the individual's overall mentalizing and of the potential imbalances between different dimensions underlying mentalizing, including whether such imbalances manifest in specific contexts and relationships.

Although an increasing number of well-validated measures are available for systematically assessing mentalizing, a more clinical approach is often needed to challenge "cold" and "offline" mentalizing in the context of a new attachment relationship (i.e., with an assessor), to provide a valid estimation of an individual's mentalizing capacities. As mentalizing is a quintessential human capacity, another human being—specifically, someone trained in the mentalizing approach—is needed to map the subtleties that are often involved in mentalizing and the impairments in this capacity. In this context, there is also a pressing need for more observer-rated scales of mentalizing to be devised, given the particular combination of strengths and sensitivities of the human mind in understanding others, as well as the many pitfalls involved in this capacity.

REFERENCES

Abbass A: Reaching Through Resistance: Advanced Psychotherapy Techniques. Kansas City, Seven Leaves Press, 2015

Allen JG, Fonagy P, Bateman AW: Mentalizing in Clinical Practice. Washington, DC, American Psychiatric Press, 2008

Arnsten AFT: The biology of being frazzled. Science 280(5370):1711–1712, 1998 9660710

Baer RA, Smith GT, Allen KB: Assessment of mindfulness by self-report: the Kentucky inventory of mindfulness skills. Assessment 11(3):191–206, 2004 15358875

Bagby RM, Parker JD, Taylor GJ: The twenty-item Toronto Alexithymia Scale—I. Item selection and cross-validation of the factor structure. J Psychosom Res 38(1):23–32, 1994 8126686

Bagby RM, Taylor GJ, Parker JD, et al: The development of the Toronto Structured Interview for Alexithymia: item selection, factor structure, reliability and concurrent validity. Psychother Psychosom 75(1):25–39, 2006 16361872

Bailey CA, Pendl J, Levin A, et al: Face Morphing Tutorial: From Models to Morphs. New Haven, CT, Yale Child Study Center, 2008

Baron-Cohen S, Wheelwright S: The empathy quotient: an investigation of adults with Asperger syndrome or high functioning autism, and normal sex differences. J Autism Dev Disord 34(2):163–175, 2004 15162935

Baron-Cohen S, Leslie AM, Frith U: Mechanical, behavioural and intentional understanding of picture stories in autistic children. Br J Dev Psychol 4:113–125, 1986

Baron-Cohen S, O'Riordan M, Stone V, et al: Recognition of faux pas by normally developing children and children with Asperger syndrome or high-functioning autism. J Autism Dev Disord 29(5):407–418, 1999 10587887

Baron-Cohen S, Wheelwright S, Hill J, et al: The "Reading the Mind in the Eyes" Test revised version: a study with normal adults, and adults with Asperger syndrome or high-functioning autism. J Child Psychol Psychiatry 42(2):241–251, 2001 11280420

Barrett LF, Quigley KS, Bliss-Moreau E, et al: Interoceptive sensitivity and self-reports of emotional experience. J Pers Soc Psychol 87(5):684–697, 2004 15535779

Bateman A, Fonagy P: Mentalization-Based Treatment for Personality Disorders: A Practical Guide. Oxford, UK, Oxford University Press, 2016

Bateman AW, Fonagy P: Psychotherapy for Borderline Personality Disorder: Mentalization-Based Treatment. Oxford, UK, Oxford University Press, 2004

Beaumont RB, Sofronoff K: A new computerised advanced theory of mind measure for children with Asperger syndrome: the ATOMIC. J Autism Dev Disord 38(2):249–260, 2008 17629782

Beeghly M, Cicchetti D: Child maltreatment, attachment, and the self system: emergence of an internal state lexicon in toddlers at high social risk. Dev Psychopathol 6:5–30, 1994

Bermond B, Vorst HC: Bermond-Vorst Alexithymia Questionnaire, 1998 [Unpublished manual]

Berthelot N, Ensink K, Bernazzani O, et al: Intergenerational transmission of attachment in abused and neglected mothers: the role of trauma-specific reflective functioning. Infant Ment Health J 36(2):200–212, 2015 25694333

Blackshaw AJ, Kinderman P, Hare DJ, et al: Theory of mind, causal attribution and paranoia in Asperger syndrome. Autism 5(2):147–163, 2001 11706863

Bosco FM, Colle L, De Fazio S, et al: Th.o.m.a.s.: an exploratory assessment of Theory of Mind in schizophrenic subjects. Conscious Cogn 18(1):306–319, 2009 18667334

Bouchard MA, Target M, Lecours S, et al: Mentalization in adult attachment narratives: reflective functioning, mental states, and affect elaboration compared. Psychoanal Psychol 25:47–66, 2008

Brass M, Schmitt RM, Spengler S, et al: Investigating action understanding: inferential processes versus action simulation. Curr Biol 17(24):2117–2121, 2007 18083518

Brown KW, Ryan RM: The benefits of being present: mindfulness and its role in psychological well-being. J Pers Soc Psychol 84(4):822–848, 2003 12703651

Brüne M, Walden S, Edel MA, et al: Mentalization of complex emotions in borderline personality disorder: the impact of parenting and exposure to trauma on the performance in a novel cartoon-based task. Compr Psychiatry 64:29–37, 2016 26350276

Carcione A, Dimaggio G, Falcone M, et al: Metacognition Assessment Scale (MAS) 3.1. Rome, Italy, Centro di Psicoterapia Cognitiva, 2007

Davis MH: Measuring individual differences in empathy: evidence for a multidimensional approach. J Pers Soc Psychol 44:113–126, 1983

Denham SA: Social cognition, prosocial behavior, and emotion in preschoolers: contextual validation. Child Dev 57(1):194–201, 1986

Diamond A, Blatt SJ, Stayner D, et al: Self-Other Differentiation of Object Representations. New Haven, CT, Yale University, 1991 [Unpublished research manual]

Diamond D, Stovall-McClough C, Clarkin JF, et al: Patient-therapist attachment in the treatment of borderline personality disorder. Bull Menninger Clin 67(3):227–259, 2003 14621064

Dimitrijevic A, Hanak N, Altaras Dimitrijevic A, Jolic Marjanovic Z: The Mentalization Scale (MentS): a self-report measure for the assessment of mentalizing capacity. J Pers Assess 100(3):268–280, 2018 28436689

Dozier M, Kobak RR: Psychophysiology in attachment interviews: converging evidence for deactivating strategies. Child Dev 63(6):1473–1480, 1992 1446563

Dziobek I, Fleck S, Kalbe E, et al: Introducing MASC: a movie for the assessment of social cognition. J Autism Dev Disord 36(5):623–636, 2006 16755332

Ensink K, Achim J: Video for Assessing Mentalizing in Preschoolers, 2016 [Unpublished instrument and coding manual]

Ensink K, Maheux J, Normandin L, et al: The impact of mentalization training on the reflective function of novice therapists: a randomized controlled trial. Psychother Res 23(5):526–538, 2013 23964813

Ensink K, Berthelot N, Bernazzani O, et al: Another step closer to measuring the ghosts in the nursery: preliminary validation of the Trauma Reflective Functioning Scale. Front Psychol 5:1471, 2014a 25566146

Ensink K, Fonagy P, Target M: The Affect Task for Children, 2014b [Unpublished instrument and coding manual]

Ensink K, Bégin M, Normandin L, et al: Maternal and child reflective functioning in the context of child sexual abuse: pathways to depression and externalising difficulties. Eur J Psychotraumatol 7:30611, 2016a 26822865

Ensink K, Berthelot N, Biberdzic M, et al: The mirror paradigm: assessing the embodied self in the context of abuse. Psychoanal Psychol 33:389–405, 2016b

Ensink K, Target M, Duval J, et al: The Child and Adolescent Reflective Functioning Scale, 2016c [Unpublished coding manual]

Ensink K, Leroux A, Normandin L, et al: Assessing reflective parenting in interaction with school-aged children. J Pers Assess 99(6):585–595, 2017 28151016

Ensink K, Borelli J, Duval J, et al: The Reflective Functioning Questionnaire for Children, 2018a [Unpublished instrument]

Ensink K, Borelli J, Roy J, et al: Costs of not getting to know you: lower levels of parental reflective functioning confer risk for maternal insensitivity and insecure infant attachment. Infancy 2018b doi: 10.1111/infa.12263 [Epub ahead of print]

Fonagy P, Luyten P: A developmental, mentalization-based approach to the understanding and treatment of borderline personality disorder. Dev Psychopathol 21(4):1355–1381, 2009 19825272

Fonagy P, Leigh T, Steele M, et al: The relation of attachment status, psychiatric classification, and response to psychotherapy. J Consult Clin Psychol 64(1):22–31, 1996 8907081

Fonagy P, Target M, Steele H, et al: Reflective-Functioning Manual, version 5.0, for Application to Adult Attachment Interviews. London, University College London, 1998

Fonagy P, Luyten P, Allison E: Epistemic petrification and the restoration of epistemic trust: a new conceptualization of borderline personality disorder and its psychosocial treatment. J Pers Disord 29(5):575–609, 2015 26393477

Fonagy P, Luyten P, Moulton-Perkins A, et al: Development and validation of a self-report measure of mentalizing: The Reflective Functioning Questionnaire. PLoS One 11(7):e0158678, 2016 27392018

Fonagy P, Luyten P, Allison E, et al: What we have changed our minds about: Part 1. Borderline personality disorder as a limitation of resilience. Borderline Personal Disorder Emotion Dysregul 4:11, 2017a 28413687

Fonagy P, Luyten P, Allison E, et al: What we have changed our minds about: Part 2. Borderline personality disorder, epistemic trust and the developmental significance of social communication. Borderline Personal Disorder Emotion Dysregul 4:9, 2017b 28405338

Fredrickson BL: The role of positive emotions in positive psychology. The broaden-and-build theory of positive emotions. Am Psychol 56(3):218–226, 2001 11315248

Ghiassi V, Dimaggio G, Brune M: Dysfunctions in understanding other minds in borderline personality disorder: a study using cartoon picture stories. Psychother Res 20(6):657–667, 2010 20737351

Golan O, Baron-Cohen S, Hill JJ, et al: The "Reading the Mind in the Voice" test-revised: a study of complex emotion recognition in adults with and without autism spectrum conditions. J Autism Dev Disord 37(6):1096–1106, 2007 17072749

Golan O, Baron-Cohen S, Golan Y: The "Reading the Mind in Films" Task [child version]: complex emotion and mental state recognition in children with and without autism spectrum conditions. J Autism Dev Disord 38(8):1534–1541, 2008 18311514

Gratz KL, Roemer L: Multidimensional assessment of emotion regulation and dysregulation: development, factor structure, and initial validation of the Difficulties in Emotion Regulation Scale. J Psychopathol Behav Assess 26:41–54, 2004

Greenberg DM, Kolasi J, Hegsted CP, et al: Mentalized affectivity: a new model and assessment of emotion regulation. PLoS One 12(10):e0185264, 2017 29045403

Grienenberger JF, Kelly K, Slade A: Maternal reflective functioning, mother-infant affective communication, and infant attachment: exploring the link between mental states and observed caregiving behavior in the intergenerational transmission of attachment. Attach Hum Dev 7(3):299–311, 2005 16210241

Ha C, Sharp C, Ensink K, et al: The measurement of reflective function in adolescents with and without borderline traits. J Adolesc 36(6):1215–1223, 2013 24215968

Happé FGE: An advanced test of theory of mind: understanding of story characters' thoughts and feelings by able autistic, mentally handicapped, and normal children and adults. J Autism Dev Disord 24(2):129–154, 1994 8040158

Hausberg MC, Schulz H, Piegler T, et al: Is a self-rated instrument appropriate to assess mentalization in patients with mental disorders? Development and first validation of the mentalization questionnaire (MZQ). Psychother Res 22(6):699–709, 2012 22867004

Hein G, Singer T: I feel how you feel but not always: the empathic brain and its modulation. Curr Opin Neurobiol 18(2):153–158, 2008 18692571

Hesse E: The Adult Attachment Interview: protocol, method of analysis, and empirical studies, in Handbook of Attachment: Theory, Research, and Clinical Applications, 2nd Edition. Edited by Cassidy J, Shaver PR. New York, Guilford, 2008, pp 552–558

Hill J, Fonagy P, Lancaster G, et al: Aggression and intentionality in narrative responses to conflict and distress story stems: an investigation of boys with disruptive behaviour problems. Attach Hum Dev 9(3):223–237, 2007 18058431

Insel TR, Young LJ: The neurobiology of attachment. Nat Rev Neurosci 2(2):129–136, 2001 11252992

Jolliffe D, Farrington DP: Development and validation of the Basic Empathy Scale. J Adolesc 29(4):589–611, 2006 16198409

Karlsson R, Kermott A: Reflective-functioning during the process in brief psychotherapies. Psychotherapy (Chic) 43(1):65–84, 2006 22121960

Kernberg PF, Chazan SE, Normandin L: The Children's Play Therapy Instrument (CPTI). Description, development, and reliability studies. J Psychother Pract Res 7(3):196–207, 1998 9631341

King-Casas B, Sharp C, Lomax-Bream L, et al: The rupture and repair of cooperation in borderline personality disorder. Science 321(5890):806–810, 2008 18687957

Lane RD, Quinlan DM, Schwartz GE, et al: The Levels of Emotional Awareness Scale: a cognitive-developmental measure of emotion. J Pers Assess 55(1–2):124–134, 1990 2231235

Lang PJ, Bradley MM, Cuthbert BN: International Affective Picture System (IAPS): Affective Ratings of Pictures and Instruction Manual. Gainesville, FL, University of Florida, 2008

Langdon R, Coltheart M: Mentalising, schizotypy, and schizophrenia. Cognition 71(1):43–71, 1999 10394709

Langdon R, Michie PT, Ward PB, et al: Defective self and/or other mentalising in schizophrenia: a cognitive neuropsychological approach. Cogn Neuropsychiatry 2(3):167–193, 1997 25419601

Laurent G, Hecht HK, Ensink K, et al: Emotional understanding, aggression, and social functioning among preschoolers. Am J Orthopsychiatry 2018a 30382723 doi: 10.1037/ort0000377 [Epub ahead of print]

Laurent G, Ensink K, Miljkovitz R: Measuring early mentalizing about the self and emotions like sadness, fear and anger, 2018b [Unpublished manuscript]

Lawrence EJ, Shaw P, Baker D, et al: Measuring empathy: reliability and validity of the Empathy Quotient. Psychol Med 34(5):911–919, 2004 15500311

Lenggenhager B, Tadi T, Metzinger T, et al: Video ergo sum: manipulating bodily self-consciousness. Science 317(5841):1096–1099, 2007 17717189

Levinson A, Fonagy P: Offending and attachment: the relationship between interpersonal awareness and offending in a prison population with psychiatric disorder. Can J Psychoanal 12:225–251, 2004

Levy KN, Meehan KB, Hill L: The Reflective Function Rating Scale, 2005 [Unpublished manuscript]

Lieberman MD: Social cognitive neuroscience: a review of core processes. Annu Rev Psychol 58:259–289, 2007 17002553

Lieberman MD, Eisenberger NI, Crockett MJ, et al: Putting feelings into words: affect labeling disrupts amygdala activity in response to affective stimuli. Psychol Sci 18(5):421–428, 2007 17576282

Luyten P, Fonagy P: The neurobiology of mentalizing. Pers Disord 6(4):366–379, 2015 26436580

Luyten P, Fonagy P, Lowyck B, et al: Assessment of mentalization, in Handbook of Mentalizing in Mental Health Practice. Edited by Bateman A, Fonagy P. Washington, DC, American Psychiatric Association, 2012, pp 43–65

Luyten P, Van Houdenhove B, Lemma A, et al: Vulnerability for functional somatic disorders: a contemporary psychodynamic approach. J Psychother Integration 23:250–262, 2013

Luyten P, Mayes LC, Nijssens L, et al: The parental reflective functioning questionnaire: development and preliminary validation. PLoS One 12(5):e0176218, 2017 28472162

Mayes LC: Arousal regulation, emotional flexibility, medial amygdala function, and the impact of early experience: comments on the paper of Lewis et al. Ann N Y Acad Sci 1094:178–192, 2006 17347350

Meehan KB, Levy KN, Reynoso JS, et al: Measuring reflective function with a multidimensional rating scale: comparison with scoring reflective function on the AAI. J Am Psychoanal Assoc 57(1):208–213, 2009 19270257

Meins E, Fernyhough C: Mind-Mindedness Coding Manual. Version 2.2. York, University of York, 2015

Meins E, Fernyhough C, de Rosnay M, et al: Mind-mindedness as a multidimensional construct: appropriate and nonattuned mind-related comments independently predict infant-mother attachment in a socially diverse sample. Infancy 17:393–415, 2012

Mikulincer M, Shaver PR: Attachment in Adulthood: Structure, Dynamics, and Change. New York, Guilford, 2007

Mikulincer M, Dolev T, Shaver PR: Attachment-related strategies during thought suppression: ironic rebounds and vulnerable self-representations. J Pers Soc Psychol 87(6):940–956, 2004 15598116

Muñoz Specht P, Ensink K, Normandin L, et al: Mentalizing techniques used by psychodynamic therapists working with children and early adolescents. Bull Menninger Clin 80(4):281–315, 2016 27936899

Murray HA: Thematic Apperception Test. Cambridge, MA, Harvard University Press, 1943

Neumann ID: Brain oxytocin: a key regulator of emotional and social behaviours in both females and males. J Neuroendocrinol 20(6):858–865, 2008 18601710

Pichon S, de Gelder B, Grèzes J: Two different faces of threat. Comparing the neural systems for recognizing fear and anger in dynamic body expressions. Neuroimage 47(4):1873–1883, 2009 19371787

Rimes KA, Chalder T: The Beliefs about Emotions Scale: validity, reliability and sensitivity to change. J Psychosom Res 68(3):285–292, 2010 20159215

Rudden MG, Milrod B, Target M: The Brief Reflective Functioning Interview. New York, Weill Cornell Medical College, 2005

Rudden M, Milrod B, Target M, et al: Reflective functioning in panic disorder patients: a pilot study. J Am Psychoanal Assoc 54(4):1339–1343, 2006 17354509

Rudden MG, Milrod B, Meehan KB, et al: Symptom-specific reflective functioning: incorporating psychoanalytic measures into clinical trials. J Am Psychoanal Assoc 57(6):1473–1478, 2009 20068250

Rutimann DD, Meehan KB: Validity of a brief interview for assessing reflective function. J Am Psychoanal Assoc 60(3):577–589, 2012 22589408

Salovey P, Grewal D: The science of emotional intelligence. Curr Dir Psychol Sci 14:281–285, 2005

Schechter DS, Coots T, Zeanah CH, et al: Maternal mental representations of the child in an inner-city clinical sample: violence-related posttraumatic stress and reflective functioning. Attach Hum Dev 7(3):313–331, 2005 16210242

Shamay-Tsoory SG, Aharon-Peretz J, Perry D: Two systems for empathy: a double dissociation between emotional and cognitive empathy in inferior frontal gyrus versus ventromedial prefrontal lesions. Brain 132(Pt 3):617–627, 2009 18971202

Sharp C, Fonagy P: The parent's capacity to treat the child as a psychological agent: constructs, measures and implications for developmental psychopathology. Soc Dev 17:737–754, 2008

Sharp C, Fonagy P, Goodyer IM: Imagining your child's mind: psychosocial adjustment and mothers' ability to predict their children's attributional response styles. Br J Dev Psychol 24:197–214, 2006

Shill MA, Lumley MA: The Psychological Mindedness Scale: factor structure, convergent validity and gender in a non-psychiatric sample. Psychol Psychother 75(Pt 2):131–150, 2002 12396760

Shmueli-Goetz Y, Target M, Fonagy P, et al: The Child Attachment Interview: a psychometric study of reliability and discriminant validity. Dev Psychol 44(4):939–956, 2008 18605826

Slade A: Parental reflective functioning: an introduction. Attach Hum Dev 7(3):269–281, 2005 16210239

Slade A, Patterson M: Addendum to Reflective Functioning Scoring Manual (Fonagy, Steele, Steele, and Target, 1998) for Use With the Pregnancy Interview (Slade, Grunebaum, Huganir, and Reeves, 1987; Slade, 2004). New York, City College of New York, 2005

Slade A, Aber JL, Berger B, et al: The Parent Development Interview—Revised. New York, City University of New York, 2004

Slade A, Bernbach E, Grienenberger J, et al: Addendum to Reflective Functioning Scoring Manual for Use With the Parent Development Interview, Version 3.0. New York, City College and Graduate Center of the City University of New York, 2007

Sonnby-Borgström M, Jönsson P: Dismissing-avoidant pattern of attachment and mimicry reactions at different levels of information processing. Scand J Psychol 45(2):103–113, 2004 15016264

Szecsödy I: A single-case study on the process and outcome of psychoanalysis. Scand Psychoanal Rev 31:105–113, 2008

Target M, Fonagy P, Shmueli-Goetz Y: Attachment representations in school-age children: the development of the Child Attachment Interview (CAI). J Child Psychother 29:171–186, 2003

Taubner S, Kessler H, Buchheim A, et al: The role of mentalization in the psychoanalytic treatment of chronic depression. Psychiatry 74(1):49–57, 2011 21463170

Tessier VP, Normandin L, Ensink K, et al: Fact or fiction? A longitudinal study of play and the development of reflective functioning. Bull Menninger Clin 80(1):60–79, 2016 27028339

Tottenham N, Tanaka JW, Leon AC, et al: The NimStim set of facial expressions: judgments from untrained research participants. Psychiatry Res 168(3):242–249, 2009 19564050

Vrouva I, Fonagy P: Development of the Mentalizing Stories for Adolescents (MSA). J Am Psychoanal Assoc 57:1174–1179, 2009

Vrticka P, Andersson F, Grandjean D, et al: Individual attachment style modulates human amygdala and striatum activation during social appraisal. PLoS One 3(8):e2868, 2008 18682729

White S, Hill E, Happé F, et al: Revisiting the strange stories: revealing mentalizing impairments in autism. Child Dev 80(4):1097–1117, 2009 19630896

Wilhelm O, Hildebrandt A, Manske K, et al: Test battery for measuring the perception and recognition of facial expressions of emotion. Front Psychol 5:404, 2014 24860528

CHAPTER 4

MENTALIZING, RESILIENCE, AND EPISTEMIC TRUST

Peter Fonagy, Ph.D., FBA, FMedSci, FAcSS

Elizabeth Allison, D.Phil.

Chloe Campbell, Ph.D.

Mentalizing is an imaginative process. We have often referred to an awareness of the opacity of other people's minds as being a central element of the mentalizing stance: we humans cannot know for sure what others are thinking, and as a result, there must (or perhaps should) be an element of tentativeness in our inferences about others' states of mind. The constant human work of reading other people in order to attempt to relate to, successfully interact with, and productively cooperate with them has made possible extraordinary social complexity. An awareness of the limitations and the artifice of individuals' attempts to reach conclusions about the content of others' thoughts is bound up with the human capacity for and interest in artistic and fictional exploration, as well as with considerable levels of uniquely human angst. In this chapter, we will explore the idea of mentalizing as an act of imagination and discuss what the idea of the human social imagination (of which mentalizing is one aspect that is directed toward imagining the mental states that underlie behavior) can contribute to the understanding of psychological resilience. We consider the notion that psychopathology may be the evolutionary flip side of the achievement of human social-cognitive complexity, in particular the capacity for imaginative thought, and discuss the implications of this hypothesis for the role of psychological therapy. In Chapter 10 ("Therapeutic Models"), we will continue this line of thinking about the social imagination and psychopathology to explore its implications for models of treatment.

WHAT IS RESILIENCE?

Resilience has been an area of highly active research and policy discourse in recent years, with some of its more popular manifestations perhaps unhelpfully (and, at worst, in a potentially blaming or punitive way) appearing to be yet another achievement that individuals in distress can be led to feel they have failed to attain. Furthermore, resilience research is well known to have been hampered by a highly confusing collection of definitions, contexts, designs, populations, and data-analytic strategies that may make the advisability of adopting the construct of resilience in an account of general psychopathology questionable, to say the least (for a useful account of these issues, see Luthar et al. 2000). However, in the face of this cacophony of constructs, some of the major contributors have brought coherence and an overarching frame to the field (Cicchetti 2016; Kalisch et al. 2015; Masten and Cicchetti 2016; Masten and Labella 2016). For all its complexities, as well as the risk of oversimplification and circularity in explanation it carries, we suggest that the construct of resilience may be of great value in helping to explore the nature of mental disorder and, more pragmatically, formulate what might underpin effective treatments (Kalisch et al. 2017).

Diverse accounts of resilience, often advanced at radically different levels of explanation, from the socioeconomic to the genetic level, have been compellingly unified within the *positive appraisal style theory of resilience* (PASTOR) conceptual framework presented by Kalisch et al. (2015). The proposed framework describes resilience as a cognitive process. A potentially stressful stimulus is perceived and mentally represented by the individual. The mental representation is then appraised using higher-order cognition and understood in terms of an ensemble of psychological mechanisms and phenomena, including executive function, attention, general intelligence, and self-awareness. This appraisal, in turn, determines the emotional response of the individual—that is, his or her resilience. Thus, according to this formulation, resilience is the outcome of the top-down cognitive appraisal of a stressful stimulus. The external and social factors that have been associated with resilience, such as social support or a secure attachment history, affect resilience either directly or indirectly, in that they shape the individual's appraisal approach or minimize exposure to stressors. This is not to deny the role of socioenvironmental factors in determining an individual's resilience, or the importance of interventions at a social or community level; it is to suggest that the mechanism by which these distal social factors affect an individual's resilience is via their impact on the individual's appraisal style.

As described above, the appropriate functioning of higher-order cognition crucially depends on appropriate judgments about social contexts. Kalisch et al. (2015) describe the following three underpinning appraisal mechanisms that determine resilience: 1) positive situation classification, 2) retrospective reappraisal of threat, and 3) inhibition of retraumatizing triggers.

Positive Situation Classification

Positive situation classification refers to the manner of immediate appraisal of a situation at the moment of encountering it (e.g., "*What is that person who is approaching me carrying in his hand?*"). Where there is no threat, a positive appraisal style enables the individual to interpret the situation as safe. Clearly, in the context of an adverse event, a negative appraisal and stress response are called for; in such situations, resilience can be subsequently promoted through the second and third forms of appraisal (described in the next two subsections). Difficulty arises when an individual misreads a situation as threatening when it is not. The mentalizing profile typically associated with individuals with borderline personality disorder (BPD), for example, tends to lean toward the automatic, nonreflective, and emotional poles on the mentalizing dimensions (see Chapter 1, "Introduction"). Individuals with BPD have been found to be more likely to view characters and behaviors as negative or aggressive (Barnow et al. 2009); to identify negative affect (such as anger or disgust) less accurately and misattribute emotion to neutral faces (Daros et al. 2013); and to react with hostility to neutral social interactions (Domes et al. 2008). This body of findings could all be interpreted within the PASTOR model as constituting a negative appraisal style (Kalisch et al. 2015). The mentalizing profile characteristic of an individual with BPD, in sum, results in an oversensitivity to possibly difficult social interactions (because distortions in mentalizing are more likely to result in mistaken interpretations of others' behavior and motivation).

Retrospective Reappraisal of Threat

Whether a traumatic event results in posttraumatic stress disorder (PTSD), for example, depends on how it is retrospectively reappraised. This, as Kalisch et al. (2015) describe, "shifts the emphasis from the external situation (or changes in the situation) to the individual's ability to flexibly adjust a current negative appraisal or to implement new, more positive appraisals and then to maintain those appraisals. Both processes have to occur in the face of interference from automatic and uncontrolled negative appraisals and the accompanying aversive emotional states" (p. 14). Patients with BPD have a specific problem in relation to reappraisal because they find it challenging to generate second-order representations of mental states that might be modified to constitute more positive reappraisals of experiences, or to mitigate (adjust) negative appraisals. In the absence of being able to mentalize in a balanced way, an event or a relationship can be endlessly discussed and dissected in an apparent attempt at reappraisal, but such attempts have an unreal quality. Complicated inferences about mental states might be made that have little connection with reality. We term this *pseudomentalizing* or, in extreme cases, *hypermentalizing* (described in Chapter 1). In the aftermath of a challenging or stressful interaction, it is difficult for the individual to make sense of, contextualize, or put aside potentially upsetting memories of experiences, leaving the individual more vulnerable to emotional storms. A capacity for explicit, reflective mentalizing in particular serves a dual interpretive (appraisal-strengthening) and self-regulatory role. The absence of this capacity deprives the individual of a fundamental tool to reduce stress.

Inhibition of Retraumatizing Triggers

This mechanism enables the individual to inhibit the threat-associated sensations that might be experienced when remembering a traumatic event. Not being able to limit this threat response can perpetuate and generalize the perception of threat. Individuals with BPD have been shown to have serious limitations in areas associated with the capacity to inhibit conflictive negative appraisals and emotional reactions that interfere with information processing (Barnow et al. 2009; Domes et al. 2009; Koenigsberg et al. 2009a, 2009b). They cannot cognitively inhibit retraumatizing triggers, leaving them vulnerable to threat-associated sensations when they remember a traumatic event. These sensations serve to reinforce the sense of threat. It is not possible for these individuals to access mentalizing if the self is overwhelmed by negative interference that impairs normal cognitive function (see Chapter 5, "Mentalizing and Trauma").

The framework for resilience provided by Kalisch and colleagues' (2015) reappraisal model can thus readily be "translated" into mentalizing processes, giving us a useful structure for understanding the different demands on mentalizing that are required to support the development of psychological resilience. In the rest of this chapter, we describe recent developments in our model of psychopathology, which seeks to locate the problem of mental health and resilience in a wider context of the human imagination, the affects associated with social relatedness, and the exigencies of the social environment.

MENTALIZING, RESILIENCE, AND THE "p" FACTOR

While the field of resilience research has been fast developing, there has been a parallel emergence of fruitful research around the concept of a general factor for psychopathology, known as the *p factor*. A serious challenge for our thinking about psychopathology arises from the fact that for many individuals, their psychiatric history over their life course rarely follows the discrete, symptom-defined and diagnosis-led categories that are used (e.g., in DSM-5; American Psychiatric Association 2013) to conceptualize specific disorders. This lack of specificity may relate to compelling evidence presented by Caspi et al. (2014) suggesting that there is, in fact, one general psychopathology factor in the structure of psychiatric disorders. In their longitudinal study based in Dunedin, New Zealand, Caspi et al. (2014) examined the structure of psychopathology from adolescence to midlife, examining dimensionality, persistence, co-occurrence, and sequential comorbidity. The study found that psychiatric disorders were more convincingly explained if the existence of one general psychopathology factor (labeled the p factor as a conceptual parallel to the g factor, the well-established dimension by which general intelligence is understood) was assumed to exist alongside clusters of symptoms (internalizing, externalizing, and psychosis) and individual psychiatric disorders (e.g., schizophrenia, generalized anxiety disorder, and depression). A higher p-factor score is associated with increased severity of impairment, more developmental adversity, and greater biological risk. The p-factor concept may help to explain why research in this field has found it so difficult to identify isolated causes, consequences, or biomarkers, or to develop specific tailored treatments for psychiatric disorders.

Work on a general factor of psychopathology has also been extended to childhood and adolescence. For instance, a longitudinal study of 2,450 girls ages 5–11 years has further indicated the criterion validity of the p-factor construct and found it to be a significantly better fit than a correlated two-factor (internalizing and externalizing) model (Lahey et al. 2015). These findings weaken the argument that the p factor is a statistical artifact and reinforce the importance of further consideration of what the p factor might substantively represent (Lahey et al. 2015). In a large community-based sample of 23,477 adolescents ages 11–13.5 years, Patalay et al. (2015) investigated 1) the traditional two-factor (internalizing and externalizing) model and 2) a bifactor model with a general psychopathology higher-order model. Both models were found to fit the data well; however, the general psychopathology model better predicted future psychopathology and academic attainment 3 years from the time of the original assessment, with individuals with high p-factor scores being 10 times as likely to have a diagnosable disorder 3 years from assessment than those with lower p-factor scores (see also Laceulle et al. 2015).

More specifically in relation to personality disorders (PDs), Sharp et al. (2015) have considered the question of whether a general factor for psychopathology exists in the context of PD diagnosis. In a series of exploratory factor analyses based on a sample of 966 inpatients, only four (avoidant, schizotypal, narcissistic, and antisocial) of the six PDs examined formed factors with 75% of the criteria that mark their respective factors. Half the obsessive-compulsive PD criteria loaded with the narcissistic PD criteria, and the other half split across two other factors. However, Sharp et al. (2015) found that 1) a BPD factor included primary loadings from just over half (55.6%) of the BPD items, of which three had notable cross-loadings, each on a different factor; 2) nearly half (44.4%) of the BPD items loaded most strongly on three non-BPD factors (although two had notable cross-loadings on the BPD factor); and 3) the BPD factor was also marked by a narcissistic PD item and had notable additional cross-loadings by other narcissistic as well as avoidant and schizotypal PD items. The same study evaluated a bifactor model of PD pathology in which a general factor and several specific factors of personality pathology accounted for the covariance among PD criteria. In the bifactor model, all BPD criteria loaded only on to the general factor. Other PDs loaded either on to both the general and a specific factor or largely only on to a specific factor. The implication of this finding is that BPD criteria may capture the core of personality pathology or may be most representative of all PDs.

The p factor has therefore been identified in these bifactor studies as a statistical construct. This of course raises the question of what psychological process this construct represents. Reviews of the candidate mechanisms underpinning psychopathology have consistently proposed that executive function might act as a critical determinant of the p factor (Caspi et al. 2014; Castellanos-Ryan et al. 2016; Martel et al. 2017). Executive function encompasses a range of cognitive processes essential to healthy functioning, namely, self-regulation, decision making, sequencing of actions, planning, prioritizing, and navigating new tasks (Banich 2009). These cognitive processes serve to maintain goal-directed behavior through three mechanisms: 1) inhibition, including self-control and interference control; 2) working memory; and 3) cognitive flexibility or shifting (Diamond 2013; Macdonald et al. 2016). Deficits in executive function characterize a wide range of mental disorders, from the most serious psychotic disorders (Forbes et al. 2009; Fusar-Poli et al. 2012) to attention-deficit/hyperactivity disorder (Barkley 1997) and conduct problems (Sergeant et al. 2002). Furthermore, both self-reported and informant-based assessments of executive function correlate positively with both internalizing and externalizing dimensional scores (e.g., Snyder et al. 2015; Vasey et al. 2013). Why should this be the case? There are a few predominant explanations: 1) a general dysfunction that forms a criterion of all mental disorders, which may involve the inability to control attention and direct it to goal-relevant information; 2) the dysfunction may be more specific to emotional challenges, such as shifting attention away from threatening stimuli (Drabick et al. 2010); and 3) the dysfunction may be concurrently specific to the control of behavioral impulses (Demeyer et al. 2012). Thus, weak core executive function potentially exposes the individual to impulsivity (Fino et al. 2014), aggression (Seguin and Zelazo 2005), worry (Snyder et al. 2014), and rumination (Demeyer et al. 2012).

In particular, the critical component of executive function is poor constraint in the presence of emotion (Berg et al. 2015; Carver et al. 2017; Fischer et al. 2008). To clarify, when we discuss impulsivity of emotional response in this context, we are not referring to hypersensitivity of psychophysical reaction to an emotional stimulus. The response we are concerned with in this model relates to the individual's understanding of his or her reaction and capacity to interpret it, which can then serve to either escalate or de-escalate his or her affect (in keeping with Kalisch and colleagues' [2015] framework, discussed in the earlier section "What Is Resilience?"). Following on from the developmental work of Gergely and Watson (1996), we relate this process to the second-order representation of emotions that the infant may have experienced in the marked mirroring of his or her affect by the caregiver. The response is not necessarily connected to the intensity or content of the current experience. For example, a sense of rejection in response to a perceived social slight may be more difficult to inhibit because it is experienced as unsymbolized and more immediate—the affect has not been reflected upon and manageably represented by the other. Positive emotions such as pleasure, although probably less often left unreflected upon and therefore unsymbolized, can create analogous problems by being experienced as needing immediate address, leading to antisocial behavior. Subsequent studies have demonstrated that the caregiver's capacity to mirror the experience of the child is a predictor of later adjustment, as well as the immediate response of parent and child to the emotional trigger (Bernier et al. 2014; Kok et al. 2015). To extend this concept, we are suggesting that the success of the child in internalizing sensitive responsiveness by the caregiver is at the foundation of the individual's capacity to exercise cognitive control as opposed to autonomic control over affect. This model is not developmentally deterministic, as we assume that the development of this capacity is not rendered immutable by either heredity or early experience. Heredity must have a major role, as some child–caregiver pairs find it more difficult to achieve contingent marked mirroring than others. Furthermore, there is a developmental cascade that undoubtedly amplifies difficulties for the child in achieving response inhibition or control and a modulating response to emotional stimuli. Lack of control over responding to emotion, operationalized as *urgency*, has been shown in longitudinal studies to be a good predictor of a range of adverse mental health outcomes (Doran et al. 2013; Kaiser et al. 2016; Pearson and Smith 2015; Webb Hooper and Carver 2016; Zapolski et al. 2009).

In describing differences in individuals' impulsive responsivity to emotion, Carver et al. (2017) draw on a well-established literature to delineate a dichotomy between a reflexive, basic, emotion-responsive mode and a reflective, deliberative mental function. They point to a large family of theories, including those of Kahneman (2011), Evans and Stanovich (2013), Rothbart et al. (2003), and Toates (2006), that implicitly or explicitly share this dichotomy. Carver et al. (2017) claim that a shared characteristic of the reflexive mode is relative simplicity of and responsiveness to affect (Metcalfe and Mischel 1999; Strack and Deutsch 2004). Helpfully, they acknowledge a link to the computational models evolved by Peter Dayan and colleagues (Daw et al. 2005; Dayan 2008; Dolan and Dayan 2013), in which the term "model-free learning" is used to describe how information is acquired through a process of association. In contrast to a reflective or deliberative mode, the reflexive mode of functioning employs automatic habits and relatively automatic responses. "Model-based learning" (a reflective mode of functioning), by contrast, involves taking more information into account and making decisions on the basis of a larger set of considerations. Learning in this context is described as model-based in the sense that it is aimed at creating a coherent picture of the world within which the organism functions (Otto et al. 2013). None of the authors proposing such dual-process models imagine that these processes function independently. Nevertheless, it is fair to assume that the processes compete for influence and that any particular output of cognition reflects the result of the competition between the two (Buckholtz 2015). Carver et al. (2017) suggest that a reflexive mode of functioning may be better adapted to environments dominated by uncertainty where "the reflexive mode brings a spontaneity to a person's experience that can be desirable" (p. 881).

MENTALIZING AND THE SOCIAL IMAGINATION

The idea that the p factor is associated with difficulties in executive function in the area of impulsivity of emotional reactivity, caused by operating in a reflexive mode, is congruent with mentalizing theory and also with Kalisch et al.'s (2015) reappraisal model—that is, the idea that a lack of balanced, reflective mentalizing obstructs the ability to recalibrate stressors in an adaptive manner. However, particularly in the context of more severe or persistent disorder, it is clear that there are distortions of cognition that more profoundly impair an individual's capacity to function than emotional impulsivity alone. We propose that a reflexive default mode becomes associated with serious impairment in mental health—what might be thought of as a high p factor—when it is found alongside disruptions in another aspect of higher-order cognition: the social imagination. We are thus proposing a two-factor model for general vulnerability to mental disorder.

- The first factor relates to an oversensitivity to peremptory emotional cues and a failure to robustly inhibit reflexive responses based on model-free associative learning.
- The second component entails an overreliance on a system that underpins human imagination, probably evolutionarily developed as one of the critical capacities that define adaptation in the human species: the capacity for inventive model building, to a large measure independent of external cues, is what makes creativity possible.

As Vygotsky (2004) pointed out, everything that was made by human hands—including all aspects of human culture—is the product of human creativity and imagination. A well-established literature with a highly distinguished history has linked biological (genetic) risk for mental disorder to higher levels of creative, divergent, or imaginative thinking (for reviews, see Kaufman 2014; Kyaga et al. 2013; Ruiter and Johnson 2015; Zabelina et al. 2015).

Viewing imagination through the lens of mentalizing can help clinicians to understand why imaginative capacity and the propensity to mental disorder should be so closely linked, and why the emergence of mental disorder in the course of the lifespan is not the exception but the rule. If epidemiological figures are to be relied on, only one in five people will go through life without experiencing a diagnosable mental health condition (Schaefer et al. 2017). Looking at such prevalence figures from the perspective of natural selection, it is clear that whatever the neural systems are that underpin mental disorder, they must have other functions that are advantageous for survival. In particular, mental disorder, which invariably incorporates an imagined version of reality that is dysfunctional in the circumstances in which it is being applied, may be the price to pay given the wider benefits of human imagination: it is essential for mentalizing, and hence for the transmission of culture. Psychopathology, we argue, is an evolutionary by-product of the human imaginative capacity.

Thus, we are suggesting that for mental disorder to develop, two factors must play a part. Common to mental disorders is a failure of imagination, which may arise as a consequence of neurobiological vulnerability associated with environmental or genetic causes, or the interaction of the two. The presence of a failure of imagination does not in itself create mental disorder without concurrent failure of the gating mechanism that is required to be in place to preclude erroneous reflexive responding. It is highly likely that failures of imagination of the kind we are proposing are very common; indeed, such failures may even have adaptive significance in producing original or novel thought. It is also likely that normally giving voice to reflexive thinking is adaptive and generates a wide range of highly valued cultural products. It is the coincident failure of two systems, each of which may be crucial to human survival, that generates maladaptation.

For most individuals, the potential to experience mental disorder has a selective advantage because it is this potential that provides humans with the creative capacities that are crucial to success as a species. Mental disorders entail beliefs, entire narratives, and actions justified by the imagined version of reality they incorporate, as described above. Individuals calibrate their social imagination in response to parameters they encounter in their early social environment. The generally accepted developmental psychopathology model shows that children are most at risk of mental disorder when they grow up in environments that are harsh, and thus within our model we need to demonstrate how individuals may achieve better, fitness-relevant outcomes if a reflexive imaginative function more readily finds expression. We argue that when children live in harsh, dangerous social contexts, high-risk life strategies (Del Giudice 2016), as generated by imaginative solutions that may bear little on objective reality, could be more advantageous than solutions reached through more exhaustive logical inference. Along with others, we have suggested that the quality of family relationships in an attachment context in early life may provide the child with information about the safety or predictability of his or her environment (Chisholm 1999). There is independent evidence that emotional responsivity mediated by executive function reflects the quality of the child's attachment environment. There is also evidence that processes entailed in imagination reflect the child's early attachment contexts. We are not arguing that attachment is a primary—or even an important—mediator of psychopathology, but merely that the evolutionary mechanisms are in place by which adaptation may be optimized through prioritizing input from a system based on imagination even at the expense of potential cost given the high potential failure rate of this capacity. Creative solutions inevitably entail high risk and are most likely to be adaptive in the context of unpredictable environments (Frankenhuis and Del Giudice 2012). This dynamic is simply a reflection of how natural selection shapes developmental strategies that in turn give rise to phenotypes adapted to a local ecology (Panchanathan et al. 2010). A possible general model for psychopathology is provided by the notion of a developmental mismatch (Gluckman et al. 2011). The argument advanced by developmental evolutionary psychologists lays claim to a developmental mechanism that uses indications from the environment to generate an appropriate level of responsivity (Del Giudice et al. 2011; Glover 2011). A change of environment might create problems of a developmental mismatch. Thus, the prioritization of reflexive cognition indicated by hostile early environmental conditions might actually generate maladaptive responses under more favorable conditions. Given the probabilistic nature of the sampling of environmental cues, it is likely that rather than favoring phenotypes that irreversibly commit the organism to a particular adaptation, natural selection would favor a "dimensional" approach that increases the likelihood of a particular type of solution for that environment. The model we propose represents exactly such a fine-tuning mechanism that enables the child to adapt incrementally to the local ecology (Frankenhuis and Panchanathan 2011).

EPISTEMIC TRUST

How does this proposed model of mental disorder fit within our wider thinking about mentalizing and epistemic trust? We have previously developed the idea that *epistemic trust*—defined as openness to the reception of social communication that is personally relevant and of generalizable significance—underpins the capacity for social learning that enables the individual to benefit from his or her social environment, creating a process of salutogenesis (Fonagy et al. 2015). We have posited that many, if not all, types of psychopathology may be associated with a breakdown of epistemic trust and the consequence this breakdown has for the social learning process that epistemic trust allows (Fonagy et al. 2015). If an infant does not experience being adequately mentalized by his or her caregiver, the infant's own emerging mentalizing capacity may become vulnerable to disruption in contexts that generate emotional arousal or stress. A further possible impact will be that owing to the importance of mentalizing as an ostensive cue, a child's naturally occurring epistemic vigilance will not be replaced by the development of epistemic trust that opens the child to taking on the social knowledge that will guide the child through his or her social environment (Fonagy and Luyten 2016). Many forms of psychopathology have the shared feature of apparent rigidity and an incapacity to adapt to changes in and learn about the social world (Fonagy et al. 2015). All people seek social knowledge, but without the reassurance and support of trusted caregivers, family, or peers, the content of communications can be confusing, and they may be rejected as a result of perceived hostile intent. We suggest that many manifestations of mental disorder may be underpinned by an inability to benefit from social communication due to epistemic mistrust or outright *epistemic freezing* (or *epistemic petrification*). The outcomes of these disruptions in epistemic trust can include the individual's reluctance to modify his or her beliefs and expectations, even in the face of social experiences that clearly indicate the value of doing so. Individuals who have experienced severe trauma and/or have PD may be almost completely unable to trust others as sources of knowledge about the social environment. For example, an individual who has been maltreated may justifiably come to regard his or her caregivers as unreliable or malintentioned sources of information about the world, and as a result the individual may learn to reject communications from others that are inconsistent with his or her preexisting beliefs. This is an adaptive response to a hostile or threatening social environment, but in a clinical setting, such an individual may be considered "hard to reach."

To explain the relationship between epistemic mistrust and clinicians' experience of individuals as interpersonally inaccessible, we need to consider how epistemic trust is generated in any particular instance in adult communication. All individuals have a personal narrative, an imagined sense of self, evidenced by their experiences—which phenomenologists have long recognized (Sass et al. 2017)—and the biological reality of this has been impressively demonstrated by the program of work summarized by Northoff and Huang (2017). The understanding of the individual's personal narrative by another person creates a potential for epistemic trust, and the individual's perception of that understanding in the other generates epistemic trust. As it is a *perception* of understanding, genuine understanding may not be necessary, and the illusion of understanding may suffice.

It is clear that the absence of epistemic trust would deeply disadvantage an individual in most social contexts. These individuals would fail to update their understanding of potentially rapidly changing social situations and would appear inflexible or even rigid in the face of social change. Why would an individual fail to experience epistemic trust even in situations where trust was warranted—that is, where his or her personal narrative was appreciated? There are two obvious reasons. First, adversity and deprivation, when tantamount to trauma, can generate chronic mistrust by inhibiting imagination, creating an overarching avoidance of mentalizing and an almost phobic avoidance of mental states, leaving the individual deeply vulnerable in most social situations. Even in the absence of such a pervasive failure of imagination, inadequate mentalizing may lead traumatized individuals to be biased in their perception of social reality (Cicchetti and Curtis 2005; Germine et al. 2015; Kay and Green 2016; Pears and Fisher 2005) and misrepresent how others represent them, leading them to feel persistently misunderstood and to experience an intense and consistent sense of (epistemic) injustice. Secondly, the long-term outcome of epistemic isolation secondary to the failure of imagination we describe here may create problems for individuals who have distorted personal narratives that generate inaccurate views of the self, so that even an accurate perception of their personal narrative by others is not experienced as a match, and a painful experience of interpersonal alienation persists. Unless a therapist is able to recognize this distorted personal narrative and reflect it back to the patient, epistemic mistrust will persist. Conversely, in yet other instances, deprivation and trauma may generate inappropriate trust. We understand such excessive epistemic credulity to be triggered by a hyperactive or unmoored imagination generating a personal narrative that is too diffuse to provide an accurate sense of differential awareness of others' capacity to perceive the individual. Excessive credulity results because all personal narratives feel as if they "fit" sufficiently for trust to be generated, making the person vulnerable to exploitation. Of course, limited imagination may cause profound misperceptions of the other's representations of the individual's personal narrative, and an illusory fit is created where none in reality exists. There may be many other possibilities. We suggest that in all these permutations an individual's social experience leads him or her to encounter problems in learning from others, which in turn creates significant problems in adaptation when the individual attempts to adjust to a frequently challenging and changing social world. To put this succinctly, the absence of resilience is the dysfunction of the process of generating appropriate epistemic trust.

To return to the role of the imagination, we suggest that individuals functioning in a state of heightened epistemic mistrust will not benefit from the access to other people's minds that could serve to regulate their own imaginative activity. Without the social metric that epistemic trust enables, the imagination may "run riot," and go substantially beyond a shared reality that people ultimately must agree on in order to collaborate. What we aim to describe here may appear to be a paradox almost verging on self-contradiction. The system of transferring trusted knowledge that humans have evolved requires imagination to establish trust; however, the transmission of knowledge that follows places a constraint on the imagination to ensure that there is an agreed version of reality. Being able to mentalize one another makes it possible to have a collectively agreed imagination (e.g., organizations talk about a "shared vision" for a reason), which in turn makes human cooperation possible (Tomasello 2018). From a developmental perspective, infants' early experiences of their knowledge of the world will be in the form of the sensations of their physical needs. When this knowledge is confirmed and validated through an appropriate caregiver response (i.e., through the meeting of those physical needs), the channel for the communication of knowledge between the self and the other is opened. It creates a sense that there is a "shared vision" of what is happening to the infant and in the world around the infant. Significant discontinuity between the infant's physical needs and the caregiver's response (e.g., through neglect) may constitute the first experience of "meaninglessness," and the unmooring of imagination in trying to make sense of what is happening (Fonagy and Campbell 2017). The value of epistemic trust in relation to our model of psychopathology is therefore that it enables the individual to align his or her social imagination with the prevailing social reality in an adaptive way.

What does this broad theory of resilience bring to an understanding of the mentalization-based approach to mental disorder? We suggest that mentalizing matters because it is the everyday social-cognitive tool that all people use to both regulate and benefit from the power of social imagination. Hypermentalizing and hypomentalizing represent different ways in which the social imagination has become unmoored. The mentalizing therapeutic approach responds to each of the two factors that we suggest work together to generate psychopathology: 1) the predominance of the reflexive mode of executive function (Carver et al. 2017) and 2) social-imaginative chaos or collapse. Vulnerability to psychopathology (i.e., the inverse of resilience) is, as has been suggested by many (e.g., Masten 2014), a construct that bridges social and individual perspectives and may lie precisely in the failing connection between the intrapsychic and the interpersonal. Building a social network is the primary task of childhood and adolescence. When the capacity to form bonds of social trust is shaky and susceptible to breakdown, the interpersonal learning network is lost and social expectations are not updated. It is the capacity to learn from social experience that enables people to respond effectively to adversity and challenge.

Distortions in social imagination may make it difficult for individuals to recognize that someone else is able to understand them: this undermines resilience because the shared understanding of personal narratives creates the interpersonal syntax that makes social communication possible and intelligible to all partners. It is what makes cooperation and the salutogenic building of interpersonal networks possible. In therapy, a clinician may accurately understand and reflect back a patient's personal narrative, but this will be of little value if the patient is unable to understand or recognize the image of himself or herself that is being revealed in the clinician's mind. The channel of social communication will remain closed, and the social "learning" of therapy cannot unfold. Alternatively, if patients' unbridled social imagination leads them to misread the image of their own personal narrative that the clinician is trying to reflect back to them, social communication will become obstructed by confusion and inaccurate mentalizing. The persistence of mental disorder, or a chronic lack of resilience, is the outcome of the breakdown of the individual's ability to benefit from experiencing his or her imagined sense of self (or personal narrative) as being identified and satisfyingly aligned with a trusted other's understanding of the individual's imagined self. Perceiving this lack of imaginative alignment will, probably for sound adaptive reasons, close down epistemic trust, rendering the individual unable to benefit from the interpersonal process the clinician is trying to generate because epistemic trust will not be triggered. It is the balance of imagination and epistemic trust, maintained within an appropriate band, that ensures the resilience of the individual. Too much imagination, which might manifest as hypermentalizing (discussed in Chapter 17, "Borderline Personality Pathology in Adolescence"), undermines the capacity to evolve learning relationships through excessive epistemic credulity (in which any idea is possible, but none is more meaningful or grounded in reality than another), which in turn undermines adaptation; too little imagination will compromise trust and generate epistemic isolation. Naturally, there is situational and temporal variation within and between people, which makes this field so challenging to research empirically.

REFERENCES

American Psychiatric Association: Diagnostic and Statistical Manual of Mental Disorders, 5th Edition. Arlington, VA, American Psychiatric Association, 2013

Banich MT: Executive function: The search for an integrated account. Curr Dir Psychol Sci 18:89–94, 2009

Barkley RA: Behavioral inhibition, sustained attention, and executive functions: constructing a unifying theory of ADHD. Psychol Bull 121(1):65–94, 1997 9000892

Barnow S, Stopsack M, Grabe HJ, et al: Interpersonal evaluation bias in borderline personality disorder. Behav Res Ther 47(5):359–365, 2009 19278670

Berg JM, Latzman RD, Bliwise NG, et al: Parsing the heterogeneity of impulsivity: a meta-analytic review of the behavioral implications of the UPPS for psychopathology. Psychol Assess 27(4):1129–1146, 2015 25822833

Bernier A, Matte-Gagné C, Bélanger ME, et al: Taking stock of two decades of attachment transmission gap: broadening the assessment of maternal behavior. Child Dev 85(5):1852–1865, 2014 24611791

Buckholtz JW: Social norms, self-control, and the value of antisocial behavior. Curr Opin Behav Sci 3:122–129, 2015

Carver CS, Johnson SL, Timpano KR: Toward a functional view of the p factor in psychopathology. Clin Psychol Sci 5(5):880–889, 2017 29057170

Caspi A, Houts RM, Belsky DW, et al: The p factor: one general psychopathology factor in the structure of psychiatric disorders? Clin Psychol Sci 2(2):119–137, 2014 25360393

Castellanos-Ryan N, Brière FN, O'Leary-Barrett M, et al; IMAGEN Consortium: The structure of psychopathology in adolescence and its common personality and cognitive correlates. J Abnorm Psychol 125(8):1039–1052, 2016 27819466

Chisholm JS: Attachment and time preference: Relations between early stress and sexual behavior in a sample of American university women. Hum Nat 10(1):51–83, 1999 26197415

Cicchetti D: Socioemotional, personality, and biological development: illustrations from a multilevel developmental psychopathology perspective on child maltreatment. Annu Rev Psychol 67:187–211, 2016 26726964

Cicchetti D, Curtis WJ: An event-related potential study of the processing of affective facial expressions in young children who experienced maltreatment during the first year of life. Dev Psychopathol 17(3):641–677, 2005 16262986

Daros AR, Zakzanis KK, Ruocco AC: Facial emotion recognition in borderline personality disorder. Psychol Med 43(9):1953–1963, 2013 23149223

Daw ND, Niv Y, Dayan P: Uncertainty-based competition between prefrontal and dorsolateral striatal systems for behavioral control. Nat Neurosci 8(12):1704–1711, 2005 16286932

Dayan P: Simple substrates for complex cognition. Front Neurosci 2(2):255–263, 2008 19225599

Del Giudice M: The life history model of psychopathology explains the structure of psychiatric disorders and the emergence of the p factor. Clin Psychol Sci 4:299–311, 2016

Del Giudice M, Ellis BJ, Shirtcliff EA: The Adaptive Calibration Model of stress responsivity. Neurosci Biobehav Rev 35(7):1562–1592, 2011 21145350

Demeyer I, De Lissnyder E, Koster EH, et al: Rumination mediates the relationship between impaired cognitive control for emotional information and depressive symptoms: a prospective study in remitted depressed adults. Behav Res Ther 50(5):292–297, 2012 22449892

Diamond A: Executive functions. Annu Rev Psychol 64:135–168, 2013 23020641

Dolan RJ, Dayan P: Goals and habits in the brain. Neuron 80(2):312–325, 2013 24139036

Domes G, Czieschnek D, Weidler F, et al: Recognition of facial affect in borderline personality disorder. J Pers Disord 22(2):135–147, 2008 18419234

Domes G, Schulze L, Herpertz SC: Emotion recognition in borderline personality disorder—a review of the literature. J Pers Disord 23(1):6–19, 2009 19267658

Doran N, Khoddam R, Sanders PE, et al: A prospective study of the Acquired Preparedness Model: the effects of impulsivity and expectancies on smoking initiation in college students. Psychol Addict Behav 27(3):714–722, 2013 22686965

Drabick DA, Ollendick TH, Bubier JL: Co-occurrence of ODD and anxiety: shared risk processes and evidence for a dual-pathway model. Clin Psychol (New York) 17(4):307–318, 2010 21442035

Evans JS, Stanovich KE: Dual-process theories of higher cognition: advancing the debate. Perspect Psychol Sci 8(3):223–241, 2013 26172965

Fino E, Melogno S, Iliceto P, et al: Executive functions, impulsivity, and inhibitory control in adolescents: a structural equation model. Adv Cogn Psychol 10(2):32–38, 2014 25157298

Fischer S, Smith GT, Cyders MA: Another look at impulsivity: a meta-analytic review comparing specific dispositions to rash action in their relationship to bulimic symptoms. Clin Psychol Rev 28(8):1413–1425, 2008 18848741

Fonagy P, Campbell C: What touch can communicate: Commentary on "Mentalizing homeostasis: the social origins of interoceptive inference" by Fotopoulou and Tsakiris. Neuropsychoanalysis 19:39–42, 2017

Fonagy P, Luyten P: A multilevel perspective on the development of borderline personality disorder, in Developmental Psychopathology Vol 3: Maladaptation and Psychopathology, 3rd Edition. Edited by Cicchetti D. New York, Wiley, 2016, pp 726–792

Fonagy P, Luyten P, Allison E: Epistemic petrification and the restoration of epistemic trust: a new conceptualization of borderline personality disorder and its psychosocial treatment. J Pers Disord 29(5):575–609, 2015 26393477

Forbes NF, Carrick LA, McIntosh AM, et al: Working memory in schizophrenia: a meta-analysis. Psychol Med 39(6):889–905, 2009 18945379

Frankenhuis WE, Del Giudice M: When do adaptive developmental mechanisms yield maladaptive outcomes? Dev Psychol 48(3):628–642, 2012 21967567

Frankenhuis WE, Panchanathan K: Balancing sampling and specialization: an adaptationist model of incremental development. Proc Biol Sci 278(1724):3558–3565, 2011 21490018

Fusar-Poli P, Deste G, Smieskova R, et al: Cognitive functioning in prodromal psychosis: a meta-analysis. Arch Gen Psychiatry 69(6):562–571, 2012 22664547

Gergely G, Watson JS: The social biofeedback theory of parental affect-mirroring: the development of emotional self-awareness and self-control in infancy. Int J Psychoanal 77(Pt 6):1181–1212, 1996 9119582

Germine L, Dunn EC, McLaughlin KA, et al: Childhood adversity is associated with adult theory of mind and social affiliation, but not face processing. PLoS One 10(6):e0129612, 2015 26068107

Glover V: Annual Research Review: Prenatal stress and the origins of psychopathology: an evolutionary perspective. J Child Psychol Psychiatry 52(4):356–367, 2011 21250994

Gluckman PD, Low FM, Buklijas T, et al: How evolutionary principles improve the understanding of human health and disease. Evol Appl 4(2):249–263, 2011 25567971

Kahneman D: Thinking, Fast and Slow. New York. Farrar, Straus, & Giroux, 2011

Kaiser A, Bonsu JA, Charnigo RJ, et al: Impulsive personality and alcohol use: bidirectional relations over one year. J Stud Alcohol Drugs 77(3):473–482, 2016 27172580

Kalisch R, Müller MB, Tüscher O: A conceptual framework for the neurobiological study of resilience. Behav Brain Sci 38:e92, 2015 25158686

Kalisch R, Baker DG, Basten U, et al: The resilience framework as a strategy to combat stress-related disorders. Nat Hum Behav 1:784–790, 2017

Kaufman J: Creativity and Mental Illness. Cambridge, UK, Cambridge University Press, 2014

Kay CL, Green JM: Social cognitive deficits and biases in maltreated adolescents in U.K. out-of-home care: relation to disinhibited attachment disorder and psychopathology. Dev Psychopathol 28(1):73–83, 2016 25851172

Koenigsberg HW, Fan J, Ochsner KN, et al: Neural correlates of the use of psychological distancing to regulate responses to negative social cues: a study of patients with borderline personality disorder. Biol Psychiatry 66(9):854–863, 2009a 19651401

Koenigsberg HW, Siever LJ, Lee H, et al: Neural correlates of emotion processing in borderline personality disorder. Psychiatry Res 172(3):192–199, 2009b 19394205

Kok R, Thijssen S, Bakermans-Kranenburg MJ, et al: Normal variation in early parental sensitivity predicts child structural brain development. J Am Acad Child Adolesc Psychiatry 54(10):824.e1–831.e1, 2015 26407492

Kyaga S, Landén M, Boman M, et al: Mental illness, suicide and creativity: 40-year prospective total population study. J Psychiatr Res 47(1):83–90, 2013 23063328

Laceulle OM, Vollebergh WAM, Ormel J: The structure of psychopathology in adolescence: replication of a general psychopathology factor in the TRAILS study. Clin Psychol Sci 3:850–860, 2015

Lahey BB, Rathouz PJ, Keenan K, et al: Criterion validity of the general factor of psychopathology in a prospective study of girls. J Child Psychol Psychiatry 56(4):415–422, 2015 25052460

Luthar SS, Cicchetti D, Becker B: The construct of resilience: a critical evaluation and guidelines for future work. Child Dev 71(3):543–562, 2000 10953923

Macdonald AN, Goines KB, Novacek DM, et al: Prefrontal mechanisms of comorbidity from a transdiagnostic and ontogenic perspective. Dev Psychopathol 28(4pt1):1147–1175, 2016 27739395

Martel MM, Pan PM, Hoffmann MS, et al: A general psychopathology factor (P factor) in children: structural model analysis and external validation through familial risk and child global executive function. J Abnorm Psychol 126(1):137–148, 2017 27748619

Masten AS: Ordinary Magic: Resilience in Development. New York, Guilford, 2014

Masten AS, Cicchetti D: Resilience in development: progress and transformation, in Developmental Psychopathology Vol 4: Risk, Resilience, and Intervention, 3rd Edition. Edited by Cicchetti D. New York, Wiley, 2016, pp 272–333

Masten AS, Labella MH: Risk and resilience in child development, in Child Psychology: A Handbook of Contemporary Issues, 3rd Edition. Edited by Balter L, Tamie-LeMonda C. New York, Routledge, 2016, p 423

Metcalfe J, Mischel W: A hot/cool-system analysis of delay of gratification: dynamics of will-power. Psychol Rev 106(1):3–19, 1999 10197361

Northoff G, Huang Z: How do the brain's time and space mediate consciousness and its different dimensions? Temporo-spatial theory of consciousness (TTC). Neurosci Biobehav Rev 80:630–645, 2017 28760626

Otto AR, Gershman SJ, Markman AB, et al: The curse of planning: dissecting multiple reinforcement-learning systems by taxing the central executive. Psychol Sci 24(5):751–761, 2013 23558545

Panchanathan K, Frankenhuis WE, Barrett HC: Development: evolutionary ecology's midwife. Behav Brain Sci 33(2–3):105–106, 2010 20546654

Patalay P, Fonagy P, Deighton J, et al: A general psychopathology factor in early adolescence. Br J Psychiatry 207(1):15–22, 2015 25906794

Pears KC, Fisher PA: Emotion understanding and theory of mind among maltreated children in foster care: evidence of deficits. Dev Psychopathol 17(1):47–65, 2005 15971759

Pearson CM, Smith GT: Bulimic symptom onset in young girls: a longitudinal trajectory analysis. J Abnorm Psychol 124(4):1003–1013, 2015 26595477

Rothbart MK, Ellis LK, Rueda MR, et al: Developing mechanisms of temperamental effortful control. J Pers 71(6):1113–1143, 2003 14633060

Ruiter M, Johnson SL: Mania risk and creativity: a multi-method study of the role of motivation. J Affect Disord 170:52–58, 2015 25233239

Sass L, Pienkos E, Skodlar B, et al: EAWE: Examination of Anomalous World Experience. Psychopathology 50(1):10–54, 2017 28268224

Schaefer JD, Caspi A, Belsky DW, et al: Enduring mental health: Prevalence and prediction. J Abnorm Psychol 126(2):212–224, 2017 27929304

Seguin JR, Zelazo PD: Executive function in early physical aggression, in Developmental Origins of Aggression. Edited by Archer J, Tremblay RE, Hartup WW, Willard W. New York, Guilford, 2005, pp 307–392

Sergeant JA, Geurts H, Oosterlaan J: How specific is a deficit of executive functioning for attention-deficit/hyperactivity disorder? Behav Brain Res 130(1–2):3–28, 2002 11864714

Sharp C, Wright AG, Fowler JC, et al: The structure of personality pathology: both general ('g') and specific ('s') factors? J Abnorm Psychol 124(2):387–398, 2015 25730515

Snyder HR, Kaiser RH, Whisman MA, et al: Opposite effects of anxiety and depressive symptoms on executive function: the case of selecting among competing options. Cogn Emotion 28(5):893–902, 2014 24295077

Snyder HR, Miyake A, Hankin BL: Advancing understanding of executive function impairments and psychopathology: bridging the gap between clinical and cognitive approaches. Front Psychol 6:328, 2015 25859234

Strack F, Deutsch R: Reflective and impulsive determinants of social behavior. Pers Soc Psychol Rev 8(3):220–247, 2004 15454347

Toates F: A model of the hierarchy of behaviour, cognition, and consciousness. Conscious Cogn 15(1):75–118, 2006 15996485

Tomasello M: Great apes and human development: a personal history. Child Dev Perspect 12(3):189–193, 2018

Vasey MW, Harbaugh CN, Lonigan CJ, et al: Dimensions of temperament and depressive symptoms: replicating a three-way interaction. J Res Pers 47(6):908–921, 2013 24493906

Vygotsky LS: Imagination and creativity in childhood. J Russ East Eur Psychol 42:7–97, 2004

Webb Hooper M, Carver CS: Reflexive reaction to feelings predicts failed smoking cessation better than does lack of general self-control. J Consult Clin Psychol 84(7):612–618, 2016 27077692

Zabelina DL, O'Leary D, Pornpattananangkul N, et al: Creativity and sensory gating indexed by the P50: selective versus leaky sensory gating in divergent thinkers and creative achievers. Neuropsychologia 69:77–84, 2015 25623426

Zapolski TC, Cyders MA, Smith GT: Positive urgency predicts illegal drug use and risky sexual behavior. Psychol Addict Behav 23(2):348–354, 2009 19586152

CHAPTER 5

MENTALIZING AND TRAUMA

Patrick Luyten, Ph.D.
Peter Fonagy, Ph.D., FBA, FMedSci, FAcSS

In this chapter we present an update of the mentalizing approach to the conceptualization and treatment of trauma, building on our previous work in this area (Allen 2005, 2013; Allen et al. 2012; Fonagy and Target 2008; Fonagy et al. 1994, 2017a, 2017b). A broad range of research findings are summarized showing that trauma can be best considered as a transdiagnostic factor that is implicated in a wide variety of emotional and (functional) somatic disorders and problems. Then we present ideas about how to conceptualize trauma and understand its impact on psychological function from a mentalizing perspective. What is it that makes trauma potentially such a disruptive experience and so difficult to treat? There are three related issues in answer to this question.

1. The **impact of traumatic experiences** on the attachment system as a basic biobehavioral system that plays a key role in the regulation of distress.
2. There is an effect of such experiences on **subsequent problems in mentalizing**.
3. The impact of trauma may contribute to **epistemic mistrust**—that is, the closing off of the mind to the possibility of accessing other people's minds as safe and reliable sources of knowledge about how to navigate the social environment (Fonagy et al. 2015).

We close the chapter with a consideration about how an understanding of these three factors leads to treatment principles that are useful for clinicians using a mentalizing approach to treatment.

At the outset of this chapter, it is important to address three potential misunderstandings related to the mentalizing approach to trauma: 1) the role of the absence of resilience rather than the presence of vulnerability, 2) the lack of consideration of the cumulative effect of prior trauma, and 3) the inadequacy of a sole treatment focus on anxiety-related symptoms of trauma. Trauma can be situated on a continuum ranging from impersonal trauma (e.g., a natural disaster) to interpersonal trauma (e.g., being abused by a colleague or stranger) and attachment trauma (e.g., being abused by an attachment figure) (Figure 5–1). The focus of the mentalizing approach—and thus of this chapter—is interpersonal trauma and attachment trauma in particular. This focus should not be interpreted as a limitation of the mentalizing approach, as interpersonal and attachment trauma have been shown to be related to increased vulnerability to psychopathology. It is easily forgotten that the normative response to single, isolated types of trauma is in fact resilience, or better, so-called minimal impact resilience, meaning that most people actually experience only temporary distress after such events. Furthermore, others show relatively quick improvement, and another group of individuals shows a return to healthy functioning after a somewhat longer period. These individuals, together with others who show delayed improvement or chronic and continuous impairments after discrete traumatic events, often have pre-existing vulnerabilities that increase the probability of maladaptation after experiencing an isolated traumatic event. Research findings have confirmed that only a subset of individuals develop enduring trauma-related emotional problems as a result of experiencing or witnessing a single extreme or life-threatening event (Type I trauma) (Bonanno and Diminich 2013; Southwick et al. 2014). This has been shown for victims of terrorist attacks and individuals who have lost their job, divorced, been bereaved, experienced a natural disaster, undergone a life-threatening medical procedure, or been deployed in military operations (for a review, see Bonanno and Diminich 2013). Importantly, prospective studies have shown that those who develop more chronic maladjustment typically have a history of previous trauma and/or poor social support and emotion regulation strategies (Denckla et al. 2018; Orcutt et al. 2014).

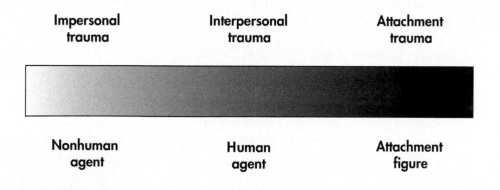

FIGURE 5–1.   Types of trauma.
Source.   Adapted from Allen 2005.

Hence, we argue in more detail below that rather than assuming that trauma leads to maladaptation, it is necessary to explain why some people show lasting maladaptation in the aftermath of traumatic experiences, and particularly single traumatic experiences. This leads us to reverse the perspective that until now has largely governed research on trauma. The essence of understanding the relationship between trauma and maladaptive development lies not in invoking the idea of *vulnerability* (defined as the presence of certain factors that render individuals vulnerable to emotional problems in the aftermath of trauma) but in emphasizing the *absence of resilience*.

This brings us to a second potential misunderstanding of the mentalizing approach. In the literature, trauma is typically associated with the notion of posttraumatic stress disorder (PTSD). However, as noted, single experiences of trauma normatively lead to adaptation; for those who develop serious problems in the aftermath of trauma, comorbidity is the rule rather than the exception. Therefore, a transdiagnostic and person-centered (instead of PTSD-focused, disorder-centered) approach is more appropriate in the study of trauma and its treatment (Luyten et al. 2008). There is increasing evidence that maladaptation after single experiences of trauma is related to a previous history of trauma. For example, military personnel who develop persistent trauma-related problems after combat exposure are much more likely to have been exposed to adverse conditions earlier in life. Thus, later-life trauma appears to trigger the cumulative effect of prior trauma in these individuals, leading to persistent symptoms and complaints (Afari et al. 2014).

Finally, the evidence base for the effectiveness of mentalization-based treatment (MBT) for trauma may be considered to be still limited; as of this writing, there have been no studies of MBT focusing on PTSD defined as an anxiety disorder marked by intrusive thoughts about trauma. Yet, in our opinion, it is considerably misguided to consider PTSD to be an "anxiety disorder." Similarly, we consider it rather unhelpful to categorize psychological disorders related to trauma as anxiety disorders, particularly when complex trauma is involved. The notion of *complex trauma* refers to types of trauma that occur repeatedly and cumulatively, and typically also occur in the context of close relationships, often with caregivers; hence, the term complex trauma is also often used interchangeably with the notion of attachment trauma. The focus in treatment should be not only on anxious intrusions and fear but also on the often "toxic" shame, guilt, anger, and disgust typically associated with trauma. Even more important, seeing trauma-related problems as an anxiety problem misses the consequences that complex trauma typically has for issues related to sexuality and aggression, its impact on mentalizing capacities (often leading to serious distortions and/or defensive inhibition of mentalizing), and particularly the tendency of many individuals with a trauma history—even those who have experienced a single, discrete episode of trauma—to reenact these traumatic experiences. This may also explain the limited effects of what are often considered to be evidence-based treatments for trauma, such as prolonged exposure (Foa et al. 2018), as they fail to address these issues. It is here that MBT may be particularly indicated and effective because of its focus on both restoring the process of mentalizing and understanding the dynamics associated with a tendency for reenactments (or externalization of nonmentalized experiences) in relationships, including the therapeutic relationship. Indeed, as discussed in more detail later in this chapter, victims of trauma often show a tendency to unwillingly recreate experiences of neglect and abuse. This tendency also seriously compromises psychotherapy, with resulting high dropout and relapse rates. Consistent with this assumption, MBT has shown considerable effectiveness in disorders that are characterized by high levels of (complex) trauma, such as borderline personality disorder (BPD). Indeed, there are very high rates of childhood trauma in individuals with personality disorders, with different studies reporting that up to 90% or even more of patients with BPD have experienced some form of abuse or neglect in childhood (Ball and Links 2009; Chanen and Kaess 2012). Individuals with BPD, in particular, have been found to be four times as likely to have suffered early trauma than normal control subjects (Johnson et al. 1999) and to have higher rates of childhood maltreatment than people with any other personality disorder (e.g., Baird et al. 2005; Buchheim et al. 2008). Similarly, the emerging evidence for MBT in mood disorders (see Chapter 23, "Depression") is another case in point, as studies suggest high rates of trauma in patients with mood disorders. For instance, a study in a large sample of chronically depressed patients found that 75% of these patients had a history of substantial trauma, and emotional and sexual abuse in particular (Negele et al. 2015). Although the future may bring the development of trauma-focused mentalization-based therapies (as discussed in more detail later in this chapter), currently a focus on (complex) trauma is part and parcel of all types of MBT.

DEVELOPMENTAL PSYCHOBIOLOGY OF TRAUMA

Consistent with the approach taken in this chapter, research concerning the sequelae of trauma has been instrumental in the move away from a search for the causes of discrete disorders toward a transdiagnostic view of psychopathology (Figure 5–2). Trauma is implicated in a wide variety of disorders, while rates of trauma differ considerably among patients who meet criteria for any single disorder. Trauma can be best considered as an *ecophenotype* associated with a number of typical features, such as an earlier age at onset of psychopathology, greater symptom severity, higher levels of comorbidity, a greater risk for suicide, and a poorer response to treatment (Teicher and Samson 2013). The transdiagnostic importance of trauma should not be underestimated, as early adversity alone has been shown to account for 30%–70% of the population-attributable risk fractions for common mental disorders such as depression and anxiety (Anda et al. 2006; Teicher and Samson 2013). Comorbidity between common mental disorders is therefore the norm rather than the exception, and the interaction between trauma and other biological, social, and psychological factors most likely determines the final phenotypic expression (i.e., *multifinality*).

Three sets of findings have emerged from the by now considerable body of research on trauma in both humans and animals (Heim and Binder 2012; Lupien et al. 2009). First, early traumatic experiences, defined as experiences that go beyond the average expectable environment, have been related to dysfunctions in the human stress system, including the hypothalamic-pituitary-adrenal (HPA) axis and the parasympathetic system. Such experiences appear to have long-lasting consequences for the response of the stress system and associated biological systems and biomediators, including neurotransmitter systems, the immune system, and, importantly, pain-processing systems. In interactions with other environmental and biological factors, this leads to increased vulnerability for psychological, somatic, and functional somatic disorders (see Figure 5–2). Again, the extensive impact that (complex) trauma may have becomes obvious from this body of research.

Second, the impact of early adversity is in part dependent on a critical time window in the development of the stress system. In human beings (and in some other animal species) this period, characterized by adaptive hyporesponsivity of the stress system in response to adversity, extends into early adulthood and is largely determined by the quality of attachment relationships (Gunnar and Quevedo 2007, 2008).

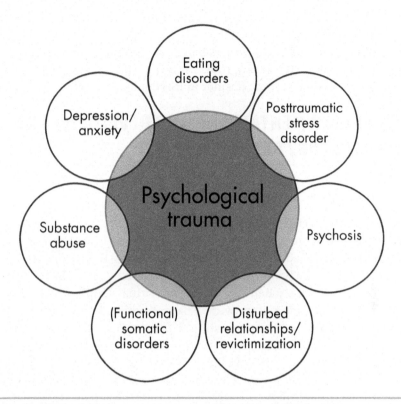

FIGURE 5–2. Psychological trauma as a nonspecific vulnerability factor.

High levels of adversity during this critical period, in combination with low levels of secure attachment, have been associated with HPA axis overactivity (i.e., a constant state of fight/flight), which, because of the wear and tear of chronic stress, typically switches to HPA hypo(re)activity (i.e., a freeze/faint state) (McEwen 2007; Miller et al. 2007). The key role of attachment figures in this context is of paramount importance in the context of this chapter, as it not only provides an explanation for the role of attachment-related trauma in particular in vulnerability to psychopathology in later life (Allen 2013), but also raises the question of what it is that explains vulnerability when faced with such events. Stated otherwise: what happens in the context of secure attachment relationships that not only buffers the effects of adversity but also has a protective function when the individual is faced with adversity later in life? This question is discussed in the next section.

The third and final set of findings that has emerged from research on trauma concerns the role of broader environmental factors in this area and their interaction with genetic vulnerability. Studies suggest that early and later adversity do not tend to occur in isolation but rather are part of a broader "risky environment" in which individuals grow up and live (Cicchetti and Toth 2005). In this context, there is also increasing interest in active and passive person–environment and gene–environment correlations, meaning that individuals may unwittingly contribute to such a risky environment because of certain personality and/or genetic features. We will return to this issue later, when we discuss reenactments in the context of trauma. Gene–environment interactions (i.e., the synergistic effects of genes and environment) and the potential role of epigenetic effects (the effects of positive and negative environmental features on gene expression) (Belsky and Pluess 2013; Dick et al. 2015; Gluckman et al. 2009) have also received increasing attention in research.

Clearly, research on trauma suggests that both vulnerability to trauma and resilience in the face of adversity have strong roots in development, with attachment-related trauma being a primary factor to consider in this context.

TRAUMA FROM A MENTALIZING AND DEVELOPMENTAL PSYCHOPATHOLOGY PERSPECTIVE

Trauma and Attachment

How then can the impact of trauma, and attachment trauma in particular, be understood? Attachment trauma can lead to serious impairment in the capacity to seek help from others in times of need because it typically involves a breach of trust with attachment figures (Teicher and Samson 2013), which then may generalize to others (Table 5–1). This mistrust seriously hampers these individuals' ability to seek help effectively in times of need. This may provide a partial explanation for the findings summarized in the previous section suggesting that a single episode of trauma may be associated with long-lasting emotional problems in a subset of individuals. As summarized in detail in other chapters in this volume (e.g., Chapter 17, "Borderline Personality Pathology in Adolescence"), when faced with attachment trauma (e.g., neglect or abuse), individuals begin to excessively rely on secondary attachment strategies, such as attachment hyperactivating or deactivating strategies, or a combination of both (such as in individuals with disorganized attachment). These insecure attachment strategies first develop in childhood as adaptation strategies in a particular environment marked by inconsistency in the availability, or the unavailability, of attachment figures. Whereas attachment deactivating strategies are a typical response to the (perceived) unavailability of attachment figures, attachment hyperactivating strategies characteristically develop as an attempt to elicit support, love, and care from attachment figures who are inconsistently available. However, attachment trauma also often involves the particularly pernicious situation in which the caregiver is the source both of security, love, and care and of abuse and neglect. As a result, the child becomes trapped in an approach–avoidance conflict for which there is no solution. Hence, attachment trauma closes the individual off from, or at least seriously limits, the capacity to turn to others when confronted with adversity.

Trauma and Mentalizing

Trauma not only disrupts the attachment system; it also impairs mentalizing. Indeed, research has suggested that there is an inverse relationship between arousal and mentalizing (Arnsten 1998; Mayes 2000). With increasing arousal, there is a switch from brain functioning involving flexible but relatively slow, prefrontal executive functions, to more rapid, automatic, and habitual responses that are mediated by posterior cortical and limbic structures (as described in more detail in Chapter 3, "Assessment of Mentalizing." Stated otherwise: when controlled mentalizing goes offline, defensive (fight/flight/freeze) automatic mentalizing comes online. From an evolutionary perspective, this switch from more controlled to automatic mentalizing has clear adaptive

TABLE 5–1.	Mentalizing approach to trauma
Systems/capacities impacted by trauma	**Consequences**
Attachment behavioral system	Increasing reliance on unhelpful secondary attachment strategies: risk of increasing dysregulation of the stress response, leading to a sense of isolation, abandonment, and/or neglect
Mentalizing capacities	Tendency for prementalizing modes to dominate subjective experience, leading to feelings of hopelessness and dread (psychic equivalence), increasing the risk for self-harm (teleological mode) and/or dissociation (pretend mode), combined with a pressure to externalize unmentalized experiences ("alien-self states"), as well as reenactment of traumatic experiences
Capacity for epistemic trust	Erosion of epistemic trust and, depending on the severity and chronicity of early adversity, development of epistemic mistrust, epistemic hypervigilance, or epistemic freezing; impairment in social communication and salutogenesis, precluding the recalibration of the mind and increasing feelings of isolation and dread

value, as it promotes rapid responses to imminent danger. Hence, in response to a discrete, single traumatic event, this response is primarily adaptive (*"First things first, let's make sure we survive!"*). Yet, the kind of automatic mentalizing that characterizes defensive responses to single episodes of trauma quickly becomes unhelpful when the individual is faced with chronic trauma, as he or she is increasingly left with unmentalized frightening experiences that are associated with a constant pressure to externalize these experiences (in self-harm or reenactments; see below and Table 5–1).

Yet, somewhat paradoxically, research has shown that the threshold for the switch from controlled to automatic mentalizing is related to exposure to early adversity and the use of attachment deactivating and hyperactivating strategies in particular (Luyten and Fonagy 2015). Hence, again, individuals with attachment trauma appear to be more vulnerable for later adversity, as they have an increased tendency to respond defensively to later stress and adversity. Consistent with these views, there is considerable evidence for an "amygdalocentric" model of trauma, with the prefrontal cortex, and the medial prefrontal cortex (mPFC) in particular, playing a key modulating role in times of stress and adversity (Rauch and Drevets 2009). As outlined in Chapter 2 ("Contemporary Neuroscientific Research"), the amygdala is activated in response to threat, whereas the mPFC plays a central role in extinction and top-down regulation of fear responses and is a key brain structure in the capacity for controlled mentalizing (Luyten and Fonagy 2015).

From a more phenomenological perspective, this view translates into the notion that attachment trauma typically impairs the capacity to frame and particularly to reframe overwhelming experiences. Individuals with attachment trauma have problems with relying on others in adaptive ways to help them understand and digest traumatic experiences. As a result, they have less or no access to the process of what we have termed *relational referencing*—that is, the process by which a person can meaningfully reframe adverse experiences and begin to mentalize what could not be mentalized before. Indeed, what is typical of trauma—regardless of the type of trauma—is that it overwhelms the individual's capacity for mentalizing, at least temporarily. Hence, the normative response to adversity appears to involve the recovery of mentalizing, by which thoughts and feelings that were previously unmanageable become more manageable.

From a mentalizing perspective, then, adversity becomes traumatic only when it is compounded by the individual's sense that his or her mind is alone and is unable to think the unthinkable and feel what cannot be felt in the first instance. In such cases, the presence of another mind that provides the social referencing that enables the person to reframe an overwhelming experience is typically called for. Being able to rely on another person's mind in such situations not only provides a sense of security and support (i.e., the attachment "secure base" function) but also makes it easier for the individual to recalibrate his or her own subjective experience.

Hence, when the mind is overwhelmed by a traumatic event, it experiences a particular need for *marked mirroring*, a key developmental process in the emergence of the capacity for mentalizing. Marked mirroring involves someone else reflecting back in a marked (i.e., digested) way what is difficult or even impossible for the person faced with trauma to mentalize. Marking such experiences involves reflecting back in a modulated and at the same time validating and caring way what the person is unable to think and feel. It typically involves a gradual and sympathetic process characterized by trial and error to arrive at what it is that the person is unable to think and feel. Hence, this back-and-forth process largely depends on the capacity of the other person (typically an attachment figure) to adequately mentalize the mind of the individual who is overwhelmed by traumatic experiences. This experience of being held in mind by another person may restore a sense of agency and control; a recalibration of the mind ensues.

It is here that a consistent mentalizing focus may show its therapeutic power. Indeed, like all effective treatments for trauma, fostering mentalizing promotes top-down regulation. Yet, overcontrol of emotion, such as that observed in the dissociative subtype of PTSD, similarly requires maintaining a focus on mentalizing and fostering mentalizing of dissociated/defended-against emotional states, strengthening so-called *mentalized affectivity* (Fonagy et al. 2002; Jurist 2005)—the individual's capacity to feel and to simultaneously reflect on his or her feelings.

Yet, trauma typically impairs mentalizing, and when faced with trauma, individuals increasingly begin to rely on nonmentalizing modes of experiencing subjectivity (see Chapter 1, "Introduction"). In psychic equivalence mode, everything becomes too real, and talking about the trauma leads the person to relive the trauma. For the individual, there is no hope and no way out; the traumatized individual feels stuck in the painful past and present. These painful feelings, which in many cases are merged with the "toxic" shame typical of attachment trauma, often give rise to teleological functioning, in which the person increasingly feels that only actions can bring relief. This typically leads to self-harm (e.g., cutting, excessive drinking) in an attempt to regulate extremely painful feelings. Ruminating about past events, in combination with intrusive thoughts, may lead to pretend mode functioning, in which the individual loses contact with reality and becomes lost in endless rumination. In the extreme, dissociative states emerge to protect against feelings of inner badness or worthlessness.

Problems with keeping mentalizing online in the face of trauma are often compounded by the fact that poor mentalizing leads to further poor mentalizing. That is, the minds of other people interacting with the traumatized individual tend to freeze (this may be thought of as "vicarious traumatization"), which further contributes to the traumatized person's painful feeling of being isolated and beyond any help. As a result, the mind of the traumatized person is dominated by dread.

Hence, having attachment figures with a robust capacity for mentalizing is of crucial importance, and this is evidenced by research findings. For instance, Berthelot et al. (2015) found that mothers who had high levels of reflective functioning (RF) with regard to their trauma history were just over half as likely to have children with disorganized attachment (37% of children) compared with mothers with low RF (67% of children). Indeed, adding maternal RF in relation to trauma explained twice as much of the variance in disorganized attachment (22% vs. 41%) as a model containing maternal unresolved trauma as the only predictor. Similarly, Fonagy et al. (1996) found that the combination of trauma and low RF was typical of patients with BPD.

The negative impact of attachment trauma on the development of the capacity for mentalizing has also been amply demonstrated. Children with a history of attachment trauma have been shown to engage in less symbolic and less child-initiated dyadic play (Alessandri 1991; Valentino et al. 2011), to show less empathy when witnessing distress in other children (Klimes-Dougan and Kistner 1990), to refer less to internal mental states when describing their own actions or those of others (Shipman and Zeman 1999), and to have more problems with understanding emotional expressions in others (During and McMahon 1991), even when verbal IQ is controlled for (Camras et al. 1990; Shenk et al. 2013). In this context, it is of particular importance to note that children with a history of maltreatment have a tendency to inaccurately ascribe anger to others (Camras et al. 1996; Cicchetti and Curtis 2005). Unsurprisingly, therefore, early adversity has been associated with delayed understanding of theory of mind (Cicchetti et al. 2003; Pears and Fisher 2005; Toth et al. 2000). Interestingly, a study (Ensink et al. 2015) found that children who had experienced intrafamilial abuse had significantly lower levels of RF compared with children with a history of extrafamilial abuse, again attesting to the negative impact of trauma that involves close attachment figures. In this study, the mothers' RF was again related to the development of RF in their children (Ensink et al. 2015). Hence, the extent to which caregivers may be able to mentalize in general (and mentalize traumatic experiences in particular) may be crucially important (Berthelot et al. 2015). This is not always easy, as is demonstrated by another study showing that mothers with children who had been sexually abused tended to show reduced RF, more negativity, and less affection in relation to their children compared with mothers whose children had no history of abuse (Ensink et al. 2017). These effects may be more pronounced in relation to boys, who may, on average, trigger more experiences related to (sexual) abuse and maltreatment than girls. However, overall, studies have consistently shown that mentalizing mediates the relationship between attachment and/or adversity and adult functioning (Bouchard et al. 2008; Chiesa and Fonagy 2014; Fonagy and Bateman 2006; Fossati et al. 2009, 2011; MacIntosh 2013; Stein and Allen 2007; Taubner and Curth 2013).

REENACTMENT

In this context, the issue of *reenactment* deserves special attention. Reenactment is a central feature in most, if not all, patients experiencing trauma-related pathology. The notion of reenactment refers to the generalization of experiences that have been learned in previous relationships. It is a core tenet of attachment theory and most other social-cognitive theories that individuals develop internal working models or cognitive–affective schemas of self and others based on previous experiences, which provide templates for future interactions. Reenactment of trauma, and particularly attachment trauma, should be seen in the same light. Here, we distinguish three types of reenactment of trauma (see Table 5–2).

TABLE 5–2. **Types of reenactment associated with (attachment) trauma**

Type of reenactment	Typical features
Revictimization	The individual unwillingly seeks out relationships characterized by physical, emotional, and/or sexual abuse, often also involving rejection, abandonment, and/or neglect.
Reenactment of neglect	The individual is hypersensitive to any signs of neglect, and constantly tends to construe interpersonal situations in terms of neglect; righteous vindication and aggression may follow, and/or the individual may become even more convinced that others are indeed neglectful.
Reenactment of attachment trauma in parenting behavior/ childhood maltreatment	Emotional states in the individual's child trigger unmentalized mental states related to the individual's own traumatic history, and these are acted out in relation to the child.

The most common and best-known form of reenactment is **revictimization**. Both prospective and retrospective studies have amply demonstrated that individuals with a history of attachment trauma are at increased risk for entering into new abusive relationships later in life (Cloitre et al. 1997; Widom 1999). While this may perhaps be counterintuitive, being in an abusive relationship as a child not only creates considerable anxiety and distress but also intensifies attachment needs, as the attachment system is typically activated as a response to threat. Thus, the relationship with an abusive attachment figure is paradoxically often strengthened, particularly if that abusive figure is also a source of comfort, support, and/or love. This pattern is then repeated in later relationships; for example, in romantic relationships with a jealous, possessive, and abusive partner (Allen 2001). This relationship is the continuation of the disorganized/disoriented attachment pattern (Main and Hesse 1990) acquired earlier in life, involving a pattern of traumatic bonding characterized by a profound and unsolvable approach–avoidance conflict.

There are two other forms of reenactment that have received less attention in the literature and are therefore often overlooked. However, they are extremely common. The first involves **reenacting the experience of neglect**. Individuals with a history of neglect typically become highly sensitized to any type of perceived or real emotional neglect. Even what seem to be minor misunderstandings, disagreements, or conflicts are met with often extreme dysphoria and/or aggressive or self-harming behavior. One of the core criteria of BPD, for instance, involves "frantic efforts to avoid real or imagined abandonment" (American Psychiatric Association 2013, p. 633), which can be seen as a posttraumatic reexperiencing of previous neglect (Allen 2001). In the teleological mode, the individual may engage in self-harm, which may lead to a vicious cycle wherein others increasingly feel that they have to distance themselves (because they feel increasingly "traumatized"), confirming the traumatized individual's worst fear—namely, that others are indeed unavailable and thus neglectful. Yet, a state of righteous vindication may also ensue, as the victim of the neglect feels he or she has every reason to retaliate because of the neglectful behavior of others (Clarkin et al. 1999). Because aggression typically helps to achieve a sense of coherence and protects the individual against even more painful feelings of sadness and anxiety, such vindictive states of mind may be very persistent. As a result, these individuals often become "addicted" to others who are (perceived as) neglectful or abusive, because aggression in response to (perceived) neglect and abuse has become a habitual response to unmentalized states of mind for these individuals. Hence, they seem to be in constant need of an enemy to establish and maintain a certain level of stability, however precarious.

Finally, **reenactments of attachment trauma** are also quite common in perpetrators of childhood maltreatment. These reenactments can be seen as a special case of the presence of "ghosts in the nursery" (Fraiberg et al. 1975)—that is, the persistent and often unconscious influence of these individuals' own history with attachment figures on the relationship with their own children. For instance, there is ample evidence for the intergenerational transmission of trauma, as is also evidenced in studies linking unresolved/disorganized Adult Attachment Interview classifications in parents to infant disorganization (Cyr et al. 2010). For these parents, observing emotional distress in their children—or, conversely, seeing their children being happy—may trigger their own past traumatic experience of neglect and/or abuse. Unmentalized experiences involving envy, anger, and sadistic lust are then acted out, repeating the traumatic behavior of the parents' own traumatizing caregiver in relation to their own children.

Again, these examples illustrate that considering trauma-related disorders as anxiety disorders, as is done in much of the PTSD literature, is often unhelpful. Labels such as *traumatic developmental disorder* and *complex trauma*, emphasizing the close link with the interpersonal world, are much more appropriate. Indeed, even single traumas often lead to a pressure in the individual to reenact what has happened (e.g., by relentless accusations against health authorities who have purportedly neglected the individual who experienced a traumatic event), or to a persistent urge to relate the traumatic experience to others, who then have no choice but to feel what the victim of trauma feels. Here, there is a real danger of secondary or vicarious traumatization and for subsequent reenactment in relationships with others. This is also the fate of many clinicians treating patients with a history of trauma, which emphasizes the need for training and continuing supervision when treating these patients. Hence, trauma is associated with a pressure to externalize what cannot be mentalized, what cannot be thought of. All effective psychotherapies have in common that they help the individual to think about and feel what he or she previously was unable to think about and feel. In addition, all effective psychotherapies appear to offer a safe context and preferably a relationship with another person, so the traumatized individual does not have to "go it alone." Such a safe haven also opens up the individual to new experiences, which brings us to the topic of resilience and the role of social communication.

Trauma, Communication, and Resilience

Because of its impact on attachment and mentalizing, attachment trauma characteristically has a negative impact on the capacity for epistemic trust and, as a result, also on the capacities for social communication and salutogenesis, both of which are rooted in epistemic trust. Specifically, attachment trauma leads to a closing of the mind to the communication of personally relevant knowledge (Fonagy et al. 2015).

Resilience is the normative response to adversity (Fonagy et al. 2017a, 2017b) and is discussed in more detail in Chapter 4, "Mentalizing, Resilience, and Epistemic Trust," and Chapter 10, "Therapeutic Models." In summary, building on the comprehensive positive appraisal style theory of resilience (PASTOR; Kalisch et al. 2015), resilience involves three central mechanisms: 1) positive situation classification, 2) retrospective reappraisal of threat, and 3) inhibition of retraumatizing triggers. These three mechanisms all rely on the ability of the individual to recalibrate his or her mind when faced with adversity. Developmentally, the roots of the individual's capacity to recalibrate his or her mind lie in social communication, which requires epistemic trust. Attachment figures play a key role in this context, as they are the first to use particular communicative signals, known as *ostensive cues*, to put the infant into a so-called learning mode. Experimental studies have indeed suggested that the use of ostensive cues triggers epistemic openness to knowledge in the infant (Csibra and Gergely 2009). Ostensive cues communicate that the attachment figure recognizes the autonomy and agency of the recipient of the communication. The use of ostensive cues also signals that the knowledge that is conveyed is of use to the recipient (i.e., personally relevant and generalizable to other contexts and situations). Hence, ostensive cues provided by an attachment figure (and, later on, other individuals who are perceived as trustworthy) provide a much-needed counterweight to epistemic vigilance, the default mode of infants toward knowledge offered by others. Indeed, from an evolutionary perspective, vigilance and even distrust toward knowledge offered by others seem to serve the survival of the species; indiscriminate trust in others would soon lead to unwanted consequences, such as being misled or coerced.

Trauma (particularly attachment trauma) typically impairs the capacity for the kind of selective epistemic trust and the openness to ostensive cues that is needed to foster social learning and salutogenesis. Epistemic mistrust in relation to the communication of social knowledge becomes (and in a sense remains) the default mode. Attachment trauma typically leads to the individual feeling unrecognized as an independent agent and lacking in experiences of marked mirroring that typically engender epistemic trust, opening up the "epistemic superhighway" that allows the fast transmission of knowledge about the self, others, and the world that is provided by attachment figures. In the case of maltreatment, ostensive cues are typically absent and/or undermined by fear or confusion. As a consequence, there is no relaxation of epistemic vigilance, and epistemic mistrust—and, in extreme cases, outright epistemic hypervigilance and epistemic freezing—may occur because the infant is largely or even completely deprived of the experience that his or her caregiver's mind may be a benign, reliable, and sympathetic source of knowledge. For children and young people faced with violence and abuse in attachment relationships, even thinking about the minds of other people might be defensively blocked, as thinking about the intentions of others leads to re-experiencing frightening and confusing events. Unfortunately, as a result, their minds become closed to processing new information, particularly when it is offered by others who claim that they can be trusted (e.g., teachers, the police, or mental health professionals).

Hence, complex trauma disorder should be seen from this perspective as a form of social understanding in which epistemic hypervigilance, mistrust, or outright epistemic freezing is adopted as an adaptive strategy in response to a given social environment. This strategy, although initially adaptive, progressively compromises social learning and salutogenesis, making these individuals particularly "hard to reach."

CLINICAL IMPLICATIONS: MENTALIZATION-BASED TREATMENT AND BEYOND

A history of attachment trauma is associated with decreased responsiveness to any psychotherapeutic intervention (Fonagy et al. 2015; Teicher and Samson 2013). To increase the effectiveness of psychotherapy with these individuals, it is therefore crucial to consider not only the "what" but also the "how" of social communication—that is, how individuals who have become closed off from the evolutionary prewired capacity for social recalibration may open up again to this process. For most of these patients, as in normal development, the establishment of an attachment relationship is a critical prerequisite for change. While patients with less severe (attachment) trauma may benefit from a range of interventions because their capacity for social communication and thus salutogenesis has remained relatively intact, for the most severely affected patients, an attachment relationship with a therapist that is able to re-establish (and often develop for the first time) epistemic trust is needed. This realization has led us to the position that effective treatment of individuals with severe attachment trauma requires an understanding of the role of attachment and mentalizing in the process. Specifically, three systems of communication that function together are responsible for therapeutic change in these patients, regardless of the type of treatment offered. The communication systems are discussed in more detail in Chapter 10, where it is argued that effective treatment activates all three systems in a sequential but cyclic manner. They are summarized briefly here in relation to the treatment of trauma.

Communication System 1

TEACHING AND LEARNING OF CONTENT

All effective types of psychotherapy for patients with (complex) trauma seem to have in common the fact that they offer the patient a convincing model for understanding his or her mind—that is, the patient feels that certain features of his or her experiences are mirrored in a marked way by the therapist. This provides the patient with not only a sense of validation but also a feeling of agency and control, which in turn lowers the patient's epistemic vigilance and/or freezing. Within MBT, this marked mirroring is provided by the therapist's careful and consistent modeling, empathic supporting, and scaffolding of the patient's mentalizing. The therapist first and foremost models an attitude that conveys that he or she is not afraid of the patient's states of mind, but is genuinely interested in them, even if they are excruciatingly painful and often unbearable. Stated otherwise: the therapist implicitly and at times explicitly communicates that his or her mind is available and able to tolerate, contain, and reflect on feelings and thoughts that are unbearable for the patient—that the patient's mind is "not alone." This has been the key feature of MBT from its inception, when it was first developed as a treatment for patients with severe BPD, who often have a history of complex developmental trauma. MBT interventions typically seek out the switch points when mentalizing collapses into nonmentalizing modes (as discussed in Chapter 1), which usually happens in the context of a discussion of close and problematic attachment relationships, including reenactments of abuse and neglect. The focus in MBT, particularly in the early phases, is not so much on the content of the dynamics that emerge in these situations, but on fostering the process of mentalizing in order to improve affect regulation, epistemic trust, and, ultimately, interpersonal relationships.

Exposure therapy (Foa and Rothbaum 1998); stress inoculation therapy (Meichenbaum 1994; Meichenbaum and Novaco 1985); other cognitive therapies, including cognitive processing therapy (Resick and Schnicke 1992, 1993); and eye movement desensitization and reprocessing (Foa et al. 2009) most likely similarly lead to an experience of marked mirroring for patients. All of these treatments involve some kind of cognitive restructuring that provides the patient with a sense of being recognized and a sense of agency as his or her trauma narrative becomes more coherent, leading to the reestablishment of feelings of control and autonomy. As is the case in MBT, this fosters in the patient not only epistemic trust but also curiosity as to what else the therapist may be able to "teach" the patient.

Communication System 2

REEMERGENCE OF ROBUST MENTALIZING

The unfolding process of increased understanding and framing of the trauma the patient has experienced, and its consequences, restores the patient's sense of agency and subjectivity. Robust mentalizing emerges (regardless of the type of treatment offered) if this unfolding process becomes one of collaborative social communication, as occurs in normal development. The patient opens up again to social communication and shows increased interest in the therapist's mind, just as the therapist becomes increasingly interested and surprised by the mind of the patient. This process fosters the emergence of robust mentalizing: the patient increasingly begins to apply the knowledge acquired in the consulting room to his or her life outside the consulting room. Different therapies differ in terms of the extent to which they support the process of translating knowledge acquired in the therapeutic setting to the outside world, but all effective treatments involve the reemergence of the capacity of the patient to reflect in increasingly sophisticated and differentiated ways about himself or herself and others. In MBT, this is a central aim of the treatment, so as to allow the individual to increasingly manage his or her emotional states and navigate interpersonal relationships in more adaptive ways.

Communication System 3

REEMERGENCE OF SOCIAL LEARNING

The relaxation of epistemic hypervigilance in combination with more robust mentalizing also leads to the reemergence of the prewired capacity for social communication and salutogenesis. The patient becomes increasingly interested in the mind of others, learns from others outside the consulting room, and is able to form more stable relationships with others who are (ideally speaking) epistemically trustworthy; this helps the patient to open up further to positive influences that are present in the outside world. This often long and painstaking process largely depends on the ability of the patient to rely on and/or create a benign social environment. In its later stages, treatment may be primarily aimed at helping the patient to change his or her environment (e.g., through ending specific relationships, experimenting with new ways of relating to others, finding a job or changing career). Such change is often a long and difficult process for individuals with attachment trauma, as they have learned not to trust anyone and/or have always been in relationships marked by abuse and neglect. Again, different psychotherapeutic treatments widely differ in the extent to which they attend to this third communication system. MBT, after the acute treatment phase, typically involves a tailored stepped-down care program aimed at maintaining and further enhancing mentalizing skills and supporting and stimulating social reintegration.

Principles of Mentalization-Based Treatment of Trauma

MBT follows a number of principles in the treatment of trauma (see Box 5–1). First, it is essential to develop a trusting relationship within a physically and psychologically safe and containing environment. Second, the patient needs to learn to manage anxiety and actively avoid dissociation before the content of trauma is discussed. The patient cannot explore trauma alone; as one patient said, the traumatized mind is a *"dangerous place, and no one wants to go there alone."* So, a core feature of MBT from the start of treatment is for the clinician and patient to work collaboratively toward formulating specific aims of treatment. Collaboratively formulating these aims has a holding and containing function, as it fosters a sense of agency, communicates realistic hope, and, above all, implies that even the most terrifying thoughts and feelings can be discussed with an empathic and validating therapist. Treatment goals also typically include goals that are directly related to traumatic experiences, such as decreasing self-harm, as well as avoidance of revictimization. Collaborative formulation is also an essential component of crisis management, another key feature of the initial phase of MBT for patients with severe psychopathology. To summarize, the following steps are followed in MBT when addressing trauma-related symptoms.

BOX 5–1. MBT principles in the treatment of trauma

- Develop a trusting relationship.
- Manage anxiety and dissociation.
- Formulate aims collaboratively.
- Provide psychoeducation about trauma and mentalizing.
- Validate and normalize feelings in relation to trauma.
- Mentalize traumatic experiences ("microslice" events) and their personal impact.
- Improve emotional regulation.
- Address interpersonal relationships.

1. **Psychoeducation.** The nature of complex trauma and its impact on mentalizing, problems with emotion regulation, and interpersonal relationships in particular, is discussed with the patient. This discussion fosters mentalizing and a sense of agency.

2. **Validation and normalizing feelings.** These are essential components of psychoeducation and later therapy sessions: *"You are not alone, and what you feel is very understandable given what you have been through."* They form a core interactional process of the MBT approach to trauma more generally. Many patients have grown up with the paradoxical feeling that what they have experienced is so beyond anything that other people have experienced that they dare not speak about it (further reinforced by feelings of shame and anxiety). In contrast, they often consider the circumstances in which they have grown up as "normal" and/or have the feeling that they have to be able to bear these experiences, however traumatic they have been (*"I thought it was normal to be always criticized and scolded"*). Validating the patient's feelings concerning these experiences as understandable responses to trauma often has a dramatic impact on various levels: it reinforces a sense of emotional connection and mutual understanding between the patient and therapist, and thus the therapeutic bond, and leads to the reemergence of mentalizing (*"We can speak about this"*) and epistemic trust, the feeling that someone may be truly concerned about the patient and is able to truly understand him or her.

3. **Mentalizing traumatic experiences and their impact.** The validation and normalizing of feelings in step 2 typically lead to the next component of the MBT approach to trauma, which is helping to mentalize traumatic experiences and their impact. In MBT, the focus is typically on fostering the process of mentalizing rather than on the traumatic content itself, although both process and content become increasingly intertwined. This approach also leads to a more solid grounding of the patient in reality and to the patient developing alternative and more adaptive ways of looking at his or her past and its influence on the present. It is recommended that specific traumatic events be "microsliced," with only small elements discussed rather than whole events, the latter of which can create excessive anxiety. MBT is concerned about the relationship of anxiety and mentalizing, so while the patient is mentalizing the traumatic experiences, the clinician monitors arousal levels carefully and helps the patient modulate his or her anxiety while maintaining a focus on the experience of trauma.

4. **Improving emotion regulation strategies.** This essential component of the MBT approach to trauma further fosters improved mentalizing. In the process of mentalizing trauma, alternative and more adaptive emotion regulation strategies can be discussed. With increased mentalizing capacities, what could not be mentalized before can be increasingly thought about, and thus the need for maladaptive emotion regulation strategies related to the pressure to externalize alien-self experiences (see Chapter 1) disappears.

5. **Fostering changes in interpersonal relationships.** Improved mentalizing and emotion regulation strategies allow a greater focus on fostering changes in interpersonal relationships. As the pressure to repeat traumatic experiences decreases, the patient can begin to experiment with new relationships. Efforts made by the patient to establish and maintain more adaptive relationships are actively supported by the therapist. Such support also includes helping the patient manage the ending of less

adaptive relationships, a task that is often unavoidable for patients, especially those with complex trauma, who are characteristically entangled in problematic relationships.

CONCLUSION

In this chapter, we offer the most recent information about the mentalizing approach to the conceptualization and treatment of complex trauma. Central to this approach is the view that the impact of potentially traumatic experiences can be understood only by considering the disruptive effect of these experiences on the attachment behavioral system, mentalizing capacities, and the capacity for epistemic trust. Importantly, we now argue that the effects of trauma, and of complex trauma in particular, can be understood only if we consider the impact of traumatic experiences on the disruption of an evolutionary prewired capacity of human beings to trust others as a source of knowledge about themselves, others, and the world. The disruption of this capacity closes individuals off from the ability to recalibrate their minds in the aftermath of traumatic experiences. This not only renders these individuals vulnerable to maladaptation when faced with new adverse experiences later in life; it also leads them to be perceived as "difficult to treat" or "hard to reach." Particularly in the most severely affected individuals, an attachment relationship (as in normal development) is needed to (re)establish these individuals' capacity for epistemic trust, opening them up again to the possibility of recalibration of the mind in the context of a relationship with another mind—first in the therapeutic relationship and then in the real world. Only through this process can their state of "aloneness" be ended. The consistent modeling and scaffolding of mentalizing by the therapist in a way that recognizes the patient as an agent plays a key role in this context, regardless of the specific type of treatment. Although these speculations await confirmation by more research, given their potential importance, it is hoped that this chapter will contribute to the further systematic empirical evaluation of these views.

REFERENCES

Afari N, Ahumada SM, Wright LJ, et al: Psychological trauma and functional somatic syndromes: a systematic review and meta-analysis. Psychosom Med 76(1):2–11, 2014 24336429

Alessandri SM: Play and social behavior in maltreated preschoolers. Dev Psychopathol 3:191–205, 1991

Allen JG: Traumatic Relationships and Serious Mental Disorders. Chichester, UK, Wiley, 2001

Allen JG: Coping With Trauma: Hope Through Understanding, 2nd Edition. Washington, DC, American Psychiatric Publishing, 2005

Allen JG: Mentalizing in the Development and Treatment of Attachment Trauma. London, Karnac Books, 2013

Allen JG, Lemma A, Fonagy P: Trauma, in Handbook of Mentalizing in Mental Health Practice. Edited by Bateman AW, Fonagy P. Washington, DC, American Psychiatric Publishing, 2012, pp 419–444

American Psychiatric Association: Diagnostic and Statistical Manual of Mental Disorders, 5th Edition. Arlington, VA, American Psychiatric Association, 2013

Anda RF, Felitti VJ, Bremner JD, et al: The enduring effects of abuse and related adverse experiences in childhood. A convergence of evidence from neurobiology and epidemiology. Eur Arch Psychiatry Clin Neurosci 256(3):174–186, 2006 16311898

Arnsten AFT: The biology of being frazzled. Science 280(5370):1711–1712, 1998 9660710

Baird AA, Veague HB, Rabbitt CE: Developmental precipitants of borderline personality disorder. Dev Psychopathol 17(4):1031–1049, 2005 16613429

Ball JS, Links PS: Borderline personality disorder and childhood trauma: evidence for a causal relationship. Curr Psychiatry Rep 11(1):63–68, 2009 19187711

Belsky J, Pluess M: Genetic moderation of early child-care effects on social functioning across childhood: a developmental analysis. Child Dev 84(4):1209–1225, 2013 23432522

Berthelot N, Ensink K, Bernazzani O, et al: Intergenerational transmission of attachment in abused and neglected mothers: the role of trauma-specific reflective functioning. Infant Ment Health J 36(2):200–212, 2015 25694333

Bonanno GA, Diminich ED: Annual Research Review: positive adjustment to adversity—trajectories of minimal-impact resilience and emergent resilience. J Child Psychol Psychiatry 54(4):378–401, 2013 23215790

Bouchard MA, Target M, Lecours S, et al: Mentalization in adult attachment narratives: reflective functioning, mental states, and affect elaboration compared. Psychoanal Psychol 25:47–66, 2008

Buchheim A, Erk S, George C, et al: Neural correlates of attachment trauma in borderline personality disorder: a functional magnetic resonance imaging study. Psychiatry Res 163(3):223–235, 2008 18635342

Camras LA, Ribordy S, Hill J, et al: Maternal facial behavior and the recognition and production of emotional expression by maltreated and nonmaltreated children. Dev Psychol 26:304–312, 1990

Camras LA, Sachs-Alter E, Ribordy SC: Emotion understanding in maltreated children: recognition of facial expressions and integration with other emotion cues, in Emotional Development in Atypical Children. Edited by Lewis MD, Sullivan M. Mahwah, NJ, Lawrence Erlbaum, 1996, pp 203–225

Chanen AM, Kaess M: Developmental pathways to borderline personality disorder. Curr Psychiatry Rep 14(1):45–53, 2012 22009682

Chiesa M, Fonagy P: Reflective function as a mediator between childhood adversity, personality disorder and symptom distress. Pers Ment Health 8(1):52–66, 2014 24532555

Cicchetti D, Curtis WJ: An event-related potential study of the processing of affective facial expressions in young children who experienced maltreatment during the first year of life. Dev Psychopathol 17(3):641–677, 2005 16262986

Cicchetti D, Toth SL: Child maltreatment. Annu Rev Clin Psychol 1:409–438, 2005 17716094

Cicchetti D, Rogosch FA, Maughan A, et al: False belief understanding in maltreated children. Dev Psychopathol 15(4):1067–1091, 2003 14984138

Clarkin JF, Kernberg OF, Yeomans F: Transference-Focused Psychotherapy for Borderline Personality Disorder Patients. New York, Guilford, 1999

Cloitre M, Scarvalone P, Difede JA: Posttraumatic stress disorder, self- and interpersonal dysfunction among sexually retraumatized women. J Trauma Stress 10(3):437–452, 1997 9246651

Csibra G, Gergely G: Natural pedagogy. Trends Cogn Sci 13(4):148–153, 2009 19285912

Cyr C, Euser EM, Bakermans-Kranenburg MJ, et al: Attachment security and disorganization in maltreating and high-risk families: a series of meta-analyses. Dev Psychopathol 22(1):87–108, 2010 20102649

Denckla CA, Mancini AD, Consedine NS, et al: Distinguishing postpartum and antepartum depressive trajectories in a large population-based cohort: the impact of exposure to adversity and offspring gender. Psychol Med 48(7):1139–1147, 2018 28889814

Dick DM, Agrawal A, Keller MC, et al: Candidate gene-environment interaction research: reflections and recommendations. Perspect Psychol Sci 10(1):37–59, 2015 25620996

During SM, McMahon RJ: Recognition of emotional facial expressions by abusive mothers and their children. J Clin Child Psychol 20:132–139, 1991

Ensink K, Normandin L, Target M, et al: Mentalization in children and mothers in the context of trauma: an initial study of the validity of the Child Reflective Functioning Scale. Br J Dev Psychol 33(2):203–217, 2015 25483125

Ensink K, Leroux A, Normandin L, et al: Assessing reflective parenting in interaction with school-aged children. J Pers Assess 99(6):585–595, 2017 28151016

Foa EB, Rothbaum BO: Treating the Trauma of Rape: Cognitive Behavioral Therapy for PTSD. New York, Guilford, 1998

Foa EB, Keane TM, Friedman MJ, et al: Effective Treatments for PTSD: Practice Guidelines From the International Society for Traumatic Stress Studies. New York, Guilford, 2009

Foa EB, McLean CP, Zang Y, et al; STRONG STAR Consortium: Effect of prolonged exposure therapy delivered over 2 weeks vs 8 weeks vs present-centered therapy on PTSD symptom severity in military personnel: a randomized clinical trial. JAMA 319(4):354–364, 2018 29362795

Fonagy P, Bateman AW: Mechanisms of change in mentalization-based treatment of BPD. J Clin Psychol 62(4):411–430, 2006 16470710

Fonagy P, Target M: Attachment, trauma, and psychoanalysis: where psychoanalysis meets neuroscience, in Mind to Mind Infant Research, Neuroscience, and Psychoanalysis. Edited by Jurist EJ, Slade A, Bergner S. New York, Other Press, 2008, pp 15–49

Fonagy P, Steele M, Steele H, et al: The Emanuel Miller Memorial Lecture 1992. The theory and practice of resilience. J Child Psychol Psychiatry 35(2):231–257, 1994 8188797

Fonagy P, Leigh T, Steele M, et al: The relation of attachment status, psychiatric classification, and response to psychotherapy. J Consult Clin Psychol 64(1):22–31, 1996 8907081

Fonagy P, Gergely G, Jurist EL, et al: Developmental issues in normal adolescence and adolescent breakdown, in Affect Regulation, Mentalization, and the Development of the Self. New York, Other Press, 2002, pp 317–340

Fonagy P, Luyten P, Allison E: Epistemic petrification and the restoration of epistemic trust: a new conceptualization of borderline personality disorder and its psychosocial treatment. J Pers Disord 29(5):575–609, 2015 26393477

Fonagy P, Luyten P, Allison E, et al: What we have changed our minds about: Part 1. Borderline personality disorder as a limitation of resilience. Borderline Personal Disorder Emotion Dysregul 4:11, 2017a 28413687

Fonagy P, Luyten P, Allison E, et al: What we have changed our minds about: Part 2. Borderline personality disorder, epistemic trust and the developmental significance of social communication. Borderline Personal Disorder Emotion Dysregul 4:9, 2017b 28405338

Fossati A, Acquarini E, Feeney JA, et al: Alexithymia and attachment insecurities in impulsive aggression. Attach Hum Dev 11(2):165–182, 2009 19266364

Fossati A, Feeney J, Maffei C, et al: Does mindfulness mediate the association between attachment dimensions and Borderline Personality Disorder features? A study of Italian non-clinical adolescents. Attach Hum Dev 13(6):563–578, 2011 22011100

Fraiberg S, Adelson E, Shapiro V: Ghosts in the nursery. A psychoanalytic approach to the problems of impaired infant-mother relationships. J Am Acad Child Psychiatry 14(3):387–421, 1975 1141566

Gluckman PD, Hanson MA, Bateson P, et al: Towards a new developmental synthesis: adaptive developmental plasticity and human disease. Lancet 373(9675):1654–1657, 2009 19427960

Gunnar M, Quevedo K: The neurobiology of stress and development. Annu Rev Psychol 58:145–173, 2007 16903808

Gunnar MR, Quevedo KM: Early care experiences and HPA axis regulation in children: a mechanism for later trauma vulnerability. Prog Brain Res 167:137–149, 2008 18037012

Heim C, Binder EB: Current research trends in early life stress and depression: review of human studies on sensitive periods, gene-environment interactions, and epigenetics. Exp Neurol 233(1):102–111, 2012 22101006

Johnson JG, Cohen P, Brown J, et al: Childhood maltreatment increases risk for personality disorders during early adulthood. Arch Gen Psychiatry 56(7):600–606, 1999 10401504

Jurist EL: Mentalized affectivity. Psychoanal Psychol 22:426–444, 2005

Kalisch R, Müller MB, Tüscher O: A conceptual framework for the neurobiological study of resilience. Behav Brain Sci 38:e92, 2015 25158686

Klimes-Dougan B, Kistner J: Physically abused preschoolers' responses to peers' distress. Dev Psychol 26:599–602, 1990

Lupien SJ, McEwen BS, Gunnar MR, et al: Effects of stress throughout the lifespan on the brain, behaviour and cognition. Nat Rev Neurosci 10(6):434–445, 2009 19401723

Luyten P, Fonagy P: The neurobiology of mentalizing. Pers Disord 6(4):366–379, 2015 26436580

Luyten P, Vliegen N, Van Houdenhove B, et al: Equifinality, multifinality, and the rediscovery of the importance of early experiences: pathways from early adversity to psychiatric and (functional) somatic disorders. Psychoanal Study Child 63:27–60, 2008 19449788

MacIntosh HB: Mentalizing and its role as a mediator in the relationship between childhood experiences and adult functioning: Exploring the empirical evidence. Psihologija (Beogr) 46:193–212, 2013

Main M, Hesse E: Adult lack of resolution of attachment-related trauma related to infant disorganized/disoriented behavior in the Ainsworth strange situation: linking parental states of mind to infant behavior in a stressful situation, in Attachment in the Preschool Years: Theory, Research, and Intervention. Edited by Greenberg MT, Cicchetti D, Cummings EM. Chicago, IL, University of Chicago Press, 1990, pp 339–426

Mayes LC: A developmental perspective on the regulation of arousal states. Semin Perinatol 24(4):267–279, 2000 10975433

McEwen BS: Physiology and neurobiology of stress and adaptation: central role of the brain. Physiol Rev 87(3):873–904, 2007 17615391

Meichenbaum D: A Clinical Handbook/Practical Therapist Manual for Assessing and Treating Adults With Post-Traumatic Stress Disorder (PTSD). Waterloo, Ontario, Canada, Institute Press, 1994

Meichenbaum D, Novaco R: Stress inoculation: a preventative approach. Issues Ment Health Nurs 7(1–4):419–435, 1985 3854020

Miller GE, Chen E, Zhou ES: If it goes up, must it come down? Chronic stress and the hypothalamic-pituitary-adrenocortical axis in humans. Psychol Bull 133(1):25–45, 2007 17201569

Negele A, Kaufhold J, Kallenbach L, et al: Childhood trauma and its relation to chronic depression in adulthood. Depress Res Treat 2015:650804, 2015 26693349

Orcutt HK, Bonanno GA, Hannan SM, et al: Prospective trajectories of posttraumatic stress in college women following a campus mass shooting. J Trauma Stress 27(3):249–256, 2014 24819209

Pears KC, Fisher PA: Emotion understanding and theory of mind among maltreated children in foster care: evidence of deficits. Dev Psychopathol 17(1):47–65, 2005 15971759

Rauch SL, Drevets WC: Neuroimaging and neuroanatomy of stress-induced and fear circuitry disorders, in Stress-Induced and Fear Circuitry Disorders: Refining the Research Agenda for DSM-V. Edited by Andrews G, Charney DS, Sirovatka PJ, et al. Arlington, VA, American Psychiatric Association, 2009, pp 215–254

Resick PA, Schnicke MK: Cognitive processing therapy for sexual assault victims. J Consult Clin Psychol 60(5):748–756, 1992 1401390

Resick PA, Schnicke MK: Cognitive Processing Therapy for Rape Victims: A Treatment Manual. London, Sage, 1993

Shenk CE, Putnam FW, Noll JG: Predicting the accuracy of facial affect recognition: the interaction of child maltreatment and intellectual functioning. J Exp Child Psychol 114(2):229–242, 2013 23036371

Shipman KL, Zeman J: Emotional understanding: a comparison of physically maltreating and nonmaltreating mother-child dyads. J Clin Child Psychol 28(3):407–417, 1999 10446690

Southwick SM, Bonanno GA, Masten AS, et al: Resilience definitions, theory, and challenges: interdisciplinary perspectives. Eur J Psychotraumatol 5:5, 2014 25317257

Stein H, Allen JG: Mentalizing as a framework for integrating therapeutic exposure and relationship repair in the treatment of a patient with complex posttraumatic psychopathology. Bull Menninger Clin 71(4):273–290, 2007 18254687

Taubner S, Curth C: Mentalization mediates the relation between early traumatic experiences and aggressive behavior in adolescence. Psihologija (Beogr) 46:177–192, 2013

Teicher MH, Samson JA: Childhood maltreatment and psychopathology: a case for ecophenotypic variants as clinically and neurobiologically distinct subtypes. Am J Psychiatry 170(10):1114–1133, 2013 23982148

Toth SL, Cicchetti D, Macfie J, et al: Narrative representations of caregivers and self in maltreated pre-schoolers. Attach Hum Dev 2(3):271–305, 2000 11708220

Valentino K, Cicchetti D, Toth SL, et al: Mother-child play and maltreatment: a longitudinal analysis of emerging social behavior from infancy to toddlerhood. Dev Psychol 47(5):1280–1294, 2011 21744951

Widom CS: Posttraumatic stress disorder in abused and neglected children grown up. Am J Psychiatry 156(8):1223–1229, 1999 10450264

PART II

Clinical Practice

CHAPTER 6

INDIVIDUAL THERAPY TECHNIQUES

Anthony Bateman, M.A., FRCPsych

Brandon Unruh, M.D.

Peter Fonagy, Ph.D., FBA, FMedSci, FAcSS

The primary aim of mentalization-based treatment (MBT) is to improve the stability and functionality of an individual's mentalizing in those contexts in which his or her mentalizing is prone to collapse into ineffective mentalizing modes or is used inappropriately. MBT was originally organized in terms of its structure and recommended interventions to meet this aim for people with borderline personality disorder (BPD); this treatment "package" is well known and described in detail elsewhere (Bateman and Fonagy 2016). Here we discuss in more detail some interventions in individual MBT that promote mentalizing for people with personality disorder but that clinicians find problematic to deliver.

MBT ADHERENCE SCALE

The MBT model is a complex psychosocial model that specifies not only what needs to be done in sessions to address mentalizing problems, but also how the treatment program should be implemented (e.g., in terms of socialization of the patient to the model, discussion of the formulation with the patient, crisis intervention, managing suicide attempts, and supervision of the clinician). MBT has been (and is still being) modified for use as a therapeutic intervention for a range of disorders. This has led to clearer division of the basic model into general components that are relevant irrespective of which disorder is being treated, and specific components that are exclusive to treating a specific disorder (e.g., BPD, antisocial personality disorder [ASPD], eating disorders). The effectiveness of MBT partly depends on the structured process within which the sessions themselves are implemented (see Chapter 12, "Partial Hospitalization Settings").

Since 2005, clinicians and researchers have been assessed for adherence to the MBT model in terms of whether their delivery in clinical practice is in line with the theoretical understanding of a specific disorder, such as BPD or ASPD (see Chapter 20, "Antisocial Personality Disorder in Community and Prison Settings"), and the intended clinical interventions for the disorder as specified in the manual, *Mentalization-Based Treatment for Personality Disorders: A Practical Guide* (Bateman and Fonagy 2016). Building on a prototypical adherence scale (Bateman and Fonagy 2006b) and an earlier scale (Karterud and Bateman 2011; Karterud et al. 2013), a new scale has been developed for use in research projects based on the clinical interventions specified in the manual (Bateman and Fonagy 2016). This is useful for supervisors to assess clinicians delivering MBT in their daily practice. This scale is freely available for clinicians and researchers on the website of the Anna Freud National Centre for Children and Families (https://www.annafreud.org/training/mentalization-based-treatment-training/mbt-adherence-scale). It can be used to support supervision and learning by all clinicians. Formal training to ensure reliability is necessary for research purposes.

The adherence scale is based on the six core domains of MBT: 1) the sessional structure, 2) the "not-knowing" stance (an attitude of authentic curiosity about mental states), 3) mentalizing process, 4) nonmentalizing modes, 5) mentalizing affects and interpersonal and significant events, and 6) relational mentalizing. Each domain is subdivided into a number of component items. These components are interventions delivered by the clinician, which indicate work in the domain and inform the rating of the domain. A summary sheet outlining the scale can be found at the Anna Freud National Centre for Children and Families website mentioned earlier. A trained rater or supervising clinician not only rates the work in the domain in terms of its frequency (F) and extensiveness (E), but also decides on the level of skill with which the clinician intervenes; these ratings address the "how" of implementation. In addition, skill is defined according to whether clinicians actively avoid using a domain, perhaps appropriately—for example, avoiding the use of relational mentalizing when the patient is highly aroused—or whether clinicians fail to intervene in a domain when they should. In the former case, the absence receives a positive rating for skill, and in the latter case it receives a negative rating.

From examining adherence ratings, it has become apparent that clinicians tend to use some interventions frequently and skillfully after training, and others less skillfully: they are good at using supportive statements, managing mentalizing process, and working with affect and interpersonal and significant events, but fail to engage in relational mentalizing when appropriate and often miss addressing the nonmentalizing pretend mode. Yet, it is likely that intervention in these domains is essential in treatment for personality disorder to increase the patient's epistemic trust—or at least decrease his or her excessive epistemic mistrust—of the world around him or her.

The low frequency of implementation of relational mentalizing may be related in part to the focus of training itself, when practitioners are cautioned about intervening at the level of relational mentalizing if patients are not currently able to take a meta-perspective about themselves in relation to others. This state of ineffective mentalizing is so common in BPD that clinicians may feel that the conditions are never right to work on relational mentalizing. Therefore, naive (and even experienced) practitioners need a clearer scaffolding on which to base their interventions at the level of relational process. In the case of pretend mode, the first issue is to recognize pretend mode itself in the clinical process. Pretend mode is very often mistaken for good therapy by the clinician; the patient–clinician dialogue seems to be coherent and thoughtful. It is only when others observe the session that it becomes more obvious that pretend mode is being used by patient and clinician alike.

We contend that both relational mentalizing and pretend mode can be addressed effectively only if the patient and clinician are sensitized to recognizing them through adequate preparation. The first preparatory step in MBT is the introductory group. It is here that clinicians set the scene for future work. They collaborate with the patient on defining the model in patient-centered terms. In particular, they establish the pattern of relational processes activated in the patient's personal interactions and generate an understanding of how ineffective mentalizing processes, including the potential for pretend mode, interfere with the patient's adaptation to a relational and social world that they distrust.

MBT INTRODUCTORY GROUP (MBT-I)

The primary purpose of the introductory phase of MBT is to ensure that patients entering long-term treatment do so with reasonable understanding of the process they are engaging in, that they are aware of the focus of treatment, and that they appreciate the expectations placed on them and the expectations they can have about treatment. Patients with BPD have 10–12 sessions in an introductory group to introduce them to treatment and to socialize them to the model; people with ASPD have 6–8 sessions. The absolute number of sessions is not the essential factor of MBT-I. Imparting knowledge, increasing understanding and motivation through empowerment, and developing a therapeutic alliance with clear goals are more important. We now add two further purposes of MBT-I: first, for the clinician to facilitate epistemic trust in the patient about the model the clinician holds, and secondly, to delineate the attachment strategies of the patient that are activated in his or her personal and intimate relationships. The patient and clinician together generate what we have termed a "relational passport," which the patient carries across treatment from assessment to individual and group therapy.

RELATIONAL MENTALIZING

The Relational Passport

The patient and clinician identify the interpersonal patterns activated when the patient forms relationships with others. These are summarized jointly by the patient and clinician and written down in a relational passport, which is a part of the overall formulation. While these interpersonal patterns have their origins in childhood and early attachment relationships, these origins are not the concern in MBT. The MBT clinician is more concerned with identifying the attachment patterns as they are played out in the patient's current daily life. In MBT-I, all patients are asked to map their own attachment patterns after being given some understanding of attachment processes. Some clinicians use an instrument such as the Attachment Style Questionnaire (Bartholomew and Horowitz 1991) to focus the discussion. In essence, two main factors of attachment style can easily be identified: *attachment anxiety* and *attachment avoidance*. The anxiety factor can be considered to be a model of the self, while the avoidance factor is a model of others. Thus, clinicians can build a personal model with patients that shows the balance between a positive or negative view of themselves and a positive or negative view of others. Some patients have a negative view of themselves and a positive view of others, and become preoccupied in their interactions. Others, meanwhile, have a positive view of themselves but a highly negative view of others; unsurprisingly, they tend to be dismissive in their relationships. Patients with a negative view of both the self and others exhibit obvious fearfulness and avoidance of social relationships.

A personal map is drawn so the patient becomes increasingly aware of his or her patterns as they play out in everyday life. Relationships are identified and the interactional roles defined. Interest is focused on any relationship that "bucks the trend" and seems to challenge the normal pattern.

For example, one patient described dismissive attachment processes with some self-aggrandizement and general contempt for others. But, when asked if there was any relationship he valued, he mentioned one with a male friend whom he respected. Contrasting this friendship with his other relationships facilitated the patient's mentalizing to the extent that he became more aware of his own narcissism and more doubtful about his belief in himself and his distrust of others. To create the patient's personal map, four quadrants were drawn and populated with the patient's relationships, showing a concentration in the quadrant of high avoidance with dismissive attitudes and low anxiety, and only one relationship in a more preoccupied pattern but with higher anxiety (Figure 6–1). This map becomes the first part of the relational passport.

The second part of the passport focuses on the consequences in the patient's life of his or her attachment strategies. In the example given here, the obvious consequence was loneliness. The patient was distrustful in all his interactions, often felt threatened, and spent a considerable proportion of his time alone trying to manage his anxiety. Sharing with others was not an option. This led him to despise emotional closeness between people, seeing it as showing weakness. Exploring this relationship pattern naturally exposed his isolation and his strong sense of being alone. Inevitably, he dismissed this as being of little importance, allowing the clinician to point out that he was then reflexively engaging in his dismissive processes to manage his anxiety about himself. From this perspective the clinician was in a position to develop the final part of the passport.

Identifying the possible ways in which the patient's attachment strategies might manifest in treatment forms the final component of the passport. Using the example above, it is likely that the patient will be dismissive, for example, toward the model of treatment ("*It does not fit me. I don't think much of this. It is too simplistic*"), toward the clinician ("*You don't really look old enough to be able to understand my issues*"), and toward the other patients in the group ("*No. I don't think you are getting what I am saying really. Let me explain it again in simpler terms*"). All these statements were made by this patient early in treatment and were predictable in their style if not their content. For both clinician and patient, "forewarned is forearmed," as the following example illustrates.

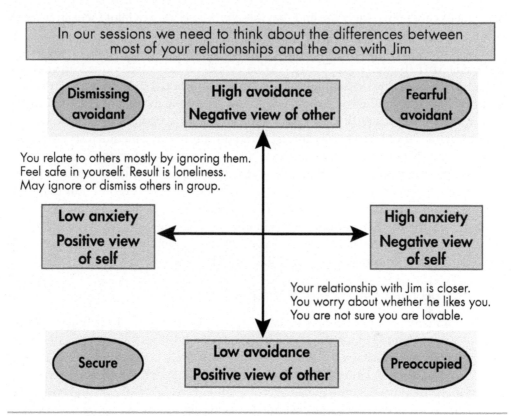

In our sessions we need to think about the differences between most of your relationships and the one with Jim

Dismissing avoidant

High avoidance
Negative view of other

Fearful avoidant

You relate to others mostly by ignoring them.
Feel safe in yourself. Result is loneliness.
May ignore or dismiss others in group.

Low anxiety
Positive view of self

High anxiety
Negative view of self

Your relationship with Jim is closer.
You worry about whether he likes you.
You are not sure you are lovable.

Secure

Low avoidance
Positive view of other

Preoccupied

FIGURE 6–1. Example of a personal map that forms part of the relational passport.

Case Example

A patient outlined her relationship with her current boyfriend during the assessment phase, when the clinician and patient were exploring her relationships. She described her current partner as loving and demonstrably solicitous of her happiness. However, she was constantly concerned that he did not love her "really" and was play-acting, to the extent that she continually and frequently asked him if he really loved her. When he affirmed his love for her, she felt calm for a short period of time, only to find that her torment returned and she had to ask him again. Not surprisingly, he became irritated by her question, feeling that he could never satisfy her doubt. She was a person who needed to be reassured. Her self-mentalizing processes were unstable so she sought a view of herself from others. In her relational passport it was predicted that she might worry between sessions and seek reassurance from the clinician if she became anxious. Access to her own internal states was limited, and so she naturally sought affirmation from others. In fact, shortly after treatment began she contacted the clinician frequently between sessions, seeking reassurance and support for everyday concerns. In the sessions themselves, she asked the clinician if he thought she was doing well in therapy. Having identified this process before the start of treatment, the clinician was able to focus quickly on the mentalizing failure that resulted in the patient's relational behavior rather than increasing her level of support and reassurance.

Use of the Relational Passport

The primary purpose of the relational passport is to ensure that the patient and clinician collaboratively develop and reflect on an understanding of the attachment strategies the patient uses in his or her life and that these processes form a joint focus in therapy. The secondary aim of the passport is to organize the mind of the clinician, who all too often can become trapped in a relational interaction that remains ill-defined. In the first outline of MBT (Bateman and Fonagy 2006a), we described a technique known as the "affect focus" as a way to highlight the implicit interactional process between patient and clinician, not in terms of the meaning or origins of the interaction, but in terms of descriptors of the process between them. While this helped clinicians to focus the mentalizing of the patient on complex interactions and stimulated a mental move in the patient from implicit to explicit mentalizing—that is, a contrary move (the use of contrary moves is described in detail in Bateman and Fonagy 2016)—use of an affect focus did not engage both patient and clinician in the more detailed exploration of relational mentalizing. The explicit development of the relational passport and its use in therapy concentrates the clinician's mind on relational mentalizing, which we hope will improve long-term outcomes in interpersonal function, a domain known to have only moderately good outcomes following MBT for BPD (Bateman and Fonagy 2008).

Relational Mentalizing in Clinical Practice

Relational mentalizing—in practice, using the relational passport in clinical interactions—may be defined in terms of what it is and what it is not. It is not the same as interpretation of the transference, which is a major technique in psychodynamic therapy and psychoanalysis. Relational mentalizing also is not linking the current pattern of behavior in the treatment setting to patterns of relationships in childhood and current relationships outside the therapeutic setting. For example, a clinician might well point to similarities in patterns of relationships within the therapy and in childhood or currently outside of the therapy, but does so without aiming to provide patients with an explanation (insight) that they might be able to use to control their behavior pattern. Relational mentalizing is *not* identifying and naming or interpreting a defense mechanism being activated to manage anxiety related to unconscious process. Far more simply, it is just one other puzzling phenomenon that requires thought and consideration, part of the clinician's general inquisitive stance that aims to facilitate the recovery of mentalizing within a complex interactional and emotional process. The clinician focuses on the relational aspect of the interaction in the moment and is *not* concerned with causality and insight.

The aim of relational mentalizing is to create an alternative perspective by focusing the patient's attention on another mind—the mind of the clinician—and to assist patients in the task of contrasting their own perception of themselves with how they are perceived by another, by the clinician, or indeed by members of a therapeutic group; hence the need for the clinician to ensure that patients discuss the content of their relational passport when starting in the group (see Chapter 7, "Group Therapy for Adults and Adolescents"). The emphasis is on using the relationship patterns identified in the passport to explore how these patterns play out in the patient's life.

Indicators for Relational Mentalizing

A number of indicators can suggest that the clinician should consider relational mentalizing. First, any break in the mentalizing process in a session may indicate that the patient and clinician should stop to think about what happened. Did the interaction suddenly jar? Was there a sudden change in topic? To start relational mentalizing in this context, the clinician may simply say *"Was there something in how I said that which made your mind jump on to something else?"* Second, the attachment strategies outlined in the passport and agreed as relevant to the patient's relationships may be apparent in a session or over a number of sessions. Commonly, and as mentioned earlier, an intervention at the level of relational mentalizing in this context will start with defining the affect focus. Third, the clinician may have a persistent counterrelationship feeling, for example, feeling stuck or useless. Again, the recognition of this feeling may begin with elaboration of an affect focus. Finally, the patient may be describing something of his or her current experience of the clinician. In this case, relational mentalizing takes place in the immediacy of the session.

Process of Mentalizing the Relationship

We define four main steps of relational mentalizing to be taken by the clinician and patient.

VALIDATE THE EXPERIENCE OF THE PATIENT

The first step is the *validation of the experience of the patient*. The clinician must be authentic in this task. For example, it is not acceptable for the clinician to say that *he or she understands that the patient feels that the clinician does not understand,* thereby immediately invalidating the reality of the patient's experience; such a statement is very likely to alienate a client with BPD. The clinician must find out exactly what he or she is failing to understand. For example, the individual who is functioning in psychic equivalence and feels that the clinician is persecuting him or her is not helped by the experience being "interpreted away" as part of a distortion. In this situation, the patient will experience the clinician as failing to understand his or her experience. In psychic equivalence, the internal is felt to be equivalent to the external, so the patient who feels persecuted is *being* persecuted; reference to a victim–victimizer type of dyadic relationship at this point, based in past relationships, will not generate reflection.

Thus, the first step of mentalizing the relationship is *ensuring that the patient feels that his or her experience is being taken seriously* and that it *is* real and legitimate, in the sense that there must be good reasons, normally to be found in the actions and comments of the clinician, why the patient experiences the clinician in a specific way.

Patient (a man): I have never thought that women can understand men at all. You have no idea what it is like for me, do you?

Clinician (a woman): I am not sure about *all* women, but you are right that I do not have a sense of what it is like for you when your partner goes out with a friend and you think she is two-timing you with another man.

Patient: You cannot trust women.

Clinician: Shall we have a look at that? It was in your relational passport that we discussed at the beginning of treatment. You get into a relationship with someone and then become trapped in thinking about him or her as being deceitful. That seems to be what is happening now with your girlfriend. It is this that you say I am not understanding. It seems that I cannot do so because I am a woman. This needs a bit more thought.

Patient: I had a row with her when she came back, and she told me I was stupid and refused to say anything else about it. She told me to speak to her friend who would tell me that nothing happened. But her friend would say that anyway.

The clinician is trying to explore the reality of the patient's current relationship with his girlfriend and is also indicating that she herself is not understanding, while pointing out that this is an area the patient and clinician had agreed to explore and had identified in the relational passport. She is, however, questioning that the reason she is unable to understand is because she is a woman—this seems an unlikely explanation!

> Clinician: Tell me what that is like for you then in terms of your relationship with her overall. How does it go for you when this is in the background all the time?

This is a move away from addressing the immediate context of the jealousy directly and broadens the frame for exploration.

> Patient: I look for other evidence a lot of the time. She shouldn't go out without me really. I make sure we spend most of our time together so I can keep check on whether she likes other men or not.
> Clinician: That sounds like hard work if you are looking all the time to see if she might like other men. Can you relax with her?
> Patient: I suppose I am tense a lot of the time, and I know that she doesn't think much of me when I am so suspicious. She feels it shows that I don't trust her. I don't think she understands how much I care about her.
> Clinician: I can see that there is quite a thing about trust here. And this is the second time you have come up with whether women understand you; we started out with me and now it is your girlfriend. Can you describe what you would like her to understand?
> Patient: I want her to realize that I do care about her. She should know that. But she does not seem to listen.

EXPLORE THE PROBLEM

The second step of relational mentalizing is *exploring the problem* using the moments of the current interpersonal interaction to highlight the detail of the relational concern being presented, either in its form (e.g., the patient's dismissive attitude toward the clinician because she is a woman) or in its content (e.g., wishing to be understood but in fact not being able to create the circumstances for better understanding). For the patient in this example, feeling understood can be experienced only through becoming aware in his own mind of the mind of the clinician accurately recognizing his own state of mind. It is this higher-level representation that would allow him to have a sense of being understood and would open up epistemic trust, which in turn would enable learning within the therapeutic relationship.

ACCEPT CLINICIAN ENACTMENT

The third step, which is really a subcomponent of the second step, is *accepting enactment*. Most of the patient's experiences about the clinician are based on reality, even if on a partial connection to it or an exaggerated component. This may mean that the clinician may be drawn into the interaction and may act in some way that is consistent with the patient's perception of him or her. The clinician should explicitly acknowledge his or her own contribution to the interpersonal problem as an inexplicable involuntary action for which he or she accepts agency. Drawing attention to such actions may be particularly significant in modeling to the patient that an individual can accept agency for involuntary acts and that such acts do not invalidate the general attitude that the clinician tries to convey. This understanding may be essential in overcoming a patient's teleological stance, where only actions are felt to be meaningful.

In the following sequence, the clinician lets the patient know that during their exchange, she lost concentration at times and her mind wandered, which resulted in her not fully understanding what the patient was trying to convey. At this point it is possible to consider what makes her mind wander at points in the session.

> Clinician: You saying that your girlfriend does not listen brings to my mind that this might be important here, because it is possible that your recognition that I do not understand is related to the fact that at times when you are talking about this my mind wanders. I think it has something to do with it being repeated a lot and our views seem so fixed.
> Patient: I am fixed about it. She ignores my frustrations.
> Clinician: Perhaps that is what we are struggling with as well, then. You are frustrated that I will not accept your view. I keep questioning it, leaving you with a clear sense that I do not understand, and you are intent on getting me to realize that you are right.

COLLABORATE TO ARRIVE AT AN ALTERNATIVE PERSPECTIVE

If the clinician and patient now seem to concur and have a shared view, the fourth step of relational mentalizing—*collaboration in a process to arrive at an alternative perspective*—becomes possible. This alternative perspective must be arrived at in the same spirit of collaboration as any other form of joint mentalizing. The metaphor we use in training is that the clinician must imagine sitting side by side with the patient, not opposite him or her. Patient and clinician sit side by side, looking at the patient's thoughts and feelings, both adopting an inquisitive stance. Thus, in the case example above, the patient's disquiet about the clinician's inability to understand him, and his default to explaining this on the basis that the clinician is a woman, becomes the focus of joint inquiry. The question the clinician is asking now is not about whether the perception is a distortion or not, but more about what it matters to the patient that he is not understood and that his experience is that women are unable to appreciate the hurt that he feels in not being listened to.

SUMMARY

In summary, intervention at the level of relational mentalizing starts in the initial phase of treatment. Without careful identification of the attachment patterns and exploration of relational processes to populate the content of the relational passport, it is more likely that the patient and clinician will miss important opportunities to elaborate on interpersonal mentalizing, which is the very area that leads to rapid instability and collapse into ineffective mentalizing for patients with BPD. Relational mentalizing may also require careful use of counterrelational mentalizing. In the example above, the clinician was aware that she had lost concentration and that it was the interaction between her and the patient that had led to that; it was not solely the patient creating it. She was able to identify and express her own state of mind and accept responsibility for it.

The gravest danger in this whole process is the development of pretend mode. This is the second area of MBT that we will discuss here in terms of mentalizing interventions in individual therapy.

PRETEND MODE

The concept of pretend mode is discussed in Chapter 1, "Introduction." In clinical practice a patient may be functioning in pretend mode when there is excessive rationalization and intellectualization, when there is disconnection in the dialogue between patient and clinician, and when explanations of symptoms and personal relationships seem trite and even take a textbook form. Attributing complex motives to others without evidence and/or the use of labyrinthine reasoning of motives without any connection to reality may occur, leading others to be perplexed about how these can be justified—a state of *hypermentalizing* (see Chapter 17, "Borderline Personality Pathology in Adolescence"). The inevitable result for the clinician is that he or she experiences a sense of not being in the room with the patient, of finding it difficult to engage meaningfully with the patient, and of not having a subjective sense of personal interaction. There is a disconnection between self and other, with the clinician becoming increasingly unable to follow the convoluted inferences of the patient's understanding of others' motives. The patient in pretend mode is talking to himself or herself and not to the clinician. As a result, the clinician's mind state has no link to the patient's mind state. It is an uncomfortable position for the clinician.

In treatment, pretend mode can become embedded, and when it does, therapy becomes static. No progress is possible; discussion becomes endless, circular, and fruitless, with damaging effects on positive change. It is essential for the clinician to dismantle pretend mode actively. We have tended to recommend the use of challenge as the main technique to undermine pretend mode and stimulate more effective mentalizing. But, in fact, it is often better to approach pretend mode with stealth rather than a full assault (see Box 6–1).

BOX 6–1.   Interventions for pretend mode

- Focus on the self–other dimension of mentalizing: who is representing whom?
- Redirect current content.
- Identify the process of the session explicitly.
- Work in the current reality of the session.
- Challenge.

First, the clinician tries to get into the dialogue through a *contrary move* along the self–other dimension of mentalizing (see Chapter 1). The aim is to activate a representation of other minds in the mind of the patient. Can the patient consider how the clinician is thinking and see that as different from his or her own mind, or does the patient simply incorporate the clinician's ideas and thoughts into his or her own reflections? If the latter, the patient will even agree with opposing perspectives and ideas, seemingly unaware that both are unlikely to be correct.

The second intervention is to direct the conversation away from content full of generalizations and quasi-explanatory reflection by *focusing on the immediate process of the session*. The aim here is to make the patient less able to obfuscate and dissemble, although this may continue if the process of pretend mode simply attaches to the new content. However, if it does, the counterrelational experience of the clinician can be used to intervene more vigorously by increasing the focus on the experiences of the clinician—that is, rebalancing the patient's focus on his or her own internal states with exploration of the clinician's internal state. We have suggested that in MBT the clinician should initially "quarantine" his or her feelings about the patient; when the clinician presents these feelings to the patient, they are for joint consideration and *not* to highlight unconscious feelings arising in the patient—that is, counterrelational elements are marked as arising from the *clinician's* current mental state. So, we recommend talking about the clinician's feelings openly but in a way that shows it is the clinician's mind that is the subject of scrutiny—to what extent he or she is reacting to the context, content, and process of treatment. Is this the clinician, at least to some extent, and is this relevant to the patient's way of functioning? It has not been our experience that patients take these statements about counterrelational process as permission to ask personal questions about the clinician's life; nor is it authorization for the clinician to indulge in self-disclosure in the sense of talking about his or her life and problems. Done skillfully, discussion centered on some of the experience of the clinician is instructive and heightens the sensitivities of the patient to interpersonal process and may pull the patient out of pretend mode.

The final intervention for pretend mode functioning is *challenge.* Challenge requires the clinician to think laterally, outside the normal therapeutic frame. The clinician has to be compassionate about the rut that he or she and the patient are in, and authentic in recognizing the negative effects it is having on treatment and wanting to make progress. It is from this position that the clinician can disrupt the rigidity of pretend mode.

Case Example

A patient began talking about his adolescent son as he and the clinician walked down the corridor to the consulting room. As they sat down, the clinician asked if that was what he wanted to talk about today, because improving his relationship with his son was a long-term aim of treatment.

> Patient: I will come to that. I want to talk about whether I come here with something to talk about or if I really let things arise spontaneously and momentarily. I follow what comes into my mind rather than focus on a particular topic. So I will come back to my son if my mind stumbles on it again. If I do come here with something to talk about, then I am not fully aware of it when I arrive. My mind meanders and wanders, stopping and looking at things as it goes, with some things seemingly being important but then becoming unimportant.
>
> Clinician: Are you talking about what we call stream of consciousness?
>
> [*This is the first error of the clinician. One principle that clinicians follow in MBT is to ensure that they do not join with nonmentalizing. This drives any nonmentalizing process faster and in particular intensifies pretend mode. This use of a technical term from psychodynamic therapy suggests the clinician has already added to pretend mode processing.*]
>
> Patient: I suppose I am, but it is not really a conscious process. It happens to me when I am here and then I talk about what is important. As I meander and follow myself, each thought can become important. I choose one and then see if it brings something more to how I think.

The patient then talked for a few minutes about his thoughts about what he would talk about when he was on his way to the session but how they now seemed to be of little importance.

> Clinician: I am not going to follow you if you carry on. Can we just focus on how you are feeling at the moment?
> [*This is a better intervention to begin a challenge to pretend mode. The clinician is trying to insert himself into the session by stating his current counterresponsiveness.*]
> Patient: Yes. I will talk about how I feel, but that will depend on the subject I am talking about. You see, if I talk about my relationship with my son, am I really talking about my relationship with my father? When I was talking to my son this week I found myself thinking that I was really talking as my father. If I was my father, then who am I talking to when I am talking to my son? Am I being my father to me, or me as a father to my son? It could be either.

The patient has not answered the question that the clinician asked. So, technically, the clinician should try to keep the focus of the session on the current interaction if pretend mode is to be tackled. For example, he could say, "*Can we just concentrate on my question for a moment about how you feel?*" or "*When I ask you something, to me you seem to veer off the topic and not answer. Am I right, do you think, or am I being too sensitive?*" The latter intervention is perhaps better to the extent that it is marked as the clinician's mental state, asks the patient to consider the process of the moment, can be said humorously with some self-deprecation, and places the clinician into the interaction.

In fact, the clinician said nothing at this point, so the patient continued to talk about father–son relationships and how his own relationship with his father was possibly interfering with his relationship with his own son. Although this may make some psychological sense in a complex way, the error for the clinician is to try to make sense of it at this point and to follow the topic as if it is meaningful. The clinician needs to be sure that the patient is using pretend mode functioning, and, if so, challenge is necessary.

In this session, the clinician inadvertently added more complexity to the dialogue by asking about the patient's father. The patient happily talked about his father and had many views about his strengths and weaknesses. It was then that the clinician realized that pretend mode was becoming increasingly embedded, and so he challenged this more directly. Nevertheless, this example illustrates how easy it is to be drawn into and join with pretend mode. Clinicians are persuaded that the content of the dialogue is meaningful when in fact it is "spinning in sand" and going nowhere.

> Clinician: I want to ask something, and please do not take this as being critical in any way. But at the moment I keep thinking that you are somehow talking to yourself and not me.

The patient stopped for a moment and then laughed, saying that he was caught up with himself.

> Clinician: I know—what about this—take this paper and pen and in no more than three words write down what you have been trying to tell me.

The patient started to talk again, so the clinician stopped him and took control of the session, asking him not to say anything but to write down three words that summarized his point about being a father. The clinician also picked up some paper.

> Clinician: I will do the same. I will write down words if I can that I think capture what you have been trying to tell me. We can then see if we get the same areas of importance.

The structure of the session has now been changed; this in itself may undermine pretend mode. The interaction is now outside the normal therapy process and thus less familiar to the patient. Furthermore, the clinician has taken control and brought both himself and the patient into the process so the isolationist effect of pretend mode is challenged. To some extent, the clinician remains joined with the content of pretend mode, but the form of the interaction between clinician and patient has changed. This shifts the patient's mind state so that the clinician has a chance to move the mental content to a topic more grounded in the real world. In this session, the clinician wrote down some words but then crossed them out, explaining to the patient that as he wrote them down he then thought that they were wrong because he was aware that he had no idea what the patient was trying to get across to him. This allowed the clinician and patient to discuss the form their interaction had taken—that is, the patient becoming trapped in his own ruminative thinking while the clinician was excluded and his muddle ignored by the patient. This was more based in reality, being grounded in what was happening between them in the session, and was relevant to the patient's interactional patterns with others, including his son.

CONCLUSION

Using relational mentalizing to highlight interpersonal sensitivities and recognizing and intervening in pretend mode are two domains of MBT that clinicians find hard to implement skillfully. This chapter emphasizes the importance in MBT of doing adequate groundwork early in treatment so that interventions to promote mentalizing are more likely to be used and may be more effective in terms of promoting robust mentalizing. In principle, both patient and clinician need to recognize the importance of relationships and the tendency to default to pretend mode as a way of managing interpersonal anxieties right from the beginning of treatment. The best place to start with this is in the introductory phase, with the development of a relational passport to be carried by the patient and discussed in individual and group MBT sessions throughout treatment.

REFERENCES

Bartholomew K, Horowitz LM: Attachment styles among young adults: a test of a four-category model. J Pers Soc Psychol 61(2):226–244, 1991 1920064

Bateman A, Fonagy P: Mentalization-Based Treatment for Borderline Personality Disorder: A Practical Guide. Oxford, UK, Oxford University Press, 2006a

Bateman A, Fonagy P: Self-rating of MBT adherence, in Mentalization-Based Treatment for Borderline Personality Disorders: A Practical Guide. Oxford, UK, Oxford University Press, 2006b, pp 175–176

Bateman A, Fonagy P: 8-year follow-up of patients treated for borderline personality disorder: mentalization-based treatment versus treatment as usual. Am J Psychiatry 165(5):631–638, 2008 18347003

Bateman A, Fonagy P: Mentalization-Based Treatment for Personality Disorders: A Practical Guide. Oxford, UK, Oxford University Press, 2016

Karterud S, Bateman A: Manual for Mentaliseringsbasert Psykoedukativ Gruppeterapi (MBT-I) [Manual for Mentalization-Based Psychoeducational Group Therapy (MBT-I)]. Oslo, Norway, Gyldendal Akademisk, 2011

Karterud S, Pedersen G, Engen M, et al: The MBT Adherence and Competence Scale (MBT-ACS): development, structure and reliability. Psychother Res 23(6):705–717, 2013 22916991

CHAPTER 7

GROUP THERAPY FOR ADULTS AND ADOLESCENTS

Anthony Bateman, M.A., FRCPsych

Mickey Kongerslev, M.Sc., Ph.D.

Sune Bo Hansen, Cand.Psych.Aut., Ph.D.

In this chapter we outline the historical development of mentalization-based group therapy (MBT-G) and discuss the core components and essential interventions of MBT-G with adults and adolescents diagnosed with borderline personality disorder (BPD). Importantly, MBT-G is not considered a treatment for all; MBT-G is modified according to the patient group.

At its inception, mentalization-based treatment (MBT) was developed as a combination of individual and group therapy (Bateman and Fonagy 2004) within a research and treatment program (Bateman and Fonagy 1999). Since then, MBT has been implemented as individual treatment only or as group treatment only, leading some practitioners to suggest that a lack of combined—or, more technically, conjoint—treatment is not "true" MBT. Certainly, it is not MBT in its original research form, but a combination of individual and group therapy never formed the essential definition of what is core to MBT in terms of therapeutic aims and principles. Indeed, there is no research to show whether individual MBT without group therapy, or vice versa, is more or less—or perhaps even equally as—effective in the treatment of BPD or any other disorder. In other complex psychosocial treatments, the combination of treatment modalities seems to be based more on theoretical reasoning than on empirical evidence regarding its ability to improve outcomes (Linehan et al. 2015). More generally, recent findings indicate equivalence in terms of outcomes for individual versus group therapy across a wide range of disorders (Burlingame et al. 2016a, 2016b). The same may be true for MBT. Research is needed on MBT-G as a treatment in its own right; it cannot be subservient to, or stand only in combination with, MBT individual therapy.

The initial discussion of MBT-G proposed specific and detailed interventions in common clinical situations when treating people with BPD (Bateman and Fonagy 2004). Nevertheless, there was less focus on defining MBT interventions in group therapy than in individual therapy. To some extent, this has been remedied (Karterud 2015a). However, there has been some loss of clarity about the core components of an MBT group in terms of structure and intervention because of variation in the way MBT-G—and even MBT as a combined treatment—is taught, practiced, and implemented. Accordingly, a further aim of this chapter is to clarify the MBT-G approach.

HISTORICAL ORIGINS

A number of theoretical and practical influences on the thinking behind the development of MBT-G are relevant to the development and current understanding of the core components of MBT-G. First and foremost, at a practical level, in the 1970s and 1980s clinicians were advised in the literature to be cautious about having too many people with BPD in a group. Nearly a decade after MBT was first developed, textbooks were still advising clinicians to compose their groups in a "balanced" way by having no more than a few BPD patients in a group (Rutan et al. 2007). Expert opinion was generally pessimistic about groups composed of only BPD patients or, at least, recommended that such groups had to be modified significantly—a view with which we agreed.

Second, group analysis and group psychodynamic therapy had contributed substantially to advances in the understanding of groups and group process over more than a century. The influence of the findings on understanding group process is unassailable; the relevance in clinical practice of the discoveries from group analysis applies equally to the management of psychoeducation and skills groups as it does to insight-oriented groups. All clinicians need an understanding of group process to manage any type of group effectively. But what does a clinician do, technically, with inevitable interactional processes—ignore them, avoid them, or harness them? In line with group analysis and other psychodynamic group therapies, MBT attempts to harness the interpersonal interactions within a group of people, in an organized way, using a structured framework.

Third, some of the developers of MBT were trainers in *interpersonal psychotherapy* (IPT) (Weissman et al. 2000) and were implementing IPT for the treatment for depression while at the same time developing ideas about how to use IPT in treating BPD (Bateman 2012). The focus and structure of group IPT (IPT-G) seemed to be applicable to people with BPD even though interventions in IPT and IPT-G were specific to depression and required modification in terms of their focus for BPD. Contemporaneously, the same clinicians were working on an idea that the core issue in BPD might be conceptualized as disordered mentalizing (Fonagy 1995). It was the combination of these conceptual and clinical frames that led to the formulation of mentalizing groups for BPD and, indeed, to the more recent operationalized mentalizing approach to depression (Lemma et al. 2011; see also Chapter 23, "Depression").

In IPT-G, the clinician is tasked with undertaking specific actions: maintaining overall authority for keeping to task, identifying each patient's depressive focus, managing the group discussion around a shared focus, summarizing the group and each patient's contribution to the discussion, and personalizing feedback (Wilfley et al. 2000). Many of these aspects of managing the group are easily identifiable in MBT-G, and these are summarized in Box 7–1.

BOX 7–1. **Common components of MBT-G and IPT-G**

- Clinician actively identifies and elaborates a patient's central problems when the patient starts in the group.

- Clinician maintains control and authority for keeping the group to task.

- Clinician presents a summary of the previous group at the beginning of the next session.

- Patients contribute to the summary of the previous group at the beginning of each session.

- Clinician ensures a shared focus is generated in each group.

- Clinician defines a period of reflection toward the end of each group on the group process.

Patients usually find it a relief to realize that the group has manageable tasks, that the clinician takes a firm lead in these tasks, and that the group focuses on problems that relate to them.

MBT-G combines an understanding and use of process from group analytic ideas with structure from IPT and other more cognitively oriented groups; it can be considered as being neatly positioned between these two somewhat opposing perspectives. This position brings advantages and disadvantages. The MBT clinician—an active participant with an authentic attitude of curiosity about mental states—manages the group, openly states the principles that are to be followed, maintains the primary task of stimulating scrutiny of the problems the patients bring, and explores the interactions between participants in terms of their mental states to highlight what is behind interpersonal interactional processes. Herein lies a central issue of MBT-G and its pluralistic origins. How is this done? Like IPT-G and some other integrative therapies, MBT-G is currently practiced in two ways—more from an "analytic" perspective or more from a "cognitive" perspective—leading to variation in terms of the balance between process, structure, and content. Neither of these ways has a monopoly on "correctness" as long as the primary aim is to facilitate more robust and flexible mentalizing ability in the participants, rather than to increase knowledge, implant specific skills, or facilitate experiential learning from participation in the group. MBT requires organized "balancing" of emerging relational processes and structured learning, which is facilitated by the clinician.

Unsurprisingly, many writers with experience of working with a range of group therapies argue that *all* group therapy takes this approach and that differentiating MBT-G from, for example, group analysis (Karterud 2015b) requires a specific reading of what group analysis really is (Lorentzen 2015). There is some merit in this argument. Mentalizing is a common factor of psychotherapy process, and an adequate level of mentalizing is necessary for patients to use psychotherapeutic interventions constructively (Fonagy et al. 2015). Still, MBT-G is also a specific approach that first and foremost targets dysfunctional mentalizing. The bottom line is that there are many roads that lead to Rome—in this case, of facilitating mentalizing capacities.

Mentalizing as a Common Process in Groups

All psychotherapy creates change in part through stimulating mentalizing; mentalizing is thus a common factor of psychotherapies. Indeed, an argument has been made that improvements in mentalizing are necessary if change in psychotherapy is to take place at all. This has led to an argument that MBT-G is not a new paradigm and treatment shift in its own right, but more a focus on and refinement of particular components of group analysis or group psychodynamic therapy (Potthoff and Moini-Afchari 2014). However, the question remains whether MBT-G is simply "old wine in new bottles" and represents normal clinical sensitivity and sensible techniques that are already in use when groups comprise only people with personality disorder—or, to put it another way, whether MBT-G is no more than mentalizing-informed group analysis and that differentiating the two is a false dichotomy. However, specific adherence to MBT-G is currently being studied, and differentiation is ultimately an empirical question for future research to address (Folmo et al. 2017).

Rather than set up straw men of group analysis or other group methods to undermine, we describe here the features of MBT-G that we think are specific (Bateman and Fonagy 2006, 2016). We leave it to the reader to decide whether these features differ enough from other forms of group treatment in terms of focus (as discussed above), structure, process, and technique to warrant differentiation. First, we briefly summarize some of the research on MBT-G as a specific treatment in its own right.

RESEARCH ON MBT-G

Adults

Research on MBT-G alone in the treatment of adults with personality disorders is in its infancy. Studying a predominantly group-oriented program for adults with BPD, Kvarstein et al. (2015) compared the outcomes for BPD patients before and after an MBT program was implemented. The patient group enrolled in the former psychodynamic treatment program had comparable baseline severity and impairments of functioning to the group that received MBT. BPD patients in MBT showed a very low dropout rate (2%), significantly lower than that associated with the former treatment, indicating that MBT adaptations managed patients' excess anxiety and prevented fight/flight responses. Improvements in symptom distress and interpersonal, global, and occupational functioning were significantly greater for MBT patients; reductions in suicidal or self-harming acts, use of medication, and hospitalizations were evident over the course of both treatments. The reason for the significant and important findings of reduced dropout and improved symptoms is unclear. The fact that MBT was delivered as a conjoint (group + individual) treatment with a focus in individual therapy on how a patient manages and uses the group—a structure and process not present in the earlier psychodynamic program—may be one of a number of factors (Kvarstein et al. 2017).

Petersen et al. (2010) treated a cohort of 22 patients with personality disorders with once-weekly mentalization-oriented group therapy for up to 3 years following a stabilization phase in a day treatment program. There were no dropouts from treatment. Significant improvements were observed on symptoms, interpersonal function, social adjustment, and vocational status, and there was significant reduction in use of services.

MBT-G has been compared with psychodynamic group therapy (PDGT) in a randomized process–outcome study (*N*=211) (Brand et al. 2016). The results on a range of outcomes in patients with mixed anxiety and mood disorders suggest that MBT-G in a heterogeneous population in a day clinic is not superior to PDGT but increases mentalizing of the self more than PDGT.

A further process–outcome study from the same authors comparing the group relationships in PDGT and MBT-G after each group session showed differences. There were higher conflict scores at the beginning of the group in MBT-G, while in PDGT there was more avoidance during the course of therapy. The group conflicts of the patients benefiting the most from PDGT showed strong and ongoing fluctuations during the therapy process, whereas among those benefiting more from MBT-G, the fluctuations of the conflicts in group relationships were much shorter (Hecke et al. 2016). These differences suggest that the different therapeutic stances create a different matrix, which may be important when treating patients with severe personality disorder, in whom unresolved conflict tends to lead to dropout.

Adolescents

For many decades, it has been recognized both by researchers and by practitioners that working with adolescents in groups (Teicher 1966) is consistent with their developmental focus on peer interaction and is effective. Moderate to large effect sizes have been demonstrated when comparing group treatment for adolescents with waiting-list and placebo control groups (Hoag and Burlingame 1997). Furthermore, the research literature suggests that outcomes of group and individual treatment for adolescents do not differ in terms of general effectiveness (Hoag and Burlingame 1997), which indicates that group treatment may be more cost-effective overall.

However, few studies have been conducted in regard to treating personality disorders in adolescents, and even fewer have investigated group treatment (Kongerslev et al. 2015). This paucity of studies can partly be explained by studies showing iatrogenic effects of group psychotherapy for adolescents with conduct disorders and substance abuse difficulties (Macgowan and Wagner 2005) and research underscoring how neurobiological development in adolescence can complicate group processes. For example, some findings have demonstrated that adolescents have difficulties recognizing and naming facial expressions due to late maturation of certain brain structures (Vetter et al. 2013). Other findings emphasize that when attention is unconstrained, adolescents are more sensitive than adults to emotional components of social stimuli, resulting in elevated activation of the amygdala and a reduced capability to reflect (Monk et al. 2003). Another study has shown that, compared with adults, adolescents engage in significantly more risk behavior when they are with peers than when they are alone (Steinberg 2005), indicating high vulnerability to peer pressure.

These normative neurodevelopmental issues can complicate, or at least require an adjustment of, the general group treatment techniques and structure described for adults. However, notwithstanding these neurodevelopmental issues and the challenges they bring for group treatment, it is possible to conduct MBT-G treatment for adolescents with BPD. A recent feasibility study reported favorable outcomes of an

MBT-G program for adolescents diagnosed with BPD (Bo et al. 2017a). MBT-G was delivered for 1 year to 34 girls ages 15–18 years. Of the 25 participants who completed the study, 23 displayed improvements in borderline symptoms, depression, self-harm, peer attachment, parent attachment, mentalizing, and general psychopathology. Importantly, enhanced trust in peers and parents in combination with improved mentalizing capacity was associated with a greater reduction in borderline symptoms, suggesting a mechanism responsible for the efficacy of the treatment. A larger randomized controlled trial exploring the effect of an MBT-G program versus treatment as usual in adolescents with BPD is currently under way (Beck et al. 2016).

CLINICAL PRACTICE OF MBT-G

Structure

MBT-G is delivered by one or two clinicians, with six to eight patients participating in the group. The length of each group session varies and is either 75 or 90 minutes depending on local service decisions; either length gives time for group process to develop and be used to highlight some of the relational focus of treatment. The rationale for this basic structure is discussed by Bateman and Fonagy (2016).

Entry to MBT-G is structured in terms of the patient pathway. All patients being treated with MBT progress from an assessment and collaborative formulation phase, through a phase that introduces the model, to beginning psychotherapy. At the end of the initial phase of treatment, patients will have agreed on a joint formulation of their problems with the clinician and have an understanding of personality disorder, mentalizing strengths and weakness, attachment processes, and potential pitfalls of treatment. The psychoeducation component is provided in group form and is known as *MBT-introductory group* (MBT-I) (Bateman and Fonagy 2016). The content varies according to the patient population—adolescents, people with psychosis, families of patients, and others. For example, for patients with psychosis, four topics are covered: understanding motives, understanding attitudes, understanding emotions, and understanding what makes me "me" (Lana et al. 2015); for patients with antisocial personality disorder, sessions cover mentalizing, violence, forms of relationships, and emotions. These groups are discussed in Chapter 25, "Psychosis," and Chapter 20, "Antisocial Personality Disorder in Community and Prison Settings," respectively. For adolescents, six sessions (as opposed to 12 sessions for adults) are provided in the initial phase. In addition, parents and guardians are asked to confirm that they will actively participate in facilitating the treatment program for the adolescent (e.g., helping with transportation).

At a patient's first MBT-G group, he or she is supported in 1) outlining his or her problems to the group in terms of his or her formulation, which is better thought of in this context as a "collaborative clinical agreement" that has been agreed between the patient and the clinicians; and 2) describing his or her attachment strategies as identified in the patient's relational passport (see Chapter 6, "Individual Therapy Techniques"). The clinician "sides" (see later) with the patient to support this process.

The format of each session follows a trajectory implemented by the clinician, as outlined in Box 7–2.

BOX 7–2. Trajectory of each MBT-G session

- Summary of previous group.
- Problem round for all patients in the group.
- Work toward synthesis of problems between group members.
- Exploration of problems by group members, facilitated by clinician.
- Closure.
- Postgroup discussion.

First, the clinician gives a summary about the previous group formed from the postgroup discussion between clinicians after the previous session, outlining the topics discussed and interpersonal issues identified, including any unresolved issues in the group. It is recommended that the summary has a positive tone, indicates ways of addressing problems, and identifies the patients involved. It is especially important that all members of the group are mentioned in the summary, even if they did not attend the previous session, to stimulate inclusion and to facilitate cohesion and continuity.

Summary of Previous Group

Hello, Mary-Ann. I am sorry that you could not get here last week. Jen, Sarah, Tom, Peter, and Clare—last week, I thought the main topic was about never managing to meet other people's expectations. We ended up not quite deciding if people expected too much of us or if we tended to expect too much of ourselves and we misread what others want from us. We all thought we could be rather self-punishing when we felt we did not match up. Sarah, you were particularly caught up with this, and it was creating tension between you and your boyfriend. But Peter, although you could see this, you thought that if people expected things from you that the best thing to do was to "fuck off" and not bother with them. This has some sense, as it made you feel better, but it also means that you end relationships quickly. We then brought up what is expected of us all here and if we ask too much or too little of each other. I'm not sure we concluded anything about that. Certainly, I felt sometimes that things were expected of me that I could not deliver, and that was a problem for me. Perhaps we could come back to the whole topic today at some point. Does anyone remember anything else about this? There may be other things?

There was also a discussion about expecting someone else to join the group. Jen, you were anxious about this, as you feel the group is comfortable at the moment and that it would be messed up by having someone else added who we all would have to get to know. So, we need to keep that in mind as Jonathan starts in 2 weeks' time.

Does anyone have any other points?

Patients then indicate if they have problems that they would like to address in the group on that day; following this, balanced turn-taking has been recommended as a possible strategy. This is not individual therapy within the group, but a focus by the group on designated patients and their current intersubjective and emotional problems (Karterud 2015a). Alternatively, the MBT clinician can negotiate a synthesis of problems so that a few patients are identified as the main protagonists to start working on the problem areas and to provide concrete and individualized examples of the problems in order to avoid pseudomentalizing (see subsection "Ineffective Mentalizing Modes" later in this section). The patients are asked to talk together to identify shared emotional states, impulsive urges, or interpersonal anxieties. Toward the end of the group there is a closure phase in which the patients consider together what they have achieved and identify any unresolved issues. This phase helps the patients gain separation from their problems and promotes emotional regulation before leaving the group (Bateman and Fonagy 2016). In groups for adolescents, examples of constructive mentalizing that occurred in the group session are highlighted at the end of every session, to elaborate on feelings of "we-ness" and group cohesion.

The purpose of these structural elements is to ensure that the clinician retains a level of authority in the group to maintain interpersonal dialogue about the subjective experience of mental states, which is consistent with the primary aim of facilitating mentalizing and preventing collapse into ineffective mentalizing modes. Moreover, this regular structure also imposes structure within the minds of the patients and provides them with a sense of security that is necessary for them to be able to begin more robust mentalizing. Allowing the trajectory of the group to unfold by following the patients, rather than leading them, is more likely to lead to ineffective mentalizing due to overstimulation of emotional and attachment processes. Groups for people with BPD that place greater emphasis on emerging relational processes have been shown to have high dropout rates, probably for this reason (Marziali and Munroe-Blum 1994, 1995). In contrast, groups that focus solely on skills and the identification of set goals related to relationship schemas, and that reduce the focus on intersubjective experience and exploration of emotional states in significant interpersonal interactions within and outside the group, show low dropout rates (Farrell et al. 2009).

Ideally, MBT-G strives to create a balance between these emerging processes and emphasis on problems specific to the patient group while avoiding the Scylla of uncontrolled process and the Charybdis of overcontrol. This requires the clinician to manage group structure and processes to maintain a safe level of stimulation of attachment process and to keep arousal at a level that facilitates rather than undermines mentalizing discourse between participants, and reduces the likelihood of ineffective mentalizing interactions. The form of the structure is less important than its aim; clinicians need to show they are actively managing the group structure and focus, not primarily or passively following the group. As emphasized earlier, in the case of MBT-G for adolescents, the clinician takes an even more active stance compared with the clinician working with an adult group. This active stance also includes being a strong role model for proper mentalizing for the group members and thereby paving the way to mentalizing for the group. Although the MBT-G clinician takes the lead in general, when the group is engaging in mentalizing dialogue, the clinician "withdraws" and allows the group to work. Adolescents listen to adolescents—often more than they listen to their clinician—and this potential for adolescent-to-adolescent learning is actively built on and supported when such learning occurs.

Process

The key feature of MBT-G is facilitating mentalizing process around the problems defined by the patients and clinicians, with priority given to interpersonal events and emotional identification and regulation. The clinician's role is to keep the conversation focused and to manage the interactions. In order to carry out this role and attain the primary aim of "focused mentalizing" between participants, the clinician asks about factual narrative information but is primarily active and questioning about mental states, using the not-knowing stance. In adolescent treatment, the clinician in many cases has to be very helpful when trying to establish a coherent narrative, because adolescents often find it very difficult to provide a coherent narrative account of an event or scenario. The MBT clinician is not a passive listener; he or she is a participant, managing arousal in the group and bringing his or her own mental state, experience, and perspective to the discussion, ensuring that all patients are involved in the process of stimulating alternative perspectives around synthesized problems. Above all, the clinician is *involved*. He or she listens carefully for ineffective mentalizing process, as will the other patients; for example, in the MBT-I phase, patients are "taught" to be sensitive to their own and others' collapse into ineffective mentalizing dialogue. This is distinctly different from listening for group unconscious process and trying to identify and use the dynamic matrix of the group (Foulkes 1975). The clinician is not focusing on unconscious group process. Free association between group members to facilitate symbolization and more profound understanding of communication is not part of the MBT-G technique. Interpretation in terms of unconscious process and meaning implies that the clinician has abilities to see things that the patients cannot and, as such, separates him or her from the group, which is not part of MBT. In addition, patients with severe BPD have problems working at representational levels and so cannot use unconscious understanding in a personally meaningful way.

Identification of Problems for the Group

Stimulation of interaction between the members of the group is a key task for the clinician. The clinician needs to generate an atmosphere of playfulness in the group and genuine interest in one another's problems. The clinician does this partly by maintaining the group's focus on agreed problems and partly through making a synthesis of problems—that is, so a subgroup of patients recognize that they share the same concerns even if those concerns take different forms.

Problem Round

Viv mentioned at the start of the group that she had difficulties with her boyfriend. She wanted to talk about them. She identified that the main problem was that she continually felt that he did not want to be with her. She worried that he was about to leave her.

Simone asked to talk about her anxieties that she always felt like an outsider wherever she was. She said she felt different from others, and this had shown itself when she was at a dance club a few days earlier. Other people seemed to enjoy themselves and feel relaxed; she felt tense.

Peter said he didn't want to talk about much, but he could recognize what Viv and Simone were saying.

Synthesis of Problems

The clinician asked Peter to elaborate: "Can you say what you recognize in what they are saying?"

Peter: We are the sort of people who are not wanted, basically. Nobody wants us around most of the time.

Clinician: Let's keep that on hold while we finish off going around to see what work we
need to do today, and then come back to it.

Having finished the problem round and identified two other main problems to be
discussed, the clinician asked Peter to elaborate further about his recognition of Viv
and Simone's problem. The clinician's intervention and Peter's answer allowed Viv,
Simone, and Peter to consider their experiences of not being wanted. They gave many
examples, but the shared core was how anyone knows if they are wanted, if people
enjoy their company, and if people appreciate them for who they are. This began to
build on the initial problems of difficulties with the boyfriend (Viv) and isolation
(Simone and Peter) when with friends, leading to identification of problems of self-
recognition and how it plays out in relation to others. The synthesis of problems created between them was around self-esteem in terms of what they thought of themselves and whether other people saw them in the same way as they saw themselves.
This is an important mentalizing problem as it requires differentiation of the mental
states of the self and others, and an ability to reduce the impact others have on self-
states. As such, the three patients became the protagonists of this discussion.

This task of joining or synthesizing problems between group participants and
making those individuals responsible for exploring the issues often uses *triangulation*
as a strategy to achieve the aim of increasing group interaction. A third person, in this
case Peter, is asked to give his views on the problems described by others or on the
interaction between others, either from his own perspective or from his understanding of their perspective. There were three other patients in the group, and, of course,
they are neither neglected in this discussion nor allowed to withdraw. The clinician
asks them to provide an alternative understanding. In this group, they talked about
how they saw Viv, Simone, and Peter, and then they were asked to compare this with
how they viewed themselves.

Postgroup Discussion

After the group, the clinician writes a brief summary of the session, which forms the
basis of feedback to the group members the following week. If more than one clinician
is present in the group, the clinicians discuss the session—this is the postgroup discussion. Their conclusions and any differences of perspective form the basis of the
written summary and the feedback to the group the following week.

Ineffective Mentalizing Modes

A number of techniques are available to the MBT-G clinician to manage ineffective
mentalizing modes and their consequential interactions in MBT groups. The clinician
should slow the dialogue, ask for reflection, display curiosity, and provide his or her
own perspective for consideration. On occasions the clinician stops the group and
asks for a pause. This is essential if psychic equivalence (see Chapter 1, "Introduction") is dominating the group interaction. In this state of mind, the patients hold
their ideas with certainty and rigidity, believing that what they think is a fact. If someone presents a different perspective, that person is wrong. To address this, a "linked
diversion" is made—that is, the clinician steers the dialogue away from the immediate topic that is associated with the nonmentalizing mode in the hope of turning on

some effective mentalizing, before returning to the topic that triggered ineffective mentalizing. The clinician actively looks for the patient or patients in the group who *are* mentalizing and brings them into the discussion— that is, the clinician "seeks the source(s) of mentalizing in the group."

> Jenny, a 19-year-old BPD patient, had had a row with her father after he had found out that she was engaging in sex work by offering "sexual conversations" on the web. She was no longer talking to him, saying that dialogue was a waste of time. He thought her work was degrading and shameful, whereas she thought it was a good way to earn money. The other group members agreed with her that it was harmless as long as she did not meet the men, and one patient thought she herself might start doing it. The clinician gauged this as an ineffective mentalizing interaction, not because of the content, but because of the lack of reflection and the rigidity with which the patient had decided her father's view was insensitive and wrong and she was right. She was unable to see the situation from any perspective other than her own, and the other patients engaged in reinforcing her view rather than asking about it. Noting that one patient was silent but manifestly listening, the clinician wondered whether she had been uninfluenced by the lightheartedness and not accepted the situation as simply being a good way to earn "easy money." So the clinician suggested (based on his own external focus of mentalizing) that this patient seemed to be thinking something else: "Sarah, you look to me like you have some other thoughts about this" *(this is an example of triangulation)*. Sarah said that she was thinking about how she would never "sell herself" in sex talk to "dirty men" and thought the whole incident with the father was about how Jenny found his disapproval difficult. Jenny denied this initially, so the clinician asked her to think a bit more about her feelings, using it as a diversion from the polarized argument of whether "sex talk" was OK or not OK: "What were things like between you and your father before this took place?" This allowed for a broader discussion related to Jenny's feelings that her father had always seen her as a wayward, uncontrollable child and an immoral person. He was ashamed of her. She was the black sheep of the family.
>
> The clinician then eventually actively slowed the process by asking if any of the more reflective dialogue the group was now engaged in was having any effect on people's thinking about the situation—"Is dialogue useful?" This is done not to disrupt reflective dialogue, but to add to the mentalizing process by asking the patients to reflect on their reflection as it progresses. The patient had said that dialogue with her father was useless and she was no longer speaking to him. But dialogue is the currency of change, and so the clinician wanted to establish with the group members whether talking about things between people was useful. This exemplifies the MBT-G clinician's direction and management of the group and illustrates how he or she asks the patients to take a meta-representational perspective on what they have been doing in the group—thinking about experience in the context of where it is being experienced— thereby stimulating mentalized affectivity as the group progresses.

The expression of ineffective mentalizing through teleological function—that is, where mental states are understood through what is apparent in the physical world— may require the clinician to "side" with a patient or patients.

> A patient who had problems attending the group, and who commonly explained her absences as resulting from practical issues such as missing the bus or not having enough money, irritated another patient, who said, "Why don't you stop coming? You obviously don't want to be here. Otherwise you would get here. It really pisses me off that you don't turn up and we all know you don't want to see us." The nonattending patient was fragile and vulnerable and did not attend the group out of anxiety related to interacting with others. Accordingly, the remark was likely to induce panic. So, the clinician "took her side" and immediately responded to the irritated patient: "I don't

think you are right. I think Jessica wants to be here. Where did you get it from that she did not? Is it based only on her not being here?" The clinician and the irritated patient then had a dialogue around the patient understanding things only in terms of what happens rather than in terms of underlying mental states—that is, the teleological understanding she was bringing to the situation without exploring mental states. Taking the nonattending patient's side also managed the tension in the situation.

TROUBLESHOOTING PRETEND MODE

Pretend mode is another ineffective mentalizing mode that is more difficult both to recognize and to intervene in. It takes two forms: *pseudomentalizing* and *hypermentalizing* (see Chapter 1). Once recognized, it is necessary for the clinician to prevent pretend mode in either form from spreading among the group members and affecting how they talk about topics.

Pseudomentalizing.   Pseudomentalizing is akin to intellectualization and rationalization in terms of how the patients talk about issues. It tends to be ruminative and overly detailed, and the person engaged in it is excessively self-absorbed. The discussion is not grounded in reality and is divorced from personal experience in terms of complexity and affect. This does not mean the person is affectless, however; pseudomentalizing may take place with high anxiety even though the physical aspects of anxiety are not apparent.

Hypermentalizing.   Hypermentalizing is said to occur when patients attribute mental states and motivations to themselves and to others that go way beyond reasonable evidence in terms of expressed mental states and information from sensitive external mentalizing. Patients may say much about states of mind but with little true meaning or connection to reality. Attempting psychotherapy with patients who are in pretend mode can lead to lengthy but inconsequential discussions of internal experience that have no link to genuine experience. A patient who shows considerable cognitive understanding of mentalizing states but little affective understanding may often hypermentalize. This state can often be difficult to distinguish from genuine mentalizing, but it tends to involve overly long narratives that are devoid of a real affective core or a connection to reality. On first impressions, hypermentalizing can lead the clinician to believe that the group is working with impressive mentalizing capacities, but after a while the clinician discovers that he or she is unable to resonate with the feelings underlying the patients' mentalizing efforts. In addition, the dialogue does not progress; it is circular and inconsequential.

The clinician challenges the different forms of pretend mode by engaging in asymmetrical discussion: rather than taking the exploratory and not-knowing stance, the clinician is contrary, a little rebellious about accepting explanations, irreverent, or perhaps oppositional. This must be done with both skill and tact. The aim is to prevent the group from developing increasingly complex discussions about motives of self and others without questioning them.

> One patient talked about how he was trying to manage the difficult behavior of his adolescent son. He told the group that when he was talking to his son, he was not sure if he was talking to him as a father or whether he was really talking to his son as someone who reminded him of how he was as an adolescent, "in which case, I am really talking to myself." The other patients became involved in this discussion about how it was pos-

sible to "project" and see yourself in others. People could talk about themselves and see things in others when it was really they who had the problem. Inevitably, this was of little help in terms of addressing the real problem of how the patient could support his son with his school difficulties and his use of drugs. The clinician challenged the group: he put his hand up, as the discussion was rapid and without pause. A member of the group reacted to this, so the clinician then asked if he could say something. This member then asked for the group to be left alone so they could get to the point. The clinician quickly interrupted, asking "What is the point? I have not managed to get what you are saying." Another patient began to explain that the point was how we never really know who we are when we are talking. The clinician opposed this by saying that he categorically was sure who *he* was, as he was talking, and it was really inconvenient if everyone else in the group was not who they seemed to be but someone else. It seemed that John was John—and he had an issue relating to supporting his son.

This is a mild challenge. In effect, the clinician is trying to ground the group in some form of reality by expressing his own state of mind. The aim is to pull the patients in the group out of themselves. A stronger challenge might have been to suggest that the group is "disappearing into itself and producing only bullshit!"

Hypermentalizing is especially common when working with adolescents diagnosed with BPD (Bo et al. 2017b). Especially in the initial phase of the group treatment, adolescent members often misunderstand what mentalizing entails and eagerly engage in wild guessing, ascribing intentions and feelings to other group members. Here, it is important that the clinician intervenes to reduce hypermentalizing while at the same time stimulating effective mentalizing.

Interactions Within the Group

The MBT-G clinician is continually alert for interactional patterns in the group that link to similar patterns demonstrated by the patient in his or her life outside the group. One part of the case formulation is a recognition of the attachment strategies used by the patient in close relationships. These are identified and personalized in the formulation with examples from the patient's life; the patient needs to recognize them and invest them with importance. It is the relational (attachment-based) descriptions agreed between the clinician and the patient that are brought to the first group session when the patient joins.

> One patient began his first group session by talking about not wanting to be there. He said that he was nervous anyway and did not think the group could help much. The other patients tried to reassure him and normalize his anxieties. The clinician then asked the patient to talk, as much as he felt able, about his problems. He said that he could not easily make friends and led an isolated life, which he found painful as it made him feel he was different from others. After the patient had attended the group for a few weeks, it was obvious that he was isolated in the group, mostly because he avoided interaction and said little about himself. So, the clinician pointed out that when other patients asked him about himself his answers tended to close down any discussion, and he continually deferred to others at the opening of the group, saying he had nothing in particular to discuss. This was the beginning of exploring the patient's position in the group in terms of his personalized formulation and working on the anxieties that led him to engage in avoidant strategies in the group, as he had done when he first started in the group, and in his life in the world outside.

Once the detail of how the patient interacts with others in the group is established, further relational mentalizing becomes possible. Technically, the MBT clinician aims to do this in stages. First, the clinician explores how the patient relates to the group itself (in the example above, pushing people away); and second, the clinician considers how the patient relates to individual members of the group, including the clinician. There is less need to understand these patterns as repetitions from the past or as having a function for the group itself. The main purpose is to increase the patient's sensitivity to how he or she interacts with others and to improve reflection on it while it is happening in the here and now. It is engaging in this process that is significant, rather than any final endpoint in terms of understanding past antecedents and how they are played out in the present; as in individual MBT, the journey is more important than the destination. Nevertheless, if patients are able to construct a narrative about how their past continues to influence the present, and if this narrative is not held in pretend mode, this is to be encouraged. In a well-functioning MBT group, participants benefit from recognizing how their behaviors have roots in early attachment experiences, as this understanding expands the mentalizing representational frame. Similarly, recognizing that their own and others' behaviors (e.g., silence) have an effect on overall processes in the group is useful for patients to understand wider social processes and how behaviors create—as well as are created by—interpersonal patterns and reactions.

In MBT-G with adolescents, it is essential for the clinician to constantly monitor how members relate to one another and to the group as a whole. Adolescent patients are not necessarily able to link current attachment relations to earlier ones, and thus, interventions aimed at linking prior attachment experiences with parents or peers to how they function in the group are often too complicated. However, this is not a goal in itself, so the clinician should not strive for such an accomplishment, but rather focus on the relations between members here and now. This is done not only to enhance relational mentalizing but also to cultivate group cohesion and prevent or address scapegoat effects, which easily arise in groups composed of adolescents with BPD.

SUMMARY OF ESSENTIAL COMPONENTS OF MBT-G FOR ADULTS AND ADOLESCENTS

The essential elements of MBT-G can be summarized as follows:

1. **Structure.** A number of ways are recommended to ensure that the group maintains a specific trajectory, from opening the group, through the work of the group, to closure of the group. This may involve turn taking, generation of a synthesis of problem areas, and agreeing on a focus.
2. **Clinician stance.** The clinician is a part of the group, and this includes working on and expressing his or her own experiences in the group. A not-knowing stance is used to increase reflection on mental states. The clinician must maintain his or her own mentalizing before addressing ineffective mentalizing in the group.
3. **Active management of process of the group.** Arousal is managed with sensitive awareness of attachment processes stimulated in the group. The clinician controls the speed of interaction between participants, slowing the discussion down at

times and even stopping the dialogue and rewinding to reconsider what has happened or what has been said.

4. **Primary target.** The primary target of intervention is ineffective mentalizing—that is, psychic equivalence, teleological mode, and pretend mode—that arises while exploring the agreed focus. Interventions for managing these modes of mental functioning are described earlier in this chapter and in more detail elsewhere (Bateman and Fonagy 2016).

5. **Exploration of mental states and affective reactions.** Exploring mental states and affective reactions around significant events in the lives of the patients and in relation to events in the group is necessary. Events are best understood as having multiple determinants; the clinician and group members work together to increase coherence of the patient's narratives and identify detailed mental state representations of them.

6. **Relational mentalizing.** Relational mentalizing with a focus on the attachment processes identified in the case formulation is essential for all group members. Problems with intimate relationships are a core component of personality disorders, and the pattern of the patient's relationships is identified in the case formulation and agreed with the patient before he or she commences group therapy. The MBT clinician is alert to indicators in the group that the attachment patterns are being activated. These activations are specifically addressed in "real time" as they occur between group members. This facilitates the development of mentalizing within close relationships that are emotionally salient and current.

7. **Active stance.** When conducting MBT-G with adolescents with BPD or emerging personality disorder, the clinician cannot deviate from an active stance when engaging in and facilitating mentalizing dialogue in the group. The neurobiological underpinnings for mentalizing are under development in adolescence, and arousal can easily overwhelm the developing mentalizing control structures, resulting in nonmentalizing functioning. So, first, it is crucial to intervene actively and assist the group members to mentalize when reflective functioning is absent. In adults, some deviation from this active stance is acceptable and may be tolerated by the patient group, but adolescents cannot accommodate inactivity on the part of the clinician. Second, the clinician should actively engage in interventions that cultivate and maintain cohesion early in the group treatment. This has also been highlighted by Burlingame et al. (2011), who emphasize that fostering cohesion is particularly useful when working with adolescents in groups.

REFERENCES

Bateman A, Fonagy P: Effectiveness of partial hospitalization in the treatment of borderline personality disorder: a randomized controlled trial. Am J Psychiatry 156(10):1563–1569, 1999 10518167

Bateman A, Fonagy P: Psychotherapy for Borderline Personality Disorder: Mentalization-Based Treatment. Oxford, UK, Oxford University Press, 2004

Bateman A, Fonagy P: Mentalization-Based Treatment for Borderline Personality Disorder: A Practical Guide. Oxford, UK, Oxford University Press, 2006

Bateman A, Fonagy P: Mentalization-Based Treatment for Personality Disorders: A Practical Guide. Oxford, UK, Oxford University Press, 2016

Bateman AW: Interpersonal psychotherapy for borderline personality disorder. Clin Psychol Psychother 19(2):124–133, 2012 22344752

Beck E, Bo S, Gondan M, et al: Mentalization-based treatment in groups for adolescents with borderline personality disorder (BPD) or subthreshold BPD versus treatment as usual (M-GAB): study protocol for a randomized controlled trial. Trials 17(1):314, 2016 27405522

Bo S, Sharp C, Beck E, et al: First empirical evaluation of outcomes for mentalization-based group therapy for adolescents with BPD. Pers Disord 8(4):396–401, 2017a 27845526

Bo S, Sharp C, Fonagy P, et al: Hypermentalizing, attachment, and epistemic trust in adolescent BPD: clinical illustrations. Pers Disord 8(2):172–182, 2017b 26691672

Brand T, Hecke D, Rietz C, et al: Therapieeffekte mentalisierungsbasierter und psychodynamischer Gruppenpsychotherapie in einer randomisierten Tagesklinik-Studie. Gruppendyn Organberat 52:156–174, 2016

Burlingame GM, McClendon DT, Alonso J: Cohesion in group therapy. Psychotherapy (Chic) 48(1):34–42, 2011 21401272

Burlingame GM, Gleave R, Erekson D, et al: Differential effectiveness of group, individual, and conjoint treatments: an archival analysis of OQ-45 change trajectories. Psychother Res 26(5):556–572, 2016a 26170048

Burlingame GM, Seebeck JD, Janis RA, et al: Outcome differences between individual and group formats when identical and nonidentical treatments, patients, and doses are compared: a 25-year meta-analytic perspective. Psychotherapy (Chic) 53(4):446–461, 2016b 27918191

Farrell JM, Shaw IA, Webber MA: A schema-focused approach to group psychotherapy for outpatients with borderline personality disorder: a randomized controlled trial. J Behav Ther Exp Psychiatry 40(2):317–328, 2009 19176222

Folmo EJ, Karterud SW, Bremer K, et al: The design of the MBT-G adherence and quality scale. Scand J Psychol 58(4):341–349, 2017 28718968

Fonagy P: Playing with reality: the development of psychic reality and its malfunction in borderline personalities. Int J Psychoanal 76(Pt 1):39–44, 1995 7775035

Fonagy P, Luyten P, Allison E: Epistemic petrification and the restoration of epistemic trust: a new conceptualization of borderline personality disorder and its psychosocial treatment. J Pers Disord 29(5):575–609, 2015 26393477

Foulkes SH: Group Analytic Psychotherapy: Method and Principles. London, Gordon & Breach, 1975

Hecke D, Brand T, Rietz C, et al: Prozess-Outcome-Studie zum Gruppenklima in psychodynamischer und mentalisierungsbasierter Gruppenpsychotherapie in einem tagesklinischen Setting. Gruppendyn Organberat 52:175–192, 2016

Hoag MJ, Burlingame GM: Evaluating the effectiveness of child and adolescent group treatment: a meta-analytic review. J Clin Child Psychol 26(3):234–246, 1997 9292381

Karterud S: Mentalization-Based Group Therapy (MBT-G): A Theoretical, Clinical, and Research Manual. Oxford, UK, Oxford University Press, 2015a

Karterud S: On structure and leadership in mentalization-based group therapy and group analysis. Group Analysis 48:137–149, 2015b

Kongerslev MT, Chanen AM, Simonsen E: Personality disorder in childhood and adolescence comes of age: a review of the current evidence and prospects for future research. Scand J Child Adolesc Psychiatry Psychol 3:31–48, 2015

Kvarstein EH, Pedersen G, Urnes Ø, et al: Changing from a traditional psychodynamic treatment programme to mentalization-based treatment for patients with borderline personality disorder—does it make a difference? Psychol Psychother 88(1):71–86, 2015 25045028

Kvarstein EH, Nordviste O, Dragland L, et al: Outpatient psychodynamic group psychotherapy—-outcomes related to personality disorder, severity, age and gender. Pers Ment Health 11(1):37–50, 2017 27766761

Lana F, Marcos S, Mollà L, et al: Mentalization based group psychotherapy for psychosis: a pilot study to assess safety, acceptance and subjective efficacy. International Journal of Psychology and Psychoanalysis 1(2):007, 2015

Lemma A, Target M, Fonagy P: Brief Dynamic Interpersonal Therapy: A Clinician's Guide. Oxford, UK, Oxford University Press, 2011

Linehan MM, Korslund KE, Harned MS, et al: Dialectical behavior therapy for high suicide risk in individuals with borderline personality disorder: a randomized clinical trial and component analysis. JAMA Psychiatry 72(5):475–482, 2015 25806661

Lorentzen S: Comments on Karterud's "On structure and leadership in mentalization-based group therapy and group analysis," June 2015. Group Analysis 49:70–77, 2015

Macgowan MJ, Wagner EF: Iatrogenic effects of group treatment on adolescents with conduct and substance use problems: a review of the literature and a presentation of a model. J Evidence-Based Soc Work 2(1–2):79–90, 2005 20396587

Marziali E, Munroe-Blum H: Interpersonal Group Psychotherapy for Borderline Personality Disorder. New York, Basic Books, 1994

Marziali E, Munroe-Blum H: An interpersonal approach to group psychotherapy with borderline personality disorder. J Pers Disord 9:179–189, 1995

Monk CS, McClure EB, Nelson EE, et al: Adolescent immaturity in attention-related brain engagement to emotional facial expressions. Neuroimage 20(1):420–428, 2003 14527602

Petersen B, Toft J, Christensen NB, et al: A 2-year follow-up of mentalization-oriented group therapy following day hospital treatment for patients with personality disorders. Pers Ment Health 4:294–301, 2010

Potthoff P, Moini-Afchari U: Mentalization-based treatment in groups—a paradigm shift or old wine in new skin? Group Analysis 47:3–16, 2014

Rutan JS, Stone W, Shay J: Psychodynamic Group Psychotherapy, 4th Edition. New York, Guilford Press, 2007

Steinberg L: Cognitive and affective development in adolescence. Trends Cogn Sci 9(2):69–74, 2005 15668099

Teicher JD: Group psychotherapy with adolescents. Calif Med 105(1):18–21, 1966 18730009

Vetter NC, Leipold K, Kliegel M, et al: Ongoing development of social cognition in adolescence. Child Neuropsychol 19(6):615–629, 2013 22934659

Weissman MM, Markowitz JC, Klerman GK: Comprehensive Guide to Interpersonal Psychotherapy. New York, Basic Books, 2000

Wilfley DE, Mackenzie KR, Welch RR, et al: Interpersonal Psychotherapy for Group. New York, Basic Books, 2000

CHAPTER 8

WORKING WITH FAMILIES

Eia Asen, M.D.
Nick Midgley, Ph.D.

Over the past decade, mentalization-based treatment (MBT) concepts and techniques have been adopted and adapted by a considerable number of family therapists and systemic practitioners to fit their practice. At the same time, a family-focused form of MBT has emerged, and various attempts have been made to manualize this approach (Asen and Fonagy 2012b; Fearon et al. 2006; Keaveny et al. 2012). A web-based "wiki-manual" (https://manuals.annafreud.org/mbtf), which runs in existing web browsers, can easily be searched and is automatically indexed.

Given the seeming use of well-tested techniques developed by systemic practitioners, there is some debate about whether it is justified to see this way of working as a new "brand" of family therapy, or simply as a new emphasis within systemic practice, with some new (but plenty of rather familiar) techniques. As a specific model of family therapy, the approach was originally termed *short-term mentalization and relational therapy* (SMART; Fearon et al. 2006) and later renamed *mentalization-based treatment for families* (MBT-F; Keaveny et al. 2012). In this chapter, however, we will refer to *mentalization-based approaches to working with families*, recognizing that in some cases what is described may be a set of concepts and techniques that can be grafted on to other systemic approaches, whereas in others it may form a more explicit model of therapy, with its own framework, guiding principles, and therapeutic techniques. In either case, we would suggest, it may be helpful to first place its development within the broader history of systemic family therapy.

DEVELOPMENT OF MENTALIZATION-BASED APPROACHES TO WORKING WITH FAMILIES

To adopt a systemic perspective implies viewing the individual and his or her presenting problems and difficulties in the following ways: 1) in the context of the family and other close relationships and 2) within the wider sociocultural setting of which the person and his or her family are part (Bowen 1978). Adopting this lens constituted a significant shift among clinicians working with families from an intrapsychic to an interpersonal (Ackerman 1967), if not social, paradigm, with little space and place for the exploration of the individual's own state of mind or internal world.

The emergence of "second-order cybernetics" (Hoffman 1981) and the social constructionist approach (Gergen 1994) challenged the seemingly reductionist biomedical and behavioral models of mainstream psychiatry and psychology. Therapy developed into a collaborative exploration of the different meanings and beliefs held by the members of the system. The therapist's stance became characterized by an inquiring and respectful attitude and "benign curiosity" (Cecchin 1987), with an awareness of the limits of an individual's knowledge of others, thereby also questioning the "expert" position of therapists. Therapists were guided by the concept of "safe uncertainty" (Mason 1993), acknowledging that an individual can never know, but only guess, what other people are thinking and feeling. It is "safe" in that this stance does not lead to the person becoming totally perplexed or overwhelmed by what may be happening in the minds of others. Gradually, systemic practitioners began to link the intrapersonal and interpersonal worlds again (Akister and Reibstein 2004; Dallos 2006; Diamond and Siqueland 1998; Flaskas 2002; Fraenkel and Pinsof 2001) and to review ideas and concepts from the psychoanalytic world. Above all, it was the work of Bateman and Fonagy (2006) that awakened the interest of systemic therapists in the concept of mentalizing, and this led to the development of mentalization-based family approaches.

MENTALIZING DIFFICULTIES IN THE FAMILY CONTEXT

As set out more fully in Chapter 1 ("Introduction"), mentalizing is important for representing, communicating, and regulating feelings and belief states linked to an individual's wishes and desires. It enables family members to create pictures of the thoughts, feelings, and intentions of those around them and helps to make sense of their actions. However, in situations of stress, difficulties in mentalizing almost inevitably arise, and if balanced mentalizing cannot be restored, emotionally charged interactions tend to evolve in families, potentially leading to a temporary loss of capacity to think about the thoughts and feelings of others and the self in an effective way (Fonagy and Luyten 2009). Automatic mentalizing may operate, with the reemergence of prementalizing or nonmentalizing (see Chapter 1) modes of family functioning. This can result in individual family members finding it difficult to check and reflect on their own mental states, let alone align them with those of other family members.

For example, when a father is stressed, his mind might become temporarily closed to seeing his daughter from a perspective other than his own. So when she is calling out for him to come and play with her while he is cooking a meal, he might see this as her just "being difficult," and tell her to be quiet and get on with something on her own. If the child feels that she is not being meaningfully responded to, she might escalate her behavior to "get through" to the father in the hope that her experience will be responded to by the trusted parent. However, the intensification of the child's behavior is likely to further derail the father's capacity to mentalize; the father and daughter are quite likely to end up in a vicious cycle of nonmentalizing. In other words, the child's emotional need and arousal may compromise the parent's capacity to provide the psychological recognition that the child craves. This happens a lot in family life and is by no means uncommon. But when this nonmentalizing is chronic, it can lead to more serious difficulties (see Box 8–1). When mentalizing is (temporarily) absent in family interactions, violence is more likely to take place. It also undermines and destroys the sense of safety required to engage in mentalizing self and others.

BOX 8–1. Mentalizing in family relationships

- Key proposition: emotional and behavioral problems are essentially relational in nature.

- Consideration, interpretation, and appraisal of mental states (in self and others) are all essential for healthy relationships.

- Family interactions, by their very nature, are likely to provoke breakdowns in mentalizing.

- Families and individuals vary in their capacity to mentalize for a multitude of reasons (e.g., genetics, early experience, trauma, current stressors).

- Chronic problems with mentalizing can generate distressing and stressful family interactions, which further undermine mentalizing.

- These distressing and stressful interactions may give rise to relational problems that undermine family coping, creativity, and resilience.

Conversely, being mentalized in the context of attachment relationships in the family generates epistemic trust (see Chapter 1) within that family unit. Even if a parent is not able to stop what he or she is doing and go to play with the child, recognizing that the child's wish to have the parent nearby may come from anxiety, excitement, or a worry that the parent has forgotten him or her, can help to build attachments. Epistemic hypervigilance, on the other hand, manifests as oversensitivity to difficult social interactions. When family members find it difficult to interpret the reasons for the actions of others, they may not be able to set aside or put out of their mind potentially upsetting memories of experiences within the family, leaving them even more vulnerable to experiencing emotional storms. When the capacity to create bonds of trust within a family breaks down, experiences created by the family itself become exceedingly difficult for the individual to contain or process. This is commonly the immediate trigger for the experience of "losing it" and showing violence, or for a deterioration in emotional well-being expressed in some other way.

AIMS OF MENTALIZATION-BASED FAMILY APPROACHES

The major aims of mentalization-based family approaches are to engage the family in discussions of problem-relevant situations, to elicit and highlight emerging feeling states and their importance, and to promote curiosity about mental states and their connections with the behavior of the self and others. These aims apply irrespective of whether the approach is being used as a standalone intervention or as an "add-on" by clinicians who are already practicing some form of systemic family therapy. In this sense the approach is not a new brand of therapy as such, as many of its techniques are based on well-known systemic practices; however, it has a unique focus, namely, to address mentalizing processes within the family context. It focuses on both thoughts and emotions as clues to what goes on in people's minds, and it both pays attention to emotional regulation and tries to affect it. One major specific goal may be to increase the felt understanding that parents or other caregivers have for their children and—depending on the developmental stages of the children—vice versa. The main objectives of mentalization-based family approaches are shown in Box 8–2.

BOX 8–2. **Objectives of mentalization-based family approaches**

- To consider each person's involvement in and contributions to the problem behavior of the symptomatic family member(s) and/or to family problems.

- To promote awareness of and curiosity about each individual's own and other people's mental states.

- To promote awareness of when the family's mentalizing capacity is vulnerable to breaking down.

- To use mentalizing to strengthen each person's capacity to regulate his or her feelings in the family context.

- To help families and their individual members shift from coercive, nonmentalizing cycles of interaction to effective mentalization-informed discussions and interactions.

- To promote trust and better attachments between children and parents.

- To promote parents' sense of competence in helping their children develop the capacity for mentalizing self and others.

- To practice skills related to mentalizing, particularly communication and problem solving in the specific areas in which mentalizing has been impeded or inhibited, which in turn will increase the capacity to make balanced reflective decisions.

- To initiate activities and create contexts where the family, friends, peers, professionals, and relevant others can engage in mentalizing, and in which experimenting with thoughts and feelings is mutually supported.

Mentalization-focused work can start at the point of referral: for example, on the telephone. Whether the therapist speaks to a referring professional or to a family member, speculation can be invited as to what members of the family might think or feel about being seen as a family. This can be done by asking specific questions, such as *"Who should attend the first session?" "What might the child feel if he is not invited and then finds out later that the parents have met without him?" "What might be the advantages and disadvantages of the mother coming on her own, without the father?" "What might each person feel about where the first meeting should take place?"*

From the very start, the enhancement of effective mentalizing is the primary focus of mentalization-based family therapy. To this end the therapist may, for example, often ask people to tentatively speculate about or label hidden feeling states of another of the family members. Furthermore, the therapist may actively encourage family members to name their own feelings and to openly reflect on how they may be affected by their feelings and how these effects might have an impact on others. In the end, good mentalizing is not only the individual's capacity to accurately read his or her own or another's inner states of mind and feelings, but also a way of approaching relationships that reflects an expectation that the individual's own thinking and feeling may be enlightened, enriched, and changed by learning about the mental states of other people (Fonagy and Target 1997).

THE THERAPIST'S STANCE

The objectives of mentalization-based family work are best achieved if the therapist can model a specific stance (see Box 8–3); this involves being inquiring and respectful in relation to everyone's mental states, and conveying that understanding the feelings of others is important—including what those feelings might be and what thoughts, meanings, and related experiences are attached or attributed to them. The therapist communicates this to the family as a whole but at the same time assists each individual family member to focus on what feelings are experienced by each person, as well as highlighting the ways in which miscommunication or misunderstanding of these feelings contributes to interactions that maintain family problems. In practice, therapists must strike a very careful balance between 1) creating a therapeutic context that allows the family to interact "naturally," including actively eliciting habitual and possibly problematic family interactions around difficult issues; and 2) being directive and intervening at critical moments.

BOX 8–3. **The therapist's stance**

- **Inquisitive**—constantly affirming the value of mentalizing by means of a respectful, curious, and tentative inquiring attitude.

- **Holding the balance** between observing natural interactions and intervening to promote change by helping family members make sense of what feelings are experienced by each family member, as well as highlighting ways in which miscommunication or misunderstanding (or lack of understanding) of these feelings lead to interactions that maintain family problems.

- **Terminating nonmentalizing interactions** and creating a context that can help create new and different perspectives, highlighting the missing perspective for each person in the family that leads to the behavior of others not being fully understood.

- **Highlighting and reinforcing effective mentalizing** and thereby deepening the family members' ability to connect feelings, thoughts, and intentions positively, noting good examples (or episodes) of mentalizing, possibly expanding on them and their implications.

Given that mentalization-based family work postulates that nonmentalizing interactions are unlikely to produce significant changes in family interactions, merely allowing these interactions to occur in sessions is unlikely to be therapeutic. Therefore, once therapists have a clear idea of the family's core mentalizing problems and once they have appropriate examples of related interactions to work with, they can intervene and actively bring nonmentalizing interactions to a halt, often followed by a process of "pause and review," where the family is invited to explore the nonmentalizing interactions that have just taken place. One major objective is to highlight the missing perspective for each family member and how this leads to the behavior of others in the family not being fully noticed and understood.

One of the underlying assumptions of the approach is the belief that mentalizing is part of a self-righting "gyroscopic" function of family systems, and that many difficulties within families can be improved if the family members' ability to think about one another's states of mind is promoted and freed from stumbling blocks and hindrances. A major risk for therapists lies in the contagious nature of nonmentalizing. Given that therapists are also vulnerable to breaks in mentalizing, they may find themselves becoming engaged with nonmentalizing interactions when faced with the challenge of contemplating genuinely destructive and malevolent thoughts and feelings that can exist but remain (for good reasons) ignored within family systems. Taking a mentalizing approach is *not* a panacea to eradicate impossible family conflicts. Simply drawing the family's attention to putative sources of hostility within the family (in other words, the promotion of insight) is unlikely to be successful, as nonmentalizing precludes the genuine contemplation of alternative ideas. If the therapist takes this approach, the best result that can be hoped for is moving the family from concrete psychic equivalence nonmentalizing to the pseudomentalizing pretend mode (see Chapter 1). The therapist must first aim to help the family members hold on to (or reestablish) mentalizing in the face of challenges to thinking and contemplating feelings where previously they have not succeeded. For this to happen, it is essential that the therapist has a structure or framework to support a mentalizing focus. One such framework is the *mentalizing loop*.

THE MENTALIZING LOOP

The mentalizing loop (Asen and Fonagy 2012a) is both a "route map" and a tool; it is a pragmatic framework for devising mentalization-based interventions that delineates the therapist's stance and allows him or her to support both his or her own and the family members' effective mentalizing. The process of identifying mentalizing loops is shared by a range of mentalization-based treatments; for example, in mentalization-based group therapy (MBT-G) for people with borderline personality disorder (BPD), the therapist follows similar steps. The framework is a loop because the process is not a linear progression of successive steps, but a recursive process of reviewing, leading to new observations, then to checking and newly observing, and so on (Figure 8–1). In employing the mentalizing loop, attention is drawn to specific interactions and communications between family members (or group members in MBT-G; see Chapter 7, "Group Therapy for Adults and Adolescents"), such as expressions of irritation, disbelief, confusion, humiliation, or frustration. Focusing explicitly on one of these states of mind in the here and now—by "noticing and naming" it— has the effect of putting family interactions temporarily on pause.

The loop is started when the therapist puts an observation into words, that is, using his or her external mentalizing focus; for example: *"I notice that when Mum talked about all the screaming that went on last night, Dad started to look quite angry and Mary had tears in her eyes...has anyone else here noticed this?"* Highlighting this observed interaction sequence has the effect of halting what could become a cycle of nonmentalizing statements, reactions, and counterreactions. However, before proceeding any further, the therapist needs to do some "checking" of whether the family members can connect with the descriptions

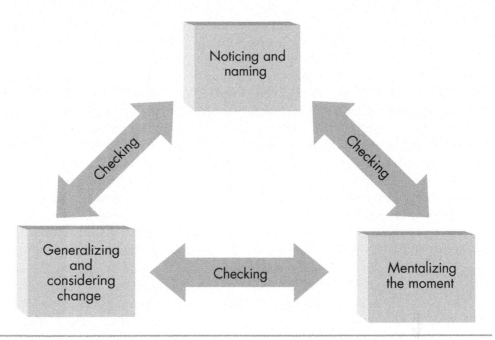

FIGURE 8–1.   **The mentalizing loop.**

he or she has given: *"Have I got that right? Do you see it that way?"* This is moving the family from the external focus of the mentalizing initiated by the therapist to an internal focus on underlying mental states. In this way, the therapist communicates that the observation and punctuation of the sequence of events was the therapist's own perspective and that it needs to now become an "object" for mutual examination by the family members, who are invited to consider what has been highlighted. If there is some recognition by them, the therapist can explicitly focus on the here-and-now processes and get family members to "mentalize the moment" by asking, for example, *"Can you put yourselves into Mary's shoes and just imagine what she might have been thinking or feeling that brought tears to her eyes? What do you think went on inside her at that point?"*

This is an invitation for the parents to mentalize their child; it is generally preferable for parents to do this before looking at their own mental states. The therapist can pursue the matter further by then getting each parent to mentalize themselves: *"And when you see Mary in that state, what feelings does that produce inside yourself?"*

When a parent speculates about what might have gone on in the child's mind—*mentalizing the moment*, as it were—it is the therapist's next task to assist the parent in checking out his or her ideas with other family members. For example, the therapist might say: *"Dad thinks that Mary is feeling happy that we are talking openly—Mum, is that what you think went on for Mary? And I wonder what her brother thinks was going on…if you could see thought bubbles coming out of your wife's head, what might be written in them?"* In this way, the therapist encourages the family members to bring in their respective perspectives, to brainstorm—or rather "mindstorm"—about states of mind, and to always check with others whether they see matters similarly or differently. The process of continuous checking—which includes the therapist—creates a loop: what has been noticed is named, and what has been named is questioned, and perceptions are checked all around (Asen and Fonagy 2017).

When family members are encouraged to rewind and review a specific sequence in this way, a metaperspective is generated, which can reignite an effective mentalizing stance. At some point, the therapist may ask a family member to connect the here-and-now mental states with similar situations that may have arisen in the course of everyday family life, and to link the specifics of the interactions occurring in the session to the more habitual patterns that unfold at home. What has been observed in the here and now of the session is "looped out" into real-life situations in an attempt to identify and address typical problem situations. This leads to family discussions of problem situations, and the focus remains on eliciting and highlighting emerging feeling states and how these express themselves in behaviors. A simple open question can achieve this: *"Have you noticed that this sort of thing is also happening at home? And if so, how might you manage it differently next time something like this happens?"* It is this shift to *generalizing and considering change* that aims to stimulate family members' own ideas and solutions. If the process leads to proposals by one family member, then it is *noticed and named* by the therapist: *"I can see that Dad thinks if this happens, Mum should take him calmly aside and not talk in front of your daughter—have I got that right?"* and the "checking" loop starts again.

It is possible to encourage individuals and families to mentalize in three different time dimensions: in the here and now (*mentalizing the moment*); retrospectively; and prospectively. This process can be termed *diachronic mentalizing*. When, for example, asking about a recent family crisis, it is possible to explore the states of mind of each family member at that time (retrospective mentalizing): *"And what do you think went on in your daughter's mind when she saw the two of you arguing?"* The states of mind of each family member at the time of the family crisis can be tracked carefully, maybe leading the therapist to then say: *"I notice that when you talk about it now, your mum looks away—what might this be about, and what does it make you feel?"* thereby bringing mentalizing back into the present. It is also possible to consider hypothetical scenarios and get family members to engage in prospective mentalizing: *"Imagine next Monday morning, you want your child not to be late for school, but you keep arguing about it—what might go on in her head, and how might this affect you?"*

In summary, it is the therapist's task to slow down the interactions between family members, questioning or expressing a specific interest in exactly what each person is feeling as interactions unfold, to temporarily pause the flow of exchanges between family members and permit further reflections all around. The aim is for the family discourse to gradually shift away from discussing a specific interaction that occurred during the session and move toward "widening the lens" and capturing more generalized understandings relating to this specific observation.

SPECIFIC TECHNIQUES TO ENHANCE EFFECTIVE MENTALIZING

Mentalization-based family work aims to identify and enhance *effective mentalizing*: this does *not* mean that the therapist has to be incessantly reflective and invite family members to mentalize explicitly at all times. There are various ingredients of effective mentalizing (see Box 8–4), and individual family members may have some of these mentalizing strengths and lack others. It is the lack of specific aspects of effective mentalizing that can be targeted via specific interventions.

For example, benign curiosity may be stimulated via reflective and circular questions that aim to awaken the interest of family members in the thoughts and feelings

BOX 8–4. **Main ingredients of effective mentalizing**

- **Benign curiosity:** Genuine interest in other people's thoughts and feelings, and respectful of the respective perspectives of others.

- **Safe uncertainty** (Mason 1993) or **opaqueness of mental states** (Leslie 1987): Open acknowledgment that the individual can never know but can only make informed guesses as to what other people are thinking and feeling.

- **Reflective contemplation:** Pursuit of how others think and feel in a way that is flexible, relaxed, and open, rather than controlled and compulsive.

- **Perspective taking:** Acceptance that the same situation or process can look very different from different standpoints.

- **Forgiveness:** Comprehension of the actions of others when understanding and accepting their mental states.

- **Impact awareness:** Appreciation of how the individual's own thoughts, feelings, and actions may affect others.

- **Trusting attitude:** Ability to have faith in others and take a nonparanoid stance.

- **Humility:** Potential for self-effacement and unpretentious modesty.

- **Inner conflict awareness:** "Tuned-in" to the individual's own opposing thoughts and feelings.

- **Playfulness and (self-mocking) humor:** Capacity to be "bouncy" and laugh with others about himself or herself.

- **Willingness to take turns:** Ability to "give and take" in interactions with family members and significant others.

- **Faith in changeability:** Belief that minds can change or be changed and a sense of optimism about the therapeutic enterprise.

- **Assuming responsibility:** Acceptance of accountability for the individual's own actions.

of their loved ones. A lack of perspective taking can be addressed by the "stepping into someone else's shoes" exercise. Here, each family member takes a piece of paper, places their feet on it, and draws the outlines of their shoes. They are asked to think about a specific problem or misunderstanding and, after a few minutes, stand up and then sit down on the chair of another family member, placing their feet into the other family member's shoe outlines. The family members are now asked to continue the discussion but to assume the perspective of the previous inhabitant of the chair. This can be repeated a few times until all positions and perspectives have been explored by each family member. Many interventions aimed at enhancing specific ingredients of effective mentalizing employ playful techniques and games, involving masks, "mind mirroring," mind-reading tools such as stethoscopes and "parento-scopes," "mind maps," and "mind scans" (Asen and Fonagy 2012b, 2017). This is partly because playfulness is an inherently mentalizing-promoting state of mind and is a fertile ground for learning about mental states (Panksepp 2007; Slade 1994).

A major goal is for family members to achieve balanced mentalizing: a balance between reasons and feelings, intuition and reflection, thinking about their own reactions and the experiences of others, and between looking inward to mental states and outward to situations. Therapeutically, this balance can be achieved by strengthening the opposite pole to the one the discourse appears to consistently favor. For example, an excessive reliance on cognition needs to be balanced by helping family members focus on the emotional impact of firmly held ideas.

There are different ways of shifting the balance, but this is often best achieved by asking questions that favor the "neglected" pole—that is, using contrary moves (see Chapter 1)—with the aim of stimulating mentalizing. Typical examples are provided in Box 8–5.

BOX 8–5. **Examples of mentalizing questions**

- What do you make of what has just happened/is happening right now?

- What were you thinking during the situation? How did you feel?

- Why do you think your child's reaction is different or similar to yours?

- What might your child have been thinking or wishing for when he or she became scared/upset/angry/argumentative?

- What do you think your child might have thought you were feeling? How might this have left him or her feeling?

- What would your child have wanted or needed from you? What do you think he or she needs now?

- If we could see "thought bubbles" coming out of his or her head, what might be written in them?

- What might the father have felt or thought when he suddenly became so irritated?

MENTALIZING APPROACHES WITH FAMILIES IN DIFFERENT CONTEXTS

The mentalization-based approach is used not only for "traditional" family work but also in other settings, such as with looked-after children where foster carers may be involved, and in a variety of different contexts, such as in nurseries, preschools, and schools.

For example, a mentalization-based approach developed from MBT-F is currently being evaluated in a small-scale feasibility clinical trial, in a specialist child mental health service in the United Kingdom for looked-after children (Midgley et al. 2017; see also Chapter 16, "Parenting and Foster Care"). The approach also includes work with the network around the child, including the social care system, which is often vulnerable to mentalizing breakdowns at a systems level (see Chapter 13, "AMBIT: Engaging the Client and Communities of Minds," and Bevington et al. 2017).

Likewise, "Adopting Minds" is an adaptation of mentalization-based work with families used specifically in the context of postadoption support. The approach recognizes the particular challenges faced by adoptive families and the significant relational risks both adopters and their adopted children often face in working together to become a family. Adopted children with past histories of abuse, neglect, and loss are more likely to misread and misinterpret their adoptive parents' intentions in trying to provide parenting; in turn, adoptive parents may have difficulty "reading" the children placed with them, who may offer confusing signals about their needs. The Adopting Minds approach pays close attention to how past history may have an impact on the here and now, and carefully monitors and manages the arousal levels of all family members to provide a "safe enough" experience of thinking together (Tasker and Wood 2016). The aim of the work is to help build trust, improve relationships, and help parents and children who have experienced trauma understand one another better. A naturalistic evaluation of this approach is currently under way, and preliminary findings (Midgley et al. 2018) suggest that this short-term intervention improves parental self-efficacy and children's emotional well-being. Qualitative data suggest that families see the service as a space for receiving support and containment, which provides a context where negative feelings are allowed and achievements praised, helping adopted children and their families to deal better with their past experiences. Two small-scale studies have examined the process by which this may be achieved: one examining how this approach can help to establish epistemic trust in families who may initially be cautious about receiving help (Jaffrani 2017), and the other exploring the way in which a therapist may draw on expert knowledge about adoption while retaining the not-knowing stance that is a key feature of this approach (Sunley 2017).

Mentalization-based therapy with families has also been adapted for use in a hospital setting with preschool-age children (Salo et al. 2016). As with older children, mentalization-based family work with infants, toddlers, and preschoolers aims to improve the stressful family interactions that are often related to young children's basic attachment needs, and to regulatory, behavioral, and socioemotional problems. As in the approach developed for school-age children, the main aim when working with younger children is to help the family members—here especially the parents—to explicitly notice and name any unhelpful interaction patterns and, by doing so, cultivate deeper understanding of each other's perspectives and needs. Compared with the approach to mentalization-based family therapy with older children, working with infants and toddlers calls for an understanding of how to work with the prementalizing modes of psychic equivalence and teleology. From a mentalizing perspective, the most important skills present in mentalization-based work with families are attention control (joint attention) and affect regulation through marked mirroring of the parents (Salo et al. 2016). Thus, much of the work also becomes more implicit or embodied (Shai and Fonagy 2013): how to help the infant attune and orient toward other family members, and how to help the infant to regulate his or her affects and start paying attention to others' emotions and—eventually—start labeling these internal states with words.

Another adaptation of mentalization-based therapeutic work with families, multi-family therapy, consists of working simultaneously with six to eight families who share similar problems and/or disorders. The work has evolved since the 1950s and has many applications (Asen 2002; Asen and Scholz 2010), including in schools (Dawson and McHugh 1994). The multifamily setting would seem to be an excellent context for practicing mentalizing (see Box 8–6).

Finally, a mentalizing intervention for families who are living with or caring for a person with BPD, Families and Carers Training and Support (MBT-FACTS; https://www.annafreud.org/training/mentalization-based-treatment-training/families-and-carers-training-and-support-programme-facts), has been developed and studied

BOX 8–6. **Multifamily therapy as a setting for practicing mentalizing**

The multifamily setting facilitates:

- Observing other families and their interactions and speculating about their mental states.

- Being exposed to multiple descriptions of the individual's own mental states provided by members of other families, and checking these with his or her own perceptions.

- Observing and experiencing attachment issues (such as seeking proximity) in other families from a "safe" distance and without increased arousal.

- Experiencing different "attachment behaviors" when being cared for briefly by another parent/when looking after the child of another parent.

- Experiencing and discussing attachment issues in a group setting.

- The individual seeing himself or herself and his or her own family "mirrored" in others who have similar problems and issues.

- Experimenting with pretend mode via playful group activities.

- Intensifying interactions and raising arousal levels, followed by affect control/regulation exercises.

- Viewing audiovisual recordings of problematic interactions made for a later video feedback session, when arousal levels are lowered.

in a randomized controlled trial (Bateman and Fonagy 2018). The intervention was delivered over five sessions by family members trained in the program to groups of family members. The research study is outlined in the next section of this chapter.

EVIDENCE BASE OF MENTALIZING WORK WITH FAMILIES

By its very nature, mentalization-based work with families encourages the therapist to invite different perspectives on the work and to engage with the views of different family members. As such, research and evaluation should be central to the approach, and there is clearly a need for more work to be done in this area. Although at least one clinical trial is currently under way (Midgley et al. 2017), to date the evaluation studies that have been carried out have been relatively small-scale and have mostly taken place in the United Kingdom.

For example, a naturalistic evaluation of the effectiveness of short-term (up to 10 sessions) MBT work with families was carried out at the Anna Freud National Centre for Children and Families (for full details, see Keaveny et al. 2012). The findings from the parent-report Strengths and Difficulties Questionnaire (Goodman 1997) suggested that the MBT approach with families led to a statistically significant reduction in behavioral and emotional difficulties in children and young people. Over the course of therapy, parents reported an overall reduction in the impact that their child's difficulties were having on both individual and family functioning. Similar results were found on therapist-report measures. However, given the relatively small sample size ($N=30$), these findings should be treated with caution.

In a small-scale qualitative study carried out in the same service (Etelaapa 2011), five families were interviewed in greater depth about their experience of the service.

Most parents spoke about their sense of "stuckness" prior to starting therapy and went on to describe the ways they felt the therapy had helped them. For example, one mother said: *"For me it was an eye-opener…When you're a mum, you tend to be involved in efficiency. It's hard to sit down with them [and say] 'Tell me about this or what does it feel?'…[The therapy] made me see her more like an individual rather than an extension of me…She has her own thoughts, own feelings, and if you don't ask her, then you lose. You miss out. You don't know her really."*

When asked to reflect on the impact of the therapies, most of the young people (ages 8–15) commented on the importance of feeling listened to and understood, and some described the way in which the sessions had affected the relationships within their family. For example, one teenage girl said: *"Now we're just like…we shout. But then after we try to calm down and then we start talking to each other…it's kinda getting resolved step by step…. And we kinda think that the meetings kinda brought us together. Like even after the meetings we felt more together"* (Etelaapa 2011).

In the MBT-FACTS trial (Bateman and Fonagy 2018), 56 family members or significant others living with and supporting individuals with a diagnosis of BPD were randomly assigned to receive either the MBT-FACTS immediately or a delayed intervention. The primary outcome was adverse incidents reported by the family member in relation to the person with BPD. Secondary outcomes included self-reported family well-being, empowerment, burden, and levels of anxiety and depression. Family members randomly assigned to the immediate intervention reported a significant reduction in adverse incidents between themselves and the identified patient in the second phase of treatment compared with those assigned to delayed intervention. Family functioning and well-being improved more in the immediate-treatment group, and changes were maintained at follow-up of up to 3 months. Interestingly, there were no differences in depression, total anxiety, and total burden; both groups showed improvement on all these measures, suggesting that the experience of joining a research trial and being offered support is itself helpful.

CONCLUSION

The small-scale evaluation studies described in this chapter indicate that families can be helped by a mentalization-based approach and that this way of working makes sense to families themselves. Further research is urgently needed, however, to explore whether a mentalization-based approach is effective either as a standalone model of therapy or as a supplement to existing approaches to working with families.

For the time being, we would argue that a mentalization-based approach can best be seen as offering an underlying rationale for focusing on mental states as part of *any* therapeutic work with families, as well as a range of pragmatic tips that we hope clinicians working with families will find useful. Fundamentally, these relate to the basic therapeutic stance that a mentalization-based approach entails: showing a genuine interest in wanting to understand family members' different perspectives (even those not currently in the room); paying careful attention to levels of arousal and noticing when family mentalizing appears to go "offline"; noticing and naming family patterns of interaction and working with them directly in the here and now; exploring ideas, needs, and emotions in a relational context; and the therapist remembering to mentalize himself or herself—in other words, the therapist paying attention to his or her own mental states and being prepared to openly explore the impact these may have on the family.

Working in this way with families can at times leave therapists feeling vulnerable, and the approach demands a commitment to being genuinely open-minded—both in the sense of the therapist being prepared to share his or her own "mental workings" with families, so that they can understand where the therapist is coming from, but also in the sense of the therapist being open to having his or her own mind changed and of coming to see things differently himself or herself. We believe that a mentalization-based approach to working with families not only stimulates clinicians and other professionals to view families and their individual members, but also provides families with an opportunity to step out of fixed patterns of relating that perpetuate difficult behaviors, and offers them new ways of being together—enriched by seeing others from the inside, and themselves from the outside.

REFERENCES

Ackerman NW: Treating the Troubled Family. New York, Basic Books, 1967

Akister J, Reibstein J: Links between attachment theory and systemic practice: some proposals. J Fam Ther 26:2–16, 2004

Asen E: Multiple family therapy: an overview. J Fam Ther 24:3–16, 2002

Asen E, Fonagy P: Mentalization-based family therapy, in Handbook of Mentalizing in Mental Health Practice. Edited by Bateman A, Fonagy P. Arlington, VA, American Psychiatric Publishing, 2012a, pp 107–128

Asen E, Fonagy P: Mentalization-based therapeutic interventions for families. J Fam Ther 34:347–370, 2012b

Asen E, Fonagy P: Mentalizing family violence. Part 2: Techniques and interventions. Fam Process 56(1):22–44, 2017 28133724

Asen E, Scholz M: Multi-Family Therapy: Concepts and Techniques. London, Routledge, 2010

Bateman A, Fonagy P: Mentalization-Based Treatment for Borderline Personality Disorder: A Practical Guide. Oxford, UK, Oxford University Press, 2006

Bateman A, Fonagy P: A randomized controlled trial of a mentalization-based intervention (MBT-FACTS) for families of people with borderline personality disorder. Pers Disord 2018 [Epub ahead of print] 29999394

Bevington D, Fuggle P, Cracknell L, et al: Adaptive Mentalization-Based Integrative Treatment: A Guide for Teams to Develop Systems of Care. Oxford, UK, Oxford University Press, 2017

Bowen M: Family Therapy in Clinical Practice. New York, Jason Aronson, 1978

Cecchin G: Hypothesizing, circularity, and neutrality revisited: an invitation to curiosity. Fam Process 26(4):405–413, 1987 3319683

Dallos R: Attachment Narrative Therapy. New York, Open University Press, 2006

Dawson N, McHugh B: Parents and children: participants in change, in The Family and the School: A Joint Systems Approach to Problems With Children, 2nd Edition. Edited by Dowling E, Osborne E. London, Routledge, 1994, pp 81–101

Diamond GS, Siqueland L: Emotions, attachments and relational reframe. J Struct Strateg Ther 17:36–50, 1998

Etelaapa K: Families' experiences of Mentalization Based Treatment for Families (MBT-F). MSc. London, University College London, 2011

Fearon P, Target M, Fonagy P, et al: Short-Term Mentalization and Relational Therapy (SMART): an integrative family therapy for children and adolescents, in Handbook of Mentalization-Based Treatment. Edited by Allen JG, Fonagy P. New York, Wiley, 2006

Flaskas C: Family Therapy Beyond Postmodernism. New York, Brunner-Routledge, 2002

Fonagy P, Luyten P: A developmental, mentalization-based approach to the understanding and treatment of borderline personality disorder. Dev Psychopathol 21(4):1355–1381, 2009 19825272

Fonagy P, Target M: Attachment and reflective function: their role in self-organization. Dev Psychopathol 9(4):679–700, 1997 9449001

Fraenkel P, Pinsof WM: Teaching family therapy-centred integration: assimilation and beyond. J Psychother Integration 11:59–85, 2001

Gergen KJ: Realities and Relationships: Soundings in Social Construction. Cambridge, MA, Harvard University Press, 1994

Goodman R: The Strengths and Difficulties Questionnaire: a research note. J Child Psychol Psychiatry 38(5):581–586, 1997 9255702

Hoffman L: Foundations of Family Therapy. A Conceptual Framework for Change. New York, Basic Books, 1981

Jaffrani A: The Creation of Epistemic Trust: A Case Study of an Adoptive Family's Experience of Mentalization-Based Therapy for Families. Research Department of Clinical, Educational and Health Psychology, University College London, 2017 [Unpublished manuscript]

Keaveny E, Midgley N, Asen E, et al: Minding the family mind: the development and initial evaluation of mentalization-based treatment for families, in Minding the Child: Mentalization-Based Interventions with Children, Young People and Their Families. Edited by Midgley N, Vrouva I. London, Routledge, 2012, pp 98–112

Leslie AM: Pretense and representation: the origins of "theory of mind." Psychol Rev 94:412–426, 1987

Mason B: Towards positions of safe uncertainty. Human Systems: The Journal of Systemic Consultation and Management 4:189–200, 1993

Midgley N, Besser SJ, Dye H, et al: The Herts and Minds study: evaluating the effectiveness of mentalization-based treatment (MBT) as an intervention for children in foster care with emotional and/or behavioural problems: a phase II, feasibility, randomised controlled trial. Pilot Feasibility Stud 3:12, 2017 28250962

Midgley N, Alayza A, Lawrence H, et al: Adopting Minds: a mentalization-based therapy for families in a post-adoption support service: preliminary evaluation and service user experience. Adopt Foster 42:22–37, 2018

Panksepp J: Can PLAY diminish ADHD and facilitate the construction of the social brain? J Can Acad Child Adolesc Psychiatry 16(2):57–66, 2007 18392153

Salo S, Fontell T, Aronen E, et al: Feasibility Study of MBT-F with Pre-School Aged Children. Psychiatric Center for Young Children, Helsinki University Central Hospital, 2016 [Unpublished manuscript]

Shai D, Fonagy P: Beyond words: parental embodied mentalizing and the parent-infant dance, in Mechanisms of Social Connection from Brain to Group. Edited by Mikulincer M, Shaver PR. Washington, DC, American Psychological Association, 2013, pp 185–203

Slade A: Making meaning and making believe: their role in the clinical process, in Children at Play: Clinical and Developmental Approaches to Meaning and Representation. Edited by Slade A, Wolf D. New York, Oxford University Press, 1994, pp 81–110

Sunley T: How Does a Mentalization-Based Therapist Use Their Expert Knowledge in Work With Adopted Families? Research Department of Clinical, Educational and Health Psychology, University College London, 2017 [Unpublished manuscript]

Tasker F, Wood S: The transition into adoptive parenthood: adoption as a process of continued unsafe uncertainty when family scripts collide. Clin Child Psychol Psychiatry 21(4):520–535, 2016 27026662

CHAPTER 9

COUPLES THERAPY

Efrain Bleiberg, M.D.
Ellen Safier, M.S.W., LCSW

Marriage—or any intimate partnership—is arguably the closest experience most people have to being a patient in therapy. In a couple relationship, we face uncomfortable truths about ourselves—those aspects of our self that expose our greatest fears and vulnerabilities and feel "alien," that are not well integrated into the narrative we have constructed of ourselves. But it is also in our intimate partnerships that our deepest longings and most tender needs and expectations come to life. Evolution based not only our physical and emotional survival but also our cognitive and social survival on our attachment partner's disposition to respond to us in a timely, protective, and soothing manner. However, such reliance on another person's response leaves us vulnerable to the indifference, misunderstanding, or malevolence of others.

Arguably, the evolutionary "solution" to protect us from this inherent vulnerability, involving the risk of the humiliation that our signals of distress and bids for affiliation will not matter to the other or will leave us open to be taken advantage of, was to privilege attachment as the context in which we acquire the capacity to understand—that is, to *mentalize*—other people's intentions. Mentalizing gives us access to the emotional and psychological heart of ourselves and others. It is a capacity that anchors our subjective sense of self and our ability to decide who is trustworthy to engage in reciprocal, sustaining, effective relationships.

Adaptive functioning involves using mentalizing to ascertain when and how much to flexibly shift back and forth from more to less emotional distance and more to less trust with each person. When we "read" another person as trustworthy, the sense of emotional distance from that person decreases, and we experience a corresponding lessening of defensiveness. Importantly, the signal of trustworthiness, as Csibra and Gergely's infancy research suggests (Csibra and Gergely 2009, 2011; Gergely 2013), is to feel mentalized—that is, to feel that the other understands us "from the inside" and can put himself or herself "in our shoes." As that signal of trust is processed, some components of mentalizing are partially deactivated, and with these, the critical social judgment about the intentions, veracity, and usefulness of the other's communications. This is the process that Csibra and Gergely describe as *epistemic trust* (see Chapter 4, "Mentalizing, Resilience, and Epistemic Trust"). This crucial notion suggests that feeling understood, or experiencing that the other has our mind in mind, serves as a signal that that person is "safe" and we can "turn off" our defensiveness, allowing greater emotional and physical proximity, all the way to the experience of merging. This occurs when we fall in love, for which a partial abandonment of critical social judgment may be a necessary condition. The sense of trust thus generated allows us to believe in, internalize, generalize, and be disposed toward applying the knowledge we acquire from the other person, especially the tools to manage the feelings generated in relationships.

Mentalizing is also turned off when we feel threatened and we activate a defensive response. In those moments, it is often not safe to imagine what is in another person's mind—as is commonly seen in previously traumatized children—illustrating that defensive responses are activated not only by real threats but by our own "mentalizing holes" (see the discussion of the "alien self" in Chapter 1, "Introduction"), the legacy of adversity and vulnerability, and our efforts to cope with that legacy (see Chapter 5, "Mentalizing and Trauma"). The "holes" stem from contexts in which certain aspects of experience were not mentalized and integrated coherently into our self-representation, and are thus felt to be "alien" parts of the self, whose activation elicits a defensive response.

This defensive response involves an increase in the sense of emotional distance from the other person and a corresponding increase in arousal and the activation of the fight/flight/freeze response (Figure 9–1). As arousal and defensiveness increase, the automatic and controlled components of mentalizing (see Chapter 1) tend to uncouple, and the balance of these components, which is the hallmark of mentalizing, breaks down.

On the other hand, when that balance is restored, it is expressed in a set of attitudes—dispositions to perceive, think, feel, and respond—that correspond with the inquisitive stance we aim to model, teach, and promote in mentalization-based therapies. This stance is one of engagement, attention, optimal arousal, humility, curiosity, openness, respect, acceptance, and tolerance for not knowing that conveys a readiness to learn the other's thoughts, feelings, and intentions.

Nowhere, except perhaps in parenting, is the delicate balance between mentalizing, attachment, and defensiveness strained as severely as in the context of a couple's relationship. Divorce rates of around 50% in industrialized societies highlight the daunting odds faced by couples seeking to preserve their commitment. But, unlike parenting, which involves a legally mandated role as guardians of a dependent, marriage and commitment to living as a couple are increasingly seen as optional, resulting in bonds that, while no less significant, appear far more vulnerable.

As the containment offered to the couple by extended family and community has eroded in industrialized societies, intimate partners are left mostly with each other as the sole source of support and validation of their identity and self-worth, such that they are faced with enormous challenges to feel "seen" (Siegel 2013) and have a "secure base" (Bowlby 1988) from which to face and explore the world, a "safe harbor"

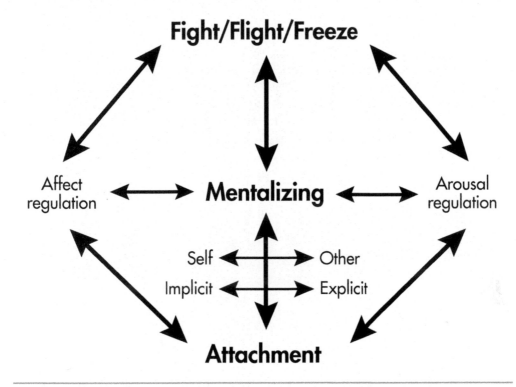

FIGURE 9–1.   Links between arousal, mentalizing, and behavior.

(Bowlby 1988) that offers soothing from the inevitable tribulations of life, and an arena in which to experience an intimate sexual relationship.

Such reliance on the other leaves intimate partners feeling vulnerable and increases the costs of being misunderstood. However, the human brain has also evolved a disposition to automatically respond with defensiveness (and a concomitant deactivation of mentalizing) to instances in which we are approached by other people showing defensive, nonmentalizing, coercive stances themselves—particularly those who are closest to us. This leads us to experience the greatest difficulty in remaining thoughtful with the people who are closest to us, not because they do not matter enough but because they matter "too much."

Transactional sequences are thus set in motion in which one member of the couple, displaying defensiveness and a loss of mentalizing, evokes a similar reaction in the other. The partner's defensive reaction, in turn, reignites nonmentalizing and fosters a vicious cycle of reactivity and dysregulation (Figure 9–2). More significantly, these cycles deprive the couple of the protective and restorative functions that intimate attachments provide, particularly epistemic trust and social learning.

At the heart of mentalization-based couples therapy (MBT-CO) is a systematic effort to stimulate and restore mentalizing and trust. The purpose is both to interrupt nonmentalizing and to help the couple use each other as a resource to update and adapt their sense of themselves, the other, and the relationship. Promoting mentalizing serves to signal the possibility of trust, which in turn opens the relationship to joint learning and exploration, mutual soothing, and the effective reciprocity that sustains in each partner a sense of coherence, hope, joy, and meaning. It replaces vicious

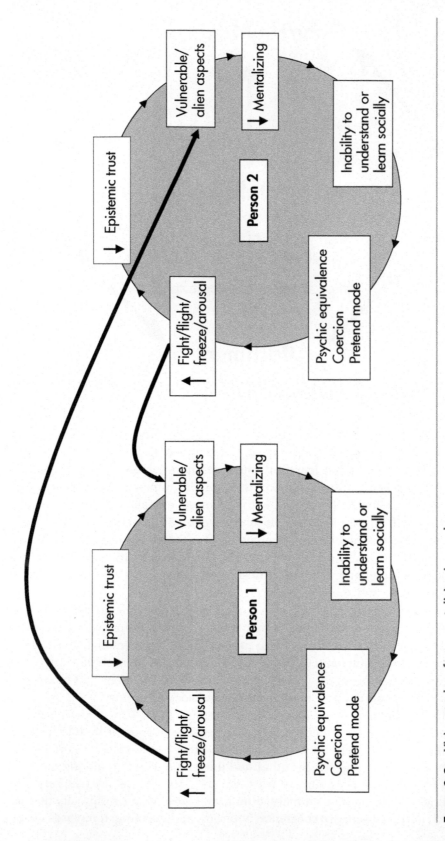

FIGURE 9–2.   Vicious cycles of nonmentalizing in couples.

with virtuous cycles in which understanding opens the opportunity for greater safety and connection.

In what follows we briefly outline the conceptual framework underlying MBT-CO as it is explicitly discussed with couples in treatment and describe the active ingredients and components.

GETTING STARTED WITH MBT-CO

The first stages of MBT-CO involve the following:

1. Educating the couple about mentalizing and epistemic trust, and how to recognize when the person himself or herself is mentalizing and trusting, and when he or she is not.
2. Assessing the couple and each member of the couple, with a particular emphasis on the following:
    a. Mentalizing strengths and vulnerabilities.
    b. How each person has an impact on the other's capacity to trust and mentalize.
    c. Specific interactional contexts in which breakdowns in mentalizing and epistemic trust occur.
    d. Coercive, nonmentalizing cycles that are generated in such contexts.
3. Sharing a formulation that explains the therapist's understanding of the couple's problems and proposes to address them by transforming nonmentalizing cycles into mentalizing conversations, particularly at the points of stress and vulnerability in which their ability to trust is most compromised.

Couple Sessions: Assessment, Education, and Mentalizing Stance

The assessment begins with a session with the couple. The therapist seeks to elicit a detailed understanding of the issues that brought them to treatment, as well as their individual histories, their history and their strengths as a couple, and their hopes and concerns about treatment.

Early in the assessment, the therapist asks each member of the couple, one at a time, to imagine his or her partner's concerns and invites him or her to check with the partner the accuracy of this understanding. Each person also is invited to consider what he or she would like to change in the relationship. Crucially, the therapist monitors his or her own mentalizing and seeks to maintain, or recover when lost, an inquisitive stance (see subsection "Maintaining an Inquisitive 'Not-Knowing' Stance" later in this chapter) that demonstrates to the couple how mentalizing is put into practice. It is particularly important for the therapist to be aware of the impact he or she has on the couple and to take responsibility for the inevitable misunderstandings that cause pain and generate defensiveness in the couple; this serves to validate the couple's experience of being misunderstood and models the path to repair of such misunderstandings.

The therapist explicitly educates the couple about mentalizing and epistemic trust, seeking opportunities to demonstrate skills and attitudes involved in understanding a person's own intentions as well as those of others and in differentiating between the person's intentions and the impact his or her behavior has on others. The couple are also asked to track their conversations between sessions and mark instances when they were effective in understanding their partner and felt understood by their partner. These moments serve to point out that for a person to feel mentalized—to experience the other as genuinely appreciating and respecting his or her thoughts, feelings, and intentions—is the key to that person feeling that trusting the other person is safe.

Concurrently, the therapist seeks to identify moments when mentalizing breaks down, and interrupts the interaction to highlight how defensiveness and nonmentalizing feel by exploring the experience of threat or misunderstanding that precedes a defensive breakdown. Each member of the couple is also asked to pay attention to how threat feels in his or her own body and how it has an impact on his or her level of arousal; this includes paying attention to physiological markers such as pulse rate. Finally, the therapist educates the couple about the various ways in which mentalizing breakdowns are manifested. These include what Gottman (2015) refers to as the "four horsemen of the apocalypse"—criticism, contempt, defensiveness, and stonewalling—as well as anger, dismissiveness, anxiety, avoidance, and detachment; dissociation and pretending to be present without conviction (pretend mode); coercive efforts to make the other person feel, think, or act in a particular way; and complete certainty about the other person's state of mind and intentions (psychic equivalence).

In summary, the therapist takes a mentalizing stance that provides the couple with the experience of feeling understood that generates epistemic trust and models mentalizing in action. Questions that the therapist, using the mentalizing stance, can employ for assessment throughout the course of treatment can include any of those outlined in Box 9–1.

INDIVIDUAL SESSION FOR EACH MEMBER OF A COUPLE

Following the joint session, an individual session with each member of the couple is scheduled. These sessions are designed to build the sense of being understood, respected, and validated. They also provide an opportunity to explore each person's attachment history and patterns, starting with his or her own parents' relationship and the impact it has had on the current relationship. Questions to ask in the individual sessions are listed in Box 9–2.

The individual sessions also offer an opportunity to assess each partner's personality traits, coping strategies, cognitive style, and patterns of communication. Last, but not least, the individual sessions make it easier to discuss individual symptoms and psychopathology, addictions, and issues such as infidelity and trauma, which are often accompanied by shame and secrecy. These issues require careful consideration of confidentiality and can call for specific remediation or referral for further assessment and treatment.

After the individual sessions, the therapist meets with the couple to share how he or she formulates their strengths and challenges and to offer recommendations. The formulation can be presented orally or summarized in writing, in common with other MBT protocols; a written summary is often helpful for the couple to use as a reference. The formulation aims to provide a model of the mentalizing approach as tentative

BOX 9–1.   Questions to assess mentalizing for the first joint interview and beyond

Trust and attunement

- How much do you feel "seen" or understood by your partner?
- Can you give me an example of when that has happened?
- How much do you imagine your partner feels "seen" or understood by you?
- How safe and trusting do you feel in your relationship with your partner?
- What have you learned about your partner over the years?
- How much do you feel you can put your guard down and trust that your partner is "on your side" or "has your back"?

Capacity for collaboration and intimacy

- How much do you feel you agree and support one another regarding children and parenting?
- What are the areas that you feel are most difficult for the two of you as parents?
- How do you collaborate in planning and managing your finances?
- What is your sexual relationship like for you? What do you imagine it is like for your partner?
- How do you express intimacy, affection, and caring to each other?
- How much do you rely on your partner for emotional soothing at times of stress?
- How do you help each other feel supported with your extended families?
- What are some challenges you have faced that you feel you handled well as a couple?

Handling conflict

- How good are you and your partner at repairing or apologizing after a disagreement or conflict?
- How much do you each take responsibility for your part in disagreements and conflicts? For example, if you each carry 10% of the responsibility for a given conflict (and "the cosmos" carries 80%), what do you imagine your part is?
- How do you and your partner handle issues of health and mental health (chronic illness, depression, or alcohol or drug abuse)?
- How easy or difficult do you think it is for you to listen to your partner when you are upset?
- What do you feel are the major stressors that are now impacting you as a couple?

Looking forward

- How much are you aware of and supportive of each other's dreams and aspirations, as well as worries and fears?
- What are some of the areas of your lives that you are particularly happy with and would not want to change?
- If we work together and things go as well as they can, how would you like your relationship to look in 6 months? What would you like to be able to change for yourself?

and humble, reflecting the therapist's impressions about the couple's experience and attachment, and the particular ways in which their vulnerabilities evoke breakdowns in mentalizing and trust.

BOX 9–2. **Mentalizing questions for the individual session of each partner**

- How did you meet and get together? What attracted you to each other?

- What do you think your relationship has been like for your partner?

- How do you imagine your partner has experienced you?

- What was your relationship like with your parents growing up?

- How do you feel that might impact your relationship with your partner now?

- Was there a history of violence or abuse or separations in your family growing up?

- How do you communicate to your partner when you feel sad, hurt, disappointed, or anxious?

- What are the situations where you are most likely to become angry, defensive, critical, contemptuous, anxious, coercive, or detached?

- What would it take to turn those conflicts into conversations in which you could hear each other's point of view?

- What do you love and cherish about your partner, and how do you let him or her know?

- How committed are you to the relationship right now, and how hopeful are you that the problems can be resolved? On a scale of 1 to 10, in which 1 is *"I am leaving this office to consult with an attorney about divorce proceedings"* and 10 is *"I can never imagine getting a divorce, no matter what,"* what number would you give yourself right now?

- What number do you imagine your partner would give?

The following case example serves to illustrate the assessment phase.

Case Example

Marcus and Jasmine have been married for 15 years and have two children—a son, age 13, and a daughter, age 11. They have come to therapy because Jasmine feels unsupported by Marcus. She feels angry and hurt and thinks that she does not matter much in his life, particularly compared with his family of origin, to whom he is very loyal. Marcus resents Jasmine's anger and wants her to be less critical. Each blames the other for the difficulties, and while they are not considering divorce, they feel stressed, unhappy, and disappointed in their marriage. They report feeling anxious in each other's presence and experience physiological symptoms: Marcus reports tachycardia and Jasmine complains of tightness in her chest.

In the first session, Marcus says he has only come because Jasmine insisted, as he is not hopeful therapy will help. He feels unsettled about Jasmine's upset with his family and cannot understand why she is so angry with him. Jasmine states that any time she tries to talk to Marcus about her own needs, he retreats emotionally and refuses to engage. He frequently works late, leaving her to deal with the children by herself, and then is surprised that she is upset. Jasmine especially resents that Marcus privileges his work over hers.

The therapist asks both of them to listen to their partner's story with some curiosity about what they each can learn from the other and without correction or rebuttal, only trying to understand the other's perspective, even if they disagree. The therapist gathers a history about what brought them together, what attracted them to each other, what they see as strengths in their relationship, how they understand the current impasses, what each would want to understand or change about themselves and their relationship, and their hopes for the therapy.

In her individual session, Jasmine reveals that she was sexually assaulted by a family friend when she was between the ages of 11 and 14. When she was finally able to tell her mother, her mother did not believe her and forbade her from telling anyone else. Mustering much courage, Jasmine told her father, who cut off contact with his friend. The issue, however, was never addressed, and Jasmine's mother never took responsibility for keeping the abuse secret. This incident and its aftermath remain a source of considerable shame for Jasmine, whose daughter is now the same age as she was when the abuse began. Jasmine is aware of feeling anxious about her daughter's well-being, and while somehow aware of the impact of her history, she does not know how to address this with her husband.

Marcus, while beloved by his parents, grew up with a mother with multiple sclerosis who was often depressed. Feeling helpless in the face of her illness and sadness, he distanced himself from her, while remaining strongly connected with his father. Marcus has some awareness of his tendency to retreat under stress but is afraid that if he lets Jasmine know this she will only become angrier.

In the joint session, the therapist introduces the concept of mentalizing, signaled by a person's capacity to be curious about his or her own intentions and those of his or her spouse, and the ability to hold two minds in mind at the same time. The therapist suggests that instead of asking *"What's wrong with you?"* to ask instead *"Can you help me understand what's going on for you?"* The therapist also suggests that when mentalizing a partner, the person should focus not on what his or her own intentions are but on how his or her behavior might have affected the partner.

Marcus and Jasmine have histories of trauma that have shaped their marriage. Each responds automatically to particular stressors in a way that leaves his or her partner feeling unseen and unsafe. Jasmine is terrified that her concerns will be silenced. For her, feeling unrecognized and invalidated is a fundamental threat that makes it impossible for her to understand or trust Marcus.

Marcus, on the other hand, survived in his family by avoiding his own feelings of helplessness. When unable to respond to someone he loves, he stops mentalizing and withdraws emotionally. But Marcus's emotional distance fuels Jasmine's sense of abandonment, exacerbating her own anxiety and mistrust, which, in turn, leads Marcus to further distance himself from her, in a cruel spiral in which each person's vulnerabilities fuel the other's defensiveness, mistrust, and loneliness. If they can understand these responses as tools for survival, they may be able to turn vicious cycles into virtuous ones and help each other feel less alone.

In closing the session, the therapist invites Jasmine and Marcus to both reflect on their experience of the process. They agree to continue in therapy, with hope that they can slow down the escalating cycles of conflict that take such a toll on their marriage and seek ways to be more attuned to and supportive of one another.

PUTTING MBT-CO INTO PRACTICE

The two core features of MBT-CO are the therapist's mentalizing stance, which helps determine *how to be* in the therapy, and the spectrum of interventions, which helps determine *what to do* in the therapy.

The Therapist's Mentalizing Stance

The therapist's stance is a fundamental component of all MBT protocols (Asen and Fonagy 2012; Bateman and Fonagy 2016). It refers to the skills and attitudes therapists deploy to model the two basic tasks: first, developing or regaining the capacity to mentalize in an important attachment relationship, and second, interrupting nonmentalizing and mistrust by pausing to consider one's own mind while being interested in understanding the mind and intentions of the other person. To promote a safe environment in which to pursue these tasks, the therapist ensures that no one talks over or interrupts the other, slows down the flow of conversation, and frequently checks to make sure he or she accurately understands what each person is conveying. The therapist also pays attention to tone and body posture, and interrupts hostile, blaming, critical, or defensive exchanges. He or she helps "warm things up" by inviting couples to talk directly to each other when they seem detached or disengaged. Conversely, the therapist helps "cool things down" by having the couple take turns talking directly to the therapist, while their partner listens, when they appear dysregulated or overwhelmed. During the course of treatment, especially at times of impasse, intense conflict, and negativity in the sessions, it is useful to schedule individual sessions with each partner to better address the underlying sources of distress. Providing each member of the couple with a validating experience may allow them to better understand themselves and their reactions, their role in the conflict, and how to communicate more effectively with each other in the couple's sessions. In individual sessions, each partner can role-play himself or herself or the partner while the therapist enacts the remaining role, to promote the person's mentalizing of himself or herself and his or her partner and to practice how to speak in ways that the other can hear.

In therapy, as in life, mentalizing constantly fluctuates. Couples therapy is designed to provide a container in which that fluidity is processed on a regular basis.

The four areas of competence for the therapist's stance are as follows:

- Maintaining an inquisitive, "not-knowing" stance.
- Holding the balance.
- Interrupting nonmentalizing.
- Highlighting and marking mentalizing.

MAINTAINING AN INQUISITIVE "NOT-KNOWING" STANCE

The therapist affirms and seeks to affirm the value of the attitudes that express a mentalizing stance: authenticity, genuineness, respect, engagement, interest, curiosity, tentativeness, and tolerance for not knowing what the other intends (Ackerman and Hilsenroth 2003). Such affirmation is expressed by an ongoing inquiry about thoughts and feelings underlying actions, and by a persistent invitation to each member of the couple to find out about their partner's subjective experience.

These inquiries are not fact-finding exercises but efforts to open conversations that track the details of each person's thoughts and feelings and how those are impacted by the meaning they attribute to each other's communications. As Lerner (2013) suggests: "The key [to connection] is to be curious, not to cross-examine. Don't act like a lawyer even if you are one."

Of particular relevance in the treatment of couples is the therapist's readiness to acknowledge his or her own mistakes, particularly those stemming from his or her own defensiveness and inability to mentalize (see the later subsection "Interrupting Nonmentalizing"). For therapists, repairing breakdowns in mentalizing and epistemic trust by taking responsibility for the impact they have on others is an important step toward transforming coercive cycles into mentalizing conversations.

HOLDING THE BALANCE

Effective mentalizing is manifested in a dynamic and flexible balance between attending to the self and paying attention to the other, between affect and cognition, between internal and external features, and between automatic (procedural, implicit) mentalizing, which is promoted by increasing stress and arousal, and controlled (representational, explicit) mentalizing, which is inhibited when arousal reaches a certain threshold (see Chapter 1, "Introduction," and Chapter 3, "Assessment of Mentalizing"). In addition to holding a balance between these dimensions of mentalizing, in MBT-CO, holding the balance involves ensuring that both members of the couple equally communicate and feel understood by their partner and the therapist.

The competencies involved in holding the balance include monitoring for imbalances in all dimensions and seeking to restore balance with "contrary moves" (Bateman and Fonagy 2016). The therapist invites a shift in perspective at a moment when affect dominates and appears overwhelming by helping the couple take a "step back" to reflect on the feelings experienced at that moment and on the sequence of interactions and subjective experiences that led to these affects. Likewise, when cognition dominates, the therapist invites the couple to recognize and name the emotions that are hidden.

Holding the balance involves an equilibrium between allowing the natural expression of habitual interactions and actively intervening to suggest alternative ways of interacting, particularly when impasses are reached and nonmentalizing dominates.

INTERRUPTING NONMENTALIZING

A basic premise of MBT-CO is that the emergence of nonmentalizing in a session is a defensive response signaling that an area of vulnerability for one or both partners has been touched. Typically, this sets in motion self-perpetuating vicious cycles, which are a clear indication for therapeutic intervention. To intervene effectively, the therapist must recognize his or her own nonmentalizing, which may be heralded by markers such as arguing with one or both members of the couple; feelings of certainty about the "true" meaning or intent of the couple's interactions; feelings of hopelessness, anger, or anxiety; and losing the ability to maintain multiple perspectives. The therapist's effort to regain his or her mentalizing can include taking a moment's break, in order to pause and reflect on what has been happening, or asking the couple for help in unpacking what has happened.

The therapist's ability to regain mentalizing when it is temporarily lost models for the couple what to do when they are feeling stuck or acting coercively. The therapist assists the couple in regaining mentalizing by asking them to pause and observe. As we discuss later, pausing is often followed by an invitation to "rewind" to the moment before the communication became problematic, allowing the therapist to tease out the subjective experiences and interactions that render the couple unable to understand one another.

The following is an example of a session in which the therapist is helping a couple by interrupting nonmentalizing.

Case Example

For married couple Robert and May, issues involving money are an immediate trigger for anger, hurt, and emotional withdrawal. May has inherited some money from her parents, who were extremely frugal and whose approval was very important to her.

Robert has experienced financial setbacks that have limited his earnings and made him dependent on May. Robert grew up in a family with a father who was chronically unemployed, struggled with alcoholism, and had difficulty supporting his family. Robert's own adult children have often needed financial assistance. When Robert feels compelled to help them pay rent or make car payments, May becomes resentful and lashes out at Robert, who then becomes critical of May.

Noticing this pattern, the therapist suggests a pause and then checks with both members of the couple about their experience of the conversation. How much does either of them feel open and able to listen? They both report feeling as if they are in a rut, hopeless, and invalidated.

The therapist encourages the couple to signal when they become defensive by raising a hand or pushing an imaginary "pause button" while also checking what is happening with their partner. Invited by the therapist to name this particular pattern of interaction, Robert and May begin to speak of the "money landmine field," which helps them to take some distance and to recognize that each is affected differently by money issues. As they are now able to be curious about their vulnerabilities and shame, the therapist observes them having a mentalizing conversation and notes a lessening of their efforts to cajole, threaten, and otherwise coerce their partner into agreement.

HIGHLIGHTING AND MARKING MENTALIZING

The therapist actively searches for instances of good mentalizing in the couple's interactions, marking when a member of the couple is curious, respectful, interested in understanding the other's perspective, aware of the impact he or she has on the other, capable of disclosing vulnerable feelings without becoming defensive, and takes responsibility for his or her mistakes or misunderstandings and the hurt they cause the other.

The Spectrum of Interventions

The spectrum of interventions (Figure 9–3) provides the therapist with a guide to match his or her interventions to the couple's mentalizing capacity and level of defensiveness at any moment in the session, on the way to assisting the couple to rehabilitate their capacity to mentalize and trust each other in the face of intense affect and conflict. The steps in the spectrum are as follows:

- Empathy, support, and validation.
- Clarification, affect focus, and affect elaboration.
- Challenge and the therapeutic bargain.
- Repair of mentalizing and epistemic trust in the here and now of the relationship (Bateman and Fonagy 2016).

Following the use of each intervention, the therapist monitors whether there is an enhancement in mentalizing and trust (and a corresponding decrease in defensiveness). This observation helps to recognize when to move to steps in the spectrum that require a greater capacity to mentalize and trust. On the other hand, a response that signals less mentalizing and greater defensiveness suggests the need to further reduce the mentalizing demands on the couple. To do so, the therapist expresses his or her own thoughts and feelings rather than asking the members of the couple to do more mentalizing, to reduce the mental pressure on them (e.g., by the therapist acknowledging feeling confused or stuck and indicating solutions to the uncertainty).

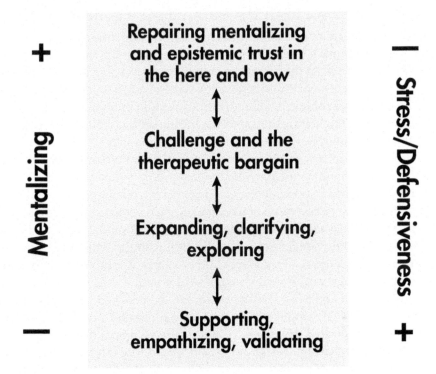

FIGURE 9–3. Spectrum of interventions in mentalization-based couples therapy.

EMPATHY, SUPPORT, AND VALIDATION

As discussed earlier, the person's experience of feeling understood and respected, and to feel that he or she is present in another person's mind, is the essential condition signaling that it is safe to trust, lower his or her guard, and listen to and learn from another. It is therefore the natural point of departure for all sessions, and the point to which the therapist returns when mentalizing breaks down and trust is eroded.

Empathic, supportive, and validating interventions include careful questioning that seeks to elicit each person's account of his or her experience and treats that account respectfully and with genuine interest and a desire to understand. Of course, respecting, understanding, and validating one person's perspective does not invalidate the perspective of the partner, but helps to expand the partner's perspective and promotes the partners' ability to validate each other.

The therapist assists the partners by asking them to hear one another "with an open heart," empathizing with their efforts to improve their relationship and the challenges of handling the space between them with compassion, kindness, and thoughtfulness.

Using the competencies described earlier in the section "The Therapist's Mentalizing Stance," the therapist seeks to identify and mark instances of effective mentalizing in the couple, judiciously praising such instances. For example, the therapist might note progress by saying, *"I had the impression that you were able to explain something very difficult in a way that your partner could hear without feeling criticized…did I get that right?"*

CLARIFICATION, AFFECT FOCUS, AND AFFECT ELABORATION

Evidence of some degree of reflectiveness, curiosity, and openness to consider other perspectives in the couple's interactions is an indication to the therapist to increase the mentalizing demands on the couple by pursuing clarification and elaboration.

This step in the spectrum of interventions involves an effort to reconstruct the emotional and interpersonal context leading to breakdowns in mentalizing and epistemic trust, including exploring the feelings and the meanings ascribed to the interactions leading to the disruption. "Rewind and reflect" is an approach in which the therapist asks the couple to track back to the last moment in which both felt they could think and interact freely without confusion, misunderstanding, or coercion.

The therapist employs a "mentalizing chain analysis," detailing how mental states, particularly affects, change as a result of the meaning each person assigns to a particular interaction. The therapist also attempts to elaborate by seeking the hidden vulnerable feelings that typically lurk behind defensive, distancing affects. This challenging intervention can help couples look at the impact on their relationship of their histories—within either their current family or their families of origin.

For example, Robert and May, mentioned earlier, were locked in battles of mutual recrimination over his "irresponsible squandering of assets" and her "demeaning comments and unsupportive stinginess." Careful reflection on hidden vulnerabilities helped May recognize that she was afraid Robert would lose interest in her if she did not provide him with the financial support he needed. Robert, meanwhile, became able to understand how desperately he needed to prove that he, unlike his father, was a caring and effective parent, and to recognize the enormous shame he associated with his inability to provide financially for his children.

The therapist then checks that both members of the couple experience a sense of ownership over the evolving narrative of the relationship that they are jointly constructing.

CHALLENGE AND THE THERAPEUTIC BARGAIN

Challenge (described in detail in Bateman and Fonagy 2016) can occur once there is a sense of enhanced collaboration and each member of the couple is working together with the other and with the therapist. Paradoxically, it is also an approach designed to surprise the couple and "trip" them to a more reflective stance, particularly when there is a predominance of the pretend mode—for example, when they ignore the "elephant in the room" of a damaging or dangerous issue such as an affair or one partner's addictive behavior.

The difficulty in facing uncomfortable, particularly shaming, experiences of vulnerability is significant.

Case Example

Paul and Helen came to therapy to address Paul's depression and the deterioration of their marriage after Paul learned that Helen had been having an affair. Barely overcoming his humiliation and despair, he decided to offer to her that they seek to rebuild their shattered trust. Helen hesitated for a moment before answering, and Paul exploded in rage, accusing her of rejecting him again, certain that she felt only contempt for him. Helen said that she felt confused, guilty, and afraid of Paul's anger when he made his request, but this did little to soothe or calm Paul.

Only in a follow-up individual session could Paul acknowledge the panic he experienced when Helen hesitated; he felt that he did not matter as much to her as she mattered to him. This reaction illustrates the understandable reluctance people experience in giving up the protection afforded by defensiveness and nonmentalizing, in spite of the pain and limitations they produce. It is a moment to reflect on the courage Paul will need to let Helen know how much she means to him and then to dare to check whether she in fact cares enough about him to try to repair their relationship.

This dilemma highlights the basic "therapeutic bargain" that treatment offers couples: choosing between, on the one hand, holding on to defensive, nonmentalizing approaches that provide an illusory semblance of control, safety, and connection, and, on the other hand, taking the risk of giving up those protections in order to trust, knowing that while there is no certainty, there is the possibility of learning how to attain real mastery and genuine attachment by identifying, communicating, and handling painful feelings.

REPAIR OF MENTALIZING AND EPISTEMIC TRUST IN THE "HERE AND NOW" OF THE RELATIONSHIP

The greatest mentalizing demand on the members of the couple is to seek to expose their vulnerabilities to each other and to maintain trust and mentalizing in the face of intense emotions. However, repairing epistemic trust and mentalizing within the session holds the greatest opportunity for awakening the salutogenic capacities of social learning and creating the foundations for a secure base and a safe haven from which to negotiate life (Fonagy et al. 2015). The capacity to repair also equips each person with a skill that can be generalized to other relationships and other contexts.

The following is a segment of a session in which the therapist works with the couple to repair mentalizing and epistemic trust.

Case Example

Maggie and Damien are discussing an argument they had when Damien came home after dropping off their 8-year-old son, Jason, at school. Damien was visibly angry because Jason had had a huge temper tantrum in the car, crying and screaming, and refused to get out until the teacher on patrol made him leave. Damien thought they had had a good morning until they got to school, when Jason realized that he had left a toy at home that he had intended to bring with him. Maggie is explaining how rude Damien was to her; how she was initially happy and excited to see him, but when he started complaining she became upset and criticized him. Damien got annoyed and left, gruffly saying good-bye. Maggie became more upset and demanded that Damien apologize, and Damien quickly refused. In describing the argument, they are both blaming and accusing each other and angrily disputing each other's account.

The therapist asks to interview each person in turn while the other listens.

Therapist (T): It sounds pretty miserable for you both. Would it be OK if I try to learn a little bit about what happened for each of you that day? [*Empathic statement to couple*]

Maggie (M) and Damien (D): Sure.

T: Maggie, when you saw Damien come home and you saw how upset he was, what did you feel? [*Focus on the person's self-experience in the context of recognizing the other's emotional state*]

M: I was angry and frustrated. I was just back from my run and was happy to see him, but when he started yelling about Jason, I got really upset.

T: Do you know what upset you?

M: He shouldn't be so angry at Jason and he shouldn't take it out on me. I needed him to apologize for being so rude to me. That's not right. *[Statement of her representation of his motivation with a judgment]*

The therapist is aware that most of Maggie's focus is on getting Damien's behavior to change and on proving that he was wrong. The therapist tries to help Maggie mentalize her own experience using a mentalizing functional analysis.

T: I get that, but if we go back to those first feelings when you were happy to see Damien and he was angry and critical of Jason, what happened then?

M: I was just upset, and I started thinking that this is hopeless. Why am I in this marriage anyway? He's never going to change.

T: So you were feeling pretty awful. I wondered, while you were talking, if you were also somewhat sad or disappointed as well, since you had come home excited to see Damien and it turned out so differently. *[Use of clarification, affect focus, and elaboration]*

M *[becoming a little tearful]*: Well yes, I was sad, and I was upset that he was so angry with Jason. I think he is not patient and I worry how that will affect our children, and I don't feel I can trust him as a parent.

Maggie is able to verbalize her fear that her children will feel unloved, like she did.

M: I try to get Damien to see what he has done and I want him to apologize for his behavior. He knows how upset I get and he should know better and at least say good-bye to me and let me know we are OK.

T: When Damien doesn't do that, what do you think might be happening for him?

M: Right then I don't really care about what's happening for him, I just want him to recognize that he was wrong and that he should apologize.

The therapist notices that Maggie is now able to be aware of times when she cannot mentalize Damien.

T: I so appreciate what you just said. That there are times when our fears are so intense that we don't have the bandwidth to think about what might be going on for anyone else.

M: Yeah, I just get afraid he's going to stay angry at me and I can't stop thinking about it and I want it to be over, and if he would just apologize then I could stop worrying.

T: I wonder what it's like for you to remember that moment as we are talking about it now?

M: Well it makes sense. I'm not even aware of how I'm feeling at the time. I don't think about being sad, I just think about getting Damien to apologize so I can be OK, but it never really works.

T: Do you think that Damien might still care about you even if he can't apologize at that moment?

M: As we are talking about it right now I do, but at the time I can't think that far.

T: What's it like to be having this conversation?

M: It's good but it makes me feel very vulnerable, like maybe Damien would use this against me.

T: Is it OK if I check with Damien and see how he understands what you said?

M: Sure.

T: So, Damien, are there any parts of what Maggie has said that you can understand? *[Checking out the understanding of the other member of the couple]*

D: Yeah, I can understand how scared Maggie gets. She just doesn't understand that sometimes I can't take it.

T: Would it be all right if we try to understand a little more about what was going on for you, when you got home from taking Jason to school?

D and M: Sure.

Damien is able to state how confused and embarrassed he felt when their son was having a tantrum, how critical he felt of his wife, and how concerned he was that she would think he was "screwing up" as a father.

T: So, when you got into the house you were upset and worried about how Maggie might see you, is that right?

D: Yeah, and then I told Maggie that we had to do something to get Jason under control and she said I was overreacting.

T: And what was that like for you?

D: I got angry and felt like she didn't care about something that is really important to me, and then when she wanted me to apologize, I got angrier.

T: Did Maggie know any of the things you were feeling, like that you were worried that she would be upset with you?

D: I didn't even know the things I was feeling until we are just talking about it now.

T: Would you be willing to see if Maggie can understand some of the feelings you were having?

D: Sure.

M: I do understand. I just got panicked when you were upset, but it was a rough morning for you too.

T: And I understand, Damien, you needed to get some space to think, but Maggie you were afraid that you had lost your connection with Damien and so thought if you could get him to apologize, it would mean that things were OK. Neither of you could really think about your own feelings or what might be going on for your partner. Does this make sense?

D: It does to me. I'm sorry that I couldn't handle Jason better. I feel embarrassed when he doesn't behave and I'm afraid to tell you, like you'll think I don't know what I'm doing and I'm just a failure.

M: Thank you. I know that I get panicked when you are angry, and I know that some of that is about us and some of this is about me and how I can't get control of my feelings when I think you're angry. I know that I can't make you give me an apology and that just makes it worse, it's just really hard for me to stop but I can try.

D: That would be good. I just—well, something happens to me when it feels like a demand.

The therapist notes that they are both able to look at the thoughts and feelings that escalate nonmentalizing, recognizing the impact their behavior has on their partner, and beginning to work on apologies and repair.

REFERENCES

Ackerman SJ, Hilsenroth MJ: A review of therapist characteristics and techniques positively impacting the therapeutic alliance. Clin Psychol Rev 23(1):1–33, 2003 12559992

Asen E, Fonagy P: Mentalization-based therapeutic interventions for families. J Fam Ther 34:347–370, 2012

Bateman A, Fonagy P: Mentalization-Based Treatment for Personality Disorders: A Practical Guide. Oxford, UK, Oxford University Press, 2016

Bowlby J: A Secure Base: Clinical Applications of Attachment Theory. London, Routledge, 1988

Csibra G, Gergely G: Natural pedagogy. Trends Cogn Sci 13(4):148–153, 2009 19285912

Csibra G, Gergely G: Natural pedagogy as evolutionary adaptation. Philos Trans R Soc Lond B Biol Sci 366(1567):1149–1157, 2011 21357237

Fonagy P, Luyten P, Allison E: Epistemic petrification and the restoration of epistemic trust: a new conceptualization of borderline personality disorder and its psychosocial treatment. J Pers Disord 29(5):575–609, 2015 26393477

Gergely G: Ostensive communication and cultural learning: the natural pedagogy hypothesis, in Agency and Joint Attention. Edited by Metcalfe J, Terrace HS. Oxford, UK, Oxford University Press, 2013, pp 139–151

Gottman J: The Seven Principles for Making Marriage Work. New York, Harmony, 2015

Lerner H: Stop being so defensive! This 12 step program may save your marriage. November 10, 2013. Available at: https://www.psychologytoday.com/blog/the-dance-connection/201311/stop-being-so-defensive. Accessed June 7, 2018.

Siegel D: Brainstorm: The Power and Purpose of the Teenage Brain. New York, Penguin, 2013

CHAPTER 10

THERAPEUTIC MODELS

Peter Fonagy, Ph.D., FBA, FMedSci, FAcSS

Chloe Campbell, Ph.D.

Elizabeth Allison, D.Phil.

We regard this chapter as something of a sequel to Chapter 4, "Mentalizing, Resilience, and Epistemic Trust." While Chapter 4 sets out our thinking about the relationship between resilience, mentalizing, and the notion of a general vulnerability factor for psychopathology by way of epistemic trust, this chapter attempts to tease out the therapeutic implications of these ideas. In keeping with the mentalizing stance, we adopt a degree of humility and uncertainty both about the exceptionalism of any (including our own) "brand" of therapy and, more broadly, about the ambition and expectations that we can claim for any form of treatment in the context of the patient's social environment. In the light of findings in relation to a putative general psychopathology factor (the *p factor*, discussed in Chapter 4), and our current speculation about the role of social communication and social imagination in human psychopathology, we consider how we might use the notion of a general factor for psychopathology to develop a general model for therapy.

WHAT DOES THERAPEUTIC OUTCOME RESEARCH TELL US?

First, it might be useful to consider where we are now in terms of outcome research on the effectiveness of psychotherapeutic treatment. Research in this field has, over several decades, consistently found that many brands of psychotherapy are demonstrably effective compared with control conditions; however, comparative outcome studies have not made it possible to identify any particular treatment model as being consistently more effective than any other (Wampold and Imel 2015). To compound this finding, a recent meta-analysis has also found that psychotherapeutic treatments for borderline personality disorder (BPD) appear to be similar in terms of outcome

(Cristea et al. 2017; Fonagy et al. 2017c). A further substantial challenge arising from the outcome literature is the discovery—again, across different studies—of diminishing effect sizes over time for treatments (Friborg and Johnsen 2017; Johnsen and Friborg 2015; Weisz et al. 2017). This range of outcome findings highlights the generally accepted fact that by and large, it is difficult if not impossible to link mechanistic accounts of therapeutic effectiveness, which are largely based on psychopathology studies, and the mechanisms of therapeutic change at work in any particular treatment application (Kazdin 2007).

A key issue to consider in this respect is that treatment research over the past 30–40 years has focused on the remission of symptoms increasingly tightly linked to particular diagnostic categories. However, the evidence suggests, for example, that psychological treatments targeted at a single specific disorder as defined in the *Diagnostic and Statistical Manual of Mental Disorders* (American Psychiatric Association 2013) tend to lead to observable improvements in different, untargeted problems (e.g., see Allen et al. 2010; Weisz et al. 2006, 2017). Using diagnosis as a primary indicator of improvement seems less than sensible in the light of the high level of comorbidity that any treatment program is implicitly targeting. Therapists tailor interventions to treat the imagined entity of a disorder, when disorders are not natural units; rather, they are the product of a process of professional prototyping (Wittgenstein 1953). The notion of a general psychopathology factor further underlines the question of the suitability of a highly targeted diagnosis-symptom-outcome model for assessing the effects of treatment: the imperative for researchers to identify a primary outcome in mental health may be particularly ill-advised when their primary outcome is an inherently ambiguous latent entity. Yet, within current trial methodology (adopted from models of studying pharmaceutical treatments for physical health problems), research has focused on a specific measure for a particular diagnosis at a specific point in time, with little understanding of the meaning of change or the threshold attained.

What we do have is evidence that reliably identifies the significance of the patient–therapist relationship in determining outcomes (Norcross 2011)—in particular, the significance of the therapeutic alliance (Horvath et al. 2011) and its capacity to recover following difficulties (Safran et al. 2011). Further, a recent longitudinal analysis of clinical outcomes not only found that the therapist is the greatest source of variance in outcomes but also reported that therapists' effectiveness tends to diminish as their experience increases (Goldberg et al. 2016). The disparate range of findings that we refer to here have contributed to a lively debate about the common factors of effective psychotherapy (Wampold and Imel 2015). What we will attempt to do in this chapter is draw together these findings to create a model of therapeutic change that is compatible with the challenges and changes in thinking in the fast-moving field of psychopathology and the great debate about the effectiveness of psychotherapy.

A GENERAL MODEL OF PSYCHOTHERAPY FOR A GENERAL FACTOR FOR PSYCHOPATHOLOGY?

How do we envisage a therapeutic model that encompasses both a general psychopathology factor and the real subjective needs of an individual in distress? We have repeatedly made the case for the importance of tailoring treatments to meet individual needs (Fonagy 2016; Fonagy and Allison 2017). In proposing a general model, we stand by this position: we will argue that it is only through people's experience of having their—very individual—minds accurately and tolerably reflected back to them that people are primed to open their minds to absorbing new knowledge about themselves and about the world, whether this information comes from within the clinical setting or from the social context. We believe that the generality of this model takes nothing away from its fidelity to the principle of personalization.

A therapeutic model that is shaped by the concept of a general factor of psychopathology should not be one that proposes a mindlessly generic, general program for psychopathology. As we shall set out below, the model we propose is one that is predicated on recognizing individual subjectivity and psychological agency. The apparently counterintuitive finding that more experienced therapists might have less effective outcomes (Goldberg et al. 2016) might arise from the fact that less experienced therapists are more able to see the individual patient in all his or her subjective complexity rather than as a "walking diagnostic prototype."

If the patient is able to perceive that the therapist can see the world from his or her standpoint, this acts as an ostensive cue that stimulates epistemic trust in the patient (as described in Chapter 4), allowing him or her to access the social benefits of learning from and about other minds, framing and aligning the patient's social imaginative capacity in a more adaptive way. People all have their working theories about themselves; we could call these "personal narratives," or the "imagined self," a model of who individuals feel that they are, and why they feel they are the way they are, based on the evidence arising from their subjective experience. These narratives tend to shape the way people mentalize themselves; they are a kind of heuristic for the individual making sense of his or her own actions. For most people, at any moment there is one predominant working theory—that is, the most obvious straightforward way of describing themselves. Individuals also all have more subdominant narratives; these are the understandings of themselves that are more nuanced or complex and are hidden from the normal shorthand they might use to describe themselves. The dominant narrative is in the foreground, but behind it may be a range of other narratives. For example, a patient might have the dominant narrative *"I need to be admired, and to achieve that, I need to meet all the expectations you have of me"* but the subdominant narrative might be *"I'm tired of working so hard trying to please people all the time."* We believe the recognition of these subdominant narratives is a particularly potent way of establishing epistemic trust; in this example, the therapist might do this by saying something like *"I have noticed just how hard you work to make sure you meet all the needs the people around you have; you know, in your shoes I would just get exhausted trying to meet every expectation anyone might have of me."*

If individuals feel that they are understood by another person (i.e., that another person is able to mentalize them), they will be more inclined to learn from that person. This dynamic creates a special role for mentalizing. We and colleagues have suggested that the facilitation of mentalizing is an essential component of what makes psychological therapies effective (Allen 2012; Allen et al. 2008). We have more recently developed the idea, influenced by evolutionary and developmental thinking, that improving mentalizing in therapy is perhaps not an end in and of itself (Fonagy et al. 2017b). Improved mentalizing may be important because it enables the individual to achieve a more fundamental social goal, which is to be able to enhance the benefits he or she derives from social experience, to improve his or her functioning in cooperation (and in competition) with other individuals and social groups. Cooperation crucially depends on learning, acquiring new understandings and adaptations in ever-changing social situations. This in turn (as described in Chapter 1, "Introduction") depends on the rapid and effective transfer of social knowledge from trusted individuals. Mentalizing is valuable to the extent that it helps to keep epistemic channels for knowledge exchange between people fully open. It does this by 1) improving the coherence of individuals' perceptions of themselves, 2) improving individuals' more generic capacity to perceive the other person's perception of them, and 3) improving individuals' capacity to match the two. Acquiring profound insight into an individual's own self is of little use if there is a mismatch between how another person perceives him or her and how the individual sees himself or herself. Similarly, individuals can learn a lot about perceiving others, but in terms of psychological and social functioning, individuals will still have severe limitations if they cannot perceive themselves accurately. Further, individuals can have a picture of themselves and a picture of the other person's view of them, but if these are, for example, at radically different levels of sophistication, the dissonance will inhibit effective social communication.

The fundamental principle informing our therapeutic model is that the human mind is essentially social and interpersonal. Both therapy and mentalizing make sense only in terms of reintegrating the patient into the large, complex, ever-moving stream of human social communication. An emphasis on mentalizing or therapeutic insight in isolation from the imperatives of wider social functioning risks becoming meaningless. This takes us to an important qualification that we must add to our emphasis on recognizing individual subjectivity, which is that although this is a critical part of the therapeutic process, it is only the beginning. The complex higher-order cognitive capacities that are associated with the prevalence of psychopathology in humans exist for social reasons—they enable humans to access, benefit from, and potentially exploit social relationships. These complex cognitive processes primarily misfire in relation to social functioning. To be effective, therefore, therapies must also have a systemic function: they must equip the individual to adapt to and benefit from the wider social environment.

Not just mentalizing, but most higher-order cognitive functions, subserve social goals of collaboration. A recent hypothesis presented by Mahr and Csibra (2017) claimed that episodic memory principally functions to enable social communication. Memory of personal experience ensures that individuals have justifications for why they believe what they do, where they are placed in terms of obligations and commitments with others, and who they can rely on and who they should treat with caution; these are key elements of human social cooperation, competition, and the construction of a network of relationships that makes human culture possible. These elements are all dependent on episodic memory. Similarly, the theory of epistemic trust explains how and why individuals exchange knowledge about the culture that gives them the tools to function within it—not just, for example, how they might use a complicated tool or technology, but how they can get access to it or make a claim to it that their peers will respect. We have argued in the same vein that human consciousness evolved to allow individuals to share their experiences, to communicate a "shared narrative" on which relationships, social ties, and group cohesion can be built (Fonagy and Allison 2016). Individuals become conscious of aspects of the world to which they are exposed, including their internal subjective experience, which others reflect on as well (Allison and Fonagy 2016; Fonagy and Allison 2016). On an individual, developmental level, we would argue that these aspects of higher-order social cognition, which we so closely associate with being human—teaching and learning, sharing narratives, having a conscious self—while unfolding to a maturational timetable, all develop to their fullest extent in the context of early emotional experiences. In the first instance, in infancy, we see this in the growth of the child's sense of self being supported by the congruent sensitive mirroring of primary caregivers. We are arguing, therefore, that human cognitive complexity is developmentally generated by and evolved for a world of social interaction. Psychotherapy as a process draws on the close association of the development of higher-order cognitive functions and personal social experience. Therapy activates social-cognitive processes necessary for the effective navigation of the social world.

This brings us back to the idea, described in Chapter 4, of two processes working together to create vulnerability to psychopathology: 1) failures in executive function, especially unmanageable impulsivity in the face of emotional stimuli; and 2) maladaptive social imagination. The model of effective treatment that we describe in the following sections—that of the three communication systems of change—is predicated on the belief that treatment can work only if it involves recognition of, and response to, the patient's needs and perceptions. It is only through identifying, acknowledging, and appreciating the individual's mental state, beliefs, and complex subjectivity that the process by which the individual can begin to learn from the mind of the therapist can be stimulated. The therapeutic model we propose is one that opens epistemic trust, making social communication and cooperative alignment with other minds possible, through the recursive experience of recognizing the individual's own mind as being accurately represented in someone else's. This alignment can bring perspective, constraint, and modification to wilder and more damaging out-of-kilter expressions of the social imagination. Therapeutic interventions are effective because they open the person to social learning experiences, which then feed back (Benish et al. 2011) in a "virtuous cycle" that enhances social understanding and communication. We have described this as a process consisting of three interacting communication systems, which are activated in a sequential but cyclic manner during the course of treatment.

Communication System 1

USING MODEL-BASED THERAPEUTIC COMMENTARY ON THE PATIENT'S LIFE AND THE NATURE OF HIS OR HER DISORDER

The first system entails the communication by the therapist of information that indicates to the patient that the therapist has considerable knowledge as well as personal characteristics that may be highly valued by the patient. The knowledge communicated will naturally vary according to the treatment model. Analysis of the therapeutic alliance has found that the relationship between therapist and patient is supported by the therapist's empathy: the therapist conveying that he or she has a convincing understanding of the patient as an intentional agent generates a sense of self-recognition in the patient (Nienhuis et al. 2018). All evidence-based "bona fide" models of psychotherapy present models of mind, disorder, and change that are to some degree accurate and helpful to patients, and increase patients' capacity for understanding their experience. This plays a key function in overcoming the epistemic vigilance (*"not true," "not relevant to me"*) with which patients, particularly those with a trauma history, arrive to treatment. So, transmitting the content effectively involves a subtle and rich process of ostensive cueing. Therapists must present their information with mentalizing in mind, establishing a collaboration with the patient, using the model in which they are trained to demonstrate that they see the patient's problems from the patient's perspective and recognize the patient as an agent, with the attitude that communication is two-way and that the patient has things to teach the therapist. From the structural perspective we are presenting here, the therapist's attempt to apply his or her model to interactions with and experiences brought by the patient serves as an ostensive cue, which in turn gradually increases the patient's epistemic trust and thus acts as a catalyst for eventual therapeutic success. We often consider that what motivates change are the contents of these communications—which may consist of psychoeducation; normalization; the creation of a shared formulation, a plan of behavioral actions, or coping strategies that help overcome challenging issues; the delineation of traumatic personal histories; the revealing of the complexity of motives through interpretations; or the modification of expectations, beliefs, and attributions about challenging aspects of current experiences. The puzzle here is the sheer variety of contents that have been shown to be effective in bringing about psychological healing, and the fact that not all such material brings change for all people.

We suggest that Communication System 1 facilitates change to the extent that 1) the therapist is able to find and effectively transmit content that provides valuable ways for patients to understand (mentalize) themselves and their reaction to others, and 2) the process of transmission involves patients recognizing the truth and personal relevance of the content being communicated to them so that they become able to relax their epistemic mistrust.

Communication System 2

IMPROVING MENTALIZING TO INCREASE THE CAPACITY TO DISCERN TRUSTWORTHINESS

Mentalizing may be a common factor in effective psychotherapies, but not in the sense that it was originally considered to be central (Allen 2008, 2012). We would no longer wish to argue that the very fact of improving mentalizing will necessarily bring with it improved symptomatic and social adjustment status. Mentalizing has to improve for the purpose of reestablishing social communication, in particular learning from social experience. In other words, mentalizing is helpful to the extent that it enables the individual to engage in a process that engenders epistemic trust. The therapist creates a representation of the patient's self-experience. The patient acquires this representation and matches it to his or her self-experience. If the match is good, trust in (the therapist's) communication ensues, such that the patient is in a position to engage in the virtuous cycle of learning about himself or herself from the therapist, and with this increased self-knowledge improve his or her capacity to appreciate the therapist's experience—including, of course, the presentation of the therapist's own experience of the patient.

Looking at this process in a little more detail, the constant engagement of the patient by the therapist has several key features that are relevant to the restoration of epistemic trust. First, the therapist consistently recognizes the patient's agency, focuses on the patient as an actor, and negotiates from the perspective of the patient's self. Second, by marking the patient's experiences, the therapist acknowledges the patient's emotional state. Third, the therapist makes extensive use of ostensive cues to denote the personal relevance of the information he or she is transmitting, and its generalizable social value. By mentalizing the patient effectively, the therapist models mentalizing and creates an open, trustworthy, and low-arousal environment.

Structurally, a second virtuous cycle is put into motion: the therapist responds sensitively to the patient, the patient takes a step back from epistemic isolation and gradually begins to exercise his or her mentalizing skills, which, step by step, extend from the confines of the therapeutic context and generalize to his or her wider social context. This elicits an emotional reaction by the patient to the social context, giving the therapist further opportunity to respond sensitively to these experiences. This process involves a complex and nonlinear progression. Improving mentalizing is not the main goal, but the improved mentalizing that results from the process enables the patient to start to approach and learn from his or her wider social context.

Answering the question of why patients with a better capacity for mentalizing improve more in psychotherapy than those whose mentalizing is poorer helps us to understand the process. Mentalizing moderates the impact of therapeutic communications: a poorly mentalizing patient will frequently interpret the therapist's ostensive cues erroneously, and epistemic trust is thus not established. With improved mentalizing, the therapist's communications are appreciated and interpreted as trustworthy by—and have the intended influence on—the patient. The "gift" of a mentalizing process in psychotherapy is to open up or restore the patient's receptivity to broader social influence, which is a precondition for social learning and healthy development at any age.

For the individual, being able to mentalize the other person sufficiently well to recognize that he or she is being accurately mentalized by that other person is the key that unlocks an epistemic barrier—the natural conservative vigilant stance to novelty. Throughout development, the key to keeping the learning channel open is the experience of self-recognition that enables genuine learning, which in turn modifies enduring structures for representing information from the communicator. That experience is based on detecting how one is seen—what we could term the *epistemic match*. We may prefer to put it thus: 1) the patient's imagined sense of self (his or her personal narrative) is 2) imagined by the therapist and this image is 3) perceived by the patient and 4) compared with his or her personal narrative, and in the case of a match the channel for rapid, efficient knowledge transfer is opened and the reason behind the apparent rigidity is dissolved; it shifts the "hard-to-reach" patient into a more "reachable" state.

In order to generate trust, the version of a personal narrative that the patient perceives in the therapist's mind must match his or her narrative in the moment. As we noted earlier, this may be particularly powerful if it includes the patient's subdominant narratives as well as his or her more apparent preoccupations in order to capture something of the nuanced whole of the patient's sense of self. In other words, if patients perceive that the other person's mind contains a representation of their mental state that matches their own experience of that mental state, then they will feel safe enough to learn from that person and therefore will let down their defense of epistemic vigilance.

Put at its simplest: *"If I feel that I am understood, I will be disposed to learn from the person who understood me."* The act of learning also opens up patients' capacity for the further gathering of social information. In regaining epistemic trust, patients will learn about themselves, but also about others and the entire world that the patients themselves live in. Patients' acquisition of the capacity to imagine their own and others' minds facilitates self-regulation and management of their social relationships (as has previously been argued by Fonagy et al. 2002). Perhaps more importantly, it also enables patients to judge whether they are accurately perceived and thus to establish epistemic trust with others, opening the channel for effective transmission of their own knowledge to others. It is perhaps this active learning aspect of all psychotherapies that ensures that so many different forms of psychological therapies can lead to substantial change.

Communication System 3

REGAINING ACCESS TO THE SOCIAL WORLD AND THE REIGNITING OF SALUTOGENESIS

The greatest benefit from a therapeutic relationship comes from the generalizing of epistemic trust *beyond* therapy, so that the patient can continue to learn and grow from other relationships. Social learning in the context of epistemic trust is (re)established, and this leads to *salutogenesis*, the "generation of health," or, in this case, the person's capacity to benefit from positive features in his or her environment. The third communication system is a process of opening the person's mind via establishing epistemic trust (collaboration) so he or she can once again trust his or her immediate social world, having become more sensitive and accurate about how others perceive him or her. This means that it is not just what is taught in therapy that helps the patient, but that the patient's capacity for learning from social situations is rekindled in therapy. Enhanced mentalizing allows the patient to achieve improved social relationships and recognize who is a reliable and trustworthy source of information— that is, who the patient can "be friends with." The improved epistemic trust and abandonment of rigidity enable adaptation and learning from experience. Therapeutic change therefore is probably as much a consequence of how the patient comes to use his or her social environment as of what happens in therapy per se. The benefits of therapy remain contingent on what is accessible to patients in their particular social world (as we discuss in more detail in the next section). Therapeutic interventions are effective because they open the patient to social learning experiences, which feed back in a third virtuous cycle. If the environment is at least partly benign, therapy will "work." Evidence for the reinforcing effect of the wider social environment in supporting outcomes is indicated by the "sleeper effect" (e.g., see Fonagy et al. 2015), whereby the effects of an intervention continue to increase after the end of treatment. We would argue that this extended trajectory of benefit from psychotherapy reflects the salutogenic effect of ongoing social learning.

A Mentalizing Model in a Nonmentalizing System

The conceptualization of the three communication systems requires an acknowledgment of the inherent limitations of clinical interventions in cases where the patient's wider social environment does not support mentalizing. The implication is that what happens in any therapeutic intervention cannot on its own be expected to be enough to bring about a lasting significant improvement in the patient's state. Indeed, in certain circumstances it would be maladaptive for individuals to develop epistemic trust and lower their social defenses—for instance, in social environments characterized by high levels of aggression or violence, in which an external, nonreflective, rapidly responding affective focus on others (as opposed to the self) would be more valuable as a survival strategy. Epistemic vigilance is in fact an efficient adaptation (Sperber et al. 2010), and an indication that the individual is exercising appropriate caution in an environment in which cooperative social learning cannot be assumed to be a prevailing characteristic.

As implied by Communication System 3, the consolidation of therapeutic gains—and indeed any meaningful improvement in quality of life for the patient—is contingent on the patient's social environment tolerating and supporting these changes. An appreciation of the dynamic socially reinforcing cycle of adaptive social communication, which is core to our understanding of psychopathology (Fonagy et al. 2017a, 2017b), should also shape any coherent therapeutic model. We suggest that it is the impact of nonmentalizing on the system of social communication, and not the unchangeability of nonmentalizing per se, that makes severe and entrenched psychopathology so clinically challenging. One of the defining characteristics of personality disorders, for example, is that the patterns of social dysfunction shown by the patient are enduring. Indeed, BPD in particular has historically been regarded as an almost untreatable condition, considerably adding to the stigma attached to the disorder. However, effective therapies for BPD now exist: at least nine forms of treatment have been tested in at least 20 randomized controlled trials (Stoffers et al. 2012), and patients with BPD should no longer be regarded as "impossible to help." We would argue that an explanation for the apparent inconsistency that a condition has long been believed to be untreatable, yet appears to be more responsive to therapy than many other mental disorders, is to be found in the way the nonmentalizing actions of BPD patients can create nonmentalizing social systems that sustain their condition, including in the consulting room. We suggest that it is unrealistic to expect clinicians working with such patients to maintain an effective mentalizing stance in the medium to long term themselves if they are not supported adequately to maintain their capacity to mentalize, ideally by a surrounding team that is not directly exposed to (and thus protected from) the patient's dysfunctional social system (see Chapter 13, "AMBIT: Engaging the Client and Communities of Minds," for a discussion of the mentalizing team).

In principle, the patient and therapist are isolated in a room, albeit with bidirectional social influence—the therapist is, after all, in a position to enhance the patient's capacity to reflect, to question, and to focus simultaneously on self and other, internal and external. But the reality is that the therapist becomes embedded within the patient's social survival mechanism, which obliterates balanced mentalizing (normally erring on the side of being unreflective, externally focused, emotional, and dominated by resonance rather than reflectiveness). Even if the clinician's mentalizing is exceptional, it is unlikely to be sufficient to be able to deal with such highly intense emotional situations and conflicts. Therapists thus require their own system of support relationships, primarily from other clinicians, in order to scaffold their capacity to mentalize and facilitate their own epistemic trust.

The self-perpetuating cycle of sustained dysfunction associated with BPD and a nonmentalizing social system reminds us of the international variability in the prevalence of BPD. It has been observed that BPD is less common in non-Western societies, possibly because the lack of social capital and community support characteristic of many modern or modernizing societies leaves individuals more vulnerable to impulsivity and affective instability (Paris and Lis 2013). Available data suggest that Western countries with higher levels of inequality of wealth have a higher prevalence of BPD (Fonagy and Luyten 2016).

Our emphasis on the role of the social environment points to the value of thinking about ways in which a social climate can be encouraged to become more mentalizing, to support a change process. Toleration and entrenchment of high levels of social inequality is made possible by a sustained failure of social imagination, in which the minds of individuals are either discounted altogether or systematically described as "culpable" and "undeserving." Distorted social cognition is, however, necessary for people to be able to live with the vivid human capacity for social imagination and function in an inherently socially imperfect world. The angry sensitivity and imaginative appreciation of the suffering of others that can be such striking features of adolescence may perhaps be tied to a general adolescent tendency to hypermentalize, and the falling away of this active social imagination in adulthood helps individuals to tolerate the social system well enough to navigate it. A mentalizing model of treatment must follow the same developmental challenge that all humans face: that of framing our social imagination in a way that is adaptive and functional within our milieu, while allowing it the capacity for both critique and creativity.

CONCLUSION

We conclude by summarizing what we have offered in this chapter as a speculation about the way therapy works. We started by claiming that an understanding of the structure of psychopathology is not possible without the assumption of a general psychopathology factor. We assume that there is a general vulnerability to psychopathology because a naturally self-righting salutogenic (i.e., health-generating) mechanism is not working. The vulnerability is in learning from experience via social routes in which interpersonal (epistemic) trust is the critical determinant. Epistemic trust is gained through the experience of an individual's personal narrative being recognized by another. People who have experienced adversities (and perhaps also have a genetic predisposition) have problems in establishing and maintaining epistemic trust and experience epistemic isolation, leaving them unable to update their knowledge of themselves and the world around them. In good therapy, the therapist learns to recognize a patient's personal narrative and helps the patient gradually establish epistemic trust to bring him or her back from isolation. This change facilitates the main driver of improvement, which is not what happens in the consulting room but is instead related to the patient (re)joining his or her social network.

REFERENCES

Allen JG: Mentalizing as a conceptual bridge from psychodynamic to cognitive-behavioral therapies. Eur Psychother 8:103–121, 2008
Allen JG: Restoring Mentalizing in Attachment Relationships: Treating Trauma with Plain Old Therapy. Washington, DC, American Psychiatric Publishing, 2012

Allen JG, Fonagy P, Bateman AW: Mentalizing in Clinical Practice. Washington, DC, American Psychiatric Press, 2008

Allen LB, White KS, Barlow DH, et al: Cognitive-behavior therapy (CBT) for panic disorder: relationship of anxiety and depression comorbidity with treatment outcome. J Psychopathol Behav Assess 32(2):185–192, 2010 20421906

Allison E, Fonagy P: When is truth relevant? Psychoanal Q 85(2):275–303, 2016 27112740

American Psychiatric Association: Diagnostic and Statistical Manual of Mental Disorders, 5th Edition. Arlington, VA, American Psychiatric Association, 2013

Benish SG, Quintana S, Wampold BE: Culturally adapted psychotherapy and the legitimacy of myth: a direct-comparison meta-analysis. J Couns Psychol 58(3):279–289, 2011 21604860

Cristea IA, Gentili C, Cotet CD, et al: Efficacy of psychotherapies for borderline personality disorder: a systematic review and meta-analysis. JAMA Psychiatry 74(4):319–328, 2017 28249086

Fonagy P: We have hard choices to make on children's mental health. 2016. Available at: https://www.huffingtonpost.co.uk/peter-fonagy/world-mental-health-day_b_12429138.html. Accessed June 6, 2018.

Fonagy P, Allison E: Psychic reality and the nature of consciousness. Int J Psychoanal 97(1):5–24, 2016 26602060

Fonagy P, Allison E: Commentary: A refresh for evidence-based psychological therapies—reflections on Marchette and Weisz (2017). J Child Psychol Psychiatry 58(9):985–987, 2017 28836679

Fonagy P, Luyten P: A multilevel perspective on the development of borderline personality disorder, in Developmental Psychopathology Vol 3: Maladaptation and Psychopathology, 3rd Edition. Edited by Cicchetti D. New York, Wiley, 2016, pp 726–792

Fonagy P, Gergely G, Jurist E, et al: Affect Regulation, Mentalization, and the Development of the Self. New York, Other Press, 2002

Fonagy P, Rost F, Carlyle JA, et al: Pragmatic randomized controlled trial of long-term psychoanalytic psychotherapy for treatment-resistant depression: the Tavistock Adult Depression Study (TADS). World Psychiatry 14(3):312–321, 2015 26407787

Fonagy P, Luyten P, Allison E, et al: What we have changed our minds about: Part 1. Borderline personality disorder as a limitation of resilience. Borderline Personal Disorder Emotion Dysregul 4:11, 2017a 28413687

Fonagy P, Luyten P, Allison E, et al: What we have changed our minds about: Part 2. Borderline personality disorder, epistemic trust and the developmental significance of social communication. Borderline Personal Disorder Emotion Dysregul 4:9, 2017b 28405338

Fonagy P, Luyten P, Bateman A: Treating borderline personality disorder with psychotherapy: Where do we go from here? JAMA Psychiatry 74(4):316–317, 2017c 28249080

Friborg O, Johnsen TJ: The effect of cognitive-behavioral therapy as an antidepressive treatment is falling: reply to Ljòtsson et al. (2017) and Cristea et al. (2017). Psychol Bull 143(3):341–345, 2017 28230414

Goldberg SB, Rousmaniere T, Miller SD, et al: Do psychotherapists improve with time and experience? A longitudinal analysis of outcomes in a clinical setting. J Couns Psychol 63(1):1–11, 2016 26751152

Horvath AO, Del Re AC, Flückiger C, et al: Alliance in individual psychotherapy, in Psychotherapy Relationships That Work: Evidence-Based Responsiveness, 2nd Edition. Edited by Norcross JC. New York, Oxford University Press, 2011, pp 25–69

Johnsen TJ, Friborg O: The effects of cognitive behavioral therapy as an anti-depressive treatment is falling: a meta-analysis. Psychol Bull 141(4):747–768, 2015 25961373

Kazdin AE: Mediators and mechanisms of change in psychotherapy research. Annu Rev Clin Psychol 3:1–27, 2007 17716046

Mahr J, Csibra G: Why do we remember? The communicative function of episodic memory. Behav Brain Sci January 19, 2017 [Epub ahead of print] 28100294

Nienhuis JB, Owen J, Valentine JC, et al: Therapeutic alliance, empathy, and genuineness in individual adult psychotherapy: a meta-analytic review. Psychother Res 28(4):593–605, 2018 27389666

Norcross JC: Psychotherapy Relationships That Work: Evidence-Based Responsiveness, 2nd Edition. New York, Oxford University Press, 2011

Paris J, Lis E: Can sociocultural and historical mechanisms influence the development of borderline personality disorder? Transcult Psychiatry 50(1):140–151, 2013 23222803

Safran JD, Muran JC, Eubanks-Carter C: Repairing alliance ruptures, in Psychotherapy Relationships That Work: Evidence-Based Responsiveness, 2nd Edition. Edited by Norcross JC. New York, Oxford University Press, 2011, pp 224–238

Sperber D, Clement F, Heintz C, et al: Epistemic vigilance. Mind Lang 25:359–393, 2010

Stoffers JM, Völlm BA, Rücker G, et al: Psychological therapies for people with borderline personality disorder. Cochrane Database Syst Rev 8(8):CD005652, 2012 22895952

Wampold BE, Imel ZE: The Great Psychotherapy Debate: The Evidence for What Makes Psychotherapy Work, 2nd Edition. Hillsdale, NJ, Laurence Erlbaum, 2015

Weisz JR, Jensen-Doss A, Hawley KM: Evidence-based youth psychotherapies versus usual clinical care: a meta-analysis of direct comparisons. Am Psychol 61(7):671–689, 2006 17032068

Weisz JR, Kuppens S, Ng MY, et al: What five decades of research tells us about the effects of youth psychological therapy: a multilevel meta-analysis and implications for science and practice. Am Psychol 72(2):79–117, 2017 28221063

Wittgenstein L: Philosophical Investigations. Oxford, UK, Blackwell, 1953

CHAPTER 11

CREATIVE ARTS THERAPIES

Dominik Havsteen-Franklin, Ph.D.

Creativity is an intrinsic element to mentalizing. Allen and Fonagy (2006) stress that mentalizing "explicitly and creatively is not limited to language; striving to empathize, we imaginatively conjure up visual and other sensory images as we strive to see, feel, and think from others' perspectives…" (p. 17). As Allen and Fonagy suggest, mentalizing truly is an art that is underpinned by scientific rigor; it takes into account uncertainty and a "not-knowing" stance, and it provides the optimal conditions for genuine inquiry, allowing for new ideas and experiences to emerge—qualities that are also at the heart of good arts therapies practice (Havsteen-Franklin 2016; Havsteen-Franklin and Altamirano 2015). Mentalizing is also a process by which we test our imagined scenarios and creative hypotheses that develop from our earliest interactive moments (Tronick 2007).

The way in which we develop our understanding of the world around us depends on reimagining alternative scenarios that utilize an exploratory process, and this process can be enhanced through the use of arts. In other words, in a mentalization-based arts therapies model, there is a focus on the method of using the arts as a practice ground for engaging with mind-mindedness. The "arts" in arts therapies is considered in the context of exploring the relationship between self and other, beginning with what can be observed in the artistic form and moving toward the interpersonal content in a way that is similar to how parent–infant interactions are seen to develop mutually through a range of sensory experiences—sound, sight, and even motoric responses (Tronick 2008). Research regarding the facilitation of mentalizing by the arts has been emerging in recent years (Haeyen et al. 2015; Hannibal 2014; Havsteen-Franklin 2016; Havsteen-Franklin and Altamirano 2015; Springham et al. 2012; Strehlow and Lindner 2015; Taylor Buck and Havsteen-Franklin 2013; Verfalle 2016). These authors conclude that the fundamental elements of a mentalization-focused arts therapies approach are the use of a collaborative approach with the patient and implicit reworking of relational sensitivities through interactive arts engagement. Recent research suggests that patients and arts therapists experience the arts-making process in arts therapies as one that engages and helps to regulate affective states and facilitates arts-based representations of those affective states (Haeyen et al. 2015; Havsteen-Franklin et al. 2016). Some of the key outcomes relate to the ability of the arts process to facilitate a more complex, multiperspective view of self–other interactions (Havsteen-Franklin 2016).

MENTALIZATION-BASED ARTS THERAPIES: AN OVERVIEW

Arts therapists use methods of verbal and nonverbal expression and exploration, with modalities of specialization including drama, dance and body movement, music, and art. The arts modality enables a representation that reflects internal experience in the context of others and becomes a vehicle for stimulating explorations about relationships. Each arts form pays emphasis to a different sense organ, facilitating the representation of experience through an emotional and embodied aesthetic exploration. The arts therapist is technically proficient at using the arts medium as well as knowledgeable and practiced in how the arts can be used to express and explore emotional states.

Arts therapy competencies required to facilitate sustained mentalizing (Box 11–1) have been documented in recent research (Havsteen-Franklin et al. 2016, 2017). This list of competencies demonstrates that the paraverbal and imaginative use of the arts requires similar therapeutic actions to those required for verbal interventions, albeit providing a different method of engaging and working through representational systems. Where implicit nonmentalizing processes remain preconscious, art therapy has been shown to provide an opportunity for accessing treatment when verbal treatment is felt to be overwhelming (Lusebrink 2004). This issue is important to consider when thinking about referral criteria, and this treatment should be prioritized for patients in whom affect dysregulation is profoundly exacerbated by interpersonal contact.

KEEPING THE WIDER CONTEXT IN MIND

Emotional awareness, social understanding, and the development of communities are established through participation in the arts (Arts Council England 2014; Campbell et al. 1999). Historically, in every culture the arts have evolved in a way that supports a common purpose of social development. An evolutionary theory suggests that human social functioning is facilitated through the arts, which have played an essential role in imagining our "social, cultural, political and personal happenings" (Zaidel 2015, p. 281) and developing new ways of adapting to and challenging social norms.

There is an additional important point about cultural sensitivity. Directly addressing feeling states and interpersonal issues is not always sensitive to cultural and religious contexts in which rituals and folk medicine may be the predominant model of therapy (Hiscox and Calisch 1998; Hocoy 2002). However, it is evident that all communities engage in the use of images, music, and drama as part of their healing social activity that helps community members make sense of social, personal, and interpersonal experience (McNiff 1984). Studies suggest that the use of arts as part of cultural rituals and healing practices helps to establish culturally sensitive contexts. There is a strong argument that participating in nonverbal acts of joint attention (Isserow

BOX 11–1. Mentalization-based arts therapies competencies

Mentalization-based arts therapists demonstrate the following competencies through arts-based and verbal means:

- Maintaining openness, curiosity, and uncertainty.
- Perspective taking and reframing.
- Being emotionally supportive and validating.
- Facilitating engagement in the here and now and with recent events.
- Establishing conditions for joint attention.
- Monitoring transference and countertransference.
- Working with implicit and explicit mentalizing processes.
- Using metaphor.
- Having a capacity to explore the interpersonal context and explore narratives.
- Using arts-based improvisation.
- Challenging rigid perspectives.
- Working collaboratively.
- Having an understanding of arts-based aesthetics.
- Promoting emotion regulation and embodying emotional experience.

2008), mirroring (Franklin 2010), finding a shared understanding (Gallese 2003), and embodying feeling states (Twemlow et al. 2008) are central functions of the arts therapies process, and these mechanisms are also central to arts-based healing rituals in many cultures. Therefore, developing a context within the clinic that closely aligns to patients' cultural resources in order to enable imaginative navigation and reflection on emotional states is central to mentalization-based arts therapies practice.

IMPLICIT AND EXPLICIT MENTALIZING THROUGH THE ARTS

To understand the therapeutic function of arts therapies requires understanding the concept of *implicit mentalizing* as key to arts-based interactions. Essentially, the aim of arts therapies is to develop an improvised use of arts as an implicit form of mentalizing. Implicit mentalizing is the automatic and fluent capacity to feel and respond to the social context according to well-informed hypotheses of self and other mental states (Allen and Fonagy 2006; Allen et al. 2003; Davidsen and Fosgerau 2015). In contrast, *explicit mentalizing* is the act of becoming conscious of those processes and reflecting on reflecting as a metacognitive processing of experience. As will be discussed later in this chapter, an important explicit mentalizing action through the arts therapies that differs from verbal therapy is that an arts product is achieved that can be reflected on and that allows for differentiations between short-term memory and the impact of episodic memories (Atwood 1971; Cortina and Liotti 2007; Fonagy 1999), facilitating cognitive and emotional reworking of implicit misperceptions. This process can be most readily used in groups when members are not in agreement about what they perceive the art form to be and are invited to share their thoughts about what is being said and what it feels like to hear what is being stated about the arts form. The therapist models curiosity and sensitively highlights members' different perceptions while also seeking a shared language to support working together. This can enable group members to consider new ways of viewing the content within an interpersonal context with further reflection on what may be helpful to them.

The use of explicit mentalizing in groups also brings into focus the process of making the arts form in the context of a group and relates to the highly implicit process of establishing a safe space that feels reliable and well attended to, but also allows the patient to represent implicit mental processing that differs from explicit reflective capabilities. These implicit processes, which occur largely through mirroring functions, can be described as initiating safety with the same model of biofeedback as originally occurs in early development (Jurist 2006; Jurist and Meehan 2009). As the patient progresses with his or her arts form, the arts usually become less controlled, and the materials, sounds, and movements offer new ways of using arts that the patient did not anticipate (Koch and Fuchs 2011). The action associated with making the sound, marks, or movement then results in an impression that is not altogether what they may have preconceived. Usually, there is initially an intention to recreate an internal representation (e.g., a memory, feeling, or thought) using the arts, but this is altered by unawareness of psychobiological influences as well as the unknown qualities of the materials themselves. The arts form then is suggestive of the patient's experience but also something that was unpredictable and unforeseen. In the early stages of therapy, this often stimulates anxieties and the need for greater control. The therapist's task is to enable openness to the experience and product of engaging in the arts as a precursor to allowing for other perspectives within interpersonal contexts. In other words, it is possible to see the movement from implicit nonmentalizing to implicit mentalizing (Figure 11–1) with the accompanying growth of openness and interest in unpredictability and uncertainty through the arts-making process that can be perceived as good mentalizing of others as the treatment progresses. Under interpersonal stress this process can be reversed, and therefore the therapist may be required to reengage with the task of doing the arts work or being mindful, curious, and descriptive.

On the basis of social learning theory (Matias et al. 2014), it is arguable that while there is fundamental reworking that happens implicitly through sensitive and attuned engagement, this implicit process becomes galvanized through conscious reflection, validation, and praise from others. Therefore, to facilitate sustained outcomes, mentalizing arts therapists also encourage an understanding within a wider context—for example, how a group context (e.g., group therapy) can be considered to hold a range of potentially useful perspectives. The mentalizing arts therapist offers praise and validation of each participant's experience as a secondary step in the process of establishing mentalizing.

THE CREATIVE USE OF METAPHOR

The *creative use of metaphor* refers to the mapping of one representation on to another to produce a novel perspective. For example, using a landscape mapped to a person's history to represent his or her autobiography as a journey produces a novel percep-

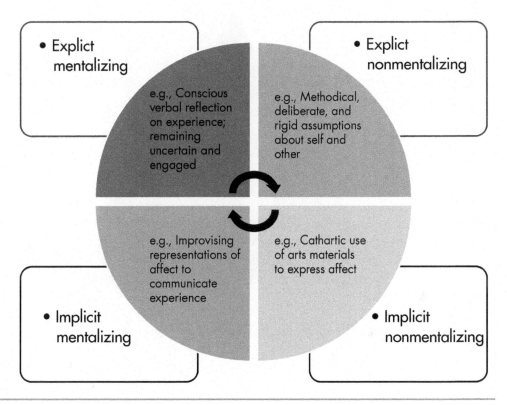

- Explict mentalizing

e.g., Conscious verbal reflection on experience; remaining uncertain and engaged

- Explict nonmentalizing

e.g., Methodical, deliberate, and rigid assumptions about self and other

e.g., Improvising representations of affect to communicate experience

e.g., Cathartic use of arts materials to express affect

- Implicit mentalizing

- Implicit nonmentalizing

FIGURE 11–1.   The mentalizing quadrant.

tion of the person's life story. Using metaphors is a process that begins early in life with the nonverbal mapping of features of the carer's communication to the infant's own experience (e.g., facial expression coupled with feeling states) (Stern 1985). This can be understood as a transition from implicit amodal experiences to more explicit reflection on affective states. The art therapist Jo Rostron describes the implicit phase of the process thus:

> This is a mysterious place where thinking and feeling are inseparable, and where sensory information is transferrable across the five senses and between therapist and client. Perceptual information is experienced—as *contours* of intensity, shape, shifts, patterns of feeling and mood tone—rather than understood or thought about as overt acts or "things" seen or touched. (Rostron 2010, p. 37)

Rostron describes amodal experiences becoming more differentiated through "exuberant" expressions that develop sensed differentiations. In other words, the mentalizing arts therapist is required to provide contingent marked mirroring responses, verbally or through the arts, in order to develop differentiations between self and other experiences (Figure 11–2). The mirroring process does not lose the qualities of the amodal perception; rather, it begins to utilize them in the service of being in a real relationship. As Gergely and Watson (1996, p. 1199) state, "The perception of this contingent relation will provide the basis for the referential interpretation and grounding of the decoupled emotion display."

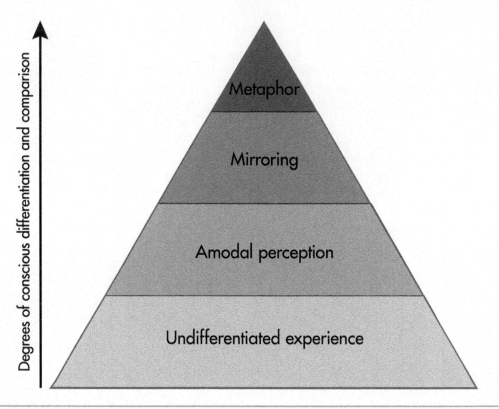

FIGURE 11–2.   Illustration of the developmental "building blocks" for metaphor comprehension.

Decoupling of undifferentiated experiences in the infant is enabled through experiencing early developmental interactions in which a caring other implicitly encourages successful comparison of emotional states, facial expression, feelings, bodily sensations, and other sensed stimuli, which evolve to generate not only a sense of relational constancy and narrative but also novel ways of understanding the self, the other, and the world.

The mirroring mechanism demonstrated in the parent–infant interaction resembles, and is the precursor to, mentalized metaphoric processes whereby the characteristics of one object are mapped to another to produce a novel perception. The cognitive mapping process of the arts representation to experience follows similar processes to the mirroring function in early development that allows for the differentiation of self and other. This early process continues and becomes manifest in increasingly articulate ways through metaphor, poetics, and other forms of symbolization. Bucci (2002) suggests that this "higher" level of articulation has a path of maturation that combines verbal and nonverbal experience as parallel processes. Therefore, rather than assuming that the patient with severe mental illness has a complete deficit in the resources available for forming metaphors, the mentalizing arts therapist assumes a lack of agency and cognitive mapping processes. This means that in nonmentalizing conditions the interpersonal decoupling process that precedes successful cognitive comparison and mapping is an area to be developed as part of being reflective about different mental states. For example, the creative process of forming metaphors about interpersonal disputes might use war, battle, the friction between surfaces, or other visual image sources, mapped to an interpersonal context, to provide the basis for describing the interpersonal struggle and the associated affect (Borbely 2009; Bucci 2002). The arts-based process of forming referential links between verbal and nonverbal language is similar to early developmental experience, where misattuned experiences can be experienced as a searching for the other, implicitly exploring separateness and separation, so that infants recognize themselves as the author of their actions and expression. This work of moving from implicit mentalizing to the metaphoric use of the arts to facilitate explicit mentalizing also has risks, in that the cognitive mapping process drawing on affect and representations as vehicles of inquiry can become unbalanced, either becoming intellectualized and developing into a pretend mode activity, or, alternatively, becoming an overwhelming and confusing imposition, experienced in a similar way to an infant being overfed by a caregiver.

Clinical Extract: Exploration of the Image as Metaphor

Amayas, a young man of Algerian descent and Muslim background, was attending group mentalization-based arts psychotherapy for 18 months, alongside further individual sessions with one of the co-therapists. As part of the mentalization-based arts psychotherapy program, individual sessions are used to reflect on experiences in the group and any encounters evoking strong responses that are too difficult to be worked through in the group context.

The following dialogue takes place 6 months into the therapy, in an individual session following a group session earlier in the week where Amayas was absorbed in making a piece of artwork but was struggling to engage with the group. Amayas had ongoing suicidal ideation, but he no longer acted on those thoughts. Nonetheless, he still found the feelings and thoughts very disturbing and could sometimes react aggressively, particularly to his family members with whom he lived, breaking furniture, including a mirror and television. The extract is from about 15 minutes into the 18th session, following a difficult experience in the group where he appeared to be very withdrawn and depressed. The numbered lines of dialogue are discussed throughout the next section, "Explicit Mentalizing and the Arts Form."

[Line 1] Arts Therapist (AT): I'm aware that we didn't have time to look at your picture in the group because of the disagreement.
[2] AT: How did you feel about that? *[Curious stance]*
[3] Patient (P): It was all right.
[4] P: I mean, I didn't really know what to say anyway. *[Looks away]*
[5] AT: Looking at the picture now, I can see that you painted it in thick black paint around the face.
[6] AT: That black paint occupies most of the space.
[7] AT: You've made some simple lines for a face in the middle. *[Mindful]*
[8] AT: An oval white face and in the center of the page...and then the expression, sad, flat, puzzled? I'm not sure...
[9] AT: It's difficult for me to see... *[Curious stance]*
[10] P: Yeah, me too. I think he's confused. Maybe sad...
[11] P: No, I think more depressed. *[Looks thoughtful]*
[12] AT: Oh, that sounds like a difficult place to be.
[13] AT: Not sad, depressed.
[14] AT: They're different kinds of feeling.
[15] AT: Why is he depressed?
[16] P: I don't know! *[Heightened feeling]*
[17] AT: I'm not sure either. Did something happen?

[18] AT: I was thinking… *[Curious stance]*

[19] P: Yeah, he's got no friends and he's isolated. He just feels like dying. *[Increased pace]*

[20] AT: So he's having a really hard time…It sounds very depressed. Is it all depressing?

[21] P: Kind of. He doesn't know what to do. *[Calmer]*

[22] AT: So there's some uncertainty about what to do next?

[23] P: Yeah. A bit stuck. *[Making eye contact]*

[24] AT: Can anyone help him?

[25] P: He seems pretty much on his own. *[Seems sad]*

[26] AT: But you said something like "He wasn't sure of what to do next, he doesn't know what to do," is that right?

[27] P: Yeah.

[28] AT: So there's some uncertainty. What are the options?

[29] P: I guess he could talk to someone, but he's pretty depressed.

[30] AT: I was just thinking, I'm not sure, but is it difficult to talk about your feelings in the group?

[31] P: Yeah, of course.

[32] AT: *[Surprised]* Oh, I didn't know that. Why is it difficult?

[33] P: Well, I just don't want to get everyone down.

[34] AT: That sounds difficult…So you feel like if you talk, you'll make everyone depressed? Was there anything that made you think that this might happen?

[35] P: No, not really.

[36] AT: This made me think of the person in the image.

[37] P: Yeah, I kind of think it's me.

[38] AT: Well, I just want to go back—I was really interested in this sense of him being uncertain about what to do next. I wonder if it's possible to imagine what he could do next?

[39] P: Maybe. I mean, perhaps he's depressed for a reason.

EXPLICIT MENTALIZING AND THE ARTS FORM

In the clinical extract above, Amayas was implicitly mentalizing through the arts, layering on thick black paint, which became a bodily enactment of an emotional state. However, Amayas also appeared to be withdrawing from the group. He found a way of representing an affective state but felt isolated in the act of doing this. Therefore, the arts-based process, which was the main focus of the work, was successful in establishing an externalization of his internal experience relatively early in the therapy. In other arts therapies, such as music therapy, the explicit interpersonal dialogue can begin through the music therapist's dialogue in the arts form. In the extract above, explicit mentalizing of an implicit process begins after the artwork has been made. The aim of bringing Amayas's attention back to the artwork he produced in the group was to reengage him with pronounced affect and explore any assumptions about the group that might be underlying his withdrawal. It is notable that before the session and within the session, a significant amount of the work depends on the implicit processing of feeling safe with another who is engaged and interested and mirrors the affect. Within the session there begins to be some movement and increased openness to exploring his experience in the group context. In terms of the attempts to make the implicit nonmentalizing processes more explicit, the image is used to facilitate reflection in a similar way to early developmental processes.

The phases of the interactions around the arts are delineated below (see also Figure 11–3), but, as can be seen in the clinical extract, this is not necessarily a linear process, and there are significant overlaps between the phases.

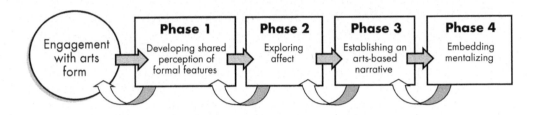

FIGURE 11–3. The four phases of mentalization-based arts therapies.

Phase 1: Developing Shared Perception of Formal Features

From a mentalization-based perspective, the content of the arts object is not known to the viewer. Feelings may be evoked—as well as sensations, memories, and bodily experiences—that offer some good hypotheses about the relationship of the content to the interpersonal context; however, the arts therapist demonstrates a curious stance where the meaning appears to remain opaque. This means that the image holds a complex array of potential possibilities, which the therapist must sensitively navigate using affective states as a focus. In the clinical extract, the arts therapist aims to establish a common ground with Amayas that assumes opaqueness of content and focuses on validating the intentions to produce an arts form and the qualities of that form (Carpendale 2015). In the extract, this occurs in lines 5–8; in those lines, the therapist focuses on the formal aesthetic properties, composition, perspective, color, line, texture, balance, and so forth. This process aims to

- Mindfully stimulate the patient's interest in the formal features.
- Develop a sense of being grounded in the here and now.
- Find a shared language for what is sensed.
- Validate mental impressions.
- Regulate interpersonal proximity.
- Establish conditions for joint attention.
- Regulate affect arousal.

The primary aim of the initial stage of the process is thus to develop a shared perception that builds the therapeutic alliance and develops an aesthetic language, providing the foundations for interpersonal exploration.

Phase 2: Exploring Affect

After the initial stage, the emotional experience of the image-making process is explored (in the clinical extract, this takes place in lines 8–15), as well as what the direct feeling states associated with the aesthetic are. The emotional qualities, associations, and impressions enable mirroring of mental states through exploring the image, as well as reflecting on emotional states that might otherwise be experienced as overwhelming. Exploring the emotional content of the work, accessed in and through the arts form, is the fundamental stage of the therapy, which helps to establish the therapeutic alliance, the focal areas of the work, and basic reflectivity. The emotions will be enveloped by affective conditions that can be traced to early experiences of attachment and separation. While the dominant affect may not be explicitly linked in the session to early development, it may become apparent to the arts therapist that the emotional state is more closely linked to early experiences that are reenacted in the clinical situation.

Once the position of being more grounded in the here and now with a shared affective focus is well established—and it may take minutes or whole sessions for patients to feel they are able to identify and name emotional states—more emotionally complex work can begin to be explored, such as the narrative associated with the content of the arts form (lines 15–29), co-occurrence of emotions (lines 20–21), nuances and blends of emotions and their relationship to the form, associations, and the group context (lines 30–37). This phase enables a sense of agentive narrative, through which relational patterns that occur in the here and now are identified, made explicit, and explored in relation to the interpersonal context.

Phase 3: Establishing an Arts-Based Narrative

The emotions as they are understood in relation to the arts form are also made sense of within the interpersonal context. For example, at the end of the clinical extract, Amayas begins to make sense of the man in the image in terms of being "depressed for a reason" (line 39), and Amayas and the therapist explore several times in the session what might happen next. Further work would include detailing recent interpersonal events that Amayas feels influenced his depression, and understanding how he and the therapist can explore different possibilities for alternative states of mind of others that change the premise of his assumptions—for example, in part of the session Amayas states that he does not know why he assumes that people will become depressed if he talks about his depressed feelings (lines 30–35).

Phase 4: Embedding Mentalizing

While the process of exploring the interpersonal narrative, being curious, and focusing on affect are fundamental principles of explicit mentalizing, for these actions to become more embedded, the arts therapist continues to offer resources to bring implicit mentalizing to the sessions, involving contingent improvisation and self-disclosure about emotional experiencing of the interactions. The emergence of collaborative conversations during which the therapist's uncertainty becomes increasingly contoured, allowing for new thoughts and feelings to emerge, begins to happen at the end of the extract, in lines 37–38, where the patient realizes that there may be a reason he is depressed that he had not been previously aware of. The therapeutic alliance was sufficiently established, and emotional states were better understood in the context of the group with the support of the individual sessions. Later in the therapy, both the patient and therapist used art materials in a way that allowed for greater ambiguity and to improvise, creating space for unpredictable qualities that added to the aesthetic. This phase is a return to implicit mentalizing, with explicit mentalizing being replaced by creative approaches to experiencing interpersonal contexts in a more open and exploratory way through improvised use of the arts. This phase also lends itself to the patient using arts in nonclinical contexts.

In all stages of the process, it is important that the patient's emotional qualities are kept in mind and that the arts therapist is sensitive to nonmentalizing states, for example, if a patient shows a detached "as if" pretend mode and begins to disengage from affective content relating to the interpersonal context. When mentalizing begins to go awry, the process may require "back-stepping" and returning to the previous phase, as illustrated in Figure 11–3.

MALADAPTIVE ATTACHMENT AND NONMENTALIZING IN ARTS THERAPIES

For arts therapies to be effective, the arts therapist must be aware of a therapeutic context that has the potential to stimulate maladaptive attachment patterns. When there is overwhelming anxiety about the relational context, this often becomes manifest in the arts form. The mentalizing arts therapist must be adept at validating the patient's experience, exploring and making sense of the situation through the use of the arts, and making the content more explicit in collaboration with the patient. The approach and the attitude of the patient in arts therapies indicate the underlying attachment pattern that is activated. These issues are summarized in Figure 11–4, which denotes a prototypical arts therapy session. The figure can be read from left to right, which represents the progress of the session. Each stage of the session can result in different maladaptive responses stimulated by the implicit or explicit demands of the arts therapy to be relational and reflective. Engagement in the arts potentially stimulates maladaptive relational patterns, resulting in nonmentalizing states of mind, which in a mentalization-based approach need to be attended to by the arts therapist. An important part of the therapy is to assist the patient with recovering from nonmentalizing positions, through slowing down the process and introducing a stance and focus that is attuned to the affective states, is validating, and provides opportunities to reconsider basic assumptions about self and other. This process is summarized with examples in the bottom row of the figure.

ARTS THERAPY AND TEAM WORKING

Most arts therapists work within a team context in mental health services. What is often asked of the arts therapist is to help assess and describe a patient's experience from another perspective, which can help to inform the overall treatment plan. While the patient may disclose helpful details about his or her experience to the therapist that can be safely shared with the treatment team, what is equally important is the arts therapist's contribution to enabling the team to mentalize the patient. The arts can have an instrumental role in enabling the patient's experience to become sensitively considered from a range of perspectives, which are stimulated through reflecting on the arts form. At times, a professional may have emotionally driven associations to the arts form, which may bypass the arts and instead focus on what the image may refer to. As illustrated in the clinical extract earlier in this chapter, slowing down the situation to digest the aes-

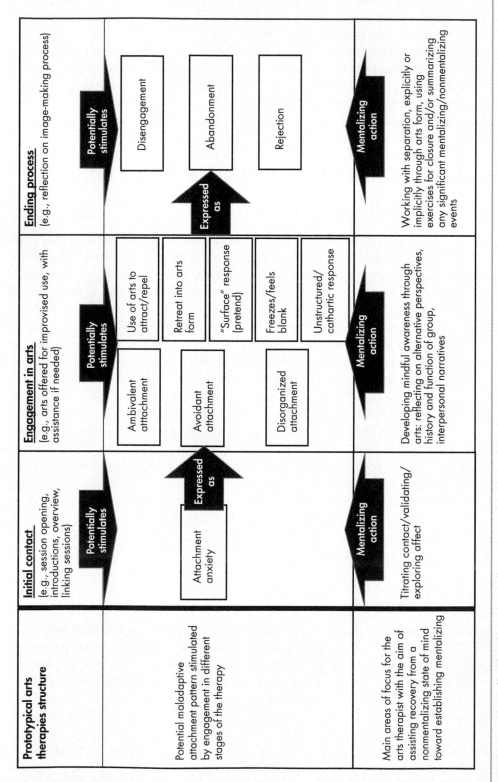

FIGURE 11–4. Mentalization-based arts therapies session process.

thetic is important to understand a range of possibilities and to form good hypotheses through dialogue with the team. This method of focusing on the arts form can also have an impact more widely in terms of professionals attuning to the emotional narrative of the patient—mentalizing nonverbal communications, associations, and images that occur for the professional group in relationship to the patient. While the optimum conditions for this kind of work are within a group supervisory context, similar processes can be initiated within team meetings and case discussions.

ARTS AND MENTALIZING BEYOND THE CLINIC

Usually, healthcare contexts provide treatment for the primary symptoms of the presenting mental health issues, allowing for discharge when symptoms such as self-harm, suicide risk, and impulsive behaviors are minimized. However, this does not mean that the work for the patient is over. There may still be interpersonal problems, social isolation, and other symptoms, including mild to moderate depression or anxiety. Because mental healthcare services discharge patients when the treatment is considered to have produced sustainable change to the levels of risk associated with the primary symptoms of the disorder, consideration needs to be given to how these persons can continue their work on regulating and sustaining mentalizing beyond their immediate social and familial context.

It is commonly the case that the patient has gained some competence in implicit mentalizing through the arts, and even creative, novel ways of understanding the content of the arts form. This process is often continued outside the clinic in the patient's own time or in the context of groups supported by non–mental health organizations. It is a central responsibility of arts therapists to support this process of social engagement where the patient can make contact with the wider community, especially in contexts in which this has proved to be difficult in the past due to nonmentalizing states disrupting social relationships. The groups with which the patient engages are unlikely to be process focused, as the patient's experience of the arts therapies groups will have been, but will allow for some similar processes to take place, including mediation of the interpersonal space through making arts, implicit processing of affect and interpersonal experiences, and allowing for permeable boundaries whereby other people's perspectives can be considered as having validity regardless of how similar or different those views are to the patient's own.

CONCLUSION

Mentalization-based arts therapies (Havsteen-Franklin 2016) are a relatively recent branch of mentalization-based practice in healthcare settings. This chapter has provided an overview of the basic tenets of this approach (see Box 11–2). The method builds on and provides a common language to many of the forms of arts therapies that have developed over recent years that are beginning to show effectiveness in healthcare contexts for patients who have difficulties resulting from nonmentalizing.

BOX 11–2.   **Mentalizing and creative arts therapies: summary**

- Arts therapists working within mental health contexts using a mentalizing-focused model have a range of interpersonal competencies that enable engagement with and reflection on the arts.

- Arts therapists have the potential to cause harm, through stimulating nonmentalizing modes; however, the facilitated recovery from these states is central to the person's overall recovery.

- A key feature of the mentalizing process is enabling the use of imagination through engaging with and reflecting on the arts form.

- Arts therapies focus on making implicit mentalizing and nonmentalizing processes explicit in the therapeutic context.

- The use of metaphor is a process of explicitly linking affect with the arts-based representation and the interpersonal context.

- The content of the arts form is opaque, requiring collaborative investigation by the patient and therapist, which begins with the formal features of the arts form.

REFERENCES

Allen JG, Fonagy P: Handbook of Mentalization-Based Treatment. New York, Wiley, 2006

Allen JG, Bleiberg E, Haslam-Hopwood T: Understanding mentalizing: mentalizing as a compass for treatment. 2003. Available at: https://www.menningerclinic.com/clinicians/clinical-resources/mentalizing. Accessed June 6, 2018.

Arts Council England: The Value of Arts and Culture to People and Society. Manchester, UK, Arts Council England, 2014

Atwood G: An experimental study of visual imagination and memory. Cognit Psychol 2:290–299, 1971

Borbely AF: The centrality of metaphor and metonymy in psychoanalytic theory and practice. Psychoanal Inq 29:58–68, 2009

Bucci W: The referential process, consciousness, and the sense of self. Psychoanal Inq 22:766–793, 2002

Campbell J, Liebmann M, Brooks F, et al: Art Therapy, Race, and Culture. London, Jessica Kingsley Publishers, 1999

Carpendale M: A hermeneutic phenomenological approach to art therapy. Can Art Ther Assoc J 21:2–10, 2015

Cortina M, Liotti G: New approaches to understanding unconscious processes: implicit and explicit memory systems. Int Forum Psychoanal 16:204–212, 2007

Davidsen AS, Fosgerau CF: Grasping the process of implicit mentalization. Theory Psychol 25:434–454, 2015

Fonagy P: Memory and therapeutic action. Int J Psychoanal 80(Pt 2):215–223, 1999 10363179

Franklin M: Affect regulation, mirror neurons, and the third hand: formulating mindful empathic art interventions. Art Ther 27:160–167, 2010

Gallese V: The roots of empathy: the shared manifold hypothesis and the neural basis of intersubjectivity. Psychopathology 36(4):171–180, 2003 14504450

Gergely G, Watson JS: The social biofeedback theory of parental affect-mirroring: the development of emotional self-awareness and self-control in infancy. Int J Psychoanal 77(Pt 6):1181–1212, 1996 9119582

Haeyen S, van Hooren S, Hutschemaekers G: Perceived effects of art therapy in the treatment of personality disorders, cluster B/C: a qualitative study. Arts Psychother 45:1–10, 2015

Hannibal N: Implicit and explicit mentalisation in music therapy in psychiatric treatment of people with borderline personality disorder, in The Music in Music Therapy: Psychodynamic Music Therapy in Europe: Clinical, Theoretical and Research Approaches. Edited by De Backer J, Sutton J. London, Jessica Kingsley Publishers, 2014, pp 211–223

Havsteen-Franklin D: Mentalization-based art therapy, in Approaches to Art Therapy Theory and Techniques. Edited by Rubin J. New York, Brunner/Mazel, 2016, 144–164

Havsteen-Franklin D, Altamirano JC: Containing the uncontainable: responsive art making in art therapy as a method to facilitate mentalization. Int J Art Ther 20:54–65, 2015

Havsteen-Franklin D, Maratos A, Usiskin M, et al: Examining arts psychotherapies practice elements: early findings from the Horizons Project. Approaches: An Interdisciplinary Journal of Music Therapy 8(Special Issue 1):50–62, 2016

Havsteen-Franklin D, Jovanovic N, Reed N, et al: Developing a shared language within arts psychotherapies: a personal construct psychology approach to understanding clinical change. Arts Psychother 55:103–110, 2017

Hiscox A, Calisch A: Tapestry of Cultural Issues in Art Therapy. London, Jessica Kingsley Publishers, 1998

Hocoy D: Cross-cultural issues in art therapy. Art Ther 19:141–145, 2002

Isserow J: Looking together: joint attention in art therapy. Int J Art Therapy 13:34–42, 2008

Jurist EL: Art and emotion in psychoanalysis. Int J Psychoanal 87(Pt 5):1315–1334, 2006 16997728

Jurist EL, Meehan KB: Attachment, mentalization, and reflective functioning, in Attachment Theory and Research in Clinical Work With Adults. Edited by Obegi J, Berant E. New York, Guilford, 2009, pp 71–93

Koch SC, Fuchs T: Embodied arts therapies. Arts Psychother 38:276–280, 2011

Lusebrink VB: Art therapy and the brain: an attempt to understand the underlying processes of art expression in therapy. Art Ther 21:125–135, 2004

Matias C, O'Connor TG, Futh A, et al: Observational attachment theory-based parenting measures predict children's attachment narratives independently from social learning theory-based measures. Attach Hum Dev 16(1):77–92, 2014 24283669

McNiff S: Cross-cultural psychotherapy and art. Art Ther 1:125–131, 1984

Rostron J: On amodal perception and language in art therapy with autism. Int J Art Ther 15:36–49, 2010

Springham N, Findlay D, Woods A, et al: How can art therapy contribute to mentalization in borderline personality disorder? Int J Art Ther 17:115–129, 2012

Stern DN: The Interpersonal World of the Infant: A View from Psychoanalysis and Developmental Psychology. New York, Basic Books, 1985

Strehlow G, Lindner R: Music therapy interaction patterns in relation to borderline personality disorder (BPD) patients. Nord J Music Ther 25:134–158, 2015

Taylor Buck E, Havsteen-Franklin D: Connecting with the image: how art psychotherapy can help to re-establish a sense of epistemic trust. ATOL: Art Therapy Online 4(1), 2013

Tronick E: The Neurobehavioral and Social-Emotional Development of Infants and Children. New York, WW Norton, 2007

Tronick E: Meaning making and the dyadic expansion of consciousness model. Paper presented at the Festschrift in Honor of Arnold Modell, Boston Psychoanalytic Society and Institute, Boston, MA, 2008

Twemlow SW, Sacco FC, Fonagy P: Embodying the mind: movement as a container for destructive aggression. Am J Psychother 62(1):1–33, 2008 18461841

Verfalle M: Mentalizing in Arts Therapies. London, Karnac Books, 2016

Zaidel DW: Neuropsychology of Art: Neurological, Cognitive, and Evolutionary Perspectives. Hove, UK, Psychology Press, 2015

CHAPTER 12

PARTIAL HOSPITALIZATION SETTINGS

Dawn Bales, Ph.D.

Originally, mentalization-based treatment (MBT) was developed and studied in a partial hospitalization setting (MBT-PH), that is, a day hospital in Europe. The first randomized controlled trial of MBT-PH showed positive effects that were discernible 5 years after treatment was completed (Bateman and Fonagy 1999, 2008). In 2004, De Viersprong, a Dutch treatment center for personality disorders, decided to replicate the partial hospitalization program developed in the United Kingdom to determine whether the favorable outcomes could be repeated by an independent institution in a naturalistic setting outside the United Kingdom. The studies provided further support for MBT-PH treatment for patients with borderline personality disorder (BPD). A prospective cohort study in the Netherlands (Bales et al. 2012) showed that manualized day-hospital MBT could indeed be effectively implemented with (at least) the same beneficial results as in the United Kingdom by an independent institute in a naturalistic setting outside the United Kingdom, strengthening the confidence that manualized day-hospital MBT is an effective treatment for patients with severe BPD. The same research group extended the evidence for long-term effectiveness of day-hospital MBT by comparing the treatment outcome of a group of BPD patients with severe comorbidity—that is, those with drug addiction and antisocial personality disorder, who are commonly excluded from other trials—with that of a carefully matched group of patients with severe BPD who received "other specialized psychotherapeutic treatments" (OPT), including dialectical behavior therapy, schema therapy, transference-focused therapy, and specialized general psychiatric management (Bales et al. 2015). Patients in the MBT group significantly improved during treatment and continued to improve in the 18-month follow-up period. Personality functioning improved largely on all five higher-order domains (i.e., self-control, identity integration, responsibility, social concordance, and relational capacities). While outcome in OPT was also favorable, the effect sizes were smaller, and the comparison between MBT and OPT indicated superior outcome for MBT patients on all outcome variables except for relational functioning.

In another independent study in Denmark, a cohort of patients treated with partial hospitalization followed by MBT group therapy showed significant improvements after 2 years on a range of measures, including global assessment of function (GAF), hospitalizations, and vocational status, with further improvement at 2-year follow-up (Petersen et al. 2010).

Because of its intensity and the related costs, partial hospitalization treatment for mental health problems has become increasingly questioned, and there is a need for more research concerning its cost-effectiveness. A current multicenter randomized controlled trial in the Netherlands (Laurenssen et al. 2014) is investigating the efficacy and cost-effectiveness of MBT-PH versus MBT-intensive outpatient (MBT-IOP) in patients with BPD. It is hoped that the study will provide more refined criteria to select patients who can be treated in an outpatient context or those who require more intensive support in a partial hospitalization program.

In the studies on the implementation of MBT in the Netherlands, the investigators found that it is one thing to investigate the efficacy of a treatment, but quite another issue to implement and/or adapt a treatment program effectively and maintain its efficacy (Bales et al. 2017a, 2017b; Hutsebaut et al. 2012). In this chapter, we consider some of these implementation issues and describe how treatment can be organized to create the optimal context within which interventions enhancing mentalizing can be delivered.

PATIENT POPULATION

The developmental model on which MBT is based suggests that constitutional vulnerabilities in interaction with early adversity (in particular emotional neglect) undermine the development of mentalizing capacities, as reflected in emotional regulation problems, self-destructive behavior, and interpersonal and social problems (see Chapter 19, "Borderline Personality Disorder"). These symptoms are characteristic of personality disorders, especially BPD, for which MBT-PH was originally developed. However, various other psychological disorders are also marked by gross deficits or considerable imbalances in and between different mentalizing capacities. Therefore, MBT is currently considered to be a transdiagnostic treatment model, aiming to increase the resilience of patients' mentalizing capacity irrespective of diagnosis. So, in contrast to many other studies of treatments for personality disorder, studies of MBT have included patients with comorbid antisocial personality disorder and other personality disorders. MBT-PH is offered only to patients with the most severe personality disorder, with high levels of comorbidity for major mental illness and personality disorders, in whom drug use and self-harm have become ingrained, and whose social function and interpersonal adaptation are severely compromised. In view of the severity of these patients' problems, a number of components of a partial hospitalization program address these issues.

TREATMENT GOALS AND TREATMENT PLANS

At the beginning of MBT-PH treatment, it is necessary to define overall treatment goals. In MBT-PH all patients work toward meeting five general treatment goals (Box 12–1).

BOX 12–1.   **General treatment goals in MBT-PH**

- Engage in therapy.

- Reduce psychiatric symptoms, particularly anxiety and depression.

- Reduce self-damaging and other behaviors that disrupt treatment.

- Improve interpersonal function.

- Improve social function.

Each of these goals is incorporated into a patient's treatment plan along with a mentalizing formulation (see also Chapter 6, "Individual Therapy Techniques," Chapter 15, "Children," and Chapter 17, "Borderline Personality Pathology in Adolescence") that is developed in the individual sessions. In the treatment plan, goals are personalized by summarizing a joint understanding between patient and clinician of the underlying problems, in terms of mentalizing and the development of the problems and their function in the patient's current life. Identified goals are linked to the components of the program in which the patient and the clinician think most of the work will be done to achieve them. All team members treating the patient need to understand the treatment plan and its implications for their work with the patient. The treatment plan serves as a guide to treatment for both patient and clinician. It guides interventions and focus in sessions. In treatment reviews with each patient, the patient is asked to report his or her views on the issues described in the treatment plan and his or her current progress toward goals. In these reviews, different views of the treatment team members are integrated into a coherent set of ideas together with the patient. The treatment reviews in themselves stimulate the mentalizing process of patient and staff alike, helping the patient to develop a coherent interpersonal and developmental narrative. A clinical example of how a treatment plan is woven into treatment itself is described by Bales et al. (2018).

At the beginning of therapy, it is important to extensively explore the patient's relationships, (self-)destructive behaviors, and previous treatments. Recognizing mental states and patterns will help the clinician know which types of interventions need to be used and will indicate the form of the relationship that is likely to develop between the patient, the clinician, and the wider treatment team. Once these patterns have been identified, they are discussed with the patient and incorporated into the mentalizing formulation and treatment plan. They offer an important opportunity to make a tentative suggestion that some of the relationship patterns may be repeated within the treatment itself.

There are a number of additional components of MBT-PH that are specific to the context of treatment and the population being treated. These include a methodically derived crisis plan, stabilization of social and behavior problems, mentalizing cognitive therapy (MCT), creative art therapy, a writing group, and explicit inclusion of family members.

Crisis Plan

Nearly all patients will experience a crisis at some point during treatment. Often, self-destructive acts by the patient in crisis are a result of overwhelming feelings and panic. Failure by mental health professionals to understand the role of self-harm in coping with unmanageable emotional states may lead to inappropriate use of medication and unnecessary hospital admissions; both of these responses remove responsibility from the patient for addressing painful affects and are potentially iatrogenic.

Agreeing on and documenting what to do in the event of a crisis is one of the very first issues discussed in the individual session at entry to the MBT-PH program. The crisis plan has two parts: 1) the individualized (process) part and 2) the practical part. From a mentalizing perspective, it is not appropriate to give the patient a plan that tells him or her what is best to do at what time. It is more in keeping with the mentalizing model to stimulate the patient to think about what situations and accompanying mental states could lead to a crisis, and what might be helpful to restabilize him or her in the event of a crisis.

In the crisis plan, ways of managing the patient's difficult emotional states related to self-destructive acts that interfere with therapy or endanger life are identified. The first part of the crisis plan is collaboratively developed between patient and clinician by stimulating discussion about different stages of mental states that precede the crisis. Each of the following stages is defined:

- 0=Feeling in control.
- 1 and 2=[Patients define these stages themselves].
- 3=In crisis or out of control.

Patients try to identify their mental states and behaviors in each of the separate stages. The clinician uses clarification and affect elaboration techniques, frequently coaxing the patient to rewind mental processes to points prior to the loss of control, thereby helping the patient to identify feelings and place them in context. Overwhelming, undifferentiated feeling states are "microsliced" into smaller, more specific mental states by using moment-to-moment exploration of the episode leading up to a crisis or act of self-harm. The emphasis is on examining feeling states and identifying possible misunderstandings or oversensitivity. The patient is helped to identify when he or she could have reestablished self-control and what could have prevented him or her from moving on to the next stage toward a crisis. Strategies that have been helpful for the patient in managing emotional crises in the past are identified, such as leaving a provocative situation, telephoning someone if trapped in a feeling of loneliness, or distracting his or her own mind by engaging in a behavioral task, such as cooking. The clinician also tries to stimulate the patient to reflect on how others might observe each stage (i.e., signals for others) and what others could do—or should not do—that might be helpful. Significant others are invited to these sessions to collaboratively work out this part of the crisis plan.

In the beginning of treatment, this part of the crisis plan is tentative. Patients often have no idea about their different mental states and about the behaviors that result from a failure of mentalizing, stating simply, *"It happens at once, and there's nothing I can do."* The plan is a work in progress, and each time certain aspects become clearer, they are added to the plan. The clinician is required to revisit the crisis plan whenever a crisis occurs. When the actions already identified in the plan fail to work, it can be helpful to stimulate the patient to think about what is missing in the plan, what mental state might not be described, what did not help, and why it did not help. In this way, the clinician is continuously pointing out the patient's own responsibility for dealing with painful and possibly overwhelming affects. At the same time, it helps to reduce the patient's perplexity about his or her emotional states, and continual clarification reduces the likelihood that the patient will need to manage his or her feelings through self-harm or other such actions.

In addition to such patient-specific plans, in the second part of the crisis plan, the clinician outlines the emergency system that is available to the patient outside office hours.

Stabilization of Social and Behavior Problems

Social and behavior problems that are most likely to interfere with treatment are identified, and ways of addressing them are organized during the initial phase of treatment. Successful stabilization and high levels of motivation are *not,* however, conditions of entering treatment; rather, they are more a focus of the pretreatment period.

Mentalizing Cognitive Therapy

In contrast to outpatient MBT, MBT-PH includes an MCT group. MCT is an explicit mentalizing group focusing on a wide range of mentalizing processes. The structured form of each MCT session is very similar to that of cognitive therapy, but there are some essential differences. Cognitive-behavioral therapy (CBT) has its roots in social learning theory, and its model of behavior does not include dynamic determinants. Thus, it is less process-oriented and more content-oriented. The MBT clinician is encouraged to think dynamically about the patient's experience; MCT is thus more process-oriented and less content-oriented. This shift of focus allows consideration of preconscious or unconscious thoughts, feelings, wishes, and desires, and of patients' struggles with these complex mental experiences in the context of the interpersonal pressures of their lives, particularly attachment relationships. The CBT clinician focuses on changing maladaptive cognitions; the MBT clinician is less interested in restructuring the content of the cognitions and more interested in changing the process by reinstating mentalizing.

MCT, unlike many forms of CBT, involves no specific use of problem-solving skills or teaching of fundamental communication skills; no attempt to delineate cognitive distortions outside the current patient–clinician relationship or to focus on behavior itself; no explicit work on schema identification; and no homework.

MCT consists of a small group that meets for 75 minutes once a week. A patient describes a situation in which he or she experienced (or is currently experiencing) overwhelming emotion or engaged in (self-)destructive behavior. The situation is represented on a whiteboard. The patient's mental state (but also the possible mental states of others, if involved) and behavior are explored, and components of the event and the associated feelings are written down. The clinician focuses on exploring the mental states broadly rather than using precise and detailed identification of thoughts, feelings, or wishes. The main focus of the session is the mentalizing process, and there is much less focus on the end-product or content of the events and interaction. If the patient wants to explore his or her (self-)destructive behavior, the clinician's main focus is to help the patient "tidy up" the behavior that has resulted from a failure of mentalizing, tracing action back to feeling, and thus stimulating mentalizing about the (recent) past. The clinician helps the patient take his or her mind back to the problematic experience, from the safety of emotional distance. In the case of overwhelming emotion, the clinician tries to help bridge the gap between the primary affective experience and its symbolic representation by helping the patient understand and label the emotional state and place it within the current context, sometimes further exploring linking narrative to the recent and remote past.

When the events and interactions have been clarified, the clinician and group help the patient by bringing in alternative perspectives. The difference from CBT is that here the alternative perspectives are not a result of a Socratic dialogue or of disputing "irrational" or "maladaptive" cognitions, but are simply alternative perspectives suggested by other patients. This helps patients question their assumptions.

Sometimes group schemas are made in which problematic interactions within the group are identified and explored in a structured way, with the mental states of several group members being highlighted, focusing on different perspectives about a turbulent issue within the group.

Creative Art Therapy

The aim of art therapy in MBT-PH is to offer an alternative way of promoting mentalizing. The use of art allows internal mental states to be expressed externally, through an alternative medium and from a different perspective. Experience and feeling are placed outside of the mind and into the world to facilitate explicit mentalizing. In these circumstances, mentalizing becomes conscious, verbal, deliberate, and reflective. Patients produce something that is part of them, yet separate. In this way, the therapy creates transitional objects, and the clinician must work at developing a transitional space within the group in which the created objects can be used to facilitate expression while maintaining stability of the self. Mentalizing in the context of art and other expressive therapies is discussed in detail in Chapter 11, "Creative Arts Therapies."

Creative therapy differs from other components of the MBT-PH program because the patient makes a concrete "product." The product gives the opportunity for the patient and group to focus specifically on a certain area of reflection. For some patients, expressive therapies are less anxiety-provoking than directly reflecting about themselves in relation to others. With their product made, an aspect of the self is outside, and is therefore rendered less dangerous, less controlling, and less overwhelming. Feelings become manageable, and the patients' understanding of themselves and others is more tolerable because of the distance created. Other patients, particularly those who function predominantly in psychic equivalence mode, can be more anxious during creative therapy. The product they make—which is now also visible on the outside and to others—makes that aspect of themselves too "real," and they become overwhelmed. Therefore, the art clinician must tailor his or her work individually with different patients at different phases of their therapy.

Art therapy is done in a small group twice weekly for 75 minutes per session. The form varies from working individually on personal goals in the group, to working individually on a group theme, to making a group project. At the start of each session, patients are helped to focus on how they are feeling at the moment and what they would like to work on. A prominent issue in the group may be brought in by the clinician or one or more of the patients. Once the form of the session (e.g., working on a theme individually or in pairs initially) has been decided, the patients choose where in the room they want to work on their project for 30 minutes.

After completing their work, the patients gather again for a group discussion of each other's work. In this discussion, as in all program components, the clinician's task is to promote mentalizing by focusing on the expression of affects, their identification, and their personal and interpersonal contexts. The clinician also should ensure that patients consider the meaning of the expressive efforts of others and can help patients recognize that others may see their work in a different way from the way they see it, helping to create alternative perspectives. The standard of the art is not important; the process of expression and discussion of the work is significant.

Clinicians must continually bring the discussion back to the agreed focus rather than follow other avenues of exploration as they might in a mentalizing group or individual therapy. This technique is necessary to increase the patients' ability to attend to a task without being diverted by other themes, to increase effortful control.

Writing Group

Writing down one's experiences, feelings, and emotions helps to bridge the gap between 1) primary experience and representation and 2) its symbolic representation, which allows the reflective process to develop and strengthens the secondary representational system. Through writing, implicit mentalizing becomes explicit mentalizing. Writing allows for reflection without the interference of other minds, and with distance in time if the patient has written about an earlier event, so less arousal occurs.

Writing therapy takes place in a small group once a week for 90 minutes, typically with two clinicians present. To begin, all the patients and the clinicians write on a piece of paper a theme that they feel is a prominent issue in the group or on the unit. All the papers are placed in a box. One of the patients picks out a paper at random, and all the patients write down the chosen theme. They then have 30 minutes to write about the theme, especially its personal meaning. Next, each patient reads aloud what he or she has written, and together, led by the clinicians, the patients explore the similarities and differences between their essays. Again, the clinicians aim to promote mentalizing by helping the patients to create alternative perspectives on what they have written. As in art therapy, what is written down is less important than the process of developing the theme, writing about it, and discussing the personal essays.

Mentalization-Based Family Therapy Module

Mentalization-based family therapy (MBT-F; see Chapter 8, "Working With Families") is a module to which patients from the different MBT programs can be referred with their families. MBT-F addresses mentalizing processes within the family context rather than focusing on specific symptoms. It aims to provide family members with tools that will enable them to initiate a self-healing process. Improved understanding within a family will improve the quality and supportiveness of family attachment relationships and strengthen the family's capacity to control and manage problems, both of which can facilitate the patient's progress in treatment.

ENDING TREATMENT

The focus of the final phase of treatment is on the interpersonal and social aspects of functioning, and on integrating and consolidating gains in mentalizing. Important goals are increasing patients' responsibility and independent functioning, focusing on affective states associated with loss, and ending treatment. Collaborative development of a follow-up treatment plan individually tailored to each patient's needs is an essential task in this final phase of treatment.

After a maximum duration of partial hospitalization treatment of 18 months, it is unlikely that patients with severe personality disorders—who often have histories of failed treatments, multiple hospital admissions, and inadequate social and relational stability—will be able to adapt and reintegrate to their new lives without further support. This is usually the case no matter how successful the treatment has been. Individual tailored follow-up treatment with stepped-down care is therefore offered. The goals of follow-up treatment are summarized in Box 12–2.

BOX 12–2. **Goals of follow-up to MBT-PH**

- Prevent relapse.

- Maintain and enhance gains made in mentalizing capacity.

- Stimulate rehabilitative changes in interpersonal interaction.

- Reintegrate the patient into the social world.

Patients continue with monthly maintenance sessions of individual therapy with the clinician they were seeing in the MBT-PH program. During these sessions the clinician continues to use mentalizing techniques to explore the patient's underlying mental states and to discuss how understanding oneself and others makes it easier to resolve problems, helping to manage both problematic areas of interpersonal or intimate relationships and the process of returning to education or employment.

In the follow-up period, the time between appointments is increased over a 6- to 12-month period to encourage greater patient responsibility. The clinician and patient decide together how long the patient will continue to be seen in this way, with a maximum duration of 18 months. The intensity and frequency of appointments in the follow-up contract are flexible, and the patient can request an additional appointment if he or she has an emotional problem that he or she is finding difficult to manage. After formal discharge, patients are still able to come back after many months or even years when they feel they are relapsing, and often only a few sessions are necessary to reinstate their mentalizing and help them restabilize. This continual follow-up with permission for self-referral means that patients experience continuity over a prolonged period. Some patients choose to be discharged after MBT-PH knowing that they can call to request an appointment at any time in the future. Others plan only a few appointments but set them far ahead with a 6-month interval; the assurance that the clinician continues to have them in mind seems to give them greater confidence and self-reliance about their ability to reintegrate.

MENTALIZING ENVIRONMENT

An important factor within the MBT-PH program structure in daily practice is how well the staff members function, how predictable they are, how consistently they implement treatment, and how clear boundaries are in terms of roles and responsibilities. Inconsistency, lack of coordination, incoherence of response, unreliability, and arbitrariness are all antithetical to structure. We discuss some of these issues here. Our research has found that the effectiveness of implementation of treatment is dependent on many of these factors.

Important nonspecific factors, such as the interrelations of the different components of the MBT program, the clinicians and their working relationship, the continuity of themes among the groups, and the consistency and coherence with which the treatment is applied over time, are likely to be key factors in effective treatment of severe personality disorders. Within MBT, this essential integration is achieved through a focus on mentalizing. How, then, does a treatment team create a framework in which mentalizing becomes and remains the focus?

Creating a Mentalizing Environment

The partial hospitalization treatment program requires patients to attend over a long time and involves considerable interaction between patients. The atmosphere created, the character of the building, and the staff and their functioning all need to be conducive to the orientation and focus of the treatment. This is the therapeutic milieu. Within MBT-PH programs, the milieu is not a treatment method in its own right, as it might be in therapeutic communities. However, establishing the best possible environment for MBT is a very important consideration when treatment is being organized. Material aspects of the milieu include the building, its location, the entrance, the style of written information provided, and the available therapy rooms, whereas nonmaterial aspects include the staff members, the quality of their working relationship, their attitude toward patients and one another, the consistency and coherence of the approach, and the management's support of the program (see Box 12–3).

BOX 12–3.   Factors optimizing MBT outcomes at organizational level

- Highly structured, project-based implementation.

- Full commitment of the board, including financial support.

- Proactive management who collaborate with supervisor and team to provide a supportive working environment.

- Active collaboration with major referral centers to provide integrated disease management across services.

- Establishment of clear pathways for referrals (including clearly defined inclusion and exclusion criteria) and rapid service access.

- Quality monitoring of treatment processes and outcomes.

- Clearly defined treatment program structure, including treatment phasing.

- Sufficient time for treatment plan review, supervision, and intervision.

- Recruitment of professionals that is based on affinity with borderline personality disorder and necessary skills and competencies.

- Team leader with the competencies to effectively build teams and to maintain a healthy and professional working environment.

In creating an optimal treatment milieu, treatment orientation and focus are the primary considerations. Within MBT, the milieu should stimulate mentalizing about the self, others, and their interactions—that is, it should be a mentalizing environment. An open, responsive, mentalizing atmosphere is not only needed for the patients but also essential for the staff. A well-functioning team will create a secure atmosphere within the treatment milieu. This allows disagreements between clinicians and patients to be used constructively; facilitates an inquisitive, curious, and open-minded culture; and encourages attempts to understand differences, generating and accepting alternative perspectives. A mentalizing milieu encourages thought over action: every action beyond protocol is first checked out with other staff members to identify possible underlying relational and counterrelational processes.

In order for the environment to remain safe and supportive, strong feelings engendered in staff members need to be contained without either using excessive protection or overstepping (therapeutic) boundaries and becoming overly permissive. When staff are able to maintain their own mentalizing amid strong emotions and confusion and can do what is necessary to reinstate mentalizing in patients and groups, the patients will experience their own emotions as less frightening and dangerous. This will ensure that patients are less likely to become overwhelmed and destabilized. Predictable and consistent staff members who are thoughtful and patient in their approach will add further stability to the system. Last, but certainly not least, setting clear boundaries in a respectful way without removing patients' own responsibility is essential to contain strong emotions, and thus is a vital part of a mentalizing milieu.

Team Functioning

Developing a secure, cohesive team is essential for effective teamwork and a well-functioning MBT unit that delivers treatment skillfully. In essence, the team has to work to generate shared representations of each patient. Any patient needs to recognize that the team has an integrated and coherent understanding of him or her. Experiencing radically different perspectives of himself or herself from different members of the team will lead to anxiety and fragmentation. Teams need to work assiduously on a shared representation of each patient so that interventions are synergistic and facilitate more robust self-representation. The development and maintenance of a mentalizing clinician in the context of a team is a primary aim of adaptive mentalization-based integrative treatment (see Chapter 13, "AMBIT: Engaging the Client and Communities of Minds").

Keeping a healthy morale when treating patients with severe personality disorders can be challenging for several reasons. First, patients with BPD are emotionally challenging, at times picking on staff members, finding their weak spots, and undermining their therapeutic zeal. Second, change in personality disorder is slow, which can lead to pessimism among members of the team. Third, splits in the team, whether arising from problems among the patients or within the team itself (which at this point may have divergent experiences and mental representations of the patients), commonly manifest themselves as disagreements that may become polarized, making it hard for individuals not to blame each other for management or treatment difficulties. Fourth, the fluctuating nature of the problems of BPD patients and their intermittent crises can lead to an onerous workload and constant anxiety about risk. Finally, in the event of a patient's death by suicide, the death has a profound effect on not only the individual clinician who was caring for the patient but also the whole team.

Sustaining and maintaining a secure, cohesive team with a healthy, enthusiastic morale can be achieved through a mixture of intervision, team supervision, and group reflections and the development of a secure atmosphere within the mentalizing milieu (see Box 12–4).

BOX 12–4. Factors optimizing MBT implementation at team and therapist level

- Maintained consistency and continuity within a coherent (MBT) framework.

- Enhancement of focused, clear, consistently applied interventions by all team members.

- Willingness of team members to improve their skills and understanding through reflection, training, and supervision.

- Optimal team size consisting of 5 to 9 therapists, with an absolute maximum of 12.

- Team consisting of active, responsive, flexible, and effective team players.

- Clearly defined roles and responsibilities and a culture in which team members help one another and address when responsibilities are not being met.

- Program supervisor who monitors and supervises clinical process and team functioning.

- Unambiguous clinical leadership.

- An appointed primary clinician for each patient who is responsible for assessment, treatment planning, and treatment coordination.

- Integration of all therapists, including the psychiatrist, into a one-team model.

- Goal-focused and process-oriented treatment approach guided by a treatment plan and monitored and revised when necessary in treatment plan evaluations.

- Crisis management protocol and a commitment protocol guiding consistent team intervention.

Intervision

The team's cohesiveness can be enhanced through staff mentalizing about themselves and one another—"practicing what they preach." This is known as *intervision* in mainland Europe. Once every 2 weeks (alternating with team supervision), the treatment staff have intervision, in which a broad range of team issues can be discussed. These issues are often more personal than in the team supervision, which is more theoretically and practically oriented. Team process is discussed in more detail in Chapter 13.

For the team to be able to work together effectively, it is very important that all members feel secure enough to talk openly with one another about their own personal emotional responses in working together and in treating the patients. This can be more important when disagreement occurs in the team, which is a danger to effective treatment because it will cause inconsistencies and undermine patients' (and clinicians') mentalizing capacity.

Disagreements in the team, often conceived of as "splitting," can have several causes. When they occur, the most important point is to try to establish their meaning.

Possible causes include the internal processes of the patient(s), poor team communication ending in fragmentation, team members' own personally unresolved relational processes, and difficulties experienced by the staff. Sometimes they have little to do with the patients. Often, the cause is a mixture of these (and other) factors. *Parallel processes* become transparent and need to be dealt with in intervision. These are elements of longer-lasting processes found in the patient group that at the same time are found in the staff and sometimes in the organization. It is often unclear where the process first originated—within the patient group or within the staff. Reinstating mentalizing about these processes and establishing their meaning help to (re)integrate the team and enable the team to offer consistency in treatment.

Different causes of splitting need different interventions. Splitting arising in the context of unresolved relational processes or because of poor communication needs teamwork (intervision) rather than patient work, but splitting caused by projections of a particular patient may need clinical discussion within the team (team supervision) followed by dialogue with the patient.

Case Example

During a period when three members of staff were on maternity leave, a member of staff was on long-term sick leave, and new staff members had joined the team because of service development, many changes occurred in the unit. The longer-employed remaining staff members had a lot of extra work covering for the staff absences and training new staff members. They felt overworked and tired and were frustrated that the three clinicians had all become pregnant around the same time. They started to isolate themselves, "trying to survive," and asked for more time off, including extra training courses. This led to fragmentation and splitting in the team—into the "committed" clinicians and the "noncommitted" clinicians—and less consistency and coherence in treatment. At the same time, patient attendance dropped dramatically, requiring more outreach work. The "diehard" patients started to form a group aligned against the non-attenders, demanding that staff do something and set stricter rules around attendance.

In team supervision, the theme was the teleological mode and how to reinstate mentalizing of patients and in the team. Staff practiced interventions with role-plays of patients demanding staff action—for example, demanding discharge of those patients who were not attending regularly. The team focused on these problems for several intervision sessions by discussing the frustrations, the splitting phenomena, and the parallel processes with the patient group.

It became apparent that the splitting and the parallel processes had arisen within the context of unresolved relational processes and because of poor communication. Tracing these processes and discussing possible interventions reinvigorated the team and reinstated a more thoughtful approach to the problems in the unit and to managing the patient demands; a mentalizing team was restored.

IMPLEMENTATION OF MBT PROGRAMS

The implementation of MBT programs in the Netherlands has been successful in many respects. However, the failure of some Dutch services to replicate good treatment outcomes found in the initial Dutch replication studies identified at the beginning of this chapter deserves scrutiny. Bales and colleagues (2017b) used a multiple case-study design to understand some of the determinants of success or failure in the implementation of seven evidence-based treatment programs for BPD. The findings demonstrate the complex nature of implementing evidence-based psychotherapy programs in regular mental health center institutions. In summary, the implementation of evidence-based MBT programs in the Netherlands has been associated with mixed outcomes at best. Implementation was clearly successful in two programs, outcomes were mixed in two programs, and implementation failed in three programs, resulting in discontinuation of those programs. Furthermore, the findings suggest that in all cases the course of implementation was influenced by multiple elements at organizational, team, and clinician level. Although each implementation trajectory constitutes its own story, involving local issues and specific team cultures, the results yield suggestive evidence for some more generic barriers and facilitators across all implementation trajectories. Facilitators include the presence of organizational support, sound financial management, strong and consistent leadership, highly structured project-based implementation, managing (negative) team processes, therapist selection, sufficient expertise, and training opportunities, whereas the absence of these elements is a barrier to implementation.

There is growing awareness of and attention being given to key factors that need to be taken into account when implementing psychological treatments for BPD. Based on an integration of these findings from the Netherlands with those from studies of treatment implementation in other health services, a range of factors can be considered to contribute to successful implementation. These can be considered at either an organizational level (see Box 12–3) or a team level (see Box 12–4). Managers and clinicians need to consider these factors if they are to deliver effective treatment services to people with personality disorders.

REFERENCES

Bales D, van Beek N, Smits M, et al: Treatment outcome of 18-month, day hospital mentalization-based treatment (MBT) in patients with severe borderline personality disorder in the Netherlands. J Pers Disord 26(4):568–582, 2012 22867507

Bales DL, Timman R, Andrea H, et al: Effectiveness of day hospital mentalization-based treatment for patients with severe borderline personality disorder: a matched control study. Clin Psychol Psychother 22(5):409–417, 2015 25060747

Bales DL, Timman R, Luyten P, et al: Implementation of evidence-based treatments for borderline personality disorder: the impact of organizational changes on treatment outcome of mentalization-based treatment. Pers Ment Health 11(4):266–277, 2017a 28703383

Bales DL, Verheul R, Hutsebaut J: Barriers and facilitators to the implementation of mentalization-based treatment (MBT) for borderline personality disorder. Pers Ment Health 11(2):118–131, 2017b 28488379

Bales D, Smits M, Luyten P, et al: Discovering how the mind works: the journey of a patient in mentalization-based treatment, 2018 [Unpublished manuscript]

Bateman A, Fonagy P: Effectiveness of partial hospitalization in the treatment of borderline personality disorder: a randomized controlled trial. Am J Psychiatry 156(10):1563–1569, 1999 10518167

Bateman A, Fonagy P: 8-year follow-up of patients treated for borderline personality disorder: mentalization-based treatment versus treatment as usual. Am J Psychiatry 165(5):631–638, 2008 18347003

Hutsebaut J, Bales DL, Busschbach JJV, et al: The implementation of mentalization-based treatment for adolescents: a case study from an organizational, team and therapist perspective. Int J Ment Health Syst 6(1):10, 2012 22818166

Laurenssen EM, Smits ML, Bales DL, et al: Day hospital mentalization-based treatment versus intensive outpatient Mentalization-based treatment for patients with severe borderline personality disorder: protocol of a multicentre randomized clinical trial. BMC Psychiatry 14:301, 2014 25403144

Petersen B, Toft J, Christensen NB, et al: A 2-year follow-up of mentalization-oriented group therapy following day hospital treatment for patients with personality disorders. Pers Ment Health 4:294–301, 2010

CHAPTER 13

AMBIT

Engaging the Client and Communities of Minds

Dickon Bevington, M.A., M.B.B.S., MRCPsych, PGCert
Peter Fuggle, Ph.D.

Adaptive Mentalization-Based Integrative Treatment (AMBIT; see later text for a full discussion of the acronym)—was initially developed as a method for working with young people with multiple complex needs who commonly reject, or are rejected by, conventional mental health services and who may yet seek help in nonconventional ways, for example, through the presentation of significant risk toward self or others. The approach is now applied to a much wider span of ages and has been extensively described in a number of publications (Bevington and Fuggle 2012; Bevington et al. 2013, 2015, 2017; Fuggle et al. 2015). In this chapter, we provide a brief overview of the main aspects of AMBIT and then focus on recent developments, in particular the dissemination of help, not only to clients but also to workers.

Note. In using the term "workers" throughout this chapter, we deliberately cast a broad net. While respecting the importance of professional expertise, we recognize also that the clients who are helped by AMBIT services do not choose where to place their epistemic trust on the basis of professional qualifications. "Workers," in the sense that we use in this chapter, refers to anyone in a relationship to a client or patient who carries a professional (or even just a "purposeful") intention to help. Examples of such workers include psychologists, youth workers, social workers, therapists, psychiatrists, counselors, or project workers.

We assert the value of the purposeful facilitation of communities that are more conducive to the development of epistemic trust (see Chapter 4, "Mentalizing, Resilience, and Epistemic Trust," and Chapter 14, "Social Systems: Beyond the Microcosm of the Individual and Family") and describe a range of approaches designed to support this. We argue that this process necessarily involves explicit attention not just to the dyadic relationships between AMBIT workers and their clients, but also to those between workers and their colleagues, and workers and those who train them.

It is a commonplace observation that there is no simple correlation between the level of expertise held by a teacher and the degree to which learners believe that the teacher's knowledge will be valuable to them in their own life. We argue for a radical approach toward understanding precisely what "expertise" is really sought by our clients. Mentalization-based approaches rely on clients perceiving their therapists as having the potential to make sense of their circumstances and states of mind. In our experience, however, the clients that AMBIT services target often see this expertise as being held by a much more diverse group than is often recognized. A significant part of the task for mental health specialists may thus be to help their clients harness this dispersed expertise (or, more simply, the available help) as fully as possible. Preservation of the workers' capacity to sustain their own mentalizing must be at the heart of their efforts.

OVERVIEW OF AMBIT

Beginning at the turn of the 21st century, and initially as a thought experiment about how to address the needs of so-called hard-to-reach adolescents with first-episode psychosis or emergent personality-based difficulties, AMBIT was originally called Integrative Multimodal Practice (IMP; Asen and Bevington 2007). We now reject the term "hard to reach" as pejorative and blaming; our clients are more often "underserved," and there are certainly many other individuals (e.g., drug dealers, pimps, unscrupulous money lenders, gangs) who do not find them hard to reach with their own offers of apparent "help."

In IMP, a new multimodal worker was envisaged—one who would be deliberately trained in a range of core skills drawn from the cognitive-behavioral, systemic, social-ecological, biological, psychodynamic, and mentalization-based frameworks. Rather than attempting to create an overarching unified field theory for the helping professions, we saw integration as happening in person, pragmatically, through the provision of a single key relationship for clients, whose attachment histories often mean that trying to engage them with more workers actually achieves less.

In practice, although an early training program in IMP at what was then the Anna Freud Centre (now the Anna Freud National Centre for Children and Families) was highly rated by participants, there was little evidence of its applicability. When one course participant raised funding for her whole team in a city in Northern Ireland to attend training, the realization that the IMP approach could only ever be implemented as a whole-team approach became obvious. Since 2005, we have only trained whole teams.

Over the course of more than 200 subsequent whole-team trainings, mentalizing began to change in relation to the array of explanatory frameworks (with their associated interventions) that were included in the emerging model, to increasingly become positioned—by trainers and trainees alike—not simply as one out of many frameworks, but as a viable integrative framework. Given the extent to which the development of mentalizing theory builds on the other frameworks mentioned earlier, mentalizing is an idea that is integrative to its core.

With this shift, IMP morphed into Adolescent Mentalization-Based Integrative Treatment, or AMBIT. The acronym is now more used as a word in itself, meaning an individual's own sphere of influence—something that workers often report as being worryingly ill-defined in their work. More recently, the A has come to stand for *Adaptive* rather than *Adolescent*. This change recognizes the fact that AMBIT is now applied far beyond its original constituency of adolescent outreach services, and now includes inpatient, residential, and secure care settings; services working with safeguarding teams; early help services for families with younger children and infants; adult personality disorder services; and adult prisons.

A typical young client may not be attending school or college, may be using substances in harmful ways, and may be in troubled family relationships, at risk of homelessness or exploitation, and perhaps drawn toward gang membership and offending. Emotion-regulation difficulties, low mood, anxiety issues, and self-injurious behaviors are common in such clients. AMBIT promotes a focus on making sense of and responding to the client's *relationship to help*, arguing that—notwithstanding responding to immediate risks of harm—mentalizing this aspect of the client's state of mind is often initially just as critical as the presenting problems he or she is struggling with. The client's reluctance to engage with offers of help may be an adaptive response to previous experiences of help (formal or informal) that were experienced as noncontingent, humiliating, or exploitative; in addition, disengagement from help increases risk to the client. Amid the complicated and individual components of a client's relationship to help, a common theme is profound mistrust of professional workers' capacity to be genuinely helpful in the problems of the client's life.

It is ironic that precisely such individuals and families often attract the involvement of a large number of agencies. Some agencies are required to offer help, in line with statutory responsibilities for the well-being of the client or the protection of the public. For example, education services are required to work with young people who are not attending school or college, regardless of whether these individuals have any wish to reengage with education. Workers are often thus obligated to offer help to young people who, paradoxically, experience this offer as a threat to their own self-agency. This effect may be attenuated in working with adult clients, in whom services are more inclined to recognize adult agency and responsibility, but there are many similar examples, for instance, when calculations of risk to the self or others pass thresholds for statutory involvement. As outsiders, professional helpers are readily perceived by clients as unlikely to ever truly understand the clients' life circumstances and relationships.

Professional meetings between multiple agencies concerned with a particular client may also include numerous workers without direct working relationships with the client (or his or her parents) but who assume significant responsibilities toward, and are often afforded significant power over, the client. It is not surprising that there is often an inverse relationship between the number of workers involved with a client and family and the degree to which any of these workers are perceived as helpful or trustworthy.

This situation is further exacerbated by what are, in our view, inevitable tensions arising between the different agencies involved. For instance, the priorities for an educational inclusion officer will be significantly different from the concerns of a social worker or a mental health professional, whose insistence on a young person's attendance at appointments within school hours directly undermines the educational inclusion officer's efforts to improve the young person's school attendance. These examples of what we term "dis-integration" are rarely anything other than conflicting good intentions, but they may not be perceived as such by different professionals in the system, let alone the client. In relation to this dis-integration across systems and between interventions, a literature is emerging that focuses on the "collective impact" (Kania and Kramer 2011, 2013) of different interventions across whole systems of help, as distinct from a focus on the effectiveness of specific, more narrowly defined (mental health or other) interventions delivered by lone professionals.

As well as holding different positions with respect to the client and family, such networks of agencies commonly hold high levels of anxiety about the well-being of the client and family, and also about the capacity of their workers to discharge their ascribed roles in such difficult circumstances. Young people who threaten self-injury, suicide, or impulsive violence create appropriate anxiety in mental health professionals, who feel a level of responsibility to their clients. In such circumstances, these workers' capacity to mentalize both their client and one another is challenged. Moreover, workers are vulnerable to feelings of professional shame about their reactions of worry or anger, which diminish their likelihood of seeking help from their professional colleagues.

Our starting point is that a level of anxiety in workers is normal and appropriate, and not an indicator of any lack of competence; the absence of worry would perhaps be more concerning, as it might indicate that a worker is in pretend mode (see Chapter 1, "Introduction") or at risk of burnout. Paradoxically, high levels of anxiety, however understandable or appropriate they may be, prevent a worker from mentalizing either the client or other workers in the network. In these conditions, decision making tends to become increasingly certain (reflecting psychic equivalence) and highly teleological and defensive, often focusing on narrowly defined professional or service remits (i.e., contractual obligations).

In working with a large number of teams from different parts of the world, we have been struck by the common observation that clients often find it easier to communicate with people who are not officially helping them, at least in specialist or directive ways. In a recent AMBIT training, one participant described how, in his adolescent inpatient psychiatric unit, it was not uncommon for the young people to seek out and spend time talking with the cook. Among all the staff of the unit, the cook was almost unique in not having a role involving the explicit encouragement of change in the young people. Such observations are not uncommon in our trainings. At the beginning of one training session in an adult women's prison, a first meeting was held with the prison officers, welfare teams, and mental health workers. One of the prison officers described how an extremely troubled inmate would seek him out to talk about the terrible events that had occurred in her early life. The prison officer found these accounts extremely distressing to listen to but was pleased that the woman herself seemed to find it helpful to share them. Paradoxically, in the same meeting, the therapist who was working with the same woman described how the inmate was relatively disengaged from the therapy process on offer from the team. In our experience, these disjunctions between workers' assigned roles and actual functions are extremely common in complex systems of help for distrustful and avoidant clients. The formal roles to which many workers bring great skill and sincerity may not match the perceived value of such a role to the client.

AMBIT has approached this common experience of frontline workers by co-constructing with them a model that aims to address the key features and challenges outlined above. The model captures these features in four key arenas:

- **Work with clients:** managing risk and nonengagement in a population that is often not conventionally help seeking.
- **Work with the team:** managing workers' experiences of anxiety, frustration, and isolation, and the risk of them experiencing professional shame and burning out.
- **Work with networks:** addressing inevitable dis-integrations across multiagency and multiprofessional networks, and the frustrations that these evoke.
- **Learning at work:** sustaining an openness to change from familiar (if frequently ineffective or exhausting) patterns of working toward the (assumed) riskiness of evaluating outcomes and trying new approaches.

These four components can be simplified into a single diagram, known as the AMBIT wheel (Figure 13–1).

The AMBIT wheel is an attempt to represent concisely and memorably the principles and key areas of practice that hard-pressed workers must struggle to keep in balance to facilitate any therapeutic progress with their clients. Applications of a mentalizing stance are translated into key techniques in each of the four quadrants of the wheel, which involves balancing four pairs of (often apparently incompatible) key principles, shown in the outer ring of the wheel. Many existing effective interventions cover these same components, but the AMBIT model insists that in order to hold the balance, equal emphasis must be given to all four aspects of the work.

The theory and knowledge around each of these domains is underpinned by the proposal that mentalizing, besides being a key component of the helping process, is not merely an individual capacity but a social process, requiring the context of a network of relationships to sustain it. The capacity to continue mentalizing self and other in stressful settings is thus dependent on the worker remaining "well-connected" to a team that works explicitly to create contexts in which its members are trusted not to evoke professional shame or amplify anxiety in one another, and in which ostensive cueing and marked mirroring (see Chapter 1) facilitate thinking or appropriate action, avoiding pretend mode or teleology.

Many AMBIT-influenced teams report their workers becoming embroiled in highly emotional, rapidly moving situations. When conducting outreach activities, and relying on phone calls or text messages, frontline workers may often find themselves absorbed in crisis and risk management, without any space for reflection and planning. Using the metaphor of a stone hitting water for the anxiety experienced by a worker in the middle of a crisis, we frequently remind teams that concentric ripples, which are predictable in their size and velocity, resolve out of the chaos at the point of impact—that is, the crisis—where the worker is commonly situated. Developing social disciplines for help-seeking conversations in such scenarios facilitates the active involvement of colleagues, who can help mark and mirror a worker's own anxious position in the middle of the chaos and offer a mentalizing glimpse from the "edge of

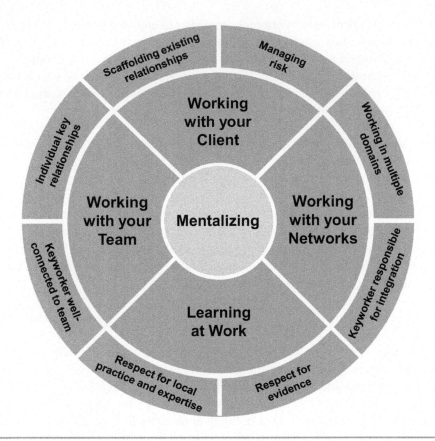

FIGURE 13–1.   The AMBIT wheel.

Source.   Reprinted from Bevington D, Fuggle P, Cracknell L, et al.: *Adaptive Mentalization-Based Integrative Treatment: A Guide for Teams to Develop Systems of Care,* Figure 1.1, p. 22. Copyright © Oxford University Press, 2017. Used with permission.

the pond," rather than simply "jumping in the water" or offering unsolicited or even unhelpful help. An explicitly ritualized approach to help-seeking between colleagues has been developed, which we call "Thinking Together" (Bevington et al. 2017). Retaining the capacity to mentalize is not equated with inaction ("pseudomentalizing"; see Chapter 1); on the contrary, the intention is to keep alive the capacity to consider new and authentic ways of helping, balancing the often-competing demands of scaffolding existing relationships and managing risk.

We find it encouraging that frontline professionals have welcomed both the pragmatism in our understanding of their work, and the willingness of the AMBIT model to value interventions that might typically fall outside formal mentalization-based approaches. Relatively brief training programs (4–5 days) in the AMBIT approach have resulted in major changes in how teams or even whole systems have begun to function. Local evaluations of these changes (Fuggle et al. 2015; Griffiths et al. 2017; Munro et al. 2017) have indicated a range of impacts on local services, including the following:

- Reductions in the frequency and length of inpatient admissions.
- Reductions in the number of young people coming into care during adolescence.

- Reductions in the number of referrals being made between agencies within a service network.
- Improvements in team and network functioning.

In addition, a doctoral study (Gelston 2015) suggested that young people treated by an AMBIT-influenced team showed enhanced mentalizing skills and improved therapeutic relationships compared with those engaged by other outreach services.

ONWARD ADAPTATION AND CHANGE

The AMBIT wheel rests upon the activity of learning at work (see Figure 13–1), and in that sense, innovation is at the heart of the program. AMBIT continues to change in the context of changing demands—including the diversification of settings where it is applied. It is no accident that learning is positioned in the lower quadrant of the wheel, at the point where traction drives forward motion. Along with changes to its name, the content of AMBIT has changed over the 15 years of its evolution, because it is designed to do so in relation to feedback from teams training in and adopting this approach.

An Open System

AMBIT, particularly in its use of online wiki technology, is an open system that is designed to develop incrementally. We have described it as an "open source" approach to the development and free sharing of evidence-based work. In the world of information technology (IT), open-source programmers share their very earliest versions of "source code" online in order to enlist real-world feedback and voluntary contributions from their open-source community. These contributions drive iterative improvements, often spawning novel applications (what computer programmers call "forks" in the developmental path of an original idea) that might not even have been envisaged by the original developer. In addition to the design advantages of this approach to development (which in the IT world is responsible for web browsers such as Firefox, or the Android mobile phone operating system), there are compelling parallels with the mentalizing stance in therapy: A half-adequate idea or understanding is released *tentatively* by the therapist, in the hope and expectation that the patient's reflections and feedback will improve on it.

In this aspect of AMBIT we have learned much from the generous community of open-source computer programmers (https://tiddlywiki.com) with whom we developed our unique online wiki platform (accessible at https://manuals.annafreud.org). A *wiki* is a user-editable website in which pages accrue in a nonlinear fashion, linked thematically with tags or directly by hyperlinks. The AMBIT wiki is arranged in what can be thought of as layers, the content of which, subject to continual updating and improvement, is curated by different groups. The foundational layer is curated by the central AMBIT program at the Anna Freud National Centre for Children and Families, and this content is shared freely. Local teams who are trained get their own local wikis in higher layers, all of which "inherit" this same foundational content; here they can record local learning and adaptations, iteratively working out and transparently sharing their current collective thinking on questions of *"How (and why) do we work effectively in this way, with this kind of problem, here, in this cultural, organizational, and geographical context?"*

Many wheels, once described locally in one setting, do not need to be reinvented in other settings; the free and open sharing of emerging best practice, or workarounds, is a key part of our aspiration for AMBIT's "community of practice" (Lave and Wenger 1991).

Some time after we had begun training teams and were successively amending and improving the AMBIT curriculum in the wiki, on the basis of the teams' real-world experience and feedback, we realized that we had stumbled on a treatment innovation methodology, already elegantly described in theory by Weisz and Gray (2008) as "deployment-focused innovation." In effect, each training acts as a new field trial to test the latest adaptations, while we iteratively record learning as we progress.

AMBIT's Approach to Learning

AMBIT's approach to learning reveals itself in three ways. First, it seeks to represent and share existing knowledge in a field in which robust evidence is thin. AMBIT especially tries to describe the challenges and difficulties of this work, in ways that are sufficiently authentic and recognizable to evoke epistemic trust in workers. The AMBIT approach seeks to share practical, evidence-oriented or evidence-based solutions for a wide array of difficulties that teams engaged in this kind of work widely report encountering in each of the four quadrants of the wheel (as described earlier in this chapter; see Figure 13–1).

Second, AMBIT aspires to act as an intelligent repository that is searchable, indexed, specific, responsive, and universally available, for new learning that supports teams and the growing community of practice. All of AMBIT's materials, training exercises, theory, and manualized interventions are freely available through the Anna Freud National Centre for Children and Families (https://manuals.annafreud.org/ambit); this rich resource includes videos, for example, of all the key didactic teaching modules, and role-plays of specific techniques.

Third, AMBIT seeks to foster teams as "learning organizations" (Senge 2006) in their own right. We see small, trusted groups of workers who share a common task (albeit individually bringing different specialist skills to the group) as the most fundamentally meaningful driver of change in health and social care. From a worker's perspective, the individual worker is almost always too puny, and the wider organization too clumsy and blind to the granularity of what is required. Senge's work on learning organizations does not explicitly mention mentalizing, but in addition to his introduction of "whole-systems thinking" for organizations involved in change or improvement, many of his methods clearly value what we would translate as a purposeful enculturation of mentalizing—valuing curiosity and the exploration of alternative perspectives, and tolerating not-knowing as a critical part of the process of coming to know.

INNOVATIONS IN PRACTICE: TOOLS TO SUPPORT COMMUNITIES OF MINDS

What follows is a description of four separate efforts to support the development of systems that can support greater mind-mindedness in those who work within them (although systems themselves will always be mindless). In turn, this supports a more mentalizing stance on the part of the workers toward their clients. The first two approaches—manualizing of learning, and the development of a community of practice—follow directly from the previous discussion on learning. The third and fourth efforts—the use of tools such as "Dis-integration grids," and the concept of the "Team Around the Worker," respectively—are more explicitly focused on helping multiprofessional networks function better.

Manualizing

As we have described in the previous section, AMBIT's open learning system is supported by the web-based team activity of *manualizing*. This fits our goal of developing communities of practice (or of practicing minds) but is also a particular example of the effort to support the development of epistemic trust in the social value of the ideas that teams might follow. In the previous section, we described the wiki in which AMBIT's manual and training resources were incubated, which has grown iteratively and incrementally by trying to absorb and respond to feedback from the experiences of successive teams and their diverse clients. Individual teams are also invited to add their own learning directly to their own local versions of the wiki. This manualizing occurs in disciplined ways, ensuring it is always a collaborative activity that represents the shared understandings of the team. Manualizing increases transparency about how professionals work and creates opportunities for teams to reflect together on their shared practices and to articulate them. Manualizing is a team-based parallel to the individual mentalizing of team members' own behavior (*"How and why do we work in this way?"*) and helps teams develop a clearer sense of identity and a shared culture. Broadcasting this material on the web adds a seriousness to the task and increases a team's sense that their work and dilemmas need not be entirely opaque to other professionals in their network.

This aspect of AMBIT—teams iteratively "blogging" their learning—still needs help. A relatively small percentage of teams that have been trained in AMBIT actively adopt regular online manualizing into their schedule. Among those who do, there is anecdotal evidence of real enthusiasm and pride in what they achieve—that is, a practical format for team reflection and learning that is traceable, not lost in the whirl of work. We suspect that manualizing in its current form is not yet contingent with the perceived needs of many teams. Many teams report wanting to do it but not having the time; for them, manualizing is perceived as another (teleological) burden. There are still technological barriers for some team members, as manualizing requires a certain confidence in working with IT (although this gets easier with experience). Social and cultural barriers exist, such as a modesty that shies away from broadcasting current understandings out of a fear of boastfulness, or that doing so will only invite criticism. Some teams report a form of "legal anxiety" that the team might be held to account if it fails to deliver on its stated aspirations. Rebadging the wiki manuals as "practice scrapbooks" has been suggested to reduce this concern. It is worth noting that teams that do regularly manualize have not reported any of these more pessimistic outcomes, despite having engaged in manualizing for a number of years.

Working Toward a Community of Practice

In a related fashion, yet not limited to online activity, AMBIT has striven to support the development of a community of practice (Lave and Wenger 1991) for AMBIT-trained teams. Capitalizing on the fact that workers in any field like to "talk shop" and share fixes to common problems, any community of practice aspires to gather these conversations so that the community becomes the holder of a "living curriculum." Online knowledge repositories offer a more realistic prospect of benefiting from pooled creativity and generosity. Over the past years, we have learned much about the requirements for implementing such aspirations, which include much more active stewarding and nurture than the simple provision of an online meeting place and repository of learning. We have a long way to go yet.

There are obvious economic advantages to introducing minds across different teams in reciprocal relationships, especially at a time when budgets for training and supervision are limited. We have tried to do this in multiteam trainings. Anecdotally, we have also recognized the value in encouraging visitors to regularly attend AMBIT team meetings, as a mechanism of change implementation. Visitors' curiosity about AMBIT-influenced practices invites the host team to explain itself (a powerful learning exercise), as well as to rehearse desired social disciplines with more conscious awareness—much as a family's manners tend to improve when a respected relative comes to dinner. Our enthusiasm for a community of practice builds on our earlier-stated understanding that mentalizing is as much a socially determined capacity as one based solely on prefrontal cortical activity and early experiences of dyadic reciprocity in attachment relationships.

Our initial and perhaps naive hope was that the online manuals would themselves support such a development relatively automatically and painlessly; teams can see what other teams are writing about and share one another's new pages, which should serve as a reinforcement of manualizing. This practice is not enough, however. Technological improvements to the online manual that are currently under way will greatly improve its facilitation of networking, but we recognize the need for much more active face-to-face contacts—both between teams and with the growing team of AMBIT trainers and facilitators.

Dis-integration Grids

In the overview of AMBIT at the start of this chapter, we described some of the features of dis-integration across complex multiprofessional networks. Just as we argue that anxiety in workers is normal, and not automatically deserving of professional shame, the same goes for dis-integration across networks, which we argue is their natural resting state.

The "Dis-integration grid" is one of a range of simple field tools or techniques that AMBIT uses to help patch the most damaging holes in a fabric that will always seem threadbare in places. It encourages a systematic approach to holding (or regaining) a mentalizing stance toward people in other parts of the wider helping system. We invite workers to mentalize each mind in the system at three levels:

1. **Explanation:** How would each player in this network describe or explain the problem that they are concerned to resolve?
2. **Intervention:** What action does each individual see as likely to help?
3. **Responsibility:** Who in the system does each individual believe should be delivering these interventions?

Creating a grid with one row for each of these three levels, and a column for each "player," enables short statements in the words of each player to be recorded. The work of imagining (i.e., mentalizing) how different players in an extended network might answer these questions (so that if they saw the suggestions they could feel understood and validated) often triggers curiosity in the worker and an interest in starting a dialogue. Many cells in these grids are often revealed to be simply unanswerable by an individual worker without engaging in respectful, inquisitive dialogue with one or more of the other "players."

Dis-integration grids help to remind us of those aspects of the work in which there are authentic shared intentions (which are easily lost in conditions of stress). Completing these grids individually (or, better still, with a client or collaboratively in a multiagency meeting) often helps to highlight one or more "connecting conversations" that could usefully be prioritized, whereby the most unhelpful dis-integrations across a system can be acknowledged and worked around rather than left implicit and unaddressed.

Here we are describing an essentially nonhierarchical process. Mentalizing is increasingly understood less as an individual power or even as a dyadic transaction, and more as a social and contextually determined activity. AMBIT encourages this shift away from the hope or expectation of creating individual "mentalizing ninjas" or "heroes" toward the purposeful creation of communities of minds that support one another's mind-mindedness and are sensitive to the fragility of mentalizing that everyone shares. There is an anarchic quality to this "making sense of one another" that sidesteps matters of technical proficiency, qualifications, professional roles, authority, or power; minds are all just minds, all subject to a fluctuating sense of being understood and of having their own understandings validated, or not. In contexts where this experience is more affirmative than negative, effective mentalizing is much more likely to be active than inactive. An AMBIT-influenced service has the goal of increasing understanding across networks as one of its core practical tasks. It is, as it were, a guerrilla approach to addressing the problem of dis-integration, rather than leaving it to structural reorganizations, which alone are unlikely to succeed.

In addition to Dis-integration grids, we have developed other techniques—such as paper-based "Pro-grams" that map networks, and "Sculpting," both described in Bevington et al. (2017)—that explore similar territory in different ways.

The Team Around the Worker: Asserting the Importance of Epistemic Trust

AMBIT invites collaboration across networks by promoting a shared interest in understanding the helping system *from the perspective of the client*. A key point of principle is that except in exceptional circumstances, AMBIT workers never form a new helping system around a client; they join an existing one. This helping system may consist of mainly informal contacts, family, friends, other non–mental health workers (e.g., teachers, probation officers), or even figures who would be judged as being far from helpful in any conventional terms (e.g., drug dealers, gang leaders) but who, from the perspective of the client, are at least providing, for example, protection or money.

We encourage an approach to developing professional networks that is complementary (not an alternative) to the conventional notion of the "Team Around the Client" (TAC). We refer to this as the "Team Around the Worker" (TAW).

The TAC approach, which places particular focus on professional roles, responsibilities, and specialist skills, is often an efficient if somewhat "industrial" model for the delivery of help. TAC relies on an accurate inventory of needs, and of available resources, and then arranges for the right people and teams to gather around the client for these resources to be delivered. This approach is generally very effective, except when there is epistemic hypervigilance (see Chapter 4), as the model does not easily take into account the demands placed on a client or family who may be struggling to create one relationship of trust, let alone multiple ones with workers from several different teams. When a TAC works well, it has often found ways to operate as a TAW.

Rather than having a primary focus on skills and responsibilities, a TAW stresses the importance of relationships and the nature of the helping process. In particular, it considers (mentalizes) the perspective of the client, asking questions like *"Where is epistemic trust currently present? Who would (or does) this client say 'gets me' at this point in time?"* In a TAW, it is this person who is the "keyworker"—the helper who is key *in the mind of the client*. The keyworker in this sense is defined differently from how it is in a TAC, where it is an organizational role that is dependent on a specific skill set and accompanied by a set of formal responsibilities. In a TAW, the keyworker could be anyone and would be expected to change across time. Indeed, the capacity for a TAW keyworking role to shift around the workers in a network might be seen as evidence of generalization in the client's capacity to open up to, accept, and use help; this would constitute a repair in the relationship to help that goes beyond improvement on a symptom checklist.

A number of features are critical for this way of working to succeed:

1. The network should be able to maintain and share awareness of where epistemic trust is currently located.
2. It avoids competitiveness between workers for this privileged relationship, but instead sees things in a whole-systems perspective; in other words, there is consideration of the collective impact of the whole helping system, rather than the helping system being subservient to, for example, the personal desires of a well-intentioned therapist or to a team's commissioned priorities as a single service.
3. The network values this epistemic trust in its own right, as a resource that can help to modulate, sequence, and introduce complex multimodal interventions without overwhelming the client, or offering noncontingent help because it is badly timed or is targeting the wrong priority.
4. It recognizes the uniquely vulnerable position into which the establishment of epistemic trust places a worker who has created such a relationship.

A TAW as a counterbalance to the TAC delivery mechanism helps to create a strong rationale for collaboration across networks: a worker who has established epistemic trust is inevitably vulnerable to feeling isolated (*"Only I really understand this client!"*) and anxious, thereby threatening his or her own mentalizing capacity, with the implications that we discussed earlier. In a TAW, a new worker who recognizes the presence of epistemic trust in another part of the helping system (i.e., an existing keyworker) might introduce himself or herself more effectively into this system by first trying to be authentically helpful *to this keyworker,* rather than insisting on a direct approach to the client. From the clients' perspective, especially if they are epistemically hypervigilant, they may be more open to another worker's approaches if they first hear not *"This person will be good for you!"* but instead—from someone in whom they already have some trust—*"This person was really helpful to me, in these ways."*

Here, we place a clear emphasis on the collective and social-contextual determinants of mentalizing. We could paraphrase it thus: *It takes a brain to create a mind; it takes a community of minds to create a mentalizer.* When we speak of the carer's mentalizing of the infant mind (see also Chapter 16, "Parenting and Foster Care"), we can only do so on the assumption that the carer's mind itself has regular access to other minds that mentalize his or her exhaustion, fears, fury, and joy. In any given dyadic relationship, a mentalizer may function like a "lighthouse," signaling its presence and illuminating the surroundings, but in reality that lighthouse is far less an independent sentinel than it is an interdependent node within a distributed network. Our argument is that to set therapists or other workers up in taxing work with very troubled clients without paying close attention to whether these workers are well connected to a team and a mentalizing network is at best an invitation to failure and at worst unethical. There are political and economic implications to this approach that we do not explore here, save to say that market competition between different providers across these complex multidisciplinary and multiagency networks seems to us unlikely to increase epistemic trust across borders.

INNOVATIONS IN IMPLEMENTATION: COLLABORATIONS AND APPROACHES TO DISSEMINATION

Collaborative and Co-constructed Trainings

Recently, the AMBIT program, with its stated aspirations for collaboration, has been challenged. AMBIT's mission is described as seeking to create contexts and conditions in teams and networks that improve effectiveness in *any* evidence-based practice (or "help," in ordinary language). In this sense, AMBIT is a service improvement model as much as it is a specific therapy in itself. Over the past few years the AMBIT program at the Anna Freud National Centre for Children and Families has been commissioned to offer a number of large, locality-wide trainings across London, specifically integrating the AMBIT curriculum with two separate evidence-based practices, neither of which is explicitly mentalization-based. In accepting these commissions, in a very real sense our bluff was called: could we work collaboratively with entirely separate models of treatment?

In one collaboration, a large number of social services and early help teams in the west and north of London had already embedded (after significant investment in training and supervision in the preceding years) the use of the Family Partnership Model (FPM; Day et al. 2011). Their enthusiasm for (we might say "epistemic trust in") FPM was unsurprising: they had already found that model to be valuable in engaging and maintaining purposeful momentum in work with families who had often previously tried and rejected (or been rejected by) more conventional helping services. FPM robustly asserts the need for partnership in its varied forms at every stage of what it defines as the "helping process," and a carefully structured range of tools and practices is used to support this partnership.

In the second collaboration, training commissioners for three boroughs in central and west London had determined that motivational interviewing (Miller and Rollnick 2012), or an adapted version of this technique, would be of value for social workers engaging with some of the most underserved families—in whom substance use is frequently one problem among many others—but they wanted to incorporate some AMBIT/mentalizing content.

Motivational interviewing, like mentalization-based work, focuses on intentionality and the importance of the worker gaining an authentic understanding of the client's present mental state. The motivational interviewing approach highlights differences between the stages of precontemplation and contemplation in relation to a potential behavior change; these stages map well to prementalistic thinking and mentalizing, respectively. Likewise, FPM focuses on an understanding of partnership—a sense of "doing with," of reciprocal understanding of each other's positions, and of mutual respect—all of which are (in the theoretical language of AMBIT) underpinned by successful mentalizing. FPM focuses on the stages of a helping process: exploration, understanding, goal setting, strategy planning, implementation, review (with or without looping back to earlier stages), and ending. Each of these stages can be achieved fruitfully only in the context of active partnership, which might take different forms at different times according to the context.

Working with FPM required two independent training teams to deliver a conjoint training program of FPM and AMBIT. It is easy to see how this training approach parallels our description of the inevitability of dis-integration across complex helping networks. For example, an obvious parallel exists between the teams coming for training and the clients or families approached by two (or sometimes more) different agencies or professionals. Both "helpers" are intent on helping, although they might have different ideas about the problem that requires help or what might work in addressing it. What we discovered, especially in our FPM collaboration, was the critical importance of our recognition of existing epistemic trust in the FPM model; we were the "newcomer" to an existing helping system, in which FPM was already (although inevitably not universally) seen as helpful by the client.

Related to this issue, during the training sessions, especially early on (we were training several hundred staff in all, so the training developed across time), we often noticed the embarrassment of "too many words." FPM and AMBIT trainers and model developers inevitably created their own "languages," marking out familiar territory in shorthand ways or jargon to create pragmatic frameworks for thinking. Learning one foreign language is hard enough for many people, but learning two simultaneously is usually too much. Workers in these trainings sometimes described feeling "overfilled."

This was not a problem of one model being "liked" and the other "disliked" by trainees; it was that the models were occasionally seen by the trainers as more important than the workers' experience of the training. The trainers' maps (the curriculum) were being mistaken for the territory (Bateson 1972/2000). As any mentalization-based worker knows, this is the very essence of the pretend mode, and we fell into it at times despite our best efforts not to. Essentially, we were struggling to find a balance between *orthodoxy* and *orthopraxis:* should we all use the same names for things, or could we find common ways to practice according to shared core guiding principles?

If a resolution was found, it was due to two factors (in an external review, Munro et al. 2017 subsequently reported large cost savings, suggesting that our synthesis was not ineffective). First (and our colleagues in FPM should be the judge of any success in this), we worked hard to create relationships of trust with the FPM training team, especially in marking the importance of their existing relationship with the commissioning body and local workers, and our enthusiasm to strengthen, not undermine, these existing relationships. We discovered that we and our FPM colleagues could be friends and could share with humor the fact that delivering our "own" training in its pure form would undoubtedly have been easier! Second, we agreed to promote a triadic approach to developing a bespoke model: AMBIT and FPM trainers explicitly tried to work in partnership with the local service, whose local expertise (about *"what might work and be applicable here, in this organizational and cultural setting"*) formed the crucial, and grounding, third position.

To the extent that the conjoint training was successful, it occurred through pragmatic adaptations and generous accommodation by all parties involved—the help that we as a conjoint training team gave was more important than the models we taught. "Working with clients" in the teams who took part in the training is now primarily organized around FPM lines, although consideration of mentalizing and its role in the creation of partnership is seen as supportive, and the approach to developing a team culture and a whole-systems approach toward collaborating across networks is primarily influenced by AMBIT but underpinned by much FPM language and process.

The parallels between working as trainers and working as therapeutic workers are instructive. Both forms of work offer help to "clients" who may be ambivalent about the extent to which they want to take the risk that accepting offers of help inevitably entails (*"Might this help simply confuse us or invalidate our existing expertise?"*). Standing before a group of trainees, just as when working with a client, there is immense pressure on workers (here, referring to trainers) to present a completely united, coherent, and expert front—but that is neither mentalizing nor partnership. The reality was messier, but ultimately more human, and—we hope, and time will tell—more helpful.

Building Epistemic Trust in Training

In the same way that AMBIT has prioritized (or rebalanced) relationships in relation to professional expertise in the process of helping our clients, we have tried to apply these principles to the process of training itself. Traditionally, training in a specific new skill or therapy is provided by those with recognized expertise in that skill or therapy. It is hard to argue with this logic; certainly, in trainings for which trainees sign up individually, the credentials of the trainer are often of critical importance. However, especially in the case of whole-team trainings, a trainer may have abundant qualifications or knowledge, but may leave some attendees feeling, *"They don't really know what it's like to do my job, in my setting."* This does not evoke epistemic trust.

Because we train whole teams, it is inevitable that some attendees will not have actively chosen this (or any) training for their work. There is a parallel here between clients who may not be seeking help, or at least not seeking the kind of help that their allocated therapist is offering. We believe that a similar risk of epistemic mistrust presents itself between some frontline workers and trainers, as it frequently does between clients and frontline workers.

In attempting to address this issue, we have successfully recruited new trainers from teams recently trained in AMBIT. These trainers frequently describe their own "AMBIT journey," which often started with a degree of epistemic mistrust toward the approach; they then go on to share and describe the changes in their own practice that have resulted from adopting AMBIT ideas. This approach has proved helpful. Consistent with the theory of epistemic trust, we believe that practitioners attending training need to be able to see that the trainers can see things from their perspective. Highly trained professionals with lofty therapeutic or academic credentials often carry little credibility with hard-pressed frontline workers managing high caseloads in uncertain service contexts. Because of this, we try to balance the training teams by recruiting trainers with experience in the service contexts with which we are working, along with trainers who have wider experience in the process of training many teams.

For example, we have recently begun a project to train workers at a residential children's home to become AMBIT trainers for other residential care staff, with the aim of establishing a center in Manchester, United Kingdom, offering AMBIT training specifically for this sector. This process mirrors our approach to working with clients, aiming to create a "team around the worker" (in this case, the residential care workers who are functioning as trainers/facilitators) that has some degree of epistemic trust with the "client" (i.e., other residential care teams).

Workers in this project demonstrate high levels of expertise and detailed knowledge of the young people with whom they work. Their capacity to establish relationships of epistemic trust with this cohort of very troubled young people is as impressive as it is remarkable that it is so often overlooked by other (more "expert") elements of the professional network. Many workers in this field remain at the frontline for many years: in one training session, the 15 attendees had a total of over 200 years of experience in this work!

More challenging for this group of workers is to gain similar levels of confidence and expertise in their capacity to deliver trainings as they have in their client-facing work. This has provoked us to rethink the basic AMBIT curriculum and materials, reducing needlessly technical language and providing greater scaffolding to facilitate such work by less experienced trainers. The principle of scaffolding workers to work just outside their main roles in adaptive ways that serve the whole system, as well as extending personal agency, has been a theme in AMBIT from the start ("scaffolding existing relationships" is one of the core practice principles of AMBIT, as shown in Figure 13–1). The process of scaffolding (Wood et al. 1976) was first described by Vygotsky (1978) as the "zone of proximal development": this is the gap between what can be achieved independently and what cannot, where continuous reciprocal feedback between the person with the primary expertise (or the parent) and the worker (or the child) who is adopting a new role enables learning and mastery. The challenge is to find ways of scaffolding such skills that meet these conditions, and to create conditions of trust that support the process. We have learned that facilitating workers to deliver training is a precarious process; as with mentalizing itself, we often get things wrong. This process is neither simple nor solved, in that we are asking people to move out of traditional roles and areas in which they feel confident and well-practiced. One of our most impressive local trainers half-jokingly refers to our training sessions as her "therapy." We have been encouraged by initial progress in this project; an evaluation of the training's acceptability and impact indicates it was highly valued, but establishing devolved local training capacity remains a work in progress.

CONCLUSION

Our aim in this chapter was to describe how we have moved away from the idea that effective help for individuals with severe and complex needs can be provided only by highly trained specialists with profound and detailed knowledge of the interventions they offer. However well-intentioned, brilliant, or even heroic such staff may be, demand for effective specialist help will always outstrip supply; moreover, it is unlikely that individual efforts have a significant impact on the complex problems these workers have been asked to address.

Sadly, there is support for this seemingly pessimistic view. In the UK, a major government initiative, the Helping Troubled Families program (Department for Communities and Local Government 2016) involved significant government investment of nearly £450 million in trying to address the needs of families similar to those described in this chapter. A national evaluation of this program (Day et al. 2016) concluded that the program had little identifiable impact on the families that had taken part. A succession of such programs have been delivered in the UK, often implemented for too brief a period but following similar patterns of top-down initiatives and placing priority on new interventions, rather than investing in and strengthening helping systems that are already functioning. We believe this approach is no longer justifiable; it may even be unethical to continue promoting the idea of individual practitioners trained in new skills following new initiatives as a credible way to address hugely significant public health matters.

In our view it is time to place two key principles at the foreground of future work. First, this work should be attempted only by workers working in teams in which attention to developing a teamworking culture is accepted as essential to the endeavor (coproducing shared values and social disciplines, with purposeful context-building to facilitate mutual epistemic trust). Second, rather than invest in the conviction that a "heroic" new skill or worker will provide the key to a process of profound change for our clients, we should instead design services in a radically different way, placing at the center the clients' knowledge of their own lives, their knowledge of what has helped them in the past, and who is helping them now. This is profoundly unsettling to the way that services are traditionally organized and delivered, and the radical nature of such an endeavor is clear to us: this is not a simple solution to an area of profound need, although it implies incremental, not revolutionary, change. As well as advocating for no more "heroes," we advocate for no more new initiatives—or, rather, for the provision of more investment in those who have already made the choice to do this difficult work. This is the task that the AMBIT program has set itself, a journey in which we are all still beginners. Progress is possible if it is based on learning from those with whom we work—our clients, and the workers whom we meet in the process of training and service development.

REFERENCES

Asen E, Bevington D: Barefoot practitioners: a proposal for a manualized, home-based Adolescent in Crisis Intervention Project, in Reaching the Hard to Reach: Evidence-Based Funding Priorities for Intervention and Research. Edited by Baruch G, Fonagy P, Robins D. Chichester, UK, Wiley, 2007, pp 91–106

Bateson G: Steps to an Ecology of Mind: Collected Essays in Anthropology, Psychiatry, Evolution, and Epistemology (1972). Chicago, IL, University of Chicago Press, 2000

Bevington D, Fuggle P: Supporting and enhancing mentalization in community outreach teams working with hard-to-reach youth: the AMBIT approach, in Minding the Child: Mentalization-Based Interventions With Children, Young People and Their Families. Edited by Midgley N, Vrouva I. London, Routledge, 2012, pp 163–186

Bevington D, Fuggle P, Fonagy P, et al: Innovations in Practice: Adolescent Mentalization-Based Integrative Therapy (AMBIT): a new integrated approach to working with the most hard to reach adolescents with severe complex mental health needs. Child Adolesc Ment Health 18:46–51, 2013

Bevington D, Fuggle P, Fonagy P: Applying attachment theory to effective practice with hard-to-reach youth: the AMBIT approach. Attach Hum Dev 17(2):157–174, 2015 25782529

Bevington D, Fuggle P, Cracknell L, et al: Adaptive Mentalization-Based Integrative Treatment: A Guide for Teams to Develop Systems of Care. Oxford, UK, Oxford University Press, 2017

Day C, Kowalenko S, Ellis M, et al: The Helping Families Programme: a new parenting intervention for children with severe and persistent conduct problems. Child Adolesc Ment Health 16:167–171, 2011

Day L, Bryson C, White C, et al: National Evaluation of the Troubled Families Programme: Final Synthesis Report. London, Department for Communities and Local Government, 2016

Department for Communities and Local Government: The First Troubled Families Programme 2012 to 2015: An Overview. London, Department for Communities and Local Government, 2016

Fuggle P, Bevington D, Cracknell L, et al: The Adolescent Mentalization-based Integrative Treatment (AMBIT) approach to outcome evaluation and manualization: adopting a learning organization approach. Clin Child Psychol Psychiatry 20(3):419–435, 2015 24595808

Gelston P: "Hard to Reach" Young People: The Role of Service Organisation and Mentalization-Based Treatments. DClinPsy Thesis. London, University College London, 2015

Griffiths H, Noble A, Duffy F, et al: Innovations in Practice: evaluating clinical outcome and service utilization in an AMBIT-trained Tier 4 child and adolescent mental health service. Child Adolesc Ment Health 22:170–174, 2017

Kania J, Kramer M: Collective impact. Stanford Social Innovation Review Winter:36–41, 2011

Kania J, Kramer M: Embracing emergence: How collective impact addresses complexity. Stanf Soc Innov Rev January:21, 2013

Lave J, Wenger E: Situated Learning: Legitimate Peripheral Participation. Cambridge, UK, Cambridge University Press, 1991

Miller WR, Rollnick S: Motivational Interviewing: Helping People Change, 3rd Edition. New York, Guilford, 2012

Munro ER, Hollingworth K, Meetoo V, et al: Ealing Brighter Futures Intensive Engagement Model: Working With Adolescents In and On the Edge of Care. London, Department for Education, 2017

Senge P: The Fifth Discipline: The Art and Practice of the Learning Organization, 2nd Edition. New York, Doubleday, 2006

Vygotsky LS: Interaction between learning and development, in Mind in Society: The Development of Higher Psychological Processes. Edited by John-Steiner V, Cole M, Souberman E, et al. Cambridge, MA, Harvard University Press, 1978, pp 79–91

Weisz JR, Gray JS: Evidence-based psychotherapy for children and adolescents: data from the present and a model for the future. Child Adolesc Ment Health 13:54–65, 2008

Wood D, Bruner JS, Ross G: The role of tutoring in problem solving. J Child Psychol Psychiatry 17(2):89–100, 1976 932126

SOCIAL SYSTEMS

Beyond the Microcosm of the Individual and Family

Eia Asen, M.D.

Chloe Campbell, Ph.D.

Peter Fonagy, Ph.D., FBA, FMedSci, FAcSS

This chapter develops some of the ideas mentioned in Chapter 10 ("Therapeutic Models"), where we discussed the role that the social system around the individual has in making beneficial outcomes possible in therapy. Mentalizing is a fundamentally intersubjective process, in its developmental origins, its evolutionary function, and its moment-by-moment unfolding. Even when an individual is mentalizing in relation to the self—attempting to make sense of his or her own actions, thoughts, or ideas—interaction and interpersonal preoccupations are normally core parts of the content. The theory of epistemic trust further reinforces the sense that developmental, attachment-based interpersonal processes are intrinsically related to learning about how best to function in the wider social system. As outlined in Chapter 4 ("Mentalizing, Resilience, and Epistemic Trust"), the evolutionary function of epistemic trust is to enable the individual to participate in the transmission of culture, and at the level of individual subjective experience, this openness to the reception of social knowledge provides individuals with the psychological heuristics to enable them to benefit from their cultural milieu. On the basis of these theoretical developments, a broader focus on social systems and their capacity to support mentalizing and the generation of epistemic trust represents a logical next step. In this chapter we explore how the theory of mentalizing and epistemic trust can be applied to thinking about social systems.

MENTALIZING SOCIAL PROCESSES

The process of socialization involves the individual encountering several extra-familial social systems, such as educational or work settings, faith-based institutions, special interest groups, or sports clubs. Functioning within the broader social environment is more difficult without developing the ability to hold other minds in mind and to engage in perspective taking. In turn, mentalizing develops and is sustained by the social system in which people live. Social systems that do not respect human subjectivity and agency (e.g., those systems that pay little or no attention to how a person is likely to feel in response to an action) re-create the evolutionary environment that demands the need for self-sufficiency—or the dismissal of subjectivity—and close down social attention to the communications of others. Mentalizing social systems, by contrast, permit imaginative thinking in relation to self and others and are thus able to further the individual's personal development and agency. In such a system, individuals are attuned to whom they can reliably relate to and whom they can—and cannot—trust. Such systems are characterized by relatively high levels of flexibility, which allow the system to accommodate challenges in effective and appropriate ways. For social systems to be successful socializing structures—that is, structures that are adequately sensitive, supportive, flexible, and responsive to the needs of the individual people within them—they must be characterized by high levels of epistemic trust: mutual and recursive understanding of the self by the other, and vice versa.

In complex postindustrial societies, it is possible that epistemic trust has become more acutely required and yet is more difficult to achieve and sustain because of larger populations and social fragmentation, and because of the larger and often more disjointed functioning of the state. Social trust is required to support social cohesion and to overcome the natural vigilance that all people feel toward ideas that are not their own. Individuals are much more likely to be able to take in and consider the novel ideas of others if they feel that their own personal narratives are regarded seriously and their agency is respected. To experience a sense of meaningful connection to the broader social community, individuals need to feel that they are recognized as having agency and that they are being mentalized by the relevant social context and those operating in it—whether educational or work settings, health and social care institutions, the justice system, or the various cultures and subcultures of which people are a part.

A cultural milieu in which political authorities and social institutions neglect citizens' needs and/or abuse their rights will close down the channel of natural pedagogy (Csibra and Gergely 2009). Cultural knowledge and expectations may be recognized and understood, but they are no longer experienced as relevant and generalizable to the individual concerned. In other words, they are stored as episodic rather than semantic memories. Social alienation is, we propose, a systemic breakdown in epistemic trust directed toward the wider environment. Dysfunctional social systems can cause the collapse of balanced mentalizing and result in highly reactive, tense, and defensive interactions that can lead to "mindless" violence and chaos. They can create fear and hyperactivate attachments, which can undermine higher-order cognition (thinking capacity) and force the system back to prementalizing modes of social functioning (see Chapter 1, "Introduction"). Such social systems can be self-reinforcing and therefore highly persistent in their instability. They undermine the very social mechanisms that could alter their character: human collaboration, negotiation, and creativity.

One of the more dramatic illustrations of this process is the social change that followed the collapse of the Soviet Union consequent on *glasnost* and the demolition of the Berlin Wall. We might anticipate that the increased personal freedom that ensued might have led to a reduction in suicidality and mental disorders. At least epidemiologically, the opposite appears to have been the case in many areas (Lester 1998; Mäkinen 2000). Why should this be the case? It seems that imposition of an unfair social system—the authorized generation of inequality by the prevailing system—generates a sense of unfairness and a pervasive sense of injustice that directly controverts personal narratives, at least in those who suffer social disadvantage. The inverse relationship between mental health and the social gradient is well known (McManus et al. 2016). For example, elsewhere we have highlighted that a linear relationship exists between the national prevalence of borderline personality disorder and the size of the income discrepancy between the top and bottom 20% of that country (Fonagy and Luyten 2016). We speculate that social systems that cultivate gross inequality in terms of income distribution are generally experienced as challenging an inherent sense of fairness that human beings all anticipate in large social groupings from around the age of 18 months (Sloane et al. 2012), and to which human beings appear biologically predisposed to respond with aggression (de Waal 2004).

Sometimes a mind–world isomorphism is created and psychic equivalence becomes institutional—it characterizes the function of a social system. George Orwell's dystopian novel *Nineteen Eighty-Four* comes close to this formulation in which thoughts and feelings acquire the significance and power of the external. If thoughts are real, it makes sense that they need to be socially as well as intrapersonally controlled. There are singular solutions to all social realities, there are no alternative ways of seeing things, and there may well be dramatic intolerance of other perspectives. However, models of minds that are simple (black-and-white thinking), schematic, and rigidly held readily generate dramatic social acts of individual prejudice. Because thoughts are close to the realm of the physical, negative ideas (any threats or images of danger) become terrifying and have to be physically defended against.

An interdisciplinary case study of the fluctuating history of homicide rates across time offers an illustration of the way in which the broader social context has a determining effect on individual violent acts (Eisner 2001, 2003). Serious interpersonal violence decreased remarkably in Europe between the mid-sixteenth and early twentieth centuries. Various explanations for the long-term decline have been offered, including the effects of the civilizing process, strengthening state powers, the Protestant Reformation, and the emergence of modern individualism. Rates of instrumental homicide, the type of homicide that fluctuates the most historically, appear to be very much influenced by whether a society is ruled by law, whether elites are trusted, whether corruption is under control, and whether socially minded services are provided; in short, they are influenced by the fair and effective functioning of social institutions and the perceived legitimacy of the state—that is, the citizens' confidence in the social and political structure (Eisner 2012). This model of political legitimacy has been tested against cross-national homicide rates and other variables and found to be a consistently strong and independent predictor. Historical research and cross-cultural criminological evidence suggest that establishing faith in the government and confidence that its legal and judicial institutions are fair and will redress wrongs and protect lives and property seems to be the most significant requirement for homicide rates to fall (Eisner and Nivette 2012). Legitimacy has its origins in political philosophy in ideas about the social contract—the notion that a government can function, and can justify its existence, only if the population has sufficient confidence in its (benign) intentions and effectiveness. Governments that break the social contract, according to this view, have already acted as agents of their own destruction (Locke 1689). We would suggest that the loss of legitimacy is driven—in terms of individual psychological mechanisms—by the failure of the state and its institutions to sustain a critical mass of epistemic trust within the population.

When the state's legitimacy is eroded, not everyone responds with physical aggression. We would suggest that one of the moderating factors that determine whether an individual is likely to act violently is his or her pre-existing capacity for mentalizing. In a situation where epistemic trust in the wider social environment has broken down, increasing strain is placed on the individual's capacity to feel a sense of agency, and this is particularly challenging for those who are already struggling to experience themselves in this way. In the absence of the organizing experience of agentive selfhood, there is a disconnection between internal experience and action. Ostensive cues are misread; other people's attempts to mentalize are scotomized. Individuals who are more prone to slip into nonmentalizing modes of subjectivity are more likely to act violently or become dysregulated (Asen and Fonagy 2017). As suggested above, in a highly noncontingent, nonmentalizing social system there may be advantages to operating in these nonmentalizing modes. To date, there has been a tendency within mentalizing theory to assume that reestablishing a capacity to mentalize is about facilitating successful adaptation to a culture in which most people are mentalizing effectively most of the time. But the reality of human experience and the social nature of a person's sense of self suggest that in order to achieve optimal outcomes for individuals, there are times when changes to the wider social environment may be required.

WORKING ACROSS CULTURES

When the clinician is working with clients and families from different backgrounds and cultures, it is essential that he or she has knowledge of different cultural systems and practices, such as kinship patterns and parenting practices, as they may well not fit neatly into normative ideas about family functioning, health, and illness that underpin mainstream trainings of clinical professionals. Cultural expertise is not routinely taught and valued in professional trainings, and this may be evidence of underlying discrimination and marginalization. When culture is attended to, it is often done so as a variable—that is, as a social category, rather than a process or meaningful system that challenges our own assumptions of what we know about the mind, mental health, emotions, and cognitions (Malik and Krause 2005). We all come from a cultural position and employ a "cultural lens" influenced by socioeconomic, historic, and political contexts, which informs the way we perceive and interpret the world.

Culture can be defined as a dynamic system of explicit and implicit rules established by groups in order to ensure their survival, involving attitudes, values, beliefs, traditions, customs, norms, and behaviors (Matsumoto and Juang 2004). Cultural norms can be explicit (e.g., enshrined in laws) or implicit (those that are characterized by conventional practices and rituals). They guide a group of people in their daily interactions and distinguish them from other groups of people. Culture could also be described as a system of knowledge shared by a relatively large group of people, passed on from one generation to the next. People are shaped by their culture, and their culture is also shaped by them. In this way culture is not static, but dynamic, changing all the time, with much of the change taking place outside our awareness, operating at a nonconscious level and influencing the automatic assumptions that we make. The term "culture" is sometimes used to refer to customs and practices from geographically "foreign" places. At other times it refers to "subcultures"—groupings of people in the same society that are viewed differently from the parent culture in which they are embedded. Subcultures develop their own norms and values regarding, for example, religious, social, and political matters.

Psychological interventions need to be meaningful within the cultural system of the client to be effective, as mental states are culturally patterned. Different cultures have different orientations and world views that can challenge compartmentalized ways of working. For example, in cultures where the body is experienced as the seat of the self, the family consists of a number of "selfs." In other cultures, the central unit is not the body or "self" of the individual, but the community and especially the family—a quasi "common body" or "family self." Seemingly individual symptoms or problems are seen as having to do with the relationships of the person with others: that is, a body disturbance signals a disharmony in the social order. Interventions therefore are often primarily somatic or "moral" rather than psychological, and Western therapeutic approaches are viewed as "psychologizing" somatic experiences.

Mentalizing-oriented clinicians need to think carefully about their own relationship with culture and how they integrate their "native" beliefs and practices with the professional cultural contexts in which they operate. They should be aware of their own position in society and, if they come from a dominant group, imagine how this may have an impact on their relationship with socially marginalized or disenfranchised clients and families. Do the clients see the clinician as privileged, belonging to an elite group or a minority? Mentalizing-oriented clinicians need to reflect on their own cultural roots and prejudices, critically examining their values and therapeutic models. This includes reflecting about their appreciation—or otherwise—of the "other," the "foreign," the "alien." They need to be curious about other cultures and their customs, without stereotyping cultural knowledge, and be interested in the models of change that their clients bring. For example, do the clinician's proposed therapeutic interventions fit with the clients' collectivist orientation? Clinicians need to think about working in conjunction with clients' natural, informal community support networks, be they neighborhood groups, churches, or spiritual healers.

Understanding and acknowledging cultural differences in this way should not blind professionals to the fact that they are also operating within their own culture—whether a school or a hospital, all social systems develop a local "culture." Culture is a profoundly important part of human experience. It is a characteristically human form of social technology, engendering a moral component with rules that buttress "the way we do things" and punishments for infraction; these rules create an acquired, not innate, distinction between insiders and outsiders. Culture has a cumulative character that builds up over time, necessitating the teaching and learning of specific content, a process that requires epistemic vigilance and the mentalizing capacity to distinguish trusted from untrustworthy informants. Those whom we perceive to recognize our unique personal narratives—that is, those who know and value us—are individuals whose knowledge is probably relevant to us in other contexts, because the fact that they recognize us in this way indicates that they have priorities, preferences, and actions that are pertinent to our shared social group. In contrast, if we do not feel personally acknowledged by another, our biological predisposition is to absorb their knowledge superficially—as relevant to that particular event and context, but not to our lives in general.

The culture of a group optimizes its members' chances of passing on their DNA. This means that it is essential for the group to survive *as a group*, as it is the specific social organization that is the conveyor of the culture. While human beings' biological need to prioritize the survival of the social organizations to which they belong is clearly an underlying factor for the evolutionary success of the species, we can understand much human misery as another consequence of the same need. This can lead to group members choosing the group's survival above other considerations, such as the actual functions of the group. Groups of people protect their culture—their commonly held beliefs—with their lives. Wars are started to protect an illusory sense of cultural belonging. We feel a need to protect organizations to which we belong, however dysfunctional they may be, even when we know that the group compromises the functions for which the organization was created. For example, there have been news reports of poorly led, dangerous hospitals that carry on operating and admitting patients because members of the organization go to extreme (and even illegal) lengths to protect it—to prioritize its survival over its intended function of saving lives. Human DNA has no knowledge of any specific culture, but codes for the vital continuity of the social group that sustains it. As a consequence, individuals working in, for example, mental health settings should not only recognize and understand other people's cultures; they also have a responsibility to be able to think robustly about their own professional cultural environment. As we explain in the sections that follow, some social systems, or cultures, are able to tolerate this better than others.

CHARACTERISTICS OF EFFECTIVELY MENTALIZING SOCIAL SYSTEMS

What are the characteristics of a social system with a capacity for effective mentalizing, and thus the potential for generating epistemic trust? The system needs to be flexible, not "stuck" in one point of view. It must be able to permit modifications of convention, at least on a temporary basis. Thus, interactions within the system should have elements of playfulness and humor that engages rather than is hurtful or distancing. There needs to be "give and take" between the various different perspectives. The system needs to listen to and value every member's experience and point of view, rather than autocratically or one-sidedly defining other people's experiences or intentions. By the same token, the social system needs to emphasize the importance of individual "ownership" of, or responsibility for, specific behaviors and actions, rather than explaining individual behaviors or actions as the result of some external force. This requires the social system to be continuously interested in and curious about each individual person's experiences and perspectives, in the belief that each individual's own views are being extended by those of others. The relational strengths of a mentalizing social system include all the important ingredients of effective mentalizing: curiosity, safe uncertainty, contemplation and reflection, perspective taking, forgiveness, impact awareness, and nonparanoid attitudes.

Being effectively mentalized by relevant social systems—as well as attempting to mentalize social systems—can contribute to better personal and family health. There is a potential virtuous cycle in relation to this process that empowers the individual by empowering the social context of that person, which ultimately feeds back at the level of the individual. If communications directed at an individual make him or her feel that his or her preferences are being taken into account, and that the individual's state of mind is a source of interest and/or concern to the person—or to the "system"—communicating with him or her, then the individual will take those communications to be relevant to organizing his or her future social behavior. For example, the individual is more likely to "learn the rules" and thus increase his or her chances of being appropriately aware of the preferences of others in the social group. Their reactions to his or her communications will, in turn, be more *deferential*—that is, they will take seriously and internalize what he or she has to say, and will more accurately perceive and reflect his or her position. Furthermore, it will also make it more likely that any future communications within the group or system will address the individual with greater relevance and make him or her feel taken seriously, and thus increase his or her sense of agency and responsiveness to social influence.

CHARACTERISTICS OF INEFFECTIVELY MENTALIZING SOCIAL SYSTEMS

Mentalizing is acquired and developed in social interactions, both in the home and in the outside world. But what if a family is operating within a much wider social system that does not value mentalizing and whose functioning depends on denying certain groups recognition of their agency and selfhood? What happens to individuals and their mentalizing capacity in societies that sanction marginalization, oppression, and persecution? In such circumstances, it may not be possible to regard representatives of social institutions—such as teachers, judges, doctors, police, and even relatives—as trustworthy. In a cultural climate where epistemic trust has broken down, it becomes increasingly difficult for individuals to experience themselves as agentive. This will become accentuated when an individual also has personal experience of the need for epistemic vigilance in the immediate social environment.

Reflective relationships, be they with children, parents, or partners, are much harder for anyone to maintain in very stressful circumstances. Nonmentalizing systems can easily become fear-driven systems: if individuals are frightened of one another, they develop a blind spot for another person's attempts to mentalize them, and are less likely to try to mentalize others. An ineffectively mentalizing system thus becomes self-perpetuating.

MENTALIZING IN SCHOOL SYSTEMS

Chaotic relationships between pupils, their parents, and the school authorities can be symptomatic of a social system that is dysfunctional. A school in which violence, aggression, and bullying are the norm is by definition a social environment that works to close down mentalizing in staff members and students. A mentalizing approach to the school system requires that the staff members involved be able to recognize the distorted power dynamics that arise as a result of the mentalizing challenges presented by individuals, whether pupils, teachers, and/or parents. In the following sections we describe mentalization-based interventions that aim to reduce bullying and improve behavior and educational attainment in schools.

Creating a Peaceful School Learning Environment (CAPSLE)

An innovative school-wide mentalization-based intervention for combating bullying, Creating a Peaceful School Learning Environment (CAPSLE), is a good illustration of this approach (Twemlow et al. 2005a, 2005b). CAPSLE has a wider focus than simply paying attention to the dysfunctional bully–victim dyad, as it also aims to change the bystanding culture (whereby others who are not directly involved as bully or victim implicitly condone this form of interpersonal violence by failing to act against it) and help students recognize that they are all agents who have played a role in the bullying. CAPSLE seeks to create a mentalizing climate and a group dynamic that can resist and limit the potency and currency carried by individual acts of violence or aggression. It is a teacher-implemented, school-wide program made up of four components: a "positive climate" campaign, a classroom management plan, a physical education program, and support programs (peer mentorship and/or adult mentorship) (see Box 14–1).

CAPSLE focuses on the power dynamics in the relationship among bullies, victims, and bystanders, and in particular the potential role of bystanders in shifting this dynamic. Bystanders are trained to act to encourage bullies, victims, and other bystanders to be aware of and move away from their "pathological" roles. This emphasis on the bystander reflects the need to create a mentalizing system around both bully and victim. In a nonmentalizing environment, the witness to a power struggle—that is, the bystander—may experience sadistic feelings of pleasure in seeing another's difficulty or suffering. This experience is possible only when the witness feels distanced from the internal world of the victim and is then able to use the victim to contain the unwanted (usually frightened) part of himself. The enjoyment and excitement that bystanding groups often show when witnessing fights or aggression in violent schools—for example, evidenced by the crowding around fights and stirring up of grudges that often take place—do not reflect a *complete* mentalizing failure: some level of empathy is necessary for this projective identification with the victim's pain to take place. However, the mentalizing that does take place is highly limited by the social setting, such that the victim's pain is not fully represented as a mental state in the bystander's own consciousness. In other words, the victim's pain is *recognized* but not *felt* by the bystander. The CAPSLE intervention constitutes a deliberate attempt to scaffold the unbalanced, fluctuating, and incompletely emerging mentalizing capacities of children and young people, as well as the teachers reacting to them, thereby creating a social environment in which

BOX 14–1. **Components of CAPSLE**

- A **"positive climate"** campaign, which uses reflective classroom discussions of immediate past experiences, in lessons led by counselors, to create a shift in the language and thinking of students and personnel.

- A **classroom management plan**, which augments the teachers' discipline skills by focusing on understanding and correcting problems at the root, rather than punishing and criticizing only the behavior that is apparent. For example, a behavior problem in a single child is conceptualized as a problem for all the pupils in the class, who, often unwittingly, participate in bully, victim, or bystander roles. This approach reduces scapegoating and creates an environment in which insight into the meaning of the behavior becomes paramount.

- A **physical education program**, derived from a combination of role-playing, relaxation, and self-defense techniques, that teaches children skills to deal with victimization and bystanding behavior. This component of the program helps children to protect themselves and others by using nonaggressive physical and cognitive strategies. For example, role-playing bully–victim–bystander interactions provides pupils with the opportunity to explore these situations and work out alternative actions to fighting.

- **Support programs**, which emphasize peer mentorship and adult mentorship. Schools may put in place one or both of these support programs. The mentoring relationships developed via these programs provide additional containment and modeling to assist children in mastering the skills and language to deal with power struggles. For example, mentors instruct children in refereeing games and resolving playground disputes and in the importance of helping others.

more balanced mentalizing can be practiced and reinforced, and its benefits experienced (Twemlow et al. 2017).

In a cluster-randomized controlled trial involving 1,345 children across nine elementary schools in a city in the United States (Fonagy et al. 2009), the CAPSLE program was found to substantially reduce aggression and improve classroom behavior. There was a reduction in children's experience of aggression and victimization. It was also found that the number of children nominated by their peers as being aggressive, victimized, or engaging in aggressive bystanding had decreased significantly. This was confirmed by behavioral observation of reduced disruptive and off-task classroom behavior in schools implementing CAPSLE. The study's findings suggested that empathic mentalizing increased in schools using the CAPSLE program.

Parental Presence in Schools: The Family Classroom Model

Another approach to dealing with disruptive pupils acting out in school and failing educationally has been to involve their parents directly and bring them into the classroom. The "Family Classroom" model, pioneered in the 1980s in London (Asen et al. 2001; Dawson and McHugh 1994), is implemented as multifamily projects sited in mainstream primary and secondary schools. Each school selects pupils who present with significant behavioral difficulties and are usually on the verge of being excluded permanently. The pupils can be of different ages and from different school years. Up to eight pupils and their parents make up a "family group," which is together for a school term and receives an average of ten 2- to 3-hour sessions at weekly intervals, delivered during normal school hours in a room within the school. Bringing families with similar issues and experiences together reduces stigma, furthers social collaboration, and equips parents and teachers with new resources to tackle problems commonly associated with academic and social exclusion. When families attend for several hours in a "real-life" context (e.g., a classroom in a mainstream school), spontaneous realistic situations and crises tend to arise, and these can be addressed on the spot. As the groups are quite structured, with tight timetables and frequent transitions from one context to another, family members need to change their roles and tasks continuously, often within the space of a few minutes. At one point they are members of a large group; a little later they can be required to be parents in charge of their children, then members of a parents-only group (or, for the pupils, a children-only group), and shortly afterward one family among six or seven other families. These continuous shifts of context generate a kind of "hothouse" effect, with families and group leaders being always on the move, having to adopt multiple positions, and experiencing multiple perspectives.

Multifamily work is a good setting to promote and practice effective mentalizing. For example, when observing other families and their interactions, group members can be encouraged to speculate about the mental states of the members of the other families. Individuals seeing themselves or their family "mirrored" in others who have similar problems is a stepping stone to self-reflectiveness. Furthermore, being exposed to multiple descriptions of their own mental states by the other participating families and their own individual family members, and then comparing these descriptions with their own perceptions of themselves, unleashes a circular process of mentalizing self and others. Adults and children with problematic attachment relationships who find it difficult to see or address these problems within their own family can spot similar difficulties in other families from a "safe" distance and without heightened levels of arousal. The technique of "cross-fostering" children for brief periods (of 1 hour or longer) to the parents of another family will give both parents and children direct experiences of different forms of child–parent interaction and prompt reflections about attachment issues (Asen and Scholz 2010).

The Family Classroom (Dawson and McHugh 2000, 2005) is run by a clinician jointly with a school-based partner, usually a teacher, teaching assistant, or special educational needs coordinator. There is a tight timetable, containing a number of different components. The Family Classroom, as the juxtaposition of these two words suggests, is a "double context" that allows the observation and addressing of classroom dynamics (between pupils and pupils; between pupils and teachers) and family dynamics (between family members of the individual's own family; between members of different families). This approach permits linking of home and school issues and leads to exploration of how these issues may affect the state of mind and behavior of the problem pupils. The structure and organization of the Family Classroom need to reflect the combined education and therapeutic context, in terms of the physical setup of the classroom, the curriculum, the timetable, and the various activities carried out. Setting a classroom context re-creates the school situation, albeit one enriched by parental presence and involvement. The behaviors that may be causing difficulty in the classroom can evolve spontaneously, in full view of the parents. The parents will be encouraged to think about and address some of these behaviors and, if possible, make links to their child's place and role in his or her family of origin. At the same time, teachers are helped to mentalize their pupils and the parents, as well as becoming more aware of their own mental states and how these are triggered during lessons. Similarly, parents are encouraged—and provided with specific tasks—to put themselves in the position of teaching staff, then mentalize the teaching staff, and then look at themselves through the teaching staff's eyes. Over time, this approach can help a mentalizing culture to develop in schools.

A study evaluating the Family Classroom approach (Morris et al. 2014) demonstrated that compared with a control group, families receiving the family group intervention benefited from it. Data on child and family social, emotional, and behavioral functioning were collected at the point of referral and at 6 and 12 months. The parents reported statistically and clinically significant improvements in their children, which were maintained at 12 months, whereas there was no change in the control group. In addition, measures of family functioning were fairly stable for the experimental group, while the control group showed significant deterioration on these measures over the same period.

MENTALIZING IN THE JUSTICE SYSTEM

The criminal justice system, with its binary model of people being found either "guilty" or "not guilty" of committing a crime, does not easily lend itself to a nuanced mentalizing approach. The polarized positions of prosecuting and defending lawyers, each of whom strategically tries to "sell" one particular version of "reality," leave it to the judge and/or jury to work out what "really" happened—and these parties will at times also attempt to mentalize, implicitly and/or explicitly, the state of mind of the accused. Rarely will they explicitly mentalize themselves.

Many individuals who have shown antisocial behavior (e.g., committing crimes such as theft, burglary, or acts of physical violence) do have expectations concerning the agency of the victim. However, these expectations are largely formulated in terms that are restricted to the physical world—meaning that, for example, protection against hostility is primarily physical, operating in the prementalizing teleological mode (see Chapter 1). Because these thoughts and feelings are so close to the material world, only what is material comes to be considered socially meaningful, and only what can be physically obtained appears to count as valuable. The gestures of others matter to the extent that they are visible and observable, but in that context only the actions, rather than any potential motives behind them, are meaningful; actions are taken to be the only true index of the intentions of the other. Because only action that has a physical impact is felt to be potentially capable of altering the mental state of others, threats of physical acts of harm or actual acts of aggression are seen as legitimate. Punishment is by payment and acts of subservience, and retributive (as opposed to restorative) justice is sought.

Restorative Justice

A good example of overcoming nonmentalizing social processes is the radical approach to criminal accountability of restorative justice (Sherman and Strang 2007). The simple expedient of confronting the offender with the victim, in the form of face-to-face conferences, victim–offender mediation, restitution, or reparation payment, forces the offender to create an image of the person he or she harmed. In many studies, offenders who receive restorative justice commit fewer repeat crimes than offenders who do not. In one study of young adult offenders in Canada, the reoffending rates after 2 years were 11% for those who had gone through a restorative justice program versus 37% for those who had served their sentence in prison (Sherman and Strang 2007). Restorative justice reduces repeat offending more consistently for violent crimes than less serious crimes, suggesting—in accordance with our hypotheses in relation to antisocial personality disorder (see Chapter 20, "Antisocial Personality Disorder in Community and Prison Settings," and also Bateman and Fonagy 2016)—that the loss of mentalizing is particularly marked in relation to acts of violence. Diversion of offenders from the traditional route of prosecution to restorative justice is a pragmatic solution because evidence suggests that it also substantially increases the odds of an offender being brought to justice. Few things turn out to be more practical than mentalizing solutions to social problems, because mentalizing underpins the way humans have evolved to function as a society.

Work With Family Courts and Social Care

Another example of applying a mentalizing approach is the joined-up work between the Family Court and Social Care systems in the United Kingdom (Asen and Morris 2016). This work has been developed to assist the outcomes of entrenched contact (visitation) and residence (custody) disputes where dependent children are caught up in their parents' chronic acrimonious relationship. In these high-conflict cases, children frequently side with the parent with whom they live and refuse to have any form of contact with the other parent, from whom they have often been alienated. Involved professionals, be they clinicians, social workers, or lawyers, are often "recruited" into the acrimonious interparental battle and take sides, becoming blind to any other perspective. Clinicians often experience the disorienting process of being "pulled back and forth" between the two parents' conflicting versions of what is "true" or "real." Forming a balanced view about what is best for the child(ren) in these scenarios is particularly difficult when dealing with such entrenched positions, which are "shored up" by the respective legal representatives of the warring parents.

To overcome such "stuck systems," a three-phase, multilevel intervention has been proposed (Morris and Asen 2018).

PHASE 1

During phase 1, the aim is to improve the parents' and involved professionals' capacity to mentalize the child (or children), each other, and also themselves. This is initially done in a network meeting, which brings together parents, their social support system, and the network of professionals. The meeting is living proof of how difficult it is to mentalize all the different minds that are in the room and how dis-integrated the system around the family is (Bevington et al. 2017). However, eliciting the different perspectives of each participant provides an immediate experience of the scope—and limitation(s)—of the mentalizing approach. The network meeting is followed by individual and joint work with the parents. A major aspect of the individual work is, again, to imagine the perspectives of other people. For example, invoking the perspective of an (imaginary) judge and asking each parent to address a number of past situations or hypothetical scenarios, as viewed through the judge's eyes, may help parents to look at themselves from the outside. Similarly, parents can be asked to view themselves and their dilemmas through the eyes of a social worker or a children's guardian. (A *children's guardian* is an independent adult who is usually appointed during legal proceedings regarding the care of children, whose role is to represent the best interests of the child: the guardian appoints a solicitor [lawyer] for the child, advises the court about the child's needs, and tells the court what he or she thinks would be best for the child, taking into account the child's feelings.) The reverse procedure can also be employed—namely, to ask the professionals in the network to look at themselves through the eyes of each parent and the child.

PHASE 2

Phase 2 consists of co-constructing with both parents (and other significant primary carers) a coherent narrative around family events, with the aim of providing this narrative to the child in an age- and developmentally appropriate way. This narrative must be acceptable to the parents as well as to the court, Social Care, and the children's guardian. This task is rarely easy, given that entrenched positions and narratives are difficult to give up. It is possible only if everyone focuses on the child and understands that the child needs to have coherence, with an agreed version of the events within the family.

PHASE 3

Phase 3 concerns the writing and submission of reports for the court or Social Care and, if requested, to give oral evidence in court. The clinician (or "expert witness") advising and reporting to the court will need to also mentalize the lawyers and judge—and help the parents to do so as well. A "mentalization-informed" report for the court will aim to see the case and the family situations through various different lenses. The report should be based on a mixture of observations—of the interactions and communications between the different family members, as well as of the family members with the social system—and also take into account the ample information contained in the large packs of documented evidence provided to the court. Having a whole range of different perspectives helps to shape the professional narrative and to balance the emerging opinions as to what might be in the child's best interest. When being cross-examined on the witness stand by a number of barristers (attorneys), each representing and defending one stance—namely, that of their respective client—the witness can quickly lose the capacity to mentalize effectively. The expert witness needs to use all his or her mentalizing capacity to understand the state(s) of mind of the cross-examining lawyer and, at the same time, consider the mind of the judge who ultimately will make decisions. Mentalization-informed reports have the recipients of the document in mind, and above all the mind of the child. These reports should be written accordingly, and also in view of the fact that they will shape the narrative with which the child grows up. An effectively mentalizing court "system" remains an aspiration that, if achieved, might contribute to a more just society.

CONCLUSION

We should add one further thought to any discussion of the concept of epistemic trust as a psychological mechanism that serves to regulate an individual's relationship with social or political institutions. We wish to highlight that although in the context of psychopathology and mental health treatment we have described epistemic trust is a positive mediator of change, epistemic trust in itself should be understood as morally neutral. Epistemic trust can be invested in any institution or figure that provides powerful and richly mentalizing ostensive cues. Critical thinking—some form of epistemic vigilance—is a highly valuable social cognitive resource. In Chapters 4 and 10 we have discussed the role of the social imagination in psychopathology. While we argue that one of the benefits of effective therapy can be to align and rein in aspects of the social imagination, we would also suggest that any robustly mentalizing social system is dependent on the presence of some degree of "wildness" of imagination. It is this that makes possible the ratcheting up of the very advances in culture that epistemic trust works to disseminate.

REFERENCES

Asen E, Fonagy P: Mentalizing family violence. Part 1: Conceptual framework. Fam Process 56(1):6–21, 2017 27861799

Asen E, Morris E: Making contact happen in chronic litigation cases: a mentalizing approach. Family Law (46):511–515, 2016

Asen E, Scholz M: Multi-Family Therapy: Concepts and Techniques. London, Routledge, 2010

Asen E, Dawson N, McHugh B: Multiple Family Therapy. The Marlborough Model and Its Wider Applications. London, Karnac, 2001

Bateman A, Fonagy P: Mentalization-Based Treatment for Personality Disorders: A Practical Guide. Oxford, UK, Oxford University Press, 2016

Bevington D, Fuggle P, Cracknell L, et al: Adaptive Mentalization-Based Integrative Treatment: A Guide for Teams to Develop Systems of Care. Oxford, UK, Oxford University Press, 2017

Csibra G, Gergely G: Natural pedagogy. Trends Cogn Sci 13(4):148–153, 2009 19285912

Dawson N, McHugh B: Parents and children: participants in change, in The Family and the School: A Joint Systems Approach to Problems With Children. Edited by Dowling E, Osborne E. London, Routledge, 1994

Dawson N, McHugh B: Family relationships, learning and teachers: keeping the connections, in Tomorrow's Schools. Edited by Best R, Watkins C. London, Routledge, 2000, pp 108–123

Dawson N, McHugh B: Multi-family groups in schools: The Marlborough Model. Contexts 79:10–12, 2005

de Waal FB: Evolutionary ethics, aggression, and violence: lessons from primate research. J Law Med Ethics 32(1):18–23, 2004 15152422

Eisner M: Modernization, self-control and lethal violence. The long-term dynamics of European homicide rates in theoretical perspective. Br J Criminol 41:618–638, 2001

Eisner M: Long-term historical trends in violent crime. Crime Justice 30:83–142, 2003

Eisner M: What causes large-scale variation in homicide rates? Working Paper. Cambridge, UK, Institute of Criminology, University of Cambridge, 2012

Eisner M, Nivette AE: How to reduce the global homicide rate to 2 per 100,000 by 2060, in The Future of Criminology. Edited by Loeber R, Welsh BC. Oxford, Oxford University Press, 2012, pp 219–228

Eisner M, Nivette A, Murray AL, et al: Achieving population-level violence declines: implications of the international crime drop for prevention programming. J Public Health Policy 37(Suppl 1):66–80, 2016 27638243

Fonagy P, Luyten P: A multilevel perspective on the development of borderline personality disorder, in Developmental Psychopathology Vol 3: Maladaptation and Psychopathology, 3rd Edition. Edited by Cicchetti D. New York, Wiley, 2016, pp 726–792

Fonagy P, Twemlow SW, Vernberg EM, et al: A cluster randomized controlled trial of child-focused psychiatric consultation and a school systems-focused intervention to reduce aggression. J Child Psychol Psychiatry 50(5):607–616, 2009 19207633

Lester D: Suicide and homicide after the fall of communist regimes. Eur Psychiatry 13(2):98–100, 1998 19698606

Locke J: Two Treatises of Government. London, Awnsham Churchill, 1689

Mäkinen IH: Eastern European transition and suicide mortality. Soc Sci Med 51(9):1405–1420, 2000 11037226

Malik R, Krause B: Before and beyond words: embodiment and intercultural therapeutic relationships in family therapy, in The Space Between: Experience, Context and Process in the Therapeutic Relationship. Edited by Flaskas C, Mason B, Perlesz A. London, Karnac Books, 2005, pp 95–110

Matsumoto DR, Juang L: Culture and Psychology, 3rd Edition. Belmont, Wadsworth/Thomson, 2004

McManus S, Bebbington P, Jenkins R, et al: Mental health and wellbeing in England: Adult Psychiatric Morbidity Survey 2014. 2016. Available at: https://assets.publishing.service.gov.uk/government/uploads/system/uploads/attachment_data/file/556596/apms-2014-full-rpt.pdf. Accessed June 8, 2018.

Morris E, Asen E: Developing coherent narratives for children of high-conflict parents. Contexts 157:8–11, 2018

Morris E, Le Huray C, Skagerberg E, et al: Families changing families: the protective function of multi-family therapy for children in education. Clin Child Psychol Psychiatry 19(4):617–632, 2014 23838692

Sherman L, Strang H: Restorative Justice: The Evidence. London, Smith Institute, 2007

Sloane S, Baillargeon R, Premack D: Do infants have a sense of fairness? Psychol Sci 23(2):196–204, 2012 22258431

Twemlow SW, Fonagy P, Sacco FC: A developmental approach to mentalizing communities: I. A model for social change. Bull Menninger Clin 69(4):265–281, 2005a 16370789

Twemlow SW, Fonagy P, Sacco FC: A developmental approach to mentalizing communities: II. The Peaceful Schools experiment. Bull Menninger Clin 69(4):282–304, 2005b 16370790

Twemlow S, Fonagy P, Campbell C, et al: Creating a peaceful school learning environment: attachment and mentalization efforts to promote creative learning in kindergarten through fifth-grade elementary school students with broad extension to all grades and some organizations, in Handbook of Attachment-Based Interventions. Edited by Steele H, Steele M. New York, Guilford, 2017, pp 360–374

PART III

Specific Applications

CHAPTER 15

CHILDREN

Nick Midgley, Ph.D.

Nicole Muller, M.Sc.

Norka Malberg, Psy.D., LPC, Ed.M., M.S.

Karin Lindqvist, M.Sc.

Karin Ensink, Ph.D., M.A. [Clin. Psych.]

It has been estimated that at any one time, approximately 1 in 10 children between ages 5 and 16 are suffering from psychological disorders (Green et al. 2005). Although there is now a wide range of evidence-based treatments available for children and families, a significant proportion of children still either drop out of therapy or are not able to make use of the treatments available (Fonagy et al. 2015). Moreover, many of the evidence-based treatments have been developed for very specific populations, making it unrealistic for psychological therapists working with children to be trained in a wide range of treatment models relevant to the entire gamut of presenting problems that may bring children to child mental health services. Paradoxically, despite the wide array of manualized therapies for specific childhood disorders, an increasingly narrow range of approaches is actually being made available to children and families, with many child mental health services primarily offering interventions based on a cognitive-behavioral therapy (CBT) approach.

Although CBT has a good evidence base for a range of childhood disorders (McLaughlin et al. 2013) and has clearly benefited many children and families, a one-size-

Some sections of this chapter are adapted from the book *Mentalization-Based Treatment for Children: A Time-Limited Approach* (Midgley et al. 2017b) and are reproduced here with permission from the American Psychological Association.

fits-all approach is always dangerous, especially when the evidence suggests that client choice and preference should be at the heart of all good clinical practice (Siminoff 2013). Moreover, many practitioners have had experiences of parents and children having difficulties using the kind of strategies that may be offered to manage their problems more effectively, often because these children and their parents do not have the affect-regulation skills or capacity to make use of guidance that is a prerequisite for benefiting from such therapeutic approaches (e.g., see Scott and Dadds 2009).

We hope that time-limited mentalization-based treatment for children (MBT-C) fills an important gap by offering a short-term, focused intervention for school-age children (roughly ages 5–12 years) that draws on traditional psychodynamic principles but integrates them with the findings from attachment theory and the empirical study of mentalizing, as well as features of other evidence-based approaches (Midgley et al. 2017b). By focusing on a core capacity that may promote resilience in a wide range of children with a variety of presenting problems, MBT-C aims to be a transdiagnostic therapy that can be adapted to the particular needs of a range of children in middle childhood.

WHAT'S NEW ABOUT TIME-LIMITED MBT-C?

With some justification, it can be said that many forms of child therapy have always included some focus on promoting the capacity to mentalize, even if this particular term has only recently been used. Empirical research has partially supported this assertion, by demonstrating that a focus on promoting reflective functioning may well be a common factor shared by both CBT and psychodynamic child therapy (Goodman et al. 2016). Nevertheless, there is a certain shift in focus, as well as in therapeutic approach, when promoting the development of mentalizing is placed at the heart of the therapeutic endeavor. In terms of individual therapy with children, Fonagy and Target's (1996) model of psychodynamic developmental therapy was perhaps the first treatment approach to be explicitly influenced by emerging ideas about mentalizing. A decade later, Verheugt-Pleiter et al. (2008) set out a model of open-ended therapy that they later described as mentalization-informed child psychoanalytic psychotherapy (Zevalkink et al. 2012). As in the work presented here, this approach moves beyond the traditional psychoanalytic approach based around interpretation and developing insight, and recognizes that helping to foster new capacities, including improved affect regulation and reflective functioning, is central to the work of child therapy. Likewise, Ensink and Normandin (2011) elaborated a mentalization-based therapy for children who had been sexually abused, incorporating child psychotherapy techniques developed by Paulina Kernberg and colleagues (e.g., Kernberg and Chazan 1991; Kernberg et al. 2000); similar models have been described in case studies by Ramires et al. (2012) and Perepletchikova and Goodman (2014). All of these approaches have been open-ended or longer-term interventions, often targeted at children with severe histories of neglect and maltreatment, and explicitly integrating mentalizing approaches with psychodynamic child therapy.

Developments in MBT have also taken place for both younger and older children. A number of teams have developed mentalization-based interventions with parents and infants (e.g., Etezady and Davis 2012; Ordway et al. 2014; Slade et al. 2005) and with adolescents (e.g., Bleiberg 2013; Fuggle et al. 2015; Malberg and Fonagy 2012; Rossouw and Fonagy 2012; Sharp et al. 2009) (see also Chapter 8, "Working With

Families"; Chapter 16, "Parenting and Foster Care"; and Chapter 17, "Borderline Personality Pathology in Adolescence"). Studies have demonstrated the value of interventions that promote mentalizing in school settings (Twemlow et al. 2005; see Chapter 14, "Social Systems: Beyond the Microcosm of the Individual and Family") and school-based psychoeducation programs (Bak 2012; Bak et al. 2015). Empirical studies examining what therapists actually do in the consulting room (looking beyond the "brand name" of therapy) have demonstrated how promoting mentalizing is a feature of psychodynamic therapy and CBT with children, as well as play therapy (Goodman et al. 2015, 2016; Muñoz Specht et al. 2016). It appears that a focus on enhancing mentalizing capacities is often an implicit element in these therapies, but in MBT-C the focus is more explicitly on promoting mentalizing *and* on understanding and repairing mentalizing breakdowns, with the assumption that being able to mentalize (and to recover the capacity to mentalize when it is lost) is at the core of being connected and attuned toward self and others. Given the links between attachment, trauma, and mentalizing, it is not surprising that a number of interesting developments have also taken place exploring how ideas about mentalizing can helpfully inform work with children in the context of fostering and adoption (e.g., Bammens et al. 2015; Jacobsen et al. 2015; Midgley et al. 2017a; Muller et al. 2012; Taylor 2012) (see also Chapter 16).

What should be made clear, however, is that the specific model described in this chapter has not yet been subjected to systematic evaluation, beyond an initial naturalistic outcome study at the Erica Foundation, Stockholm (Thorén 2014), and as such it is not yet an evidence-based approach to treatment. The particular model of MBT set out in this chapter, with a focus on time-limited work for children in middle childhood, will need to be systematically evaluated before we can say "what works, for whom, under what circumstances, and in what conditions."

AIMS OF TIME-LIMITED MBT-C

The overall aim of time-limited MBT-C is to promote mentalizing and resilience in such a way that the developmental process of the child is put back on track, and the family and child feel that they are in a position where they are better equipped to tackle the problems that first brought them to therapy. Sometimes this means that not all problems are solved, but the child and parents feel more empowered and better able to deal with their problems themselves. In doing this, MBT-C aims to increase the child's capacity for emotional regulation and to support parents to best meet the emotional needs of their children. For both parents and children, this means providing opportunities to practice good mentalizing, but also to pay attention to the situations in which mentalizing breaks down, or work on areas in which there are deficits in the capacity to mentalize. Such a focus is justified by the fact that research is increasingly demonstrating that the capacity to mentalize contributes to a positive sense of self, healthy relationships, and better emotional regulation (Ensink et al. 2014, 2016). Targeting such capacities is likely to be of value to children (and their parents) with a range of presenting problems, even if the underlying psychological symptoms are not "caused" by a failure of mentalizing.

For children who have experienced breakdowns in mentalizing due to trauma, loss, or other specific triggering situations or events, an additional aim can be to create a coherent narrative about the event, as well as exploring related thoughts, feelings, and experiences. A crucial element of this process is *mentalizing the affect* (Jurist 2005), which is at the heart of regulating emotions. By mentalizing the affect, we mean reflecting on emotions linked to traumatic events or losses and accepting the existence of feelings without being overwhelmed by them. The aim is not to create insight into the trauma, but to learn and understand in the here and now how to endure and regulate the emotions associated with the traumatic event or the impact the trauma has on the capacity to stay attached to self or others.

Alongside the direct work with the child, the fundamental aim of the work with parents is to strengthen their parental reflective functioning (Slade 2005) and capacity for assuming a reflective stance as parents (Ensink et al. 2017). This includes helping them to develop a capacity to see their child as a separate person with his or her own thoughts and feelings, with a sense that being curious about their child's experiences can help them to give meaning to behaviors. A secondary, but important, component is to help the parents develop the capacity to see their own affects and behavior from the perspective of their child, as this might have an impact on their parenting in important ways: Sometimes this could mean asking parents to literally look in a mirror and wonder out loud what kind of parent they imagine their child sees when looking at them. In this way, parents are helped to look at their own behavior and mentalize what happens inside themselves while being with, or reacting to, their child. When parents can explicitly mentalize themselves and their child, they can better respond to the child's needs and emotions in more flexible and attuned ways, and are better able to distinguish between their own needs or feelings and those of their child.

As the above description implies, the focus of MBT-C is more on process than on content. The aim is not primarily for either parent or child to gain insight into their difficulties, or to develop an understanding of where their difficulties may have come from; rather, it is to enhance their capacity to use mentalizing to manage their emotions and relationships, and to increase the child's capacity to make use of relationships for emotional learning. As such, the ultimate aim of time-limited MBT-C is to help the child to make better use of helping relationships *after the therapy has ended*, and for the parents to be better equipped to support their child's development *outside and beyond therapy*.

WHICH CHILDREN MIGHT BENEFIT FROM TIME-LIMITED MBT-C?

When children fail to develop sufficient capacity to mentalize, they are deprived of one of the most valuable tools available to the developing child: a skill that is at the heart of the capacity both to self-regulate and to manage an increasingly complex, interpersonal world. Entering middle childhood, the capacity to mentalize is for interpersonal relations what a healthy diet might be for physical health: it creates resilience in the face of hardship, and internal resources in the face of a demanding external world.

Time-limited MBT-C was developed for children ages 5–12 years presenting with a wide range of emotional and behavioral difficulties. Because of its focus on promoting a core developmental process, MBT-C has not been developed specifically for treating one type of clinical presentation. Informed by developmental research on the role of mentalizing in child psychopathology as well as our own clinical experience, MBT-C may be primarily suitable for children presenting with affective or anxiety disorders or mild to moderate behavior problems, as well as those with adjustment reactions or who need help dealing with a particular life challenge, such as parental divorce or bereavement. In some cases, as set out below, time-limited MBT-C may also be recommended for children who have experienced trauma and attachment difficulties. With regard to attachment disorders, our experience is that children with these disorders can benefit from this model. However, caution is needed when recommending time-limited MBT-C for children with more severe externalizing disorders, as well as severe attachment disorders or neurodevelopmental disorders, and in all cases a careful consideration of the child's particular circumstances should inform any treatment recommendation.

Although studies of nonbehavioral therapies generally report less successful outcomes for children with externalizing problems, there is a particular reason why we do not rule out time-limited MBT-C as a treatment for all children with behavioral problems. In many cases of externalizing and aggressive children, parents and clinicians alike often focus on the "noisy" symptoms, thereby missing co-occurring internalizing symptoms such as anxiety, depression, or low self-esteem (Goodman et al. 2012). Many children with conduct problems have received little help in understanding and integrating aspects of their temperament such as impulsivity, aggression, competitiveness, or desire for dominance, and may benefit enormously from the opportunity to think about this with someone who is curious rather than judgmental. In these cases, a therapist can help the child to develop self-awareness, and potentially explore more adaptive ways of integrating these aspects of the child's temperament or personality to help facilitate self-esteem and affect regulation.

For children with experiences of trauma or loss, the extent and severity of the trauma needs to be assessed in order to establish whether a time-limited model is suitable or sufficient. Children who have experienced severe maltreatment, trauma, or ongoing emotional neglect often evoke so much worry in the adults around them that it can be difficult to look past the adults' own reactions to the traumatic events and concerns about their possible impact to see the child. A treatment that focuses on the child's mind and experiences in a relational context may well be of benefit, although there should be no illusion that a piece of short-term work can undo the impact of severe and enduring trauma. Having said this, for some chronically traumatized children, the time limitation may help them to commit to the process, as it can make therapy appear less threatening.

Likewise, for children with multiple experiences of separations and disruptions, there may be reason to reflect on whether a time-limited model is appropriate. For most children, the separation from the therapist after a time-limited intervention is an opportunity to work through a well-prepared ending. However, for some children who have had multiple rejections (e.g., those who have had multiple moves between different foster families), ending and separating so soon after establishing a bond—perhaps for the first time—may not be therapeutic. With these children, it is recommended that the clinician makes a careful clinical evaluation and embarks cautiously on time-limited psychotherapy, with the notion that more extended treatment may be needed.

Neurodevelopmental disorders such as autism spectrum disorder are not absolute contraindications for time-limited MBT-C. On the contrary, children with these difficulties can benefit from this way of working, possibly with some modifications to the therapy. However, we want to underscore that these conditions are *not* the target for treatment, but that children should not be excluded from treatment solely on the basis of having these diagnoses. Children may be able to benefit from time-limited MBT-C despite these difficulties, and in fact may be particularly in need of help with developing some mentalizing skills around specific key issues or difficulties, while accepting that their abilities are different. For example, children with autism spectrum disorder may need help with exploring their feelings of exclusion and in considering what they may realistically be able to expect in the future, what they have to accept, and what they may be able to change, as well as developing ways in which they may address certain social deficits. For children with an intellectual disability, working in the here and now, using direct experience, and actively asking instead of "knowing" what the child feels can have positive outcomes (Dekker-van der Sande and Sterkenburg 2015). However, in setting goals, being realistic about what to expect from therapy is even more essential for children with whom there are many core issues that cannot be expected to be resolved in the course of a time-limited psychotherapy.

STRUCTURE AND FRAME OF TIME-LIMITED MBT-C

The basic time-limited MBT-C model is 12 individual sessions, with separate meetings for the parent(s) offered in parallel alongside the sessions. Although some therapists may view short-term and time-limited therapies as a "necessary evil" in the era of managed care (Salyer 2002), there is now a significant body of research suggesting that short-term interventions in child mental health can be effective (McLaughlin et al. 2013), including short-term psychodynamic interventions (Abbass et al. 2013). Likewise, a meta-analysis of attachment-focused interventions by Bakermans-Kranenburg et al. (2003) showed that most effective interventions use a moderate number of sessions (between 5 and 16) and tend to be more focused in their aims. Time-limited work, when effective, is clearly in the interests of children and families, because it allows the children to return to their daily lives without too great a disruption to their normal lives. Nevertheless, for some children, a brief intervention may not be indicated (Ramchandani and Jones 2003). In certain cases, when a longer-term intervention is appropriate (e.g., for those children whose early relational trauma or attachment insecurity makes trusting an adult a real challenge), it is possible to offer up to three blocks of 12 MBT-C sessions (i.e., up to a total of 36 sessions). These additional blocks of treatment are based on a review process that weighs the pros and cons of additional treatment, and the treatment never is open-ended in these cases, but continues to be time-limited, with a clear focus and aims.

We aim at not being overly prescriptive, as the practicalities of the treatment can be organized in several different ways, depending on the clinical setting and the severity of the problems of the child and parents. What is important is that the therapeutic contract is clear and coherent from the beginning—for the parents, as well as for the child. This is a way of creating a sense of safety and collaboration and of avoiding a scenario in which the therapist makes decisions of which the family is unaware. This transparency is part of the mentalizing stance and contributes to a sense of shared ownership of the therapeutic process.

The notion of "phases" in therapy is to some degree an artificial one, given that the underlying aims and techniques of the work continue from the beginning to the end of therapy. Nevertheless, part of the structure of time-limited MBT-C is a predictable shape to the treatment, which can be thought of in terms of key phases, each with its own particular tasks.

Assessment Phase (3–4 Meetings)

All therapeutic work with children and their families should be based on a thorough assessment leading to some provisional understanding of the presenting problem(s), as well as a formulation of how those problems may be linked to the proposed intervention (see Chapter 6, "Individual Therapy Techniques"; Chapter 17, "Borderline Personality Pathology in Adolescence"; and Chapter 22, "Eating Disorders," for further discussion of formulation). An assessment that focuses on developing a "mentalizing profile" of the child and family would include some formulation about how mentalizing difficulties may be linked to the child's presenting problems, and whether a mentalization-focused intervention is likely to be of help. If work is going ahead, a focus statement will be formulated (the "focus formulation," described later in this chapter), and the child, parents, and therapists will agree on a set of goals for the treatment. (For a more detailed account of the assessment process in MBT-C, see Muller and Midgley 2015.)

Sessions 1–3: Initial Phase

Although it can be thought of as a separate phase of treatment, much of what is done during the first few sessions of MBT-C builds on the work already done in the assessment phase and makes use of techniques that are also part of the ongoing sessions with the child. With children, the primary aim of this initial phase is to establish a therapeutic alliance, primarily by means of empathic attunement and genuine engagement with and curiosity about the child's world. Play is central to this process of engagement and is a marvelous way to socialize the child to the way that therapy works. This will include introducing the calendar (described later in this chapter) and a therapy box (containing a set of play materials) for the child, and exploring whether the child can play around the focus formulation.

With the parent(s), engagement and establishing a therapeutic alliance are also paramount, as the parents' therapist begins to support "reflective parenting" (Redfern and Cooper 2015; see also Chapter 16). Empathic attunement with the parent's experience, even when the therapist may have different views on how a parent is responding to the child, is key at this stage. By feeling seen and validated, parents experience reduced levels of stress, which in turn can enable them to become less preoccupied with their own feelings and more open to their child.

Sessions 4–8: Middle Phase

The middle phase of MBT-C is where the core work on developing the child's mentalizing capacity takes place, in relation to the focus formulation, drawing on a wide range of therapeutic techniques. Meanwhile, the sessions with the parents can increasingly focus on promoting the various elements of reflective parenting. In the work with both parents and children, if affects can be regulated in a way that make explicit mentalizing possible, then empathic attunement can increasingly be complemented by a focus on promoting perspective taking and seeing things from others' points of view. In some cases, the focus will be more on promoting the underdeveloped capacity for mentalizing and/or paying attention to the situations in which explicit mentalizing breaks down.

Review Meeting

After the first eight sessions, a review meeting is offered with the child and parents. At this meeting, the initial focus and treatment goals are reviewed, and it is decided whether the first block of sessions seems to be sufficient and therapy should be coming toward an ending, or whether further work needs to be done. Monitoring the focus formulation is often part of this process as well: Was it a good focus formulation? How has it developed? Has it been forgotten, or is it not a part of the therapy? How can this process be understood? When it is felt that the therapeutic work will need to go on for longer than the initial block of sessions, it is still possible to work in a time-limited way using an "open-ticket model." In this case, another block of 12 sessions can be offered, up to a maximum of 36 (3 sets of 12) sessions. This flexibility facilitates using the time-limited approach for children with more complex disorders, such as those who have experienced trauma or have attachment disorders. However, we would not necessarily subscribe to the idea that more complex difficulties always benefit from longer (or open-ended) therapies. Our experience is that working with a time limitation and a focus can be helpful, but that children with more complex problems often need more than one block of 12 sessions.

Sessions 9–12: Ending Phase

When therapy is due to end, the focus is on preparing for the ending and exploring how best to maintain the gains that have been made beyond the end of therapy. The time-limited nature of MBT-C means that endings are kept very actively in mind throughout the work, and the use of a calendar helps the child to be aware of how many sessions he or she has had and how many are left. Because one of the aims of MBT-C is to ensure that the child and his or her parents end the therapy with a better capacity to make use of other relationships outside therapy, a particular focus of the ending phase is on translating what has been learned in therapy to other supportive relationships.

Checking-In or Booster Sessions

At whatever point the time-limited therapy ends, the MBT-C model includes a checking-in or booster session, which is arranged any time between 3 and 12 months after finishing.

PHYSICAL SETTING FOR THERAPY

In terms of an optimal setting for MBT-C, we recommend that the therapy should be planned to take place in the same room for all sessions, and that this room does not change too much. Sometimes, however, there may be reasons for changing the room when there is reason to believe that the child needs a specific context. For example, in some settings there may be an outdoor space that is available to the therapist, or a gym in which the child is able to engage with more physical activities. Moving the therapy at certain points into such a setting can be helpful for children with attention-regulation problems, such as those who are very hyperactive or aggressive, or who are quickly overwhelmed by incentives from the outside and lack regulation capacities.

A child's therapy room does not necessarily need to contain a lot of toys or play material. On the contrary, children with regulation difficulties may become overwhelmed in rooms containing too much play material from which to choose. When the arousal level is too high, the child will not be able to play or pay attention to what he or she is experiencing. Likewise, some children may feel safer in a smaller room, whereas others may need the space of a bigger room in order not to feel restricted. Ideally, the room needs to have at least some floor space large enough for the child to move around in and play more physical games, such as looping a ball into a basket, playing mini hockey, or simply throwing and catching a ball. For some children, it can be helpful to have some personal items in the room because they might recognize aspects of the therapist in the way the room is styled, as well as creating an atmosphere that is not too institutional (Slijper 2008). At the same time, some children may feel anxious or experience feelings of rivalry toward other children when a room is too personal.

When selecting playroom material, the therapist aims to create the optimal space for children to play and express themselves. It is recommended to have some sensory play material that stimulates or awakens the senses. As Stern (1992, 2004) has pointed out, such materials are often very important for children with attention and affect-regulation problems. Suitable materials can be a sand tray or kinetic sand, clay, finger paint, water, bubbles, or different sizes and types of balls. In order to stimulate fantasy and role-play, dolls, animal figures, cars, bricks, and dress-up clothes are often used, and it is valuable to have dolls with a variety of skin tones, of different genders and ages. It is also a good idea to have a few games as part of the playroom material. Almost all therapists have some art supplies, and some therapists also have other creative materials such as musical instruments. Of course, therapists do not always have much control about what kind of space is available or what materials are provided; even so, it can be helpful to think with the child and parents about how the space may be experienced, and how it may impact on the child's behavior in sessions. The aim is for the child to feel invited and at ease to play following his or her impulses (within certain limits) and to express himself or herself freely.

TIME AS A FRAMEWORK FOR THERAPY

Time is an aspect that is addressed throughout therapy; its importance is emphasized by the time limitation, supported by the use of a calendar (as discussed later in this section). The time limitation can be a motivational factor to work with the most urgent issues and reminds the therapist and family alike that the family will need to have the capacity to address difficulties themselves in the near future. Every therapeutic intervention in MBT-C has as its ultimate aim to encourage and increase the parents' and children's ability to mentalize in a way that can help them manage their difficulties more constructively once the treatment is over. In this way, the ending is built into the process from the very beginning of therapy.

Being transparent about the time limitation and the number of sessions remaining also gives the child an opportunity to prepare for and work through the separation that will come with the end of therapy. Many children in therapy have experienced multiple separations in their lives, but they may not always have had the time to prepare and work through them, making this a new experience through which feelings about endings can be addressed together with the therapist. Because MBT-C is process-focused, the time frame also can serve as a port of entry in terms of activating relational dynamics. For example, when a child (or, indeed, a parent) complains, *"You don't give me enough time!"* this can be used to explore triggers of nonmentalizing moments, or may reflect issues of fairness for some children and families that can be helpfully explored.

Inspired by developmentally directed time-limited psychotherapy for children (Haugvik and Johns 2006; Røed Hansen 2012), one of the ways in which the MBT-C therapist actively works with the time limitation as part of the therapy is by using a calendar together with the child. The aim of the calendar is to stimulate a sense of ownership of the therapy in the child and to encourage a reflective stance, as well as helping the child to have some sense of the time-limited nature of the work (Gydal and Knudtzon 2002).

Calendars can look different but should always consist of a (preferably large) sheet of paper marked with as many rectangles or circles as there are sessions. The therapist introduces the calendar during the first session. As part of establishing the framework of the therapy, the therapist tells the child that at the end of each session, the child will be asked to draw something in the calendar, and that this is a way for them both to keep track of the sessions and reflect together on what has happened that day. A good idea may be to let the child number the spaces in the calendar in order to establish it as a way to give some sense of the length of the therapy from the beginning. The child can also decorate the back of the calendar in order to make it more personal and thereby enhance the sense that it belongs to him or her.

When there is approximately 5–10 minutes left in each session, the child is asked to draw something in the calendar. The main rule for this is that *anything is OK*. The calendar belongs to the child, and he or she decides what to draw in it. There may be times when the therapist feels an urge to help the child by suggesting certain things to draw—or even to help directly with the drawing—but unless the child explicitly asks for this, the therapist should refrain. Sometimes, however, the therapist needs to take responsibility for the calendar in the sense of not letting the child tear it apart, paint all over the different spaces, or ruin it in other ways.

Through the use of a calendar, the child and the therapist create their own story— a narrative about the therapeutic process can be created and visualized together. The calendar can also be a powerful tool for addressing the ending of the session or the therapy, and the forthcoming separation. By looking at the calendar together, the child and the therapist can keep track of the number of sessions they have left and prepare for their farewell. At the end of the therapy and in the booster session(s), the calendar can be used for looking back and reviewing the work that has been done together (Røed Hansen 2012).

FOCUS FORMULATION

Another core aspect of the therapeutic frame, also inspired by developmentally directed time-limited psychotherapy for children (Haugvik and Johns 2006; Røed Hansen 2012), is formulating a focus for the therapy, which should emerge out of carefully observing and listening to what the child conveys, verbally and nonverbally, during the assessment sessions. The focus formulation should be a short phrase or a story that is shared with the child and parents at the start of treatment, just as the formulation is shared with the patient in other mentalization-based interventions. All MBT formulations have this feature in common: they contain an outline of the patient's attachment and relational problems in language that the patient can understand, with consideration about how these problems might be activated in treatment. The formulation needs to be written in such a way that the patient is able to see himself or herself in the formulation—so it "is" him or her rather than "*about*" him or her. In a way, it can be related to Stern's (1985) concept of a "key metaphor," representing core relational and emotional themes (Johns 2008).

Case Example

A 10-year-old boy came to therapy with his parents. His mother spoke of a period in which she had hit the boy, when she was struggling with her own problems (related to, most likely, borderline personality disorder). This incident had occurred 4 years ago, but the relationship between the mother and boy was never totally restored after that. The boy had a number of problems—he was wetting his bed; he had attentional difficulties, especially at school; and he had problems in playing with other children. During the assessment, he had spoken of his love for playing computer war games and his desire to become a soldier one day. His mother had worked really hard on her own problems and could regulate her emotions much better. The boy, however, kept trying to please his mother, not speaking his mind, and being tense in the relationship. As the assessment period came to an end, the therapist and family decided to formulate a focus connected to this relational problem and the boy's love for computer games and soldiers. The therapist asked him what kind of soldier he wanted to be: A soldier who could not feel what was going on inside himself, who could not sense fear or anger, and simply tried to obey others? Or a soldier who could be firm and decisive and true to himself and others, who could feel his emotions and bodily signals to help him to stay safe, even when the going got tough? The boy loved this focus formulation, and once in therapy he worked really hard to become more connected with his body and emotions, as well as understanding himself better. At the end of the 12 sessions, the boy could talk about what had happened between him and his mother, he hardly wet his bed anymore, and he felt better attuned to peers at his school. Alongside MBT-C he also started to take medication for his attentional problems, which helped a lot at school and also improved his self-worth and self-esteem. In the therapy itself, he sometimes referred back to the questions that the therapist had asked him, and this became a way in which they continued to explore who he was and who he wanted to become.

As this example makes clear, one of the main aims of the focus formulation is to speak with the child and to convey that the therapy has something to offer him or her. Many children are brought to therapy by parents or other adults, with little notion of why they have been brought, or with a sense of being there simply in order to please the adults around them (Johns 2008). When time is limited, the task of engaging the child becomes more urgent, and the focus can be seen as functioning as an invitation to the child to engage in the therapy process. Using material from the assessment with the child in formulating the focus can strengthen the child's sense of agency in the therapy: something the child has contributed to the encounter becomes a focus for the treatment.

Another aim with the focus formulation is to stimulate mentalizing by directing the parents' attention to central experiences, thoughts, and feelings in the child—keeping the child's mind in mind and at the same time stimulating the child's self-reflection around his or her own inner states. The parents of the boy in the case example above had to be helped with mentalizing about their son being oppositional and not doing what the parents asked. In their own sessions, they spoke with their therapist about when a normally developing boy age 10 or 11 could disagree with his parents. The mother was helped with her feelings of guilt and how these feelings affected her approach to her son, and began to become more curious about what kind of man he could become, as someone separate and different from herself.

The therapist's formulation becomes a model for keeping someone else's mind in mind. The focus creates joint attention toward what the child presents as central experiences, thoughts, and feelings. It shows that the therapist has taken in something from the parents and child, and invites a meaning-creating dialogue around the problems that brought the child to therapy.

THERAPIST STANCE IN TIME-LIMITED MBT-C

Most people working in the field of psychotherapy would probably agree that any specific model of therapy—whether, for example, MBT, CBT, or interpersonal psychotherapy—is not simply a set of tools or techniques that can be "applied"; it also implies a stance (or "way of being") that informs every aspect of the therapeutic work. When researchers ask adults or children to look back on what it was like going to therapy, very few of them say much about what kind of techniques the therapist used—they do not often comment on the quality of the cognitive reframing, or whether the therapist's interpretations were accurate. Instead, they tend to begin by speaking about the person of the therapist: What was he or she like? Was he or she nice? Did they feel comfortable with him or her? Of course, this does not mean that the techniques the therapist uses do not matter—just that all such techniques always take place in the context of a relationship, and that the therapist's "way of being" may be as important as the particular techniques that he or she uses, especially when therapy is understood in terms of helping clients to overcome *epistemic vigilance* (Fonagy and Allison 2014).

As in other forms of MBT, the stance in MBT-C is not just a background to the real work of therapy; it is at the core of what the therapy is and how it works. The stance is crucial because it is both an *aim* of MBT-C, insofar as MBT-C therapists are trying to help the families they work with to develop a capacity to mentalize, and the *means* by which the therapists can achieve this aim (by trying to model this stance themselves).

The key components of the mentalizing stance include the importance of curiosity, an interest in mind (not just behavior), and an interest in exploring the perspective of others from a "not-knowing" position. Most importantly, it is vital to recognize the ways in which the therapist's own mentalizing capacity can break down. In MBT-C, therapists try to help parents and children understand themselves and each other better by offering them a therapy in which they learn a way of exploring and talking about thoughts and feelings that helps them to be better attuned. For the therapists working with this model, it is equally important to actively mentalize and to notice when their own mentalizing (inevitably) breaks down. In working with the parents, therapists explicitly identify mentalizing breakdowns, in the here and now. In working with children, the therapists also notice these moments but may sometimes hold off before intervening. Sometimes the therapist might subtitle his or her own thoughts by saying something about it (e.g., *"I feel confused when you do this and look that way"*)— or when a child is behaving so angrily that the therapist feels under attack and mentalizing stops, the therapist can address the interaction explicitly by saying, *"When you are so angry with me and try to hit me, I feel I have to respond to you right away, just to make sure we are all safe—and later on, I hope to understand what happened."*

In some clinics, therapists will be working in larger teams, whereas in other settings the therapist may work with a single colleague or even alone. Regardless of the setting, the most important factor is to create a working environment that is safe and secure to allow mental states to be explored from a curious, not-knowing position. When therapists feel safe and supported, they are usually more able to ask for help and speak freely about experiences while working with challenging clients (Muller 2009). However, a sense of safety is not always easy to maintain. Some therapists may work in an organization that sets up prerequisites for work that may not always be completely congruent with the therapists' ideals. Furthermore, different patients will challenge the therapist's capacity to remain reflective, and some children or families may trigger feelings and conflicts in the therapist, affecting his or her mentalizing capacity.

Given that most therapists work in relatively high-stress conditions, and that much of what goes on in therapy happens in physical isolation behind closed doors, it is not surprising that the mentalizing stance can be hard to sustain. As Bevington and Fuggle (2012) note, there can be "a tendency to move into non-mentalizing states such as teleological thinking (preoccupation with what to do) or with psychic equivalence (the belief that how the worker thinks/feels is actually how it is)" (p. 176). In the light of such (normal) challenges, Bevington et al. (2017) have proposed a particular format for supervision, called "Thinking Together." This approach draws on the natural ability to regain the capacity to mentalize through contact with attachment figures (in the context of therapists, their colleagues and supervisors), while avoiding the risk that supervision becomes a simple narrative of dramatic events, or an opportunity for the supervisor to demonstrate a "better" understanding of the child than the therapist has. This latter scenario, in particular, is likely to result in reduced mentalizing on the part of the therapist, even when the supervisor's insights about the child may be quite brilliant!

CONCLUSION

Time-limited MBT-C has been developed for use with children with a range of presenting problems. As such, time-limited MBT-C is a transdiagnostic approach—one that can be practiced by a wide range of clinicians in many different settings, without a large amount of additional training. We argue that this is a strength of the model. However, understanding in both heart and head what mentalizing is, and being able to translate this knowledge effectively to clinical practice with children, is a challenge, and careful thought needs to be given when considering which families should be offered MBT-C. When assessing suitability and planning the treatment, the clinician needs to undertake a comprehensive review of the child and family functioning—one that pays attention not only to symptoms and behavior but also to the nature and severity of the mentalizing deficits, to ascertain especially whether there is a global underdevelopment of mentalizing or whether the breakdowns in mentalizing are more specific or temporary.

The overarching aim of time-limited MBT-C is to foster the development and enhancement of mentalizing processes, helping the child to become aware of and regulate emotions, as well as to mentalize about difficulties that he or she might face. This in turn can help to reduce epistemic mistrust so that the child is better able to make use of supportive relationships both within and beyond therapy. The aim of the work with parents is to enhance their ability to mentalize regarding their child's experiences, including the child's experience of them, as well as the parents' own emotions related to parenting and how these influence family interactions. When these two aims can be achieved side by side, children with a range of presenting difficulties may be meaningfully helped.

The standard model for MBT-C is 12 sessions for the child with simultaneous sessions for the parents, but this model leaves room for adaptations. The use of a calendar and the focus formulation become means for the child to develop a sense of participation, ownership, and agency in the therapeutic process, as well as being helpful instruments for keeping track of time and creating coherence in the therapy. In time-limited MBT-C, structure and focus are seen as important therapeutic factors. Everybody knowing and agreeing on the setting of the therapy from the start enhances the sense that the therapeutic endeavor is a shared one, and that the therapist does not have privileged information or make decisions on his or her own. By discussing aspects of the therapeutic setting together with the family, the therapist can model a reflective stance, as well as negotiate an appropriate frame and a focus formulation for therapy. Nevertheless, many aspects of the therapeutic frame, such as working with one or two therapists, can be tailored according to the needs of the family and the preferences of the therapist(s), as well as the opportunities provided in the clinical setting.

REFERENCES

Abbass AA, Rabung S, Leichsenring F, et al: Psychodynamic psychotherapy for children and adolescents: a meta-analysis of short-term psychodynamic models. J Am Acad Child Adolesc Psychiatry 52(8):863–875, 2013 23880496

Bak PL: "Thoughts in mind": Promoting mentalizing communities for children, in Minding the Child: Mentalization-Based Interventions With Children, Young People, and Their Families. Edited by Midgley N, Vrouva I. London, Routledge, 2012, pp 202–218

Bak PL, Midgley N, Zhu JL, et al: The Resilience Program: preliminary evaluation of a mentalization-based education program. Front Psychol 6:753, 2015 26136695

Bakermans-Kranenburg MJ, van IJzendoorn MH, Juffer F: Less is more: meta-analyses of sensitivity and attachment interventions in early childhood. Psychol Bull 129(2):195–215, 2003 12696839

Bammens AS, Adkins T, Badger J: Psycho-educational intervention increases reflective functioning in foster and adoptive parents. Adopt Foster 39:38–50, 2015

Bevington D, Fuggle P: Supporting and enhancing mentalization in community outreach teams working with hard-to-reach youth: the AMBIT approach, in Minding the Child: Mentalization-Based Interventions With Children, Young People and Their Families. Edited by Midgley N, Vrouva I. London, Routledge, 2012, pp 163–186

Bevington D, Fuggle P, Cracknell L, et al: Adaptive Mentalization-Based Integrative Treatment: A Guide for Teams to Develop Systems of Care. Oxford, UK, Oxford University Press, 2017

Bleiberg E: Mentalizing-based treatment with adolescents and families. Child Adolesc Psychiatr Clin N Am 22(2):295–330, 2013 23538015

Dekker-van der Sande F, Sterkenburg P: Mentaliseren kan je Leren. Introductie in Mentaliseren Bevorderende Begeleiding (MBB) [How to Learn to Mentalize: An Introduction on Mentalization Based Accompaniment]. Doorn, Netherlands, Bartiméus Reeks, 2015

Ensink K, Normandin L: Le traitement basé sur la mentalization chez des enfants agressés sexuellement et leurs parents [Mentalization-based treatment in sexually abused children and their parents], in L'Agression Sexuelle Envers les Enfants [Sexual Abuse of Children]. Edited by Hébert M, Cyr M, Tourigny M. Montréal, Quebec, Canada, Presse de l'Université du Québec, 2011, pp 399–444

Ensink K, Berthelot N, Bernazzani O, et al: Another step closer to measuring the ghosts in the nursery: preliminary validation of the Trauma Reflective Functioning Scale. Front Psychol 5:1471, 2014 25566146

Ensink K, Bégin M, Normandin L, et al: Maternal and child reflective functioning in the context of child sexual abuse: pathways to depression and externalising difficulties. Eur J Psychotraumatol 7:30611, 2016 26822865

Ensink K, Leroux A, Normandin L, et al: Assessing reflective parenting in interaction with school-aged children. J Pers Assess 99(6):585–595, 2017 28151016

Etezady MH, Davis M: Clinical Perspectives on Reflective Parenting: Keeping the Child's Mind in Mind. Lanham, MD, Jason Aronson, 2012

Fonagy P, Allison E: The role of mentalizing and epistemic trust in the therapeutic relationship. Psychotherapy (Chic) 51(3):372–380, 2014 24773092

Fonagy P, Target M: A contemporary psychoanalytic perspective: psychodynamic developmental therapy, in Psychosocial Treatments for Child and Adolescent Disorders: Empirically Based Strategies for Clinical Practice. Edited by Hibbs ED, Jensen PS. Washington, DC, National Institutes of Health and the American Psychological Association, 1996, pp 619–638

Fonagy P, Cottrell D, Phillips J, et al: What Works for Whom? A Critical Review of Treatments for Children and Adolescents, 2nd Edition. New York, Guilford, 2015

Fuggle P, Bevington D, Cracknell L, et al: The Adolescent Mentalization-based Integrative Treatment (AMBIT) approach to outcome evaluation and manualization: adopting a learning organization approach. Clin Child Psychol Psychiatry 20(3):419–435, 2015 24595808

Goodman G, Stroh M, Valdez A: Do attachment representations predict depression and anxiety in psychiatrically hospitalized prepubertal children? Bull Menninger Clin 76(3):260–289, 2012 22988901

Goodman G, Reed P, Athey-Lloyd L: Mentalization and play therapy processes between two therapists and a child with Asperger's disorder. Int J Play Ther 24:13–29, 2015

Goodman G, Midgley N, Schneider C: Expert clinicians' prototypes of an ideal child treatment in psychodynamic and cognitive-behavioral therapy: is mentalization seen as a common process factor? Psychother Res 26(5):590–601, 2016 26169491

Green H, McGinnity A, Meltzer H, et al: Mental Health of Children and Young People in Great Britain, 2004. London, Office for National Statistics, 2005

Gydal M, Knudtzon S: Om tidsbegrenset psykoterapi med barn [Time-limited psychotherapy with children]. Tidsskr Nor Psykol foren 39:911–915, 2002

Haugvik M, Johns U: Betydningen av felles fokus i tidsavgrenset psykoterapi med barn: En kvalitativ studie av psykoterapi med barn som opplever vanskelige familieforhold [Importance of a common focus in time-limited psychotherapy with children: a qualitative study of psychotherapy with children experiencing difficult family relationships]. Tidsskr Nor Psykol foren 43:19–29, 2006

Jacobsen MN, Ha C, Sharp C: A mentalization-based treatment approach to caring for youth in foster care. J Infant Child Adolesc Psychother 14:440–454, 2015

Johns UT: "Å bruke tiden—hva betyr egentlig det?" Tid og relasjon—et intersubjektivt perspektiv ["Spending time—what does that mean?" Time and relationship—an intersubjective perspective], in Perspektiver på Musikk og Helse [Perspectives on Music and Health]. Edited by Trondalen G, Ruud E. Oslo, Norway, NMH, 2008, pp 67–84

Jurist EL: Mentalized affectivity. Psychoanal Psychol 22:426–444, 2005

Kernberg P, Chazan SE: Children With Conduct Disorders: A Psychotherapy Manual. New York, Basic Books, 1991

Kernberg PF, Weiner AS, Bandenstein KK: Personality Disorders in Children and Adolescents. New York, Basic Books, 2000

Malberg N, Fonagy P: Creating security by exploring the personal meaning of chronic illness in adolescent patients, in A Psychodynamic Understanding of Modern Medicine: Placing the Person at the Center of Care. Edited by Reilly Landry MO. London, Radcliffe Press, 2012, pp 27–38

McLaughlin C, Holliday C, Clarke B, et al: Research on Counselling and Psychotherapy With Children and Young People: A Systematic Scoping Review of the Evidence for Its Effectiveness From 2003–2011. Leicester, UK, British Association for Counselling and Psychotherapy, 2013

Midgley N, Besser SJ, Dye H, et al: The Herts and Minds study: evaluating the effectiveness of mentalization-based treatment (MBT) as an intervention for children in foster care with emotional and/or behavioural problems: a phase II, feasibility, randomised controlled trial. Pilot Feasibility Stud 3:12, 2017a 28250962

Midgley N, Ensink K, Lindqvist K, et al: Mentalization-Based Treatment for Children: A Time-Limited Approach. Washington, DC, American Psychological Association, 2017b

Muller N: MBT in organizations. Lecture at a conference organised by Triade: Dutch Organisation for Clients with a Diagnosis of BPD and their Families, Breukelen, The Netherlands, 2009

Muller N, Midgley N: Approaches to assessment in time-limited Mentalization-Based Therapy for Children (MBT-C). Front Psychol 6:1063, 2015 26283994

Muller N, Gerits L, Siecker I: Mentalization-based therapies with adopted children and their families, in Minding the Child: Mentalization-Based Interventions With Children, Young People, and Their Families. Edited by Midgley N, Vrouva I. London, Routledge, 2012, pp 113–130

Muñoz Specht P, Ensink K, Normandin L, et al: Mentalizing techniques used by psychodynamic therapists working with children and early adolescents. Bull Menninger Clin 80(4):281–315, 2016 27936899

Ordway MR, Sadler LS, Dixon J, et al: Lasting effects of an interdisciplinary home visiting program on child behavior: preliminary follow-up results of a randomized trial. J Pediatr Nurs 29(1):3–13, 2014 23685264

Perepletchikova F, Goodman G: Two approaches to treating preadolescent children with severe emotional and behavioral problems: dialectical behavior therapy adapted for children and mentalization-based child therapy. J Psychother Integration 24:298–312, 2014

Ramchandani P, Jones DP: Treating psychological symptoms in sexually abused children: from research findings to service provision. Br J Psychiatry 183:484–490, 2003 14645018

Ramires VRR, Schwan S, Midgley N: Mentalization-based therapy with maltreated children living in shelters in southern Brazil: a single case study. Psychoanal Psychother 26:308–326, 2012

Redfern S, Cooper A: Reflective Parenting. London, Routlege, 2015

Røed Hansen B: I dialog med barnet. Intersubjektivitet i utvikling og i psykoterapi [In Dialogue with the Child. Intersubjectivity in Development and in Psychotherapy]. Oslo, Norway, Gyldendal, 2012

Rossouw TI, Fonagy P: Mentalization-based treatment for self-harm in adolescents: a randomized controlled trial. J Am Acad Child Adolesc Psychiatry 51(12):1304.e3–1313.e3, 2012 23200287

Salyer K: Time limited therapy: a necessary evil in the managed care era? Reformulation Autumn(17):9–11, 2002

Scott S, Dadds MR: Practitioner review: when parent training doesn't work: theory-driven clinical strategies. J Child Psychol Psychiatry 50(12):1441–1450, 2009 19754503

Sharp C, Williams LL, Ha C, et al: The development of a mentalization-based outcomes and research protocol for an adolescent inpatient unit. Bull Menninger Clin 73(4):311–338, 2009 20025427

Siminoff LA: Incorporating patient and family preferences into evidence-based medicine. BMC Med Inform Decis Mak 13(Suppl 3):S6, 2013 24565268

Slade A: Parental reflective functioning: an introduction. Attach Hum Dev 7(3):269–281, 2005 16210239

Slade A, Grienenberger J, Bernbach E, et al: Maternal reflective functioning, attachment, and the transmission gap: a preliminary study. Attach Hum Dev 7(3):283–298, 2005 16210240

Slijper FME: Treatment in practice, in Mentalizing in Child Therapy: Guidelines for Clinical Practitioners. Edited by Verheugt-Pleiter AJE, Zevalkink J, Schmeets MGJ. London, Karnac Books, 2008, pp 179–194

Stern DN: The Interpersonal World of the Infant: A View from Psychoanalysis and Developmental Psychology. New York, Basic Books, 1985

Stern DN: Diary of a Baby: What Your Child Sees, Feels, and Experiences. New York, Basic Books, 1992

Stern DN: The Present Moment in Psychotherapy and Everyday Life. New York, WW Norton, 2004

Taylor C: Empathic Care for Children With Disorganized Attachments: A Model for Mentalizing, Attachment and Trauma-Informed Care. London, Jessica Kingsley Publishers, 2012

Thorén A: Outcome of short-term psychotherapy for children. Paper presented at the 45th International Annual Meeting of the Society for Psychotherapy Research, Copenhagen, Denmark, June 25–28, 2014

Twemlow SW, Fonagy P, Sacco FC: A developmental approach to mentalizing communities: II. The Peaceful Schools experiment. Bull Menninger Clin 69(4):282–304, 2005 16370790

Verheugt-Pleiter AJE, Zevalkink J, Schmeets MGJ: Mentalizing in Child Therapy: Guidelines for Clinical Practitioners. London, Karnac Books, 2008

Zevalkink K, Verheugt-Pleiter A, Fonagy P: Mentalization-informed child psychoanalytic psychotherapy, in Handbook of Mentalizing in Mental Health Practice. Edited by Bateman AW, Fonagy P. Washington, DC, American Psychiatric Publishing, 2012, pp 129–158

CHAPTER 16

PARENTING AND FOSTER CARE

Sheila Redfern, Ph.D.

The influence of parental, particularly maternal, mental health on infant development is well documented. With its roots in attachment theory, and particularly the importance of contingent marked mirroring during the first few months of an infant's life, mentalizing theory has an important theoretical framework to offer academics in the field. The difficulty emerges in operationalizing this for parents and for professionals working with parents. To this end, the author and her colleague developed a model of parent–child mentalizing that can be practically applied to parents, namely, Reflective Parenting (Cooper and Redfern 2016). This chapter sets out the model of Reflective Parenting and highlights the importance of working clinically with both the parental state of mind and the parents' capacity to mentalize the child. The model is then applied to the context of foster care, where it has particular relevance in trying to further our understanding of the mediating effects of early adversity on children's development. This chapter provides an overview of the application of this approach to foster carers looking after children who have experienced significant relational trauma and have deficits in perspective taking.

BACKGROUND

The impact of a parent's state of mind on infant and child development has far-reaching effects. This impact begins during pregnancy, with the mother's capacity to consider the thoughts and feelings of her baby growing in the womb—that is, to *mentalize* the baby. Throughout an infant's life, the mother's capacity to reflect back the infant's state of mind, and also concurrently her own mind reflecting on the infant's, forms the building blocks for learning about both the self and others. This in turn leads to greater emotion regulation and the capacity to understand the perspectives, thoughts, feelings, wishes, and desires of others, leading eventually to more successful social understanding and relationships. When there are significant deficits in a mother's capacity to do this, to such an extent that she experiences dissociative states, the impact on the infant is far reaching (Beebe et al. 2012). When a mother not only is not contingent with her infant but frequently reflects back a state of mind that is greatly at odds with the infant's, an "alien self" (Bateman and Fonagy 2016) is internalized in the infant, which results in the infant having a very poorly developed sense of his or her own mind. For other infants in less extreme everyday interactions, the mother can lack congruence with her infant's state of mind intermittently but frequently enough for the infant to develop significant difficulties with emotion regulation. However, in the majority of normally developing children, the process of contingent marked mirroring builds the foundations of the capacity to mentalize in the child within the context of a secure relationship.

A parent's ability to understand the child's state of mind has been referred to for more than 20 years as *reflective functioning*. This construct emerged from the well-known London Parent–Child Project study (Fonagy et al. 1991a), in which groundbreaking findings showed that there was a high level of concordance between a parent's and a child's patterns of attachment. Fonagy et al. (1991b) hypothesized that this concordance was related to the parental capacity to see the child as a separate psychological entity with a mental experience of his or her own. In addition, the parent's capacity to not only perceive but then to reflect back the mental state of the child—and then respond through the parent's own behavior—was seen as strongly linked to attachment security. This finding led to the development of the Reflective Self-Function Scale and subsequent development of the Reflective Functioning Scale (RFS; Fonagy et al. 1998), an important measure of parents' capacity to understand their own mental states. The RFS was initially applied to the Adult Attachment Interview (AAI; George et al. 1985) and led to the identification of markers that were seen as evidence of reflective functioning. This development is relevant here to parental mentalizing because these markers related not only to an awareness of mental states and their nature, but also to how the parents were able to, in their AAIs, reflect on their childhood experiences and how those experiences had affected them in the here and now (as future parents). Fonagy et al. (1991b) assumed that this ability in parents to understand and to reflect on their own as well as others' mental states originates from a parent–child relationship in their own early history in which they experienced a caregiver (usually the mother) as someone able to recognize and respond to their mental states. They assumed further that this ability of the caregiver to understand the child's mental states would not only lead to security in the attachment relationship but would in turn be vital to the child's learning to develop the same capacity. This ability to have a "reflective self" therefore is a careful interplay between reflecting on the self (parental) state of mind and turning this reflective capacity toward the developing child. This important balance is key to working to increase a parent's capacity to mentalize, as parental mentalizing is about not simply the parent's capacity to reflect on the child, but also the parent's capacity to reflect on his or her own mental activity. The mother's mentalizing of her own childhood before the birth of her child predicts the child's security of attachment (Fonagy et al. 1991a).

Suchman et al. (2010) proposed a two-factor model of parental reflective functioning. Interestingly, this study found that the parents' capacity to mentalize themselves (self-mentalizing) was more highly predictive of the quality of parental caregiving than their capacity to mentalize their child. In developing a model of Reflective Parenting for both a clinical and a nonclinical sample, it was hypothesized that the mother's ability to understand her own mental states, associated with the ability to self-regulate the related affective experience, would allow the mother to subsequently begin to mentalize her child and then respond more contingently to the child's emotional needs.

In the model of Reflective Parenting (Cooper and Redfern 2016), there is a strong emphasis on operationalizing this important reflective self in supporting parents to develop a more attuned and connected relationship with their child. Self-mentalizing plays a key role in the Reflective Parenting model and is the first step for parents in this work.

THE REFLECTIVE PARENTING MODEL

The Reflective Parenting model aims to

1. Encourage professionals to take a mentalizing stance toward parents. As a result, the parents feel understood, which then helps them begin to mentalize.
2. Increase parents' awareness of their own mind in relation to parenting.
3. Explicitly provide parents with psychoeducation in developing knowledge of how an understanding of feelings (both their own and those of their child) links to managing feelings and behavior.
4. Give parents an awareness that understanding the "inside story" to why a child behaves in a particular way leads to greater connection between parent and child.
5. Increase parents' abilities to help their child understand how he or she is feeling and why he or she feels this way.

Reflective parents do not focus solely on the external behavior of their child. Rather, they also keep a focus on the child as an individual with his or her own mind, understanding that the child often does things for reasons that are linked to how he or she is thinking or feeling—in other words, that there is an inside story. The parent frequently responds to that inside story of thoughts and feelings, rather than just reacting to the behavior.

Reflective Parenting has three key components: 1) **Professional APP** (Attention and curiosity, Perspective taking, Providing empathy: the mentalizing stance of a supporting professional); 2) the **Parent Map** (the parent's state of mind and capacity to mentalize himself or herself and others); and 3) the **Parent APP** (the parent's stance in relation to mentalizing his or her child). A tool that forms a part of the approach, referred to as the "emotional thermometer," is also used to help parents and professionals bring their level of emotional arousal into their awareness and then manage this in order to get into a more reflective, mentalizing range. These components are discussed in turn in the following subsections.

The Professional APP

Central to a Reflective Parenting intervention is the professional's stance toward the parent, especially the parent's mind. This stance is based on the core principles of mentalizing. To simplify this stance, the model developers have termed it the Professional APP, an acronym for three qualities: Attention and curiosity; Perspective taking; and Providing empathy. The mentalizing stance directly engages a parent to begin to mentalize.

In order for the therapist to connect with parents and carers in their work, it is essential that there is epistemic trust in the relationship. This is a particular type of trust in which there is a willingness on the part of parents or carers to *learn* from the therapist, as he or she is seen as a source of valuable knowledge that will help them in their most intimate relationship, that with their child. The theory of natural pedagogy and epistemic trust (Csibra and Gergely 2009; Fonagy and Allison 2014) states that the pedagogic stance is triggered by ostensive communicative cues (e.g., turn-taking contingent reactivity, eye contact); these ostensive cues indicate to the recipient that the communicator is someone to whom special attention should be paid. It is the sense of being seen psychologically and understood by another that encourages epistemic trust to develop. These experiences are central to the model, in that the stance helps to establish trust in the relationship as the therapist explicitly connects with the mind of the parent through interest and curiosity, taking the parent's perspective in explicit ways, and making empathic and validating comments.

A foster carer's capacity to mentalize his or her looked-after child is frequently compromised by the child's challenging behavior and/or difficulty in developing and maintaining relationships. When foster carers face extreme challenges in this relationship, this raises their level of arousal, thus compromising their capacity to mentalize. Inevitably, this leads to high levels of arousal being brought to the foster carer–professional relationship, which makes it even more important that the professional in this context maintains his or her own capacity to mentalize. The Professional APP is a tool to help the professional regulate his or her own and the foster carer's arousal in these moments of high affect. In the Reflective Parenting model, and also the Reflective Fostering Programme (described later in this chapter), adopting the mentalizing stance from the professional's point of view is the first essential step in working with this model with parents and carers. For it is via this stance that the professional both models the stance for the parent or carer and maintains an awareness and control over his or her own state of mind in relation to the work and the relationship with the parent or carer.

The Parent Map

Reflective Parenting makes explicit to parents how their own state of mind can be highly influential on their child's emotional state and how a greater calibration of these emotions in the parent–child relationship can lead to a greater connection between parent and child. It is increasingly understood that a parent's capacity for self-mentalizing has a significant impact on the quality of interaction between parent and child—often more so than the parent's capacity to mentalize the child (Suchman et al. 2012).

The Parent Map is a tool that is used directly with parents to help professionals explain and work through parents' own examples of interactions in which their mentalizing may have gone "offline." Professionals can validate a parent's state of mind in relation to the child, while also enabling a process that gently challenges and shifts thinking in a way that promotes mentalizing and enables the parent to take some responsibility for lapses in mentalizing by considering what influenced his or her thoughts, feelings, and responses in specific parenting situations.

Once the parent has been given the time and space to think about his or her own mind, the authors have found clinically that this is often when a parent is in a state of psychological readiness (preparedness) for mentalizing his or her child.

The Parent APP

The purpose of the Parent APP is to help to explicitly turn the parent's mind toward the child's mind—that is, to the motives, feelings, thoughts, and intentions behind the child's behavior. The Parent APP mirrors the Professional APP, and the stance is the same. The core principles of the Parent APP are to pay specific and active attention to the baby or child; this links to interventions related to child-led interactions. The parent, by paying active attention and being curious about the child, is beginning to cultivate an interest in the inside story to the child's behavior.

The Reflective Parenting approach rests on the belief that there is an important sequence to the work, namely, that the initial emphasis should be on the parent's capacity to mentalize himself or herself. A clinical focus on encouraging the parent to mentalize the child too early without first working on the parent's self-mentalizing capacity can invalidate the parent's state of mind. It also can have an impact on the therapeutic relationship and ultimately be less likely to lead to the kind of caregiving behaviors that support and encourage the child in free play and the development of behaviors associated with security.

Figure 16–1 shows the important sequence of Reflective Parenting interventions.

Challenges for Foster Carers and Looked-After Children

A sensitive parent's intimate care provides vital regulatory functions for his or her child and promotes the development of brain functions that support the child's capacity to calm distress (Schore 1994). For many looked-after children, the environment of their early years may have been characterized by a lack of the type of contingent, responsive, and sensitive care essential for accurately reflecting back their emotional states. This sensitive responding is essential to helping a child manage stress as he or she learns to self-regulate. If instead there is severe ongoing stress, this can alter the structural development of the brain and in turn affect its neural networks and biochemistry (Perry and Hambrick 2008). Such stressful experiences have a significant detrimental impact on the child's ability to manage extremes of arousal and to regulate his or her emotions when faced with such arousal.

Furthermore, higher-order cognitive abilities, including the ability to mentalize, are influenced by the complex psychological processes engendered in infancy by close proximity to and interaction with the attachment figure. Difficult or disrupted early attachment relationships can embed developmental vulnerabilities, affecting the capacity to build and sustain future relationships. Poor mentalizing abilities in childhood have been associated with reduced peer acceptance (Slaughter et al. 2015), poor school adjustment and educational attainment (Dunn 2002), and increased vulnerability to a wide range of mental health difficulties involving aggression, poor empathy, and emotional regulation (Fonagy et al. 2004; Gomez-Garibello and Talwar 2015).

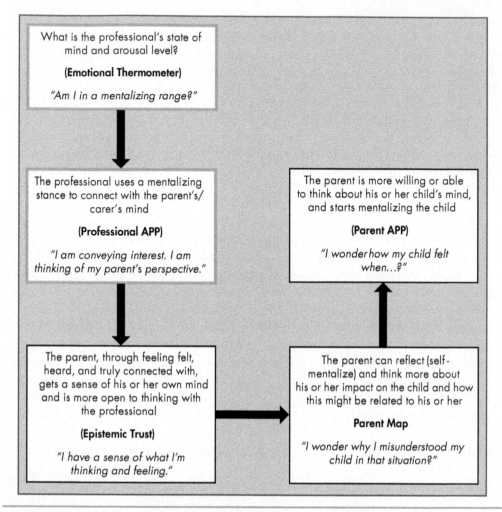

FIGURE 16–1.   The components of a reflective parenting intervention.

Note.   APP=Attention and curiosity, Perspective taking, and Providing empathy: the mentalizing stance of a supporting professional (or the parent's mentalizing stance of supporting his or her child); Parent Map=a tool that is used by professionals directly with parents to help them learn how to mentalize themselves and work out examples of interactions in which they are not mentalizing, and why.

Recent advances in neuroscience, neurobiology, and developmental psychology illuminate the impact of early adverse experiences on the susceptibility to later difficulties. For example, McCrory et al. (2013) demonstrated that maltreated children had more pronounced neural responsiveness to heightened affect in faces in the early preconscious stages of processing (i.e., before the influence of higher-order systems). Such studies help us understand how maltreated children react differently to emotionally charged social interactions, with increased threat-based responses such as freezing, dissociation, or anger. For older children, the impact of increased arousal is likely to trigger implicit automatic reflexive mentalizing, which relies on implicit templates to guide interpretations of the world and influence reactions.

When a child has a parent whose mind is extremely hard to understand, within a family where abuse and fear are ongoing, self-reflection is discouraged, which in turn impedes the development of self-agency. Children who have experienced maltreatment may have learned to inhibit their mentalizing function or may not have developed the capacity to mentalize because of the trauma they experienced to their attachment system (Allen and Fonagy 2006). Feelings and experiences are not put into language; instead, the child may shut down or become compliant or defiant.

Although these advances in research can help our understanding of the impact of early experience on children's development, they do not in themselves lessen the impact that a child's functioning can have on foster carers. Instead, children's difficulties can continue to place great demand on foster carers who have taken on what can be an extremely demanding role. Spending time understanding, with a nonjudgmental and empathic attitude, the acute and chronic impacts on a foster carer of parenting a child who has suffered maltreatment is vital to the professional's work. Often, even very experienced foster carers struggle when facing the challenging behaviors of children who have experienced relational trauma, and such challenges can affect the foster carer's parenting and reflective capacity. The emotional health of carers is positively associated with the success and stability of placements (Furnivall 2011), which is not surprising considering the central role of a foster carer in a looked-after child's life and given that this relationship is central to meeting the child's emotional needs (Simmonds 2010).

Carers' capacity to reflect on the children in their care as autonomous individuals with needs, feelings, and thoughts is crucial in order for them to understand why a child may be displaying some of the worrying or disruptive behavior witnessed. In this regard, foster carers often need specific support around this issue to help reduce the emotional impact they feel from the emotional and behavioral problems of the child, so that the carers are more able to remain present and reflective. Equally important to this relationship is carers' capacity to mentalize themselves, as the need to attend to the mental states of looked-after children requires carers to effectively and actively separate out self from other. This often becomes particularly difficult in the face of high arousal, where, again, the influence of implicit mentalizing dominates and guides quick and automatic interpretation of behavior. Foster carers' ability to mentalize is therefore vulnerable because of the often high level of externalizing behavior experienced in the home.

One study indicated that it can be difficult for foster carers to understand that their foster children's feelings and behaviors in the present moment can be a result of the children's past traumatic experiences, rather than the circumstances in which these children currently find themselves (Bunday et al. 2015). Experiences of loss and trauma are painful to acknowledge, and foster carers themselves may come into the role with their own difficulties and experiences of being parented; these in turn, in the face of traumatic presentations, can make the parenting role extremely difficult. These difficulties interfere with a foster carer's ability to be present and to think and respond in a reflective manner rather than with projections, distortions, or premature conclusions when considering motives for children's behaviors.

The challenges in foster care are associated with factors pertaining to the child, to the foster carer, and to the relationship between the two, within an often challenging context for all professionals working with looked-after children. These factors are all related to a risk of placement breakdown; reported rates range from 22% to 56% (e.g., Kufeldt et al. 1995; Rubin et al. 2007). Research indicates that once foster carers are appropriately supported, looked-after children are able to use their carer as a secure base;

a study has shown that even children who were maltreated can develop secure new attachments toward their foster parents (Joseph et al. 2014). Placement stability is supported by both child and carer commitment to the placement and by how the child relates to the carer and others in the home (Luke et al. 2014). Further, the emotional health of carers has been shown to be positively related to the success and stability of placements (Furnivall 2011). Placement stability is important in improving outcomes for looked-after children, and foster families need help to support their relationships with each other so that the children have a better chance of experiencing consistent care.

Many interventions focus on children's behaviors. Although there is a need to focus on problem behaviors, this focus might not address the actual difficulties in the relationship between the child and his or her carers, and ignores the importance of the different mental states underlying the problem behavior. Mentalization-based treatment (MBT), with its original application of supporting adults with an early history of attachment-related maltreatment in order to increase their abilities to mentalize, offers an area of treatment that the developers of the Reflective Parenting model consider to be highly relevant in clinical work with looked-after children and their carers. Two main reasons are as follows:

1. Mentalizing can act as a buffer against the expression of psychological difficulties, whereas failure of the capacity to mentalize is associated with the development of psychopathology (Bateman and Fonagy 2016). Therefore, an approach that is targeted at increasing the mentalizing capacity of children could increase resilience and prevent later difficulties.
2. Parental reflective functioning is associated with secure child attachment (Fonagy et al. 2007; Sharp and Fonagy 2008), and more specifically with positive outcomes in adoption (Steele et al. 2003) and parental tolerance of infant distress (Rutherford et al. 2013, 2015), and leads to better emotion regulation (Slade et al. 2005).

Therefore, an approach that effectively targets parental mentalizing in foster carers is likely to lead to positive outcomes.

Given the high prevalence of relational trauma experienced by looked-after children, a capacity for reflective functioning is crucial for them and their carers. Providing programs that directly target reflective functioning in foster carers is therefore a promising line of development and has gradually become the focus of several interventions with families aiming to improve the carer–child relationship (Slade et al. 2005; Suchman et al. 2008, 2011). Some preventive programs rooted in mentalizing approaches have also demonstrated efficacy in normally developing children and communities (e.g., Keaveny et al. 2012; Twemlow et al. 2011), as well as with foster carers (Adkins et al. 2018).

Two MBT programs for children in foster care have been developed by staff at the Anna Freud National Centre for Children and Families. The first is the Herts and Minds Study (Midgley et al. 2017), which draws on the work of mentalization-based treatment for families (MBT-F; see also Chapter 8, "Working With Families") and the core MBT model. This model is undergoing feasibility testing of the approach to train mental health practitioners. Following this phase of the work, the acceptability of the model as a treatment intervention for looked-after children and their families will be examined. Finally, a large-scale evaluation will assess whether the group-based psychoeducation intervention is acceptable to families, in terms of increasing foster carers' sense of competence, reducing foster carers' stress, and in improving the stability of foster placements and the relationships within them.

The second program being tested with looked-after children and their foster families is the Reflective Fostering Programme (RFP). This was developed in response to a call from the NSPCC (a major UK children's charity) to develop more effective interventions for looked-after children and their foster carers. The RFP is based largely on the Reflective Parenting model (Cooper and Redfern 2016) of self-focused mentalizing and parent–child mentalizing within a context of managing emotional arousal. It also draws on some of the thinking and activities from MBT-F, as well as the core theoretical framework of the adult model of MBT for borderline personality disorder (Bateman and Fonagy 2016).

RFP has been tested as a manualized 10-session group intervention to support foster carers, combining psychoeducation with a mentalization-based group intervention. It offers a highly collaborative approach aimed at promoting the quality of foster family relationships, supporting effective and sensitive parenting, and breaking unhelpful patterns of relating. The program has been developed as a way to improve foster carers' sense of competence and confidence in understanding themselves and their foster child, with the ultimate aim to improve foster children's relationships with their carers and, as a consequence, promote placement stability and the outcomes for children in care.

To date, this model has been tested in a group setting with foster carers, without the children present. It is also designed to be used by social care practitioners and mental health professionals with individual families. However, the model is strongly based on the premise that foster carers' sense of competence and epistemic trust will be greatly enhanced by completing this program with other foster carers. The rationale for not including children in the group comprises several reasons, but the main ones are that the program views foster carers as the main agents of change, and that the children are seen not necessarily as having mental health problems, but more as having a need for consistent and reliable care, and therefore the program focuses on enhancing the mentalizing capacity of the carers.

Foster carers are invited to practice various techniques at home in between sessions, with an emphasis on increasing mentalizing, reducing stress reactivity, and developing confidence around parenting skills. These techniques include devoting some thought and time to building a Carer Map (the foster carer equivalent of the Parent Map), which plots out their own stance as carers and all the influences that go to making them into the carers they are today. The emphasis in the group-based activities is on practicing the techniques of Reflective Fostering and going through incidents that have occurred at home in the session with the group.

CHALLENGES TO THE WORK

There are several challenges in supporting foster carers in taking up and maintaining a reflective or mentalizing stance in their relationship with their looked-after child.

Child Factors

The child's history and age can have a significant impact on how long it takes before real change is seen in the child's capacity to build trust in the relationship. Foster carers' skills and capacity to self-regulate and to send out the kind of ostensive cues that are needed for a child to learn to develop trust are highly variable, and without a supportive system, even the most experienced foster carer can quickly lose his or her capacity to mentalize and self-regulate in the face of a highly dysregulated child with a long history of mistrust and trauma before coming into placement. Maintaining commitment to a child who is hard to parent can be extremely challenging. However, direct expressions of commitment are important experiences for children, as such expressions reinforce a sense of self-worth and provide more emotional exchanges and interactions with a caregiver—which are so important in developing a child's ability to regulate his or her emotions.

However, it can be a challenge to increase enjoyment, playful positive interactions, and positive regard when a child is displaying either 1) a high level of externalizing behavior or 2) withdrawn behavior or no clear expression of "needing" a caregiver. Intervening to help caregivers understand the importance of being explicitly committed to children in their care, despite aspects of the situation that make this difficult, is vital, as is supporting caregivers to respond in nurturing ways even when children do not elicit nurturance or when nurturance does not come naturally to the carers.

The RFP results obtained to date point to the importance of helping foster carers to mentalize themselves first, to bring their arousal level down by being attentive to their current thoughts and feelings and the explanation for them, and *then* to be able to connect with the child. The important message in the RFP is to help foster carers to make their minds available to their looked-after child. Evidence suggests that for looked-after children, adversity becomes traumatic when it is compounded by the child's sense that his or her mind is alone—when under normal circumstances in a secure relationship, an accessible other mind provides the social referencing that enables a child to frame a frightening and otherwise overwhelming experience (Jacobsen et al. 2015).

Working With Foster Carers

The first challenge when working with foster carers is that of introducing the work itself. The author would recommend that any therapeutic work that aims to increase parental mentalizing has a psychoeducation component. This is consistent with both the application of MBT to adults (Bateman and Fonagy 2016) and recent research demonstrating that psychoeducation alone can have a positive impact on foster carers' capacity to mentalize, increasing their reflective functioning (Bammens et al. 2015).

There are benefits to explaining to foster carers the theory of mentalizing and its application in foster care. These include the following:

- Creating a shared language.
- Enabling a clear theory-driven formulation and shared approach to the work.
- Establishing clear treatment goals (e.g., managing arousal during difficult times or helping a child name his or her emotions) within a theoretical framework.
- Providing an "anchor" to bring clarity and focus during a session.

Despite these benefits, it can be difficult to explain the model of Reflective Parenting and mentalizing, especially the importance of the stance in the field of foster care. One of the challenges is to maintain a balance between psychoeducation and a more experiential approach. A purely academic approach may be experienced as a mini-lecture, which may be accessible for some but not all carers, whereas a purely experiential method may seem less clear and specific. Although the developers of RFP have no specific data around this, they have found that the concept of mentalizing is best explained over time, through providing a combination of information about the utility of the approach and how it helps both child and foster carer, and examples to illustrate points. Being able to name and label specific activities related to mentalizing while linking these activities to the benefits of mentalizing is an important skill.

Helping foster carers in the RFP group find their own language is extremely important. One group facilitator explained the concept of mentalizing as being like having a tool that has 1) a mirror on one side for looking at the carer's own face and showing the child's own face to the child, and 2) a magnifying glass on the other side for looking into the carer's own and the child's mind.

Through their clinical experience and the experience of training professionals in this model, the RFP developers have identified two specific challenges that may arise through this work: 1) working with foster carers in high states of arousal, where the carers are very dysregulated from dealing with high levels of externalizing and oppositional behavior; and 2) working with foster carers who seem emotionally cut off from reflecting on the thoughts and feelings of both their foster child and themselves, and are underaroused. Both of these are ineffective mentalizing positions, and the professional working with foster carers in these instances would be encouraged to use the Professional APP in order to provoke a mentalizing stance in the foster carers about both themselves and their child.

Both foster carer and clinician may feel reticent about focusing on the carer's state of mind, especially in the first stage of the work. Some of the concerns may relate to the foster parent feeling somehow accused of being "responsible" for what he or she sees as a problem in the foster child. However, the Reflective Parenting/Reflective Fostering model is not a causal one in the sense of blaming parents for a child's difficult behavior or hard-to-manage-or-understand emotions. Rather, this phase of the work is an opportunity to really connect with foster carers' experiences of parenting their foster child and understand, from their point of view, the challenges and joys of fostering and what influences their parenting. Normalizing this phase of the work is also extremely important, and making statements about the importance of the foster carers' role in their child's life is helpful—for example, *"In our work together, I hope to communicate how important I see your role is in Jessica's life. Just to emphasize this, I always start with you, thinking about you as a foster parent, what your experience on a daily basis is like, thinking about when things go how you want them to and what helps this to happen. Your thoughts and feelings are really important to this work too...."*

Assessments of foster carers routinely consider their own past histories and relationship patterns. However, this often does not include formal assessments of their state of mind regarding attachment or their mentalizing skills. Carers with insecure and unresolved attachment histories will have difficulties in their mentalizing and be more likely to be triggered negatively by their foster children's attachment needs and behaviors (Howe 2005). This triggering can in turn reactivate the childhood anxieties, traumas, and defenses of these foster parents. Unfortunately, this cascade of effects prevents them from being able to successfully attune to their foster child and challenges their sensitivity. It is vital to the work that carers be supported in becoming more aware of how their own experiences contribute to their vital role; however, some foster carers may find this aspect of the approach difficult. In the author's experience, avoiding explanations of research, and instead using the Carer Map to help a foster carer reflect on a situation and then to ask about past parenting experiences, is more effective. Having simple examples of how past experiences can impact both positively and negatively on parenting also helps normalize this process.

Often in clinical work either a foster carer or a clinician will look quickly for behavioral solutions—a response to a situation that will stop it happening or change a child's behavior. Reflective fostering requires a degree of discipline on the part of the clinician to resist the urge to respond in this way, as the work resides in thinking through, in relational terms, the states of minds relating to specific situations, wherein often relational solutions can be considered.

A foster carer may persist in asking for solutions; a useful technique in response is to try to connect with the thoughts and feelings that may be underlying the carer's insistence, and to help the foster carer mentalize himself or herself: *"Can I just stop and think with you about something? I am trying to imagine what it's like for you at the moment. I know you are a very experienced carer who has looked after many children, and I am wondering how it is for you looking after Billy, where nothing seems to be stopping this behavior? What is that like for you?"* Often carers begin to communicate frustration and a sense of disempowerment, or a sense of incompetence, which is important to discuss and understand, as these feelings can be detrimental to forming a more positive and connected relationship.

Case Example

Carol was a foster carer with over 15 years' experience of fostering children with a wide range of ages and backgrounds. When she became a connected carer to her grandchildren (her daughter's two children), she was faced with the additional difficulty of her own sense of guilt about her daughter's inability to provide consistent and reliable care for the children, Alfie and Sylvie, on top of their persistently challenging and aggressive behavior. Alfie was particularly oppositional toward Carol and had difficulties in his peer relationships at school. Carol would respond to his aggressive challenges by sending him to his room and telling him to stop being so naughty all the time. Alfie would respond by hitting Carol and was left with his feelings of shame unresolved, alone in his room, which he would frequently then trash.

Through an RFP approach, Carol used another tool of the RFP, the "emotional thermometer" (a visual aid to help carers monitor their level of arousal), along with her Carer Map to identify that she was in a high state of arousal when Alfie challenged her, because she felt guilty about her own daughter's neglect of his needs, and her own part in "failing" (in her eyes) to give her daughter the parenting skills she needed. When her arousal was lower, she was able to see that Alfie's lashing out at her was his need for control over a situation in which he felt he did not have the emotional language to say how he felt and saw his grandmother as being harsh and critical of him (he often misread her face as threatening when she was feeling stressed). Carol started to be curious and attentive to Alfie's frame of mind when he came home from school, where he had few friends, and she gave him more rather than less attention after school to show him that she was interested in him and in spending time with him. The next time he got angry with her, instead of sending him away to his room, Carol asked him if he could try to calm down and suggested that after he felt calm they could cook the evening meal together. Alfie did this and felt understood and calmer in himself over the mealtime.

Establishing Support for the Caring Team

Without ongoing supervision of foster care social workers, or regular refreshing and re-engaging of foster carers with the mentalizing stance, there is a risk that the foster carers' mentalizing will easily go offline. It can be hard for even the most experienced carer to maintain a reflective, mentalizing stance, particularly when under high stress. It is recommended that foster carers, social care staff, and the wider team around the child receive ongoing access to a consultation or supervision resource. The model of Reflective Fostering was designed to include ongoing peer support embedded within it so that foster carers, having developed an understanding of the model and a shared language, can continue to support one another. Moreover, it is hoped that some of these foster carers will become group facilitators of future Reflective Fostering programs.

REFERENCES

Adkins TE, Fonagy P, Luyten P: Development and preliminary evaluation of Family Minds: a mentalization-based psychoeducation program for foster parents. J Child Fam Stud 27(8):2519–2532, 2018

Allen JG, Fonagy P: Handbook of Mentalization-Based Treatment. New York, Wiley, 2006

Bammens AS, Adkins T, Badger J: Psycho-educational intervention increases reflective functioning in foster and adoptive parents. Adopt Foster 39:38–50, 2015

Bateman A, Fonagy P: Mentalization-Based Treatment for Personality Disorders: A Practical Guide. Oxford, UK, Oxford University Press, 2016

Beebe B, Lachmann F, Markese S, et al: On the origins of disorganized attachment and internal working models: Paper II. An empirical microanalysis of 4-month mother-infant interaction. Psychoanal Dialogues 22(3):352–374, 2012 23066334

Bunday L, Dallos R, Morgan K, et al: Foster carers' reflective understandings of parenting looked after children: an exploratory study. Adopt Foster 39:145–158, 2015

Cooper A, Redfern S: Reflective Parenting: A Guide to Understanding What's Going on in Your Child's Mind. Oxford, UK, Routledge, 2016

Csibra G, Gergely G: Natural pedagogy. Trends Cogn Sci 13(4):148–153, 2009 19285912

Dunn J: The adjustment of children in stepfamilies: lessons from community studies. Child Adolesc Ment Health 7:154–161, 2002

Fonagy P, Allison E: The role of mentalizing and epistemic trust in the therapeutic relationship. Psychotherapy (Chic) 51(3):372–380, 2014 24773092

Fonagy P, Steele H, Steele M: Maternal representations of attachment during pregnancy predict the organization of infant-mother attachment at one year of age. Child Dev 62(5):891–905, 1991a 1756665

Fonagy P, Steele M, Steele H, et al: The capacity for understanding mental states: the reflective self in parent and child and its significance for security of attachment. Infant Ment Health J 12:201–218, 1991b

Fonagy P, Target M, Steele H, et al: Reflective-Functioning Manual, version 5.0, for Application to Adult Attachment Interviews. London, University College London, 1998

Fonagy P, Matthews R, Pilling S: The Mental Health Outcomes Measurement Initiative: Report from the Chair of the Outcomes Reference Group. London, National Collaborating Centre for Mental Health, 2004

Fonagy P, Gergely G, Target M: The parent-infant dyad and the construction of the subjective self. J Child Psychol Psychiatry 48(3–4):288–328, 2007 17355400

Furnivall J: Attachment-Informed Practice With Looked After Children and Young People. Glasgow, Scotland, Institute for Research and Innovation in Social Services, 2011

George C, Kaplan N, Main M: The Adult Attachment Interview. Department of Psychology, University of California at Berkeley, 1985

Gomez-Garibello C, Talwar V: Can you read my mind? Age as a moderator in the relationship between theory of mind and relational aggression. Int J Behav Dev 39:552–559, 2015

Howe D: Child Abuse and Neglect: Attachment, Development, and Intervention. Basingstoke, UK, Palgrave, 2005

Jacobsen MN, Ha C, Sharp C: A mentalization-based treatment approach to caring for youth in foster care. J Infant Child Adolesc Psychother 14:440–454, 2015

Joseph MA, O'Connor TG, Briskman JA, et al: The formation of secure new attachments by children who were maltreated: an observational study of adolescents in foster care. Dev Psychopathol 26(1):67–80, 2014 24169078

Keaveny E, Midgley N, Asen E, et al: Minding the family mind: the development and initial evaluation of mentalization-based treatment for families, in Minding the Child: Mentalization-Based Interventions with Children, Young People, and Their Families. Edited by Midgley N, Vrouva I. London, Routledge, 2012, pp 98–112

Kufeldt K, Armstrong J, Dorosh M: How children in care view their own and foster families: A research study. Child Welfare 74:695–715, 1995

Luke N, Sinclair I, Woolgar M, Sebba J: What Works in Preventing and Treating Poor Mental Health in Looked After Children? London, NSPCC, August 2014. Available at: http://reescentre.education.ox.ac.uk/wordpress/wp-content/uploads/2014/09/onlinePoorMental Healthfullreport.pdf. Accessed June 9, 2018.

McCrory EJ, De Brito SA, Kelly PA, et al: Amygdala activation in maltreated children during pre-attentive emotional processing. Br J Psychiatry 202(4):269–276, 2013 23470285

Midgley N, Besser SJ, Dye H, et al: The Herts and Minds study: evaluating the effectiveness of mentalization-based treatment (MBT) as an intervention for children in foster care with emotional and/or behavioural problems: a phase II, feasibility, randomised controlled trial. Pilot Feasibility Stud 3:12, 2017 28250962

Perry BD, Hambrick EP: The neurosequential model of therapeutics. Reclaiming Child Youth 17:38–43, 2008

Rubin DM, O'Reilly AL, Luan X, et al: The impact of placement stability on behavioral well-being for children in foster care. Pediatrics 119(2):336–344, 2007 17272624

Rutherford HJ, Goldberg B, Luyten P, et al: Parental reflective functioning is associated with tolerance of infant distress but not general distress: evidence for a specific relationship using a simulated baby paradigm. Infant Behav Dev 36(4):635–641, 2013 23906942

Rutherford HJ, Booth CR, Luyten P, et al: Investigating the association between parental reflective functioning and distress tolerance in motherhood. Infant Behav Dev 40:54–63, 2015 26025253

Schore A: Affect Regulation and the Origin of the Self: The Neurobiology of Emotional Development. Hillsdale, NJ, Lawrence Erlbaum, 1994

Sharp C, Fonagy P: The parent's capacity to treat the child as a psychological agent: constructs, measures and implications for developmental psychopathology. Soc Dev 17:737–754, 2008

Simmonds J: The making and breaking of relationships: organizational and clinical questions in providing services for looked after children? Clin Child Psychol Psychiatry 15(4):601–612, 2010 20923906

Slade A, Grienenberger J, Bernbach E, et al: Maternal reflective functioning, attachment, and the transmission gap: a preliminary study. Attach Hum Dev 7(3):283–298, 2005 16210240

Slaughter V, Imuta K, Peterson CC, et al: Meta-analysis of theory of mind and peer popularity in the preschool and early school years. Child Dev 86:1159–1174, 2015 25874384

Steele M, Hodges J, Kaniuk J, et al: Attachment representations and adoption: associations between maternal states of mind and emotion narratives in previously maltreated children. J Child Psychother 29:187–205, 2003

Suchman N, DeCoste C, Castiglioni N, et al: The Mothers and Toddlers Program: preliminary findings from an attachment-based parenting intervention for substance-abusing mothers. Psychoanal Psychol 25(3):499–517, 2008 20057923

Suchman NE, DeCoste C, Leigh D, et al: Reflective functioning in mothers with drug use disorders: implications for dyadic interactions with infants and toddlers. Attach Hum Dev 12(6):567–585, 2010 20931415

Suchman NE, DeCoste C, McMahon TJ, et al: The Mothers and Toddlers Program, an attachment-based parenting intervention for substance-using women: results at 6-week follow-up in a randomized clinical pilot. Infant Ment Health J 32(4):427–449, 2011 22685361

Suchman NE, DeCoste C, Rosenberger P, et al: Attachment-based intervention for substance-using mothers: a preliminary test of the proposed mechanisms of change. Infant Ment Health J 33(4):360–371, 2012 23024442

Twemlow SW, Fonagy P, Sacco FC, et al: Reducing violence and prejudice in a Jamaican all age school using attachment and mentalization theory. Psychoanal Psychol 28:497–511, 2011

BORDERLINE PERSONALITY PATHOLOGY IN ADOLESCENCE

Carla Sharp, Ph.D.
Trudie Rossouw, M.B.Ch.B., FFPsych, MRCPsych, M.D. (Res)

In the previous edition of this book (Bleiberg et al. 2012, pp. 467–468), eight key assertions were made regarding mentalizing as a framework for understanding and treating borderline personality pathology (BPP) in adolescence:

1. Increasing evidence supports the perspective that the symptom constellation of borderline personality disorder (BPD) is rooted in childhood and adolescence and can be reliably assessed in adolescents with BPD, differentiating them from adolescents with other disorders.
2. Prevalence studies point to BPD becoming significantly more common during adolescence, in the context of widespread increases in vulnerability to adaptive breakdown and to psychiatric disorders.
3. Neuroscientific studies suggest an association of such increased vulnerability with neurodevelopmental changes during adolescence, which then compromise different facets of mentalizing, leading to poor integration of cognitive, explicit, controlled, internally focused mentalizing and affective, implicit, automatic, externally focused mentalizing (see Chapter 1, "Introduction").
4. Increasing evidence from multiple lines of research supports the mentalization-based approach to the development of BPD. This approach suggests that a phase-specific compromise in mentalizing during adolescence affects individuals who are vulnerable to developing BPD because of preexisting impairments, which include a low threshold for the very intense and rapid activation of the attachment system and a corresponding deactivation of controlled mentalizing. This set of core impairments leads to difficulties in differentiating self and others and to affect

    dysregulation in attachment and emotional contexts, and appears to be associated with the emergence of BPD in adolescence.

5. Adolescence appears to be a critical point for preventive and therapeutic intervention because of the increased prevalence of severe psychiatric problems and adaptive breakdown in general, and BPD symptomatology in particular, during this developmental stage. Because adolescent turmoil affects society, peers, school environments, family functioning, and ultimately the adolescents' own capacity to meet developmental tasks, it shapes lifespan trajectories, leading to the persistence of psychopathology.

6. Identifying natural protective and adaptation-promoting processes creates a framework to organize preventive and therapeutic interventions that can more effectively assist young people and families in turmoil. In this regard, the association we have noted between good and even exceptional adaptation in adults who had been affected as teenagers by severe emotional turmoil and maladjustment, on the one hand, and the capacity to mobilize mentalizing skills in the context of attachment and stress, on the other, is highly significant. These skills involve the capacities to engage in agency, reflection, and relationships.

7. In seeking to explain the decline in prevalence of BPD in adulthood, no empirical study has established a link between mentalizing skills and protection from adult BPD in adolescents with clinical presentations meeting criteria for BPD. It is compelling, however, to hypothesize that the recruitment of mentalizing skills opens a path for adolescents at risk to resiliently "come out of the woods" (Hauser et al. 2006) and avoid persistent misery and maladjustment.

8. The abovementioned hypothesis, together with the conceptual soundness and empirical support of the mentalization-based approach to BPD and its treatment in adults, provides the impetus to test a model of mentalization-based treatment for adolescents (MBT-A). This model is designed to address the specific developmental issues facing teenagers with BPD and adaptive breakdown in general.

    In this chapter, we provide new empirical evidence in support of these eight key assertions. Since the previous edition of this book, data have emerged demonstrating significant mentalizing impairments in adolescents, and MBT-A has been empirically evaluated in the context of open and randomized controlled trials. Together, these data provide compelling evidence to suggest that a mentalization-based approach to understanding adolescent BPP is useful and can guide treatment delivery in adolescent mental health services, either as the main modality of treatment or as an add-on to existing interventions.

RECENT FINDINGS IN ADOLESCENT BORDERLINE PERSONALITY PATHOLOGY

BPD has recently been identified as a novel public health priority (Chanen et al. 2017) and has been legitimized in the *Diagnostic and Statistical Manual of Mental Disorders* (DSM) and *International Statistical Classification of Diseases and Related Health Problems* (ICD) systems of diagnosis, as well as the national treatment guidelines of the United Kingdom and Australia. However, until the early to mid-2000s, the assessment, diagnosis, and treatment of personality pathology in adolescents were regarded as highly controversial. Arguments against the clinical management of personality pathology in adolescents have included the belief that 1) psychiatric nomenclature does not allow the diagnosis of personality disorder in adolescence; 2) typical features of personality pathology (e.g., impulsivity, affective instability, identity disturbances) are normative and not particularly symptomatic of personality disturbance; 3) the symptoms of personality pathology are better explained by internalizing and externalizing disorders; 4) adolescent personalities are still developing and therefore too unstable to warrant a personality disorder diagnosis; and 5) because personality pathology is long-lasting, treatment-resistant, and unpopular to treat, it would be stigmatizing to label an adolescent with a diagnosis of personality disorder (Sharp 2017; Sharp et al. 2018c).

Despite these early concerns, there has been a significant proliferation of empirical studies supporting the construct of BPP in adolescents, which has provided a firm basis for establishing early diagnosis and treatment ("early intervention") for BPD and for subthreshold BPP (Chanen et al. 2008). Specifically, research has suggested that adolescent BPP operates in function and form very similarly to adult BPP, including its phenomenology (Sharp and Romero 2007; Sharp et al. 2012b), genetic basis (Distel et al. 2008), prevalence (Bradley et al. 2005; Zanarini et al. 2011), stability (Bornovalova et al. 2009), risk factors (Gratz et al. 2009; Rogosch and Cicchetti 2005), comorbidity (Ha et al. 2014), disability and lost productivity (Chanen et al. 2007), and rates of self-injurious behavior (Gratz et al. 2012). The details of these and many other studies have been summarized in several review articles (e.g., Chanen and Kaess 2012; Sharp and Fonagy 2015). Here, we wish to highlight the evidence in support of a few key findings that together point to adolescence as a sensitive period for the development of BPP. We will then, in the next section, demonstrate how mentalizing protects against (or, conversely, facilitates) the onset of BPP.

The first finding relevant to the argument that adolescence is a sensitive period for the development of personality pathology was demonstrated in the Children in the Community (CIC) study, which showed that BPP has its onset in early adolescence, peaks in mid-adolescence, and subsequently declines into early adulthood (Cohen et al. 2005). However, the CIC study showed that approximately 21% of adolescents demonstrated an *increase* in personality pathology into adulthood. This finding suggested a normative pattern of a general decline in personality pathology and an increase in adaptive personality traits as adolescents enter young adulthood, with a subset of adolescents diverging from the norm with worsening or persisting personality pathology. More recent community-based studies have confirmed this initial finding (de Clercq et al. 2009; Wright et al. 2011). In parallel, a growing body of research began to make use of validated tools for the assessment of BPP in adolescents (see Sharp and Fonagy 2015 for a review) and demonstrated that a group of adolescents can reliably be identified whose clinical presentation meets full criteria for adult-like BPD. This group appears to constitute 11% of adolescent outpatients (Chanen et al. 2004) and one-third to half of inpatient adolescents (Ha et al. 2014; Levy et al. 1999). Approximately 3% of adolescents in the general population appear to meet full criteria for BPP (Johnson et al. 2008; Zanarini et al. 2011), mirroring the prevalence in adult samples.

The second finding that supports adolescence as a sensitive period for the development of BPP is the fact that adolescent personality pathology appears to be moderately stable—or at least as stable as in adulthood. The CIC study demonstrated rank-order stability coefficients for all adolescent personality pathology (including BPP) in the

0.4–0.7 range, similar to ranges reported for normal personality traits in both adults and children. These stability coefficients have been replicated by other community (Bornovalova et al. 2009) and clinical (Chanen et al. 2004) studies and appear to be more stable than internalizing or externalizing pathologies associated with adolescence (de Clercq et al. 2009).

The third finding is that personality pathology appears to be preceded by internalizing and externalizing pathology, but not the other way around. Stepp et al. (2016) systematically reviewed the antecedents of BPP, identifying 39 studies that considered risk factors for BPD. Nineteen of these studies examined internalizing and externalizing psychopathology as a predictor of BPD, and 16 reported either internalizing or externalizing disorder as a significant predictor. However, borderline features do *not* appear to precede internalizing and externalizing pathology (Bornovalova et al. 2013).

A fourth finding is that, while clearly being antecedents of adolescent BPP, internalizing and externalizing psychopathology appear to be distinct from BPP. The high comorbidity between BPP and other clinical syndromes in adults and adolescents (Chanen et al. 2007; Ha et al. 2014) has sometimes been used to call into question the validity of the BPP construct. However, studies in adults (Eaton et al. 2011; James and Taylor 2008) and adolescents (Sharp et al. 2018b) have demonstrated that BPP is not fully subsumed by internalizing and externalizing psychopathology. Moreover, adolescent BPP appears to be uniquely related to aspects of self–other function when internalizing and externalizing disorder are controlled for (Wright et al. 2016). This finding suggests that personality pathology is particularly important for understanding and predicting functional outcomes in the interpersonal domain. In addition, adolescent BPP has been found to provide incremental predictive power for general psychiatric severity (Chanen et al. 2007) and suicidal outcomes (Sharp et al. 2012a) over and above internalizing and externalizing pathology, suggesting that assessment of BPP is crucial to fully characterize an adolescent's prognosis.

To summarize, BPP has its onset in adolescence. While some adolescents show the normative decline in personality pathology through to early adulthood, a subset of adolescents' symptoms increase or stagnate, and a smaller proportion of these adolescents likely have presentations that meet criteria for DSM-defined BPD. BPP is moderately stable, and more stable than internalizing and externalizing pathology, which are antecedents (but not consequences) of BPP. While internalizing and externalizing pathology are comorbid with BPP, BPP appears to be uniquely associated with dysfunction (specifically in the domain of interpersonal function) and psychiatric severity. Taking these pieces of evidence together, adolescence seems to represent a unique developmental period for the onset of personality pathology. The question then arises as to why this should be the case. What is it about adolescence that causes vulnerability specifically for personality pathology? And could mentalizing play a role in buffering adolescents from these vulnerabilities?

ADOLESCENCE: THE EMERGENCE OF A COHERENT AND INTEGRATED "IDEA OF ME"

In this section, we put forward the thesis that adolescence is a sensitive period for the development of BPP because it is during adolescence that an agentic, self-determining author of the self emerges (McAdams and Olson 2010). It has been known for a long time that adolescence is a developmental period marked by psychological turmoil, impulsivity, dramatic and rapidly fluctuating mood, and heightened vulnerability to adaptive breakdown. Consistent with these accounts, empirical studies show that risk taking, novelty seeking, and hunger for stimulation increase during adolescence, together with a shift toward an increased focus on peer-directed social interactions and greater conflict with parents. For instance, 47% of adolescents reported having ever had sexual intercourse, and 34% had had sexual intercourse during the previous 3 months (Centers for Disease Control and Prevention 2016). Adolescents between the ages of 12 and 20 drink 11% of all alcohol consumed in the United States, and over 90% of this alcohol is consumed with peers (Kann et al. 2014). Similarly, 35.8% of teens report using drugs in their lifetime, 28.4% in the past year, and 17.3% in the past 30 days (Johnston et al. 2013). It has been suggested that increased impulsivity, risk taking, and peer-focused interactions may have become highly conserved because they serve to facilitate adaptive fitness. This facilitation involves an impetus for exploration and a promotion of the transition from dependent children who are reliant on caregivers to individuated independent adults who can engage in the fundamental reorganization of the self necessary to encompass physical and sexual maturation; the acquisition of sex-specific, nonincestuous attachment roles of mating and parenting; and a remarkable increase in the capacity for representing events with abstract concepts (Spear 2007; Tucker and Moller 2007).

Necessarily, this transition is associated with increased perspective-taking skills and a greater sense of self-agency (Harter 2012; Sharp et al. 2018c), but it also creates vulnerability for pathologies of self–other relatedness. Expanded cognitive skills in early adolescence facilitate self-consciousness and concern about the appraisal of others, especially in the context of peer relationships. The result of these two developments is shared reflection with peers such that the adolescent's personal goals become integrated with the goals of close others. Further, an adolescent develops an "imaginary audience," referring to the perception that others are as preoccupied with his or her behavior as the adolescent is. It has been suggested that the imaginary audience phenomenon is a function of the separation–individuation process of adolescence such that constructing an imaginary audience creates a sense of closeness and importance among peers as adolescents renegotiate relationships with their parents, which is a reflection of the expansion of intimacy and close relationships beyond the family system to peers and potential romantic partners. In balancing the perspectives of peers and parents, the adolescent is tasked with beginning the process of integrating different selves from other contexts during pre-adolescence and comparing and contrasting self-images that often seem to be contradictory to one another. By late adolescence, the ability for causal coherence is developed, and this allows adolescents to develop narratives that explain how chronological events in their life are linked—that is, the integration of an autobiographical past with an imagined future. Additionally, by middle to late adolescence, individuals are able to identify overarching themes, values, or principles that integrate different events in their life—this is called *thematic coherence*. Both causal and thematic coherence are due to an adolescent's newly acquired ability for higher-order abstractions, which is used to meaningfully integrate what previously seemed to be contradictions in self-representations, allowing identity to consolidate. Furthermore, by late adolescence, individuals start to normalize potential contradictions in self-representations, and this serves to reduce internal conflict. As adolescents move into young adulthood, they gain a greater sense of agency as they take steps to become their future selves. While the described developmental tasks are largely a result of cognitive development through adolescence, higher-level acquisitions require greater social scaffolding. Therefore, others (e.g., parents) assist adolescents in fostering new skills in order to integrate contradictory self-images and normalize potential contradictions.

The developmental toll of these transformations in self–other relatedness (individuation) appears to impose a heavy burden on some youngsters and their families. While most adolescents grow out of the normative inter- and intrapersonal conflict, confusion, distress, and instability in self-representation, others do not. We suggest that the capacity to mentalize forms a central, if not *the* central, component for the emergence and consolidation of a coherent "idea of me." Without the metacognitive capacity to self-reflect, "make meaning," or interpret the self, a coherent, agentic, self-determining author of the self cannot emerge. Accordingly, Hauser et al. (2006) followed a sample of 150 teenagers into adulthood, half of whom had been psychiatrically hospitalized in early adolescence. The authors found that a subgroup of these individuals, as adults, reported that they liked their lives and talked about them openly in a lively and fluent manner. They had lasting and satisfying relationships and were involved in work or education they found meaningful. They were interested in psychological experience and thought about themselves and about others' experience, and they felt hopeful and optimistic about the future. In short, these "surprisingly" resilient young adults showed the markers of effective mentalizing; specifically, *reflection*—that is, the capacity and willingness to recognize, experience, and reflect on their own thoughts, feelings, and motivations; *agency*—that is, a sense of themselves as effective and responsible for their actions; and *relatedness*—that is, a valuing of relationships that takes the form of openness to the other's perspective and of efforts to engage with others.

Conversely, weakened mentalizing capacity is identified as the core of BPP and theorized to develop as an interaction between constitutional vulnerabilities (interpersonal sensitivity) and attachment insecurity—be it as a result of neglect or invalidation or of the immense challenges involved in parenting a highly sensitive child. Children who reach adolescence with an enfeebled capacity to mentalize in the context of attachment are less able to withstand the developmental challenges of adolescence (Bleiberg et al. 2012). That is, they are less able to integrate a vastly changed body, to manage increased sexuality and affective intensity, and to deal with a greater capacity for abstraction and symbolization in a reorganized sense of self while also meeting the pressures for an increased focus on peer-directed norms and interactions, the psychosocial demands of achieving autonomy and separation, and the assumption of distinct adult roles. All this takes place in the neurodevelopmental context of mentalizing brain circuits that are undergoing pruning (and thus are less able to modulate affect and arousal) and a limbic system that is generating a hunger for novelty and stimulation. We have suggested that this biopsychosocial storm that takes place in adolescence converges to precipitate the adaptive collapse we identify as adolescent BPP.

EMPIRICAL EVIDENCE AND THE ROLE OF HYPERMENTALIZING

A large body of literature exists that demonstrates mentalizing failures in adults and adolescents with BPD (see, e.g., Fonagy and Luyten 2016; Sharp and Vanwoerden

2015). Mentalizing failures most reliably emerge in studies utilizing experimental tasks with high task demands (e.g., multimodal tasks requiring the integration of information across modalities) and emotionally charged stimuli. This suggests that a task's complexity or ecological validity may require a certain threshold in order for a clear BPP-related deficit to emerge. In addition, our research has shown that adolescents with BPP are more likely to *hypermentalize*, or overattribute extreme mental states to others, rather than "undermentalize" or *hypomentalize* (Sharp et al. 2011). Thus, when presented with mutually exclusive response options for no mentalizing, hypomentalizing, hypermentalizing, and accurate mentalizing, borderline features do not associate with deficits in (or lack of) mentalizing; rather they associate with an altered style of mentalizing, in the form of hypermentalizing (Sharp et al. 2011, 2013). Hypermentalizing, also referred to as *excessive theory of mind* (Dziobek et al. 2006), is defined as a social-cognitive process that involves making assumptions about other people's mental states that go so far beyond observable data that others may struggle to see how they are justified (Sharp et al. 2013). Similarly, Fonagy et al. (2015) described hypermentalizing as *making groundless inferences about mental states*. Elsewhere, we have provided rich clinical illustrations of hypermentalizing (Bo et al. 2017b), and here, we provide a short excerpt of a session to demonstrate hypermentalizing in an adolescent.

Case Example

Gina, a 17-year-old girl, had been diagnosed with BPD, attention-deficit/hyperactivity disorder, and moderate depression. She lived in an institution and had only sporadic contact with her family. At the age of 11, she had been removed from her family due to their incapacity to take care of her. Before beginning therapy, Gina had made four serious suicide attempts, and she was hospitalized for long periods each time. She had been self-harming on a regular basis for 2 years, and had a difficult time regulating her emotions in relation to both health workers and friends. Gina had expressed clear goals for her future, which included a career working with vulnerable adolescents, and at the time of her therapy she was enrolled in high-school-level courses. Gina had recently broken up with her boyfriend and was struggling to recover from the break-up.

> Therapist: So tell me about the difficult situation when you met with your ex-boyfriend…it seems to me that it was a bit frustrating for you to meet with him, is that right to put it that way?
>
> Gina: He met with me just to see that I was still in pain….
>
> Therapist: What was it like for you to meet with him?
>
> Gina: Awful…I mean…I spent 2 hours in hell…he kept telling me about his life, and that he is going out and has a lot of new friends…so annoying…
> I hate him and he doesn't respect me, just wants to bug me….
>
> Therapist: That doesn't sound nice…did you feel anything in particular in that situation?
>
> Gina: I fucking told you I HATE HIM…what is it you don't get? [*talks very loudly, and seems agitated*]
>
> Therapist: Wow…it seems to me that you are very much upset about what happened…sorry, it wasn't my intention to annoy you….
>
> Gina: You all say you're sorry, but it is a lie [*talks really loudly and very fast*]… John [*ex-boyfriend*] says he is sorry that we could not stay together…bullshit…he is not sorry about anything…Lisa [*Gina's contact person at the institution*] says she wants to help me and tries to understand me all the time…she is not trying to understand anything or help anyone…you and all this mentalizing….

Therapist: Hold on, hold on for a second Gina, this is going really fast, and I can't quite figure it all out…can we please pause for a second, and look at what happened here….

Gina: I don't want to pause anything, I know what you are up to, you want to blame me, tell me it is my own fault, that I have to work with myself, that "we should try and look at it together" [*makes a face*]…no way, you obviously don't want to help me, that is clear…you just want talk, I need action, action…Lisa doesn't like me, I know for a fact, and Carl [*head of the institution*] ignores me on purpose… [*Gina starts to cry*]

As demonstrated in this excerpt, a vicious cycle between hypermentalizing and emotional dysregulation escalates as the session proceeds. Supporting these clinical observations, we have shown hypermentalizing to be related to increased levels of emotion dysregulation, which in turn are associated with the likelihood of high levels of BPP (Sharp et al. 2011). Moreover, the tendency to hypermentalize appears to mediate the relation between attachment security and borderline symptoms and with emotion dysregulation, and hypermentalizing rather than emotion dysregulation is the key factor linking attachment security and borderline symptoms (Sharp et al. 2016). In one study in an inpatient setting, a reduction in hypermentalizing (but not other forms of mentalizing) from admission to discharge appeared to be associated with a reduction in adolescent borderline symptoms from admission to discharge (Sharp et al. 2013). The presence of hypermentalizing can also distinguish between adolescents with BPP, adolescents with other psychiatric disorders, and healthy control adolescents on the basis of self-report (Sharp et al. 2018a). Finally, mentalizing of the self (as operationalized through measures of experiential avoidance) was found to predict an increase in borderline symptomatology over the course of a 1-year follow-up period in 881 adolescents recruited from the community (Sharp et al. 2015).

That hypermentalizing can be reduced through a mentalization-based milieu approach to treatment (Sharp et al. 2009) accords well with the results of a recent study in Denmark that showed a reduction in borderline symptoms in adolescents with BPP taking part in mentalization-based group therapy (Bo et al. 2017a). The most compelling evidence in support of not only the mentalization-based model of adolescent BPP but also the efficacy of a mentalization-based treatment approach was derived from a randomized clinical trial conducted by Rossouw and Fonagy (2012). In this study, 80 adolescents (85% female) consecutively presenting to mental health services with self-harm and comorbid depression were randomly allocated to either MBT-A or treatment as usual (TAU). Adolescents were assessed for self-harm, risk taking, and mood at baseline and at 3-month intervals until 12 months. Their attachment style, mentalizing capacity, and BPP were also assessed at baseline and at the end of the 12-month treatment. Results indicated that MBT-A was more effective than TAU in reducing self-harm and depression. This superiority was explained by improved mentalizing and reduced attachment avoidance, and reflected improvement in emergent BPD symptoms and traits. We present details of MBT-A in the next section.

MENTALIZATION-BASED TREATMENT FOR ADOLESCENTS

The MBT-A program is derived from the adult MBT model with modifications based on developmental factors and the importance of the family context. MBT-A is a year-long program (Figure 17–1) involving weekly individual MBT-A sessions and monthly mentalization-based therapy for families (MBT-F; see Chapter 8, "Working With Families"). Some work has been done recently on using MBT group therapy for adolescents rather than individual therapy; this approach is discussed in Chapter 7, "Group Therapy for Adults and Adolescents." The individual MBT-A sessions are 50 minutes long and are held on a weekly basis at the same time and place. The MBT-F sessions tend to be at another consistently scheduled time and day, and the dates are known to the family well in advance to try to ensure attendance.

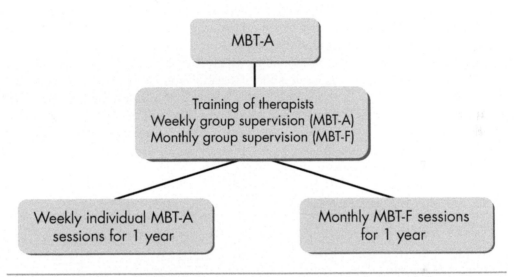

FIGURE 17–1. **Structure of mentalization-based treatment for adolescents (MBT-A).**
MBT-F = mentalization-based family therapy.

Training of the therapists is a crucial starting point of the model, but the cornerstone of the program is ongoing weekly group supervision (see Figure 17–1). Group supervision provides a platform for continuous learning; it creates a forum for containment and understanding of the patients and a structure to help with patient risk management. While MBT-A supervision is done in groups and on a weekly basis, MBT-F supervision takes place once a month. Supervision is conducted in a mentalizing framework. In the supervisory sessions, the group members reflect on their emotional experience while listening to the clinical material, seeking to mentalize what went on in the session. This mentalizing stance in supervision not only enhances continuous learning from experience about the model but also creates a nonpersecutory supervisory context that is far more facilitating of the enhancement of mentalizing in the work of all the group members. Video or audio clips of the sessions and role-plays to facilitate mentalizing of the material are used in supervision.

As detailed in the next subsection, the MBT-A treatment begins with an assessment phase, which lasts for a few sessions. These sessions conclude with the development of a formulation, which is given to the patient in writing and includes a treatment plan and a crisis plan. The formulation is not discussed with the patient's parents, but the parents do receive a copy of the treatment plan. The family therapy sessions have an assessment phase in the beginning, which is followed by feedback and educational input.

The assessment phase is followed by the initial therapeutic phase, in which great emphasis is placed on the establishment of a therapeutic alliance. The cornerstone of establishing a therapeutic alliance, both in the individual work and in the family work, is the therapist's ability to be empathically attuned with the patient and to maintain a mentalizing stance. Once the alliance is achieved, the next phase is the working (middle) phase, followed by the consolidation (final) phase before the end of treatment.

Assessment Phase

The assessment phase (Box 17–1) is used to gain an understanding of the adolescent and the difficulties he or she faces. During this phase, the therapist also hopes to get an idea of the adolescent's style of managing difficulties, the adolescent's ability to mentalize, and the particular situations in which this ability fails. This assessment usually takes two to three sessions. Results of the adolescent's psychometric tests conducted before entry into treatment are a valuable way of tracking outcomes and informing the mentalization-based formulation (see Sharp et al. 2009 for a detailed description of a mentalization-based assessment battery in this regard). In MBT-F, the therapist tries to get to know the family, the different family members, and their mentalizing ability in the first session.

BOX 17–1. **MBT-A: assessment phase**

Getting to know the

- Patient.
- Patient's history.
- Patient's relational context.
- Meaning of the reason for referral.
- Patient's coping strategies
- Patient's mentalizing abilities.

Formulation

- Background.
- Personality style.
- Engagement in therapy.
- Self-harm in context.
- Mentalizing.
- Treatment plan.
- Crisis plan.

Formulation

Once the assessment is complete, the therapist gives the adolescent the formulation to read and to discuss with the therapist. An example of a brief crisis plan for an adolescent is shown in Box 17–2, and a crisis plan for the parents is summarized in Box 17–3. An example of the formulation given to the patient is set out below.

BOX 17–2. **Example written crisis plan for an adolescent patient**

Trigger factors that you and I identified are times when you feel rejected, humiliated, or bad about yourself. As we have discussed, these feelings do not just arrive out of the blue; they are likely to have been triggered in a close relationship. When you have those feelings, you tend to rush into an action to take the feelings away.

When you feel like that again, I would like you to use the COPING SKILLS APP. STOP AND PAUSE.

Try focusing on your breathing or on one of your senses. Then try to reflect—what are you feeling? What happened before you had the feeling? Did something happen between you and someone else? Can you try to pause before you make an assumption about what the other person is feeling and thinking? Remember we cannot see into someone else's mind, and we can make mistakes when we make assumptions about what that person feels. Sometimes we are so overwhelmed with our own feelings, we assume others feel it too.

Signed:

Patient: _____

Parent: _____

Therapist:_____

Example Formulation

Background information. When you were referred to this service, you reported a 2-year history of feeling depressed and harming yourself. At times you have felt so depressed that life did not feel worth living. You thought your parents' divorce 3 years ago, your mother's subsequent depression, your father's drinking, and his recent violent relationship with his girlfriend all played a role in making you depressed. You spoke about feeling guilty as if it was your fault. Before you came to us for help, you entered into a relationship in which you allowed someone to treat you in a disrespectful manner, almost as if you were being punished. All of this made you feel terrible about yourself.

Personality style. You are a very brave young person who has coped with a lot in your life. You were also very brave to speak to me about your feelings and stuff that has happened in your life. You are kind and caring to others, and you have been a very reliable friend to your friends. It is sad to notice how you cannot see your own beautiful qualities and how you constantly expect people to dislike you. This can make you feel so anxious in social situations that you tend to withdraw yourself—but the problem with this way of coping is that it does not allow others to be close to you, and in that way it reinforces your view that they do not like you.

You also told me that in your relationships things can be up and down at times. You explained that you have a desire to be close to people, but as soon as you are close to them, you feel ripped apart by anxieties that they will let you down or reject you. This, you said, can make you feel so anxious that you can feel as if you are on a rollercoaster emotionally, with large mood swings. From our discussions, I had the impression that sometimes when you have strong feelings inside you, you cope with them either by cutting yourself or by switching your emotions off until you feel empty. Is that what happens to you?

When we spoke about you switching your emotions off, I thought about it afterward and I thought that although I can see that it feels as if this coping style helps you at the time, I did wonder whether it also makes you feel disconnected from what you or other people feel, and whether it is then difficult to understand what is going on. I wondered if it may be at times like this that you feel action is the only thing available to you—and

BOX 17–3. **Crisis plan for parents**

As we discussed, X's self-harm is often in the context of very strong feelings that she finds hard to manage. Here are three **do's** and three **don'ts** that may help you at times of risk:

Do

- Listen.
- Understand.
- Help to mentalize.

Don't

- Panic.
- Blame.
- Punish.

Don't blame her and don't blame yourself. Just try to understand what she felt before she wanted to harm herself, and help her to speak about 1) the feelings and 2) the events leading up to the feelings. If the events involved you, listen and try to understand *her* perspective without becoming defensive. You don't have to hold the same perspective, but it is important that you validate her perspective. If there was a misunderstanding between you that you contributed to, own up to it. You are here not to win battles but to restore the connection between you.

If she is very aroused, speaking too much is not helpful. Just be kind and supportive and say things like: "I am not angry with you, I am here to help you and keep you safe. Something has made you so upset. I don't know what it is and if it is something I have done, I am sorry. I really want to understand. Talk when you are ready, but until then, I will just be with you to keep you safe."

If she wants to hurt herself, you could say: "I really don't want you to hurt yourself. You deserve so much more. Let's try one of the alternatives. I will help you; shall we get a bowl of ice?"

If she is suicidal, you could say: "Killing yourself is not an option. I love you and do not want you to kill yourself. You are not alone. We will get through this together. I am going to stay here with you to keep you safe. Let's try to think of something that will help right now. Will distraction help—maybe going for a walk or watching TV?"

If all else fails, call the clinic, or if it is after hours, you may have to take her to the emergency department.

whether it may be at these times that you have a tendency to harm yourself. What do you think about that?

In listening to the way you spoke about yourself, I felt myself feeling very sad about the constantly negative ways in which you see yourself. I was also struck by how you seem to relate to other people in a self-sacrificing manner and how at times you allow them to take advantage of you. Perhaps in therapy we can work on all these aspects and help you to develop a desire to look after yourself and to allow others to look after you rather than hurt you. You are a lovely person, and you deserve more than what you currently allow yourself to have.

Sensitive mentalizing. You show a great ability to understand what is in the mind of others, such as an awareness of what your friends feel or what your mother feels, and you try to please them. You also try to understand your own thoughts and feelings, and sometimes can do it, but at other times find it harder not to fall into familiar patterns of criticizing yourself.

Problems in mentalizing. You fall into a pattern of hateful thoughts, leaving you with horrible feelings, which you manage by turning them into an action (e.g., self-harm). This means that a feeling becomes something real in the physical world; the feeling is transformed into blood, and then you or someone else provides physical care to take care of it. This is an example of how a feeling ended up as an action, but the actual feeling and what may have caused it are not understood. We need to work out what the feelings are.

Treatment plan. We propose to offer you a treatment in which we suggest a combination of individual therapy once a week and family therapy once or twice a month delivered by the community team.

Initial Phase of Treatment

Although the initial phase is described after the assessment phase, in reality many aspects of the initial phase start with the assessment, because the main focus of the initial phase is the establishment of a therapeutic alliance and engagement of the adolescent in therapy (Box 17–4). It is quite common for adolescents to have difficulties engaging in a therapeutic relationship, especially one that is sustained over the longer term. We typically find that dropout is most likely in the time between assignment to treatment and the start of treatment. Once MBT begins, the dropout rate is very low (much lower than for TAU). The mentalizing stance of the therapist—who adopts a nonjudgmental, curious, and not-knowing attitude—is emphasized throughout, but especially in the beginning.

BOX 17–4. **MBT-A: initial phase**

- Provide formulation and psychoeducation.

- Use empathy, empathy, empathy!

- Establish emotional contact.

- Establish a positive alliance.

In the model of MBT for adults (described in Chapter 6, "Individual Therapy Techniques"), once the assessment is completed, the therapist discusses the diagnosis with the patient, and this is followed by psychoeducation. Given recent data on the validity of BPP in adolescence, we feel comfortable with using this approach in adolescents, too.

With a positive therapeutic alliance in place, the rest of the initial phase follows. This involves slowly getting to know the young person's range of feelings, vulnerabilities, ways of coping, and particular nonmentalizing mechanisms deployed. It is critical to gain an understanding of the adolescent's relational context and to help him or her develop an understanding of when his or her mentalizing abilities fail and of the particular emotions that led to the failure, as well as the events and emotions that preceded the moment.

Case Example

The following is an example of a first session with a very anxious 14-year-old who presented to a service for children and adolescents with mental health difficulties, operating within the National Health Service in the UK, following a suicide attempt. She had taken an overdose in an attempt to escape from a torturous inner world dominated by anxiety, panic, and constant feelings of emptiness. The example illustrates the therapist's efforts to engage with the patient and make emotional contact with her. It also shows the therapist's efforts to ameliorate the patient's anxiety by not allowing uncomfortable silences.

Therapist: Welcome. I am glad you came; from what your mom said on the phone, it sounded as if it was difficult for you to come. So, that tells me you must have been quite brave to come.

Patient: [*silent, looking down*]

Therapist: Is it okay to be here?

Patient: It's awkward to talk to people.

Therapist: I understand that, especially now, because I am still a stranger to you. If you think, at any stage, that I say something that makes you feel that I don't understand, please tell me. Would you mind just giving me an idea of what happened and how you came to be here?

Patient: I had problems at school... [*silence*]

Therapist: I am sorry to hear that; what happened?

Patient: I was bullied by some kids, and I'm worried about the exams. I'm scared of what people think of me.

Therapist: Tell me more.

Patient: I'm worried that I will do badly in the exams and that the teacher will be angry.

Therapist: Do you have a horrible teacher?

Patient: She sometimes takes marks off just to make me feel bad so that I work harder.

Therapist: Gosh, how does that make you feel?

Patient: It upsets me, and then I feel angry, and I think I didn't work hard enough.

Therapist: It sounds to me that when the teacher does that, you get cross with yourself, but she is the one who is doing something wrong, not you, so why should you get cross with yourself?

Patient: I always get cross with myself.

Therapist: Do you think you just feel cross, or do you feel other things, too?

Patient: I think I feel sad.

Therapist: What do you think is making you sad?

Patient: I try so hard.

Therapist: Yes, I understand that. And when she takes marks off like that, do you feel as if she does not notice how hard you try?

Patient: Yes. [*cries*]

Therapist: I wonder if that feels quite cruel to you.

Patient: Yes.

Therapist: Is she just a horrible, cruel woman? Why do you think she does that?

Patient: She says she does it to help me, to motivate me to work harder.

Therapist: But that isn't the way it makes you feel, is it? It sounds to me like you feel that nothing you do is good enough.

Patient: Yes.

Therapist: Do you think she knows how you suffer?

Patient: No, I think she thinks it is a game.

Therapist: If people play games with my feelings, I sometimes get angry.

Patient: I am very bad with anger.

Therapist: What do you mean?

Patient: I get worried when I get angry that I have ruined everything.

Therapist: Do you feel like that with your family, too?

Patient: Yes, I do with my dad.

Therapist: Tell me more....

Middle Phase of Treatment

The middle phase is the longest treatment phase and contains the bulk of the work (summarized in Box 17–5).

BOX 17–5. MBT-A: middle phase

Engage in the bulk of the work:

- Address nonmentalizing.

- With patients in emotionally aroused states, pause, go back, and explore feelings and trigger factors.

- With patients in affective storms, stay calm, avoid complex or transference interpretations, keep interpretations simple and nonthreatening, stay emotionally attuned, and avoid silences.

- Address misinterpretations.

- Explore alternative possibilities.

- Open feelings up to explore more subtle feelings underneath.

- Help patients to mentalize others.

Now that the deficits in mentalizing and their particular emotional context have been understood, this phase aims to enhance the patient's mentalizing abilities. The emphasis in the initial treatment phase was on the alliance and on mentalizing the patient (i.e., opening up and exploring feelings and responses—in particular, responses in a relational context). The middle phase focuses on challenging different forms of nonoptimal mentalizing, as illustrated in the case example that follows. Throughout the excerpt, we highlight and name the different kinds of nonmentalizing modes that emerge (pretend mode, teleological mode, and psychic equivalence; see Chapter 1 for a description of these modes). The excerpt also illustrates attempts by the therapist to mentalize the patient and to stimulate mentalizing in the patient.

Case Example

Peter, a 15-year-old boy, was referred to our service with a history of cutting himself, taking overdoses, and having great difficulty managing relationships at school. Peter also had a strong history of violent outbursts and impulsive behavior, and on one occasion he had been reprimanded by the police for attacking another boy. He grew up with his mother and two half-siblings from different fathers. His mother has a history of drug abuse. Peter experienced life as unpredictable when he was growing up, surrounded by volatile relationships and inconsistent boundaries, which had left him with very little ability to manage his own feelings, and hence he frequently fell back on concrete ways of trying to reassure himself of his safety and concrete ways of managing his feelings.

> Peter: I broke up with Michelle. You remember that I wanted to see her last Friday, and she said she was busy. Later, I found out that she was only busy for one hour, and I could have seen her. So, on Saturday, *I thought I'm not having this; I may as well end it with her rather than wait around for her.* [teleological]

Therapist: What did you feel on Friday?

Peter: I sent her a text on Saturday and said, "If you don't call me by 5 o'clock, it's over." I used to think that she wasn't answering her phone because it was broken, but, funnily enough, just after I sent the text, she texted straight back saying, "I am sorry, but I am a happy person, and you are always moaning, and it brings me down." *So, I thought, okay, whatever, and just left it.* [pretend]

Therapist: Gosh, you must have felt very hurt.

Peter: No, I tried to convince myself that I felt nothing. I just don't understand; I was always happy when I was with her. *I don't see how she could say that I am always moaning. The only thing I moaned about was that she just never answered her phone. Any boyfriend would want that, right?* [psychic equivalence]

Therapist: So, when she didn't answer her phone, what did that feel like?

Peter: It felt as if she didn't care. *Jenny [another ex-girlfriend] always answered her phone, and that is how I knew she cared.* [teleological]

Therapist: And when you felt that she didn't care, how did that make you feel?

Peter: Anxious, *and then I would phone her nonstop, and I would text and leave messages* [teleological]. *It's not right to ignore me like this.* [psychic equivalence]

Therapist: So, the more she didn't answer, the more anxious you would get.

Peter: Sometimes *I would call her 20 times* [teleological], and she would ignore me. I know why. [psychic equivalence]

Therapist: And when you were anxious, what thoughts did you have, and what were you anxious about?

Peter: *I think that she's met someone else* [psychic equivalence]. And I sort of saw it coming, so Friday evening, when I went dancing, *I flirted with people* [teleological], and then I met this new girl. She's not really new; she is a sort of a friend. So, I thought that I'd like to take her out, so I pretended to be drunk, and then I told her that I would like to take her out. I thought that if I pretended to be drunk and she said no, then I would just say the next day that I was drunk and that I don't remember anything. Then I won't have to feel embarrassed. So, she didn't do that but said that she'd like to go out with me. On Saturday, *when I dumped Michelle, I already had the other one lined up, so I didn't really care about Michelle anymore* [pretend]. *Now life has moved on* [pretend], and this weekend I will go out with her for the first time. *And this week I felt really happy* [pretend]. *This girl is really special. We have so much in common; she is pretty...* [pretend]

Therapist: Can I just slow things down a bit to try and catch up?

Peter: Yes, it is a bit fast, isn't it? I always do that—I always have one in reserve. The minute I see trouble coming, I get one in reserve.

Therapist: It seems to me that all of this action about phoning her so many times and getting another girl in reserve are ways in which you try to manage a terribly anxious feeling inside you.

Peter: *Yes, but now I don't feel it because the new girl answers her phone all the time, so I know she likes me.* [teleological]

Therapist: You said that when Michelle didn't answer her phone, you got anxious. Is that all you felt, or did you have other feelings, too?

Peter: I felt anxious that she was seeing another guy *and then I phoned again and again.* [teleological]

Therapist: If I thought that someone I like was seeing someone else, it would make me feel angry.

Peter: Yes, I felt like I could smash my phone up. I wanted to break her door down.

Therapist: So, part of phoning her so many times was also an angry thing.

Peter: Yes, I suppose it was a bit smothering; maybe that is why she said that I was moaning. *But any guy would be upset if he was ignored...* [psychic equivalence]

Interrupting and repairing nonmentalizing in adolescents follows the same steps as described by Bateman and Fonagy (2016). We will not repeat these here, but we will remind the reader that the most important goal of working with adolescents is to stay emotionally in touch in the service of containment of the aroused mental state, which facilitates the return of the young person's ability to mentalize, in addition to helping the adolescent reflect on the mental states of those close to him or her. This is a slow process, and the therapist should not expect the adolescent to respond immediately to a mentalizing intervention. Repetition is needed, as in building a house, brick by brick. For MBT-F-specific techniques, readers are referred to Chapter 8.

Final Phase of Treatment

The final phase occurs in the last 2 months of treatment. The aim is to increase independence and responsibility (Bateman and Fonagy 2016), to enhance social stability, to work through the pending separation, and to consolidate the gains made during therapy (Box 17–6). In some cases, it may be best to taper the therapy by offering reduced sessions after a year, such as twice monthly for a period followed by monthly sessions. At the end of therapy, the young person receives an outcome formulation. The work in this phase is similar to the work that occurs in the last 2 months of MBT-F.

BOX 17–6.   MBT-A: final phase

- Increase independence and responsibility.

- Enhance social stability.

- Work through pending separation.

- Consolidate gains.

- Taper treatment over a longer time when needed.

- Develop an outcome formulation.

REFERENCES

Bateman A, Fonagy P: Mentalization-Based Treatment for Personality Disorders: A Practical Guide. Oxford, UK, Oxford University Press, 2016

Bleiberg E, Rossouw T, Fonagy P: Adolescent breakdown and emerging borderline personality disorder, in Handbook of Mentalizing in Mental Health Practice. Edited by Bateman A, Fonagy P. Arlington, VA, American Psychiatric Publishing, 2012, pp 463–510

Bo S, Sharp C, Beck E, et al: First empirical evaluation of outcomes for mentalization-based group therapy for adolescents with BPD. Pers Disord 8(4):396–401, 2017a 27845526

Bo S, Sharp C, Fonagy P, et al: Hypermentalizing, attachment, and epistemic trust in adolescent BPD: clinical illustrations. Pers Disord 8(2):172–182, 2017b 26691672

Bornovalova MA, Hicks BM, Iacono WG, et al: Stability, change, and heritability of borderline personality disorder traits from adolescence to adulthood: a longitudinal twin study. Dev Psychopathol 21(4):1335–1353, 2009 19825271

Bornovalova MA, Hicks BM, Iacono WG, et al: Longitudinal twin study of borderline personality disorder traits and substance use in adolescence: developmental change, reciprocal effects, and genetic and environmental influences. Pers Disord 4(1):23–32, 2013 22642461

Bradley R, Zittel Conklin C, Westen D: The borderline personality diagnosis in adolescents: gender differences and subtypes. J Child Psychol Psychiatry 46(9):1006–1019, 2005 16109003

Centers for Disease Control and Prevention: Sexual Risk Behaviors: HIV, STD, and Teen Pregnancy Prevention. 2016. Available at: http://www.cdc.gov/healthyyouth/sexualbehaviors. Accessed June 10, 2018.

Chanen A, Sharp C, Hoffman P; Global Alliance for Prevention and Early Intervention for Borderline Personality Disorder: Prevention and early intervention for borderline personality disorder: a novel public health priority. World Psychiatry 16(2):215–216, 2017 28498598

Chanen AM, Kaess M: Developmental pathways to borderline personality disorder. Curr Psychiatry Rep 14(1):45–53, 2012 22009682

Chanen AM, Jackson HJ, McGorry PD, et al: Two-year stability of personality disorder in older adolescent outpatients. J Pers Disord 18(6):526–541, 2004 15615665

Chanen AM, Jovev M, Jackson HJ: Adaptive functioning and psychiatric symptoms in adolescents with borderline personality disorder. J Clin Psychiatry 68(2):297–306, 2007 17335330

Chanen AM, Jackson HJ, McCutcheon LK, et al: Early intervention for adolescents with borderline personality disorder using cognitive analytic therapy: randomised controlled trial. Br J Psychiatry 193(6):477–484, 2008 19043151

Cohen P, Crawford TN, Johnson JG, et al: The Children in the Community study of developmental course of personality disorder. J Pers Disord 19(5):466–486, 2005 16274277

de Clercq B, van Leeuwen K, van den Noortgate W, et al: Childhood personality pathology: dimensional stability and change. Dev Psychopathol 21(3):853–869, 2009 19583887

Distel MA, Trull TJ, Derom CA, et al: Heritability of borderline personality disorder features is similar across three countries. Psychol Med 38(9):1219–1229, 2008 17988414

Dziobek I, Fleck S, Kalbe E, et al: Introducing MASC: a movie for the assessment of social cognition. J Autism Dev Disord 36(5):623–636, 2006 16755332

Eaton NR, Krueger RF, Keyes KM, et al: Borderline personality disorder co-morbidity: relationship to the internalizing-externalizing structure of common mental disorders. Psychol Med 41(5):1041–1050, 2011 20836905

Fonagy P, Luyten P: A multilevel perspective on the development of borderline personality disorder, in Developmental Psychopathology Vol 3: Maladaptation and Psychopathology, 3rd Edition. Edited by Cicchetti D. New York, Wiley, 2016, pp 726–792

Fonagy P, Luyten P, Bateman A: Translation: mentalizing as treatment target in borderline personality disorder. Pers Disord 6(4):380–392, 2015 26436581

Gratz KL, Tull MT, Reynolds EK, et al: Extending extant models of the pathogenesis of borderline personality disorder to childhood borderline personality symptoms: the roles of affective dysfunction, disinhibition, and self- and emotion-regulation deficits. Dev Psychopathol 21(4):1263–1291, 2009 19825268

Gratz KL, Latzman RD, Young J, et al: Deliberate self-harm among underserved adolescents: the moderating roles of gender, race, and school-level and association with borderline personality features. Pers Disord 3(1):39–54, 2012 22448860

Ha C, Balderas JC, Zanarini MC, et al: Psychiatric comorbidity in hospitalized adolescents with borderline personality disorder. J Clin Psychiatry 75(5):e457–e464, 2014 24922498

Harter S: Emerging self-processes during childhood and adolescence, in Handbook of Self and Identity, 2nd Edition. Edited by Leary MR, Price Tangney J. New York, Guilford, 2012, pp 680–716

Hauser ST, Allen JP, Golden E: Out of the Woods: Tales of Resilient Teens. Cambridge, MA, Harvard University Press, 2006

James LM, Taylor J: Associations between symptoms of borderline personality disorder, externalizing disorders, and suicide-related behaviors. J Psychopathol Behav Assess 30:1–9, 2008

Johnson JG, Cohen P, Kasen S, et al: Cumulative prevalence of personality disorders between adolescence and adulthood. Acta Psychiatr Scand 118(5):410–413, 2008 18644003

Johnston LD, O'Malley PM, Miech RA, et al: Monitoring the Future National Results on Drug Use: 2013 Overview of Key Findings on Adolescent Drug Use. Ann Arbor, MI, Institute of Social Research, University of Michigan, 2013

Kann L, Kinchen S, Shanklin SL, et al; Centers for Disease Control and Prevention (CDC): Youth risk behavior surveillance—United States, 2013. MMWR Suppl 63(4):1–168, 2014 24918634

Levy KN, Becker DF, Grilo CM, et al: Concurrent and predictive validity of the personality disorder diagnosis in adolescent inpatients. Am J Psychiatry 156(10):1522–1528, 1999 10518161

McAdams DP, Olson BD: Personality development: continuity and change over the life course. Annu Rev Psychol 61:517–542, 2010 19534589

Rogosch FA, Cicchetti D: Child maltreatment, attention networks, and potential precursors to borderline personality disorder. Dev Psychopathol 17(4):1071–1089, 2005 16613431

Rossouw TI, Fonagy P: Mentalization-based treatment for self-harm in adolescents: a randomized controlled trial. J Am Acad Child Adolesc Psychiatry 51(12):1304.e3–1313.e3, 2012 23200287

Sharp C: Bridging the gap: the assessment and treatment of adolescent personality disorder in routine clinical care. Arch Dis Child 102(1):103–108, 2017 27507846

Sharp C, Fonagy P: Practitioner Review: Borderline personality disorder in adolescence—recent conceptualization, intervention, and implications for clinical practice. J Child Psychol Psychiatry 56(12):1266–1288, 2015 26251037

Sharp C, Romero C: Borderline personality disorder: a comparison between children and adults. Bull Menninger Clin 71(2):85–114, 2007 17666001

Sharp C, Vanwoerden S: Hypermentalizing in borderline personality disorder: a model and data. J Infant Child Adolesc Psychother 14:33–45, 2015

Sharp C, Williams LL, Ha C, et al: The development of a mentalization-based outcomes and research protocol for an adolescent inpatient unit. Bull Menninger Clin 73(4):311–338, 2009 20025427

Sharp C, Pane H, Ha C, et al: Theory of mind and emotion regulation difficulties in adolescents with borderline traits. J Am Acad Child Adolesc Psychiatry 50(6):563–573.e561, 2011 21621140

Sharp C, Green KL, Yaroslavsky I, et al: The incremental validity of borderline personality disorder relative to major depressive disorder for suicidal ideation and deliberate self-harm in adolescents. J Pers Disord 26(6):927–938, 2012a 23281677

Sharp C, Ha C, Michonski J, et al: Borderline personality disorder in adolescents: evidence in support of the Childhood Interview for DSM-IV Borderline Personality Disorder in a sample of adolescent inpatients. Compr Psychiatry 53(6):765–774, 2012b 22300904

Sharp C, Ha C, Carbone C, et al: Hypermentalizing in adolescent inpatients: treatment effects and association with borderline traits. J Pers Disord 27(1):3–18, 2013 23342954

Sharp C, Kalpakci A, Mellick W, et al: First evidence of a prospective relation between avoidance of internal states and borderline personality disorder features in adolescents. Eur Child Adolesc Psychiatry 24(3):283–290, 2015 24958159

Sharp C, Venta A, Vanwoerden S, et al: First empirical evaluation of the link between attachment, social cognition and borderline features in adolescents. Compr Psychiatry 64:4–11, 2016 26298843

Sharp C, Barr C, Vanwoerden S: Hypermentalizing: the development and validation of a self-report measure, 2018a [Unpublished manuscript]

Sharp C, Elhai JD, Kalpakci A, et al: Criterion validity of borderline personality disorder within the internalizing-externalizing spectrum in adolescents, 2018b [Unpublished manuscript]

Sharp C, Vanwoerden S, Wall K: Adolescence as a sensitive period for the development of personality pathology. Psychiatr Clin North Am 41(4):669–683, 2018c 30447731

Spear L: The developing brain and adolescent-typical behavior patterns, in Adolescent Psychopathology and the Developing Brain. Edited by Romer D, Walker EF. New York, Oxford University Press, 2007, pp 9–30

Stepp SD, Lazarus SA, Byrd AL: A systematic review of risk factors prospectively associated with borderline personality disorder: taking stock and moving forward. Pers Disord 7(4):316–323, 2016 27709988

Tucker DM, Moller L: The metamorphosis: individuation of the adolescent brain, in Adolescent Psychopathology and the Developing Brain. Edited by Romer D, Walker EF. New York, Oxford University Press, 2007, pp 85–102

Wright AG, Pincus AL, Lenzenweger MF: Development of personality and the remission and onset of personality pathology. J Pers Soc Psychol 101(6):1351–1358, 2011 21967009

Wright AG, Zalewski M, Hallquist MN, et al: Developmental trajectories of borderline personality disorder symptoms and psychosocial functioning in adolescence. J Pers Disord 30(3):351–372, 2016 26067158

Zanarini MC, Horwood J, Wolke D, et al: Prevalence of DSM-IV borderline personality disorder in two community samples: 6,330 English 11-year-olds and 34,653 American adults. J Pers Disord 25(5):607–619, 2011 22023298

CHAPTER 18

CONDUCT DISORDER

Svenja Taubner, Prof. Dr. Phil.

Thorsten-Christian Gablonski, Dipl.-Psych.

Peter Fonagy, Ph.D., FBA, FMedSci, FAcSS

In industrialized countries, one of the major risks for early death and low quality of life is suffering from a noncommunicable disease such as a mental disorder; these tend particularly to affect minorities such as young offenders, who have a 10-fold higher risk of dying in adolescence compared with nonoffending adolescents (Patton et al. 2016). Antisocial behaviors in adolescence are common, but a small subgroup of adolescents show chronic offending. Among young offenders, conduct disorder (CD) is the most prevalent mental health disorder (e.g., reported among 44.5%–66.1% in adolescents in long-term juvenile justice residential placements; Baglivio et al. 2017). In this chapter, we suggest that the mentalization-based approach may be of value in developing both the understanding of developmental pathways to CD and its treatment options. We also present a modification of mentalization-based treatment (MBT) for CD in adolescence. Further discussion of mentalizing in adolescence and particularly its relationship to borderline personality pathology can be found in Chapter 17, "Borderline Personality Pathology in Adolescence."

DEFINITION AND FEATURES OF CONDUCT DISORDER

The essential feature of patients with CD is a repetitive pattern of behavior that violates basic rights or major age-appropriate societal norms or rules. According to DSM-5 (American Psychiatric Association 2013), for a diagnosis of CD, at least 3 of 15 criteria, spanning four domains (see Box 18–1), must be met during the past 12 months.

A childhood-onset type of CD (first symptoms before age 10 years) is differentiated from an adolescent-onset type (no symptoms before age 10 years). Furthermore,

BOX 18–1.   **Four behavioral domains for conduct disorder**

- Aggression against humans and animals (e.g., initiating physical fights, physical cruelty to animals).

- Destruction of property (e.g., deliberately destroying others' property).

- Deceitfulness or theft (e.g., burglary, shoplifting).

- Serious violations of rules (e.g., truancy).

DSM-5 includes a new subtype classification for CD, characterized by limited prosocial emotions.

Epidemiological studies have shown the prevalence of CD to be approximately 2%–10%, with higher rates in adolescence than in childhood and a prevalence sixfold greater in boys compared with girls (Ravens-Sieberer et al. 2007; Wagner et al. 2017). These prevalence rates are relatively consistent worldwide (Erskine et al. 2013).

Oppositional defiant disorder is regarded as a mild variant of or precursor to CD (Loeber et al. 2002), while CD is a risk factor for the development of antisocial personality disorder (Ridenour et al. 2002) (see Chapter 20, "Antisocial Personality Disorder in Community and Prison Settings"). Furthermore, CD may lead to anxiety disorders, depression, drug abuse, and bipolar disorders (Kim-Cohen et al. 2003). Adolescents with CD and callous-unemotional (CU) traits (discussed later in this chapter) have a more negative and often more persistent course of development (Frick et al. 2003).

ETIOLOGY OF CONDUCT PROBLEMS

It is assumed that the accumulation and interaction of biological and environmental factors increase the risk for CD (Maughan and Rutter 2001). At the same time, protective factors, such as higher intelligence or good social support, can help prevent dysfunctional development (Lösel and Bender 2003). The etiology of CD can best be understood within a transactional biopsychosocial model, which at present still does not constitute a coherent theory of causal and maintaining factors (Dodge and Pettit 2003). Among the biological factors are pre- and perinatal problems, abnormal neurotransmitter activities (e.g., low serotonin), and lower-than-normal galvanic skin response, startle response, and heart rate (Ortiz and Raine 2004), as well as hypoactivity in the prefrontal cortex (PFC) and amygdala (Fairchild et al. 2011).

Social risk factors for CD are low socioeconomic status, belonging to an ethnic minority, and low parental control (McCabe et al. 2001), as well as changing caregivers before the age of 11 years (Moffitt and Caspi 2001), belonging to a deviant peer group in adolescence, and extensive social media/computer game use as a maintaining factor (Galica et al. 2017). The strongest social predictors of CD are critical life events such as parental divorce, parental loss, and physical or sexual abuse (Loeber et al. 2002; Moffitt et al. 2002). Experiences of childhood maltreatment are particularly associated with an increased level of aggressive behavior in childhood or adolescence. Jaffee et al. (2005) suggest that early maltreatment is associated with a 24% increase in the probability of a CD diagnosis in children with a high genetic risk for the disorder. While a fuller understanding of the mechanisms linking early abuse with later violent behavior is still required, recent studies have indicated that mentalizing could be a crucial protective factor (Taubner et al. 2013, 2016).

A MENTALIZING MODEL OF CONDUCT DISORDER

Given the complexity of the cascade of factors that may result in CD, it is a particularly difficult disorder to bring into a firm theoretical framework. Here, we attempt to set out a mentalization-based developmental model of CD (see Figure 18–1) and show how this model has shaped the mentalization-based approach to treatment of CD.

Research findings have implicated impairments in different dimensions of mentalizing, ranging from bias in basic externally based mentalizing (i.e., sensitivity to social cues in facial expressions) to problems with more complex internally based social cognition and their relation to impairments in the "unlearning" of aggression (Lahey et al. 2000; Tremblay et al. 2004). We propose that different pathways in the emergence of CD involve temporary or enduring impairments in mentalizing that compromise the individual's ability to interpret others' social actions accurately and proportionately and to moderate the individual's own behavioral response to them (Sharp et al. 2008).

Before discussing these mentalizing processes further, it is necessary to distinguish between CD in the presence or the absence of CU traits. There is good evidence that a subgroup of children and adolescents with CD (15%–45%; Rowe et al. 2010) have high CU traits (Frick and Ellis 1999). These individuals tend to demonstrate low empathy, low interpersonal emotion, and callous behavior toward others (Frick et al. 1994). Although high CU traits in CD are regarded as being associated with a more severe, stable, and increasingly aggressive course of the disorder, with distinct emotional, cognitive, temperamental, biological, and social risk factors (Frick et al. 2014), etiological models need to take into account that not all individuals with high CU traits have CD (Kumsta et al. 2012).

Youths with serious conduct problems and high CU traits display distinct cognitive and emotional characteristics compared with others with CD. It has been found that individuals with CD and CU are relatively insensitive to punishment cues (Blair et al. 2001), underestimate the likelihood that they will be punished (Pardini et al. 2003), endorse values such as "aggression is legitimate," and see dominance and revenge in social conflicts as appropriate (Chabrol et al. 2011). Research has also found this group to have reduced sensitivity to others' distress (Marsh et al. 2011), to be less reactive to parental disengagement in a separation–reunion paradigm (Willoughby et al. 2011), and to have less profound heart rate change and cortisol response to experimentally induced stress (de Wied et al. 2012; Staebler et al. 2011).

CU traits have tended to be considered heritable (Viding et al. 2013) and until recently were regarded as only weakly related to parenting factors (Edens et al. 2008). The increased heritability of CD with high CU traits also raises the issue of differential susceptibility to environmental risk factors among individuals (Kochanska et al. 2015). Specifically, it is often claimed that harsh, coercive, inconsistent parenting predicts aggressive antisocial behavior more strongly in those with relatively low CU trait scores (Pasalich et al. 2012). The picture has become more complicated, as a lack of positive parenting (Kochanska et al. 2008) appears to be more strongly associated with CD in high-CU than in low-CU individuals (Kroneman et al. 2011; Pasalich et al. 2012). The current state of the evidence makes the distinction between an exclusively biological high-CU CD and a socially conditioned low-CU CD less sustainable (Waller et al. 2017). We would argue that high CU traits do not preclude individuals from benefitting from an attachment-rooted, mentalization-based therapeutic approach.

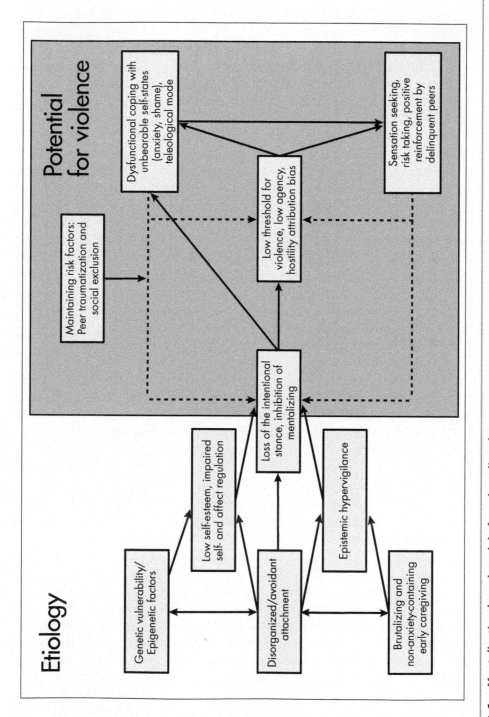

Figure 18–1. Mentalization-based model of conduct disorder.

Attachment

Attachment disruption in youths with conduct problems has been extensively documented. Meta-analyses have shown that insecure attachment (particularly disorganized attachment) has been prospectively related to the development of externalizing problems (Fearon et al. 2010), CD and oppositional defiant disorder (Theule et al. 2016), and physically aggressive and violent behaviors (Savage 2014). A pair of longitudinal studies has shown that secure attachment can diffuse anger proneness in children and, conversely, that insecure attachment, particularly in the context of power-assertive parenting, increases the risk of various conduct-related problems, including callousness (Kochanska and Kim 2012).

Further, negative parenting styles, such as poor parental monitoring, inconsistent discipline, and physical punishment (Pardini et al. 2007), as well as problems with parent–child communication in early adolescence, are prospectively related to the development of CD and psychopathic features (Pardini and Loeber 2008). A reanalysis of the National Institute of Child Health and Human Development Study of Early Child Care and Youth Development (Buck 2015) found that secure attachment mediated the interaction between maternal sensitivity and inhibitory control, but only for female participants. Sensitive parenting (assessed from 54 months to 15 years of age) predicted secure attachment at age 15 in females who were low on inhibitory control at 54 months. Among males, CU traits were reduced if the mothers were sensitive across development.

Finally, and importantly, when attachment relationships are unrewarding, and people are regarded as threatening, it is perhaps unsurprising that a person's commitment to sociocultural values, habits, and rules based on valuing closer relationships might be undermined (Pedersen 2004). This might explain why youths with CD seek alternative means to stimulate the reward system (e.g., by taking drugs or by engaging in risky sexual activities or aggression) (Foulkes et al. 2014).

Mentalizing

The findings summarized above broadly suggest that positive emotion orientation by the caregiver may be helpful in the prevention of CU traits. The cascade of processes involved in CU traits compromising socialization tends to be assumed rather than detailed. We suggest that caregivers' attention to their infants' states of mind is key to establishing openness to social learning, without which the process of socialization may be compromised (Fonagy et al. 2015). More specifically, we suggest that if a child does not feel recognized as an agent, he or she will experience limited epistemic trust (Sperber et al. 2010; Wilson and Sperber 2012) in relation to adults who attempt to teach him or her. This developmental failure may come about as the endpoint of two relatively distinct etiological paths. High CU traits may be an outcome of compromised learning resulting from limitations in the back-and-forth mirroring of emotions between caregiver and infant that might normally prevent the development of CU traits in at-risk individuals (Center on the Developing Child 2012). Children with a strong genetic predisposition to CU traits are initially likely to be hypersensitive to signs of a relatively stress-free environment and look for clear indications of positive responses to their expressions of self-agency in the context of emotional interchanges. If they do not experience such early cues, a developmental "switch" is thrown (Koós and Gergely 2001), and they adapt to their expected environment with hyporesponsiveness and (defensive) self-protection against a harsh world. Youths with CD with CU traits, instead of being hyperresponsive to the mental states of others, might develop a particular form of "mind-blindness" that prevents the unlearning of aggression. They purposely do not respond to communicational cues that indicate the inappropriateness of antisocial and aggressive behavior. Only extreme levels of focus on self-agency will provide an opportunity to reverse this; however, the process of engaging with these adolescents is compromised by the same defensively low expectation of meaning associated with any social communication.

By contrast, those with impulsive, reactive, oppositional patterns of aggression may show a more selective impairment of socialization based on a related but far more limited loss of capacity to envision mental states in those with whom they interact. Their mentalizing failure may be episodic and linked to high arousal, and the lack of impact awareness associated with this loss of mentalizing permits antisocial and aggressive behavior (Fonagy 2003, 2004). The paths to the mentalizing vulnerability in these individuals may be rooted in parenting experiences, which may themselves have been undermined by the child's behavior. This creates a cascade in which the socializing experiences that would normally ensure that balanced mentalizing develops are undermined by the child's problem behavior, which further compromises the benefit from extrafamilial social contexts (principally the child's school) that would normally facilitate the development of understanding of minds (Fonagy et al. 2009; Twemlow et al. 2008).

These speculations are consistent with evidence that physically aggressive behavior is most evident in the second and third year of life (Tremblay 2010) and then declines with age (Lahey et al. 2000; Tremblay et al. 2004), suggesting an unlearning process. However, if CD reflects problems with the unlearning of impulsivity and aggression because of impairments in social cognition, particularly mentalizing capacities, broader environmental factors beyond attachment are likely to be at least as important. In fact, any context that hampers the development of mentalizing and social learning is likely to be conducive to the development of problem behaviors, because it inhibits consideration of the impact of the individual's actions on others (Matthys et al. 2013). Further, in a context where nonmentalizing and even violence are needed for survival, mentalizing will be less firmly established and more easily abandoned in states of emotional distress or high arousal. This is likely to manifest itself in both emotional problems and conduct problems, particularly in children with a genetic predisposition, which may account for the high comorbidity between internalizing and externalizing problems. It may also explain why genetically vulnerable individuals may show stability in conduct problems: in children with less genetic vulnerability, environmental input later in development may have a significant impact through interactions with peers, teachers, and the media, for instance (Viding and McCrory 2012).

Importantly, adolescents with CU traits do not exhibit impairments in cognitive mentalizing, that is, mentalizing about others' beliefs and intentions, but do show marked impairments in specific types of affective mentalizing (i.e., the capacity to feel what others are feeling) (Jones et al. 2010). While youths with CU traits can recognize anger and disgust in others, meta-analytic reviews suggest that these youths struggle to recognize distress cues (pain, fear, and sadness) and happy expressions in others (Blair 2013; Blair et al. 2014). The emotional reactivity of youths with CU traits is modulated, in particular in terms of negative reactivity (e.g., Willoughby et al. 2011). A fa-cial electromyography study revealed that high-CU individuals were more reactive while watching aggressive social interactions, but this response was likely to reflect amusement rather than compassionate anger (de Wied et al. 2012). Decreased emo-tion recognition in response to visual (e.g., Sylvers et al. 2011) or vocal (e.g., Stevens et al. 2001) cues has been reported very frequently, but not in hypothetical emotion-recognition tasks (Woodworth and Waschbusch 2008). The latter finding suggests that "talking the talk" of emotions (Dadds et al. 2009) is easier than organizing behav-ior according to the output from emotion-processing networks. Within a mentalizing model of antisocial and aggressive behavior, such cognitive function is considered to be occurring in pretend mode (i.e., dissociated from the representation of physical re-ality; see Chapter 1, "Introduction"). Here, "islands" of high functioning are com-monly observed precisely because constraints imposed by other priorities of brain function are sacrificed—a process that has been termed *paradoxical functional facilita-tion* (Kapur 1996) or *savant syndrome* (Treffert 2014). If brain capacity for certain types of neurocognition is sacrificed (perhaps the systems underpinning emotional per-spective taking, such as the amygdala, basal ganglia, ventromedial PFC, and so on) then perhaps, because of dormant capacity, some degree of rewiring of circuitry oc-curs in systems normally recruited for cognitive perspective taking (such as the me-dial PFC, medial temporal lobe, and medial anterior cingulate cortex; see Chapter 2, "Contemporary Neuroscientific Research," for more in-depth discussion of neurobi-ology).

Social Communication

We postulate that the tendency to resort to violence is the outcome of social knowledge transmitted directly and indirectly to the child through his or her family's emotional and social environment. Whereas attachment behavior is an ancient evolutionary in-stinct that is shared by most mammals, human social communication, which enables infants and children to acquire increasingly complex and opaque social knowledge, evolved more recently (Wilson et al. 2014). The mechanism for the transgenerational transmission of knowledge (as discussed in Chapter 1, "Introduction," and Chapter 4, "Mentalizing, Resilience, and Epistemic Trust," and by Csibra and Gergely 2011), or rather the dysfunction of this social learning process, may be highly relevant in un-derstanding CD.

Findings concerning deficits in social referencing in individuals with CD may be particularly pertinent here. High-CU children might be less receptive to cues indicating that their caregiver has something relevant to communicate. Experimental demonstra-tions of this phenomenon are compelling (e.g., Egyed et al. 2013). Children generalize socially communicated information when the demonstration is preceded by eye con-tact and a social smile (Deligianni et al. 2011). Gaze following, which can be difficult for children with CD, occurs in 8-month-olds only when preceded by effective osten-sive cues (Senju and Csibra 2008). Gaze aversion not only deprives infants of emo-tional or mental-state cues; it also disrupts gaze following. Gaze following and shared attention were argued by Tomasello (2008) to be a critical component of human evolu-tion. Youths with CD might be less receptive to ostensive cues, particularly ostensive cues with regard to signs of distress in others, as is also suggested by their reduced focus on the eye region of the communicator (Blair et al. 2014; Dadds et al. 2014). The model suggests an early disruption of communication specific to social learning: reduced sensitivity to ostensive cues (whether as a consequence of deliberate avoidance of such cues or constitutional insensitivity to them) results in a barrier to learning remaining in place, and the process of socialization is disrupted.

In this regard, findings concerning the association among CD, attachment trauma, and risky environments more generally take on a quite important role, as such environments impede the capacity for not only mentalizing but also epistemic trust, and thus learning from social experience and the developmental unlearning of aggression (Latimer et al. 2012; Murray and Farrington 2010). Consistent with these assumptions, studies have shown that secure attachment experiences foster epistemic trust and override the natural tendency for epistemic hypervigilance (Corriveau et al. 2009). By contrast, a history of neglect and lack of parental warmth (Kochanska et al. 2013) may generate epistemic hypervigilance or epistemic petrification, where others are consistently not trusted as sources of knowledge about the world. This would lead to long-term impairments in the process of social learning, consequent on a failure of social communication. The strongest evidence for the close link between social communication and CD with high CU traits is the range of social influences implicated in the emergence of the disorder. The fact that it is more common for children to show a developmental decrease in CU traits than an increase is further indication that CU traits are open to socializing influences (Fontaine et al. 2011).

In summary, we suggest that while CD is a good example of equifinality (Cicchetti and Rogosch 1996)—that is, of multiple pathways arriving at the same outcome—in terms of developmental psychopathology, mentalizing as a construct has unique explanatory power in helping us understand antisocial behavior. The reason for this is that although genetic determinants are critical to conduct problems, there is overwhelming evidence, among both youths with high CU traits and those with antisocial and aggressive behavior who have low CU traits, that suboptimal early attachment patterns have a role in generating behavioral problems. While there is no implication of causality here (i.e., early manifestations of CD can disrupt mutuality in relationships), given the interdependence of attachment and the development of mentalizing, we can readily see that both emotional and cognitive difficulties in understanding self and others in mental-state terms are likely to contribute to impulsive aggression and very selective impact awareness. Further, we have seen that assuming an underlying inadequacy of mentalizing in adolescents with CD helps us understand to some degree the anomalies of social behavior in this group. As with other disorders associated with mentalizing problems, it is the persistence and inaccessibility to modification that may be the key focus for effective intervention.

MENTALIZATION-BASED TREATMENT FOR ADOLESCENTS WITH CONDUCT DISORDER

Mentalization-based treatment for adolescents with conduct disorder (MBT-CD), developed for adolescents between ages 12 and 18 years with CD, is an adaptation of MBT for borderline and antisocial personality disorder (Bateman and Fonagy 2016). The primary goals of MBT-CD are facilitating mentalizing in the adolescent and his or her family; reducing symptoms, especially aggressive and antisocial behavior; and establishing social learning to interrupt negative pathways to chronic offending and antisocial personality disorder.

Structure of MBT-CD

The therapy program lasts 12 months and consists of two psychoeducational workshops, 30 individual sessions, and 10 family sessions (Figure 18–2). Patients and their families start therapy with a psychoeducational group (see Box 18–2) that outlines core concepts and methods. Individual sessions start with an assessment of the adolescent's mentalizing capacities; family sessions begin with assessing the different perspectives of every family member on the "problem" and developing a shared crisis plan. Importantly, the initial work with the adolescent in individual sessions is to explore motivation and stimulate self-reflection about treatment, using a compassionate, not-knowing stance. Problematic behaviors are viewed as resulting from ineffective mentalizing and consequent loss of inhibition. This initiates the groundwork to formulate joint therapy goals and an early treatment focus. The initial phase ends with an individualized case formulation that summarizes and contextualizes how problem behaviors are related to mentalizing. The patient must be able to see himself or herself in the formulation and see that the clinician is recognizing the patient and his or her own personal narrative. This will enhance an alliance and help stimulate epistemic trust (see Chapter 4).

After the initial phase, the therapist follows the individual process, with the initial goal of engaging the patient and family in mentalizing and breaking coercive "loops" (see Chapter 8, "Working With Families"). There is an inevitable nonmentalizing loop between family members faced with seemingly uncontrollable and nonunderstandable behaviors. The therapist uses the classic not-knowing stance and intervention techniques such as empathic validation and mentalizing the relationship (Bateman and Fonagy 2016). Family sessions follow the format of MBT-F (see Chapter 8). After the end of therapy, three booster sessions are arranged to stabilize therapeutic success.

CLINICAL PROCESS

Clinicians need to take into account the low motivation of the patient, the patient's often lowered capacity for mental processing, avoidant attachment, trauma, and CD-specific dynamics such as hidden antisocial behavior, low trust, and the presence or absence of CU traits. Adolescents with CD are treated individually and not in groups. In a group, they may identify with and normalize the aberrant behavior and attitudes of the other group members. Patients need special engagement from the therapist and external support from other services such as their school or juvenile justice support system. Integrating services is a key part of MBT when patients are involved with other agencies (see Chapter 13, "AMBIT: Engaging the Client and Communities of Minds"; Chapter 20, "Antisocial Personality Disorder in Community and Prison Settings"; and Chapter 22, "Eating Disorders"). The majority of adolescents with CD have developed deactivating strategies to cope with attachment needs, and offering treatment thus presents a threefold problem: first, it is perceived as being counter to their desire for

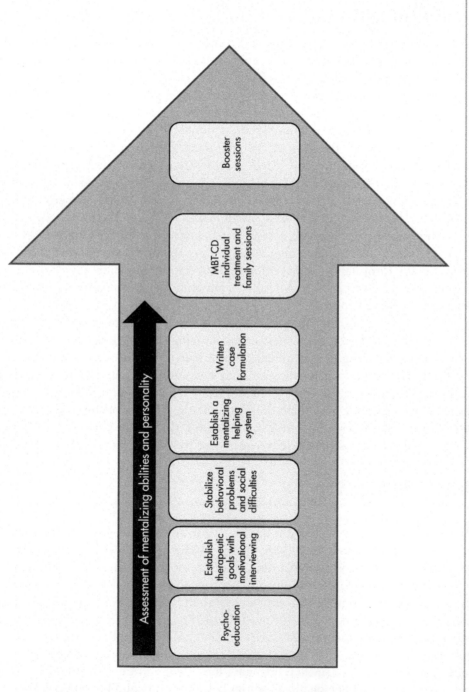

FIGURE 18–2. The process of mentalization-based treatment for adolescents with conduct disorder (MBT-CD).

BOX 18–2. **Overview of MBT-CD psychoeducational group**

Introduction: What is mentalizing?	• General group conditions, group rules. • Definition of mentalizing. • Importance of mentalizing. • Characteristics and consequences of failed mentalizing. • Mentalizing under stress (the switch model; see Chapter 3, "Assessment of Mentalizing").
Learning about emotions	Panksepp's seven basic emotions (Panksepp 1998). • Recognizing emotions. • Mentalizing and regulating emotions.

Identity and attachment	Adolescents: • Attachment and changes during adolescence. • Identity. • Social network analysis. • Emotion network analysis. • Risk behavior.	Parents: • Attachment and changes during adolescence. • Relationship to the child. • Parenting skills. • Mentalizing stance.

Conflicts and boundaries	• Resolving conflicts. • Boundaries. • A glance at the past. • Contingency plan. • A glance into the future.

maturation and autonomy; second, they are fearful of close relationships; and third, they fear a loss of "street credibility" if their peers know they are in treatment. Motivation in MBT arises if the clinician is able to identify problems as a task for the whole family rather than the individual, to be authentically interested and curious about their view, and to be actively and empathically validating about their experience. However, treatment is difficult because adolescents with CD are likely to use avoidant strategies: they may appear not interested, deny problems, and seem inarticulate—unable to speak about their thoughts and experience—or even provocatively oppositional. This might lead to anxiety or impatience in the therapist, particularly if the patient is uninterested in the emotional consequences of behavior such as bringing a knife to therapy. This can lead to a vicious circle of irritation and lack of empathy in the therapist, who feels undermined and rejected and is at risk of using interventions that are shaming and thus increase the patient's avoidance. This ultimately leads to dropout from treatment. Therefore, the therapist works hard on maintaining a mentalizing, nonjudgmental stance and being aware of his or her own mentalizing, which is crucial for a successful treatment. It is essential that the clinician is adequately supported; supervision, a core component of MBT, is essential when treating CD—with video recordings of sessions used when feasible—if the clinician is to maintain equanimity in the face of problematic counterresponsiveness from the patient. Owing to the high risk of problematic behaviors outside therapy and the need to create a mentalizing system around both clinician and patient, close collaboration with other services and the family is needed (Bevington et al. 2017; see also Chapter 13).

In order not to overwhelm a sometimes very poor mentalizing ability in people with CD, it is recommended, at least at the beginning of each session and perhaps throughout the session, that the therapist engages with something the adolescent is passionate about, and that he or she includes playful elements if possible and creative ways to establish joint attention (e.g., drawing). The aim is to re-establish the adolescent's curiosity about mental states in domains outside the core problem behavior while staying carefully attuned to the level of anxiety in the therapeutic relationship, as these patients have frequently learned to conceal their arousal. Furthermore, anxiety levels in adolescents and their families are sometimes higher than therapists expect and patients show.

Clinical Example: Luke, the Drug Dealer With Social Phobia

Luke was referred from an adolescent assessment service and came to the first session with his mother. He was 17 years old, a tall, blond, and handsome young man, wearing a dental brace and a baseball cap. His mother was a small woman, age 35 years, who was blonde and handsome, very much like her son. Instantly, she started blaming her son for being aggressive at home, not going to school, taking drugs (cannabis), and destroying her shower. Her blaming attitude was so persistent that the therapist stopped her and tried to empathically validate Luke's experience of listening to her. He glanced at the therapist and asked if it was possible to talk to her alone. She consented after having asked the mother for her permission. In our view, these are small, key moments in which the patient is testing the therapist to see if he or she is trustworthy. Recognizing these moments is crucial at the beginning of treatment if an adolescent with CD is to be engaged.

Luke was able to express his thoughts and feelings when alone with the therapist, and consented to start treatment afterward. He presented with characteristic CD that had started when he was 11 years old, together with a severe social phobia that prevented him from actively participating in school. He started abusing cannabis, became obsessed with computer games, and stopped attending school after negative remarks from teachers and pupils. At age 15, he started dealing cannabis and did poorly at school, regularly truanting and not taking exams. The school did not react to his nonattendance and gave him a basic exam pass to get rid of him. Luke's mother felt helpless and unable to control him, and this led to permanent tension and arguments at home. Sometimes his anger would lead to violent outbursts against family property or physical fights with peers. He felt deeply misunderstood by his mother and other family members, socially excluded by the school, and dreamed of getting big money by becoming a famous rapper (which would of course be difficult because of his social phobia).

His biological father had left the family when Luke's sister, who is a year younger than Luke, became pregnant. The father did not support the family in any way and was considered a bad person and a drug addict. The mother worked as a gardener, and managing financially would have been very difficult without the support of Luke's grandparents. However, living conditions were difficult—the mother had no room of her own in the small apartment and slept in the living room, which led to regular fights between her and Luke about not taking care of each other's space. Luke tried to escape his unbearable reality by smoking cannabis and dreaming of a great future. At night, when he was high, he regularly sneaked into his mother's bed to hug her and tell her that he loved her.

During sessions, he constantly bit his fingernails and contorted his whole body like a hospitalized small child. At the same time, he was very talkative and tried eagerly to convince the therapist of his worldviews—for example, that his mother had fascist attitudes and that generosity is the most important personality trait. He was sure about his thoughts and did not like other ideas or questioning of his own, both of which suggest psychic equivalence. The striking disparity between his ideas and actions, and his way of understanding self and others, was regarded as pseudomentalizing, and there was evidence of teleological mode when his emotions increased. The therapist got the impression of a small child whose needs were constantly unmet (by emotional and/or physical neglect) by a young, insecure, and inadequately supported mother.

NOT-KNOWING STANCE ON DRUG DEALING

Luke had the idea that he was fine and that others (especially his mother) needed to change. After the collection of different views of all family members at the first family meeting, he was shocked and a bit angry that his sister shared his mother's view that he had a problem. Both mother and sister identified the abuse of marijuana as one of the major behavioral problems. Thus, Luke agreed to consider the advantages and disadvantages of taking this drug. The clinician used techniques from motivational interviewing, which aim to trigger mentalizing of self and personal motivation, to assess his motive to change or maintain his behavior while empowering and affirming his struggle. The not-knowing stance is nonjudgmental, exploring, and validating, and remains exploratory as much as possible.

The interview with Luke started with the question of his interest in taking drugs and what pleasure it gave him and whether there were any problems with it. When asked about his wish to carry on with the drug and his confidence in his decision, and to rate his answers using a 0–10 scale, he chose a 5 to express the degree of his motivation to change and reduce his drug use, and a 4 to describe his confidence in doing so. The therapist expressed her surprise about the high number on change motivation, and started collecting the pros and cons of changing and sustaining on a decision matrix (see Table 18–1). (The aim of this activity is to stimulate self-reflection and build a mentalizing self: *"Do I want to change? What will I experience if I do? Will this have good or bad effects?"*)

TABLE 18–1. **Decisional matrix of a motivational interviewing session with a patient**

	Pros	Cons
Stop selling drugs	Feeling better More reality	Then I have nothing any more/ I *am* nothing anymore No respect from other people No "income" for food, drinks, cigarettes, and family Fear of becoming an adult
Selling drugs	Get to know people I'm interesting to others (boys and "bad" girls) Consumption is legal (in the jurisdiction where the patient lives) Feeling good, floating (when using it) Job that makes me happy No worries in everyday life I'm taken seriously Feels free	Exclusion from some people (e.g., "good" girls) Possession of drugs+drug selling→ prosecutable Trouble with family Has to be a secret Money debt, trouble with dealer Danger of addiction "You can be fucked" (it is dangerous) Low profit margin No time for other things

During the interview, it turned out that not only using but also selling cannabis was of central importance to Luke. He gained self-esteem from being a dealer, being respected for the first time, and being able to be generous to others. On the other hand, he realized that dealing drugs involved effort, risk, uncertain financial gain, and resentment from his family.

FAMILY INTERVENTION

To illustrate family interventions when treating someone with CD, a short transcript from an MBT-F session with Luke and his mother follows. As mentioned earlier in the first assessment session, Luke's mother was emotional and blamed him for not listening to her. In the second session, she remains angry and criticizes Luke for not wanting to come to the session.

> Mother (M): And today's appointment was exactly the same! I told him: first the drugs, but what about your [Luke's] health and being normal? This is exactly what I meant when I say that he blames others, because he then claimed that all this was my idea.
> Therapist (T): To do the therapy?
> M: Exactly!
> Luke (L): No. When? I ha— Did I really say that right then?
> M: Yes, this is exactly what you said.
> L: Mhm?! [*very aggressive*]
> M: Luke!
> L: What the fuck are you talking about?!
> M [*to the therapist*]: Do you see?
> L: Don't piss me off, I didn't say anything.
> M: You did.
> L: No, I'm not discussing this any more. [*Almost jumps from his chair but takes control by pushing his baseball cap over his face.*]
> M: This happens all the time.
> T: Does this happen often between the two of you?

> *Noticing a dysfunctional interaction in the family communication in which neither considers the other.*

> M: Yes. Yes.
> T: Okay.
> M: Happens very often.
> T: Yeah, how…
> M: It's the negativity…
> T: How often each day?
> M: Usually every day.
> T: Once a day?
> M: In the morning. It started when I woke him for school. It's immediate; "Don't piss me off" and such. Sometimes he says he's going to leave for school later, but when I get back from work I find he wasn't in school at all. It is other things as well. When I tell him to switch the light off or close the door or something like that, he says "You're telling me for the five thousandth time." Well, when I come back from work and the door is wide open and lights are on everywhere, then I have to repeat myself, because I'm of the opinion he either didn't get it or didn't listen.
> T: I thought it was pretty tense between the two of you just a moment ago. I just want to understand this a bit more. I have to take a breather as it was intense. Phew. So, what did just happen?

> *Empathic validation of the interactive tension and the therapist trying to regain mentalizing in herself while initiating it in the family to enable mentalizing the moment. Clinician focuses on the quality of the interaction rather than the content.*

[Luke reappears from behind his baseball cap and smiles.]

L: Nothing happened but it pisses me off. I did not say anything like that [*refer-ring to the statement about whose idea it was to come to therapy and to the ap-pointment*].

M: Luke, you told me, you wanted to go somewhere else instead and not come here.

L: No, I said I don't want to go to the appointment *now*. I asked if we can go at 6:00, because I had plans with Ben.

They carry on arguing until the therapist makes a "pause" intervention to focus on rekin-dling mentalizing.

T addresses L: Okay, let's take a break here. Can you tell me what is making you so furious right now?

Asks Luke to mentalize the moment.

L: The blaming! I did not blame her. She always blames me. I'm to blame for ev-erything, for the end of her relationship, all of that.

M: Luke, take a step...

L: And as to my friend, to my friends, I could accept it if she would just say no, but she says, "Your *shitty* little friends can't come over." She blames them for everything. No I don't want this. I want to live alone, to have my prop-erty, my house. And I can do everything that I want.

T: So, you and your mother blame each other or someone else for the trouble.

L: Yeah.

T: Can I add that to a list of what you and your mother share? Because this is also something you have in common then.

Low-level challenge to interrupt pseudomentalizing—Luke feels distinct from his mother, but he is also similar to her in some attributes. The challenge is an attempt to trigger a thought that he is not quite what he believes himself to be and that he shares some characteristics with his mother.

M: Can we say something about that? He is to blame for not going to school, be-cause it's his responsibility. He didn't graduate. He only received the lower secondary school degree when he wanted to do the upper one. I blame him. He didn't go to school for half a year. I'm not saying that he is to blame for my trouble, I don't know, he is only responsible for his own life, that's what I mean. That if he doesn't go to school he is not going to be able to learn anything or get an apprenticeship.

T: Can you describe what annoyed you so much just now? I was wondering why you mentioned his unwillingness to come to the appointment.

A not-knowing stance in relation to the continuing interaction with Luke.

M: He didn't say that he wasn't going to come, it's just that he knew that he had an appointment, agrees with his buddy to do something right before, and then goes wherever. We originally wanted to leave right before 4:00, left at 4:25, it's quite a bit to drive...

L: And we still made it on time...

M: And I had to call him a thousand times!

T: Whoops! I can see that it understandably makes you anxious about whether you will get all of you here in time. But you push back at him straight away there, blaming him for your worry that you will be late.

M: Well we would have been.
T: Maybe Luke can say what was important about meeting his buddy?
L: I like him. He is fun and we understand each other.

This exchange shows a typical dynamic in a family session with adolescents with CD. The arousal level is very high. Parents often shame their children without recognizing the impact. Shaming is often followed by a dysregulation of affect in the adolescent, and the parents then feel rejected and confirmed in their inability to talk to their child. The therapeutic task is to manage arousal, help the family regulate affect, and enable the family members to consider one another's perspectives. In this example, both Luke and his mother are fixed in their own understanding of how things are and unable to consider each other's perspective. The clinician tries to explore Luke's perspective in the last intervention and focuses on that in the next part of the interview, which explores whether the mother recognizes Luke's pleasure in being understood by his friend. This is a self–other exploration to trigger an alternative understanding in the mother. If this is successful, the clinician then reverses the situation and asks Luke to see things from his mother's side.

CASE FORMULATION

After a few sessions, the therapist was able to create a formulation to discuss with Luke. This contains indications related to his mentalizing profile, his use of avoidant attachment strategies, and identification of the immediate focus of sessions.

Formulation

You came to see me with your mother and sister to talk about how things were going in your life. You realized that your mom and sister and you have very different ideas about what needs to change between you. You told me that they have a very bad opinion of you, and they want you to change. They are worried that you will be a criminal. They blame you and think that you should "pull yourself together." You have to protect yourself. You are unable to communicate or to listen to each other. This goes round and round in arguments (a nonmentalizing loop).

You told me that they are very important to you, but also that you often do not feel they understand and love you. You react angrily to them and then you worry that you are no good. Understanding them and getting them to see you how you are will be a focus for us in our meetings. Even in school you do not feel comfortable; you felt rejected by teachers and don't like speaking to others. At the age of 13, you started to smoke dope and to play computer games, and you neglected your education, although it is obvious to you and others that you are intelligent. It was more comfortable to avoid your schoolmates, and you think they misunderstood you too. What makes you avoid people and close off from your family is another focus for us.

You met people who sell cannabis and for the first time felt that people respected you and saw you as an important person. But it got you into trouble. You wanted to make a lot of money from drug dealing, but this drives you further away from your family and a "normal" life. You want a girlfriend, but many girls reject your lifestyle.

You have set yourself high standards in relation to how you want to relate to others, such as being reliable and generous, which is amazing since you have never experienced anyone being generous to you. You do not understand your mother's rejection of your friends, and experience this as her rejecting you. If your mother asks you to do things and you do not feel valued by her, you can become very angry and sullen, and withdraw. Your mother sometimes seems helpless about how to talk to you; she tries to get you out of your shell, but this threatens or shames you. Then you reach a point where you feel pushed into a corner and you pull your baseball cap over your face—out of sight, out of mind. But you can become desperate because this is exactly the opposite of what you want. You want to be understood and not blamed; thought about and not dismissed; a person and not a nuisance.

In therapy, we could work out your concerns, how to let others know about them, and see if your family can see things from your point of view even if they do not agree with it. We can also see if you can understand their perspective. But what about your self-confidence as well? This is from your drug dealing. But this is about you and not what you do. What about thinking about you as a person rather than basing this on your actions?

This written understanding was shared with Luke and he agreed to talk about his experience that his mother constantly criticized him.

CONCLUSION

CD is a severe and complex mental disorder with high incidence in adolescence. Several studies have shown that adolescents with CD have pronounced deficits in mentalizing. MBT could therefore be a promising method for the treatment of adolescents with CD. MBT-CD has been used with several individuals and families and is currently being tested for efficacy in a multisite randomized controlled trial across three cities in Germany and Austria (Heidelberg, Innsbruck, and Klagenfurt).

REFERENCES

American Psychiatric Association: Diagnostic and Statistical Manual of Mental Disorders, 5th Edition. Arlington, VA, American Psychiatric Association, 2013

Baglivio MT, Wolff KT, Piquero AR, et al: Racial/ethnic disproportionality in psychiatric diagnoses and treatment in a sample of serious juvenile offenders. J Youth Adolesc 46(7):1424–1451, 2017 27665279

Bateman A, Fonagy P: Mentalization-Based Treatment for Personality Disorders: A Practical Guide. Oxford, UK, Oxford University Press, 2016

Bevington D, Fuggle P, Cracknell L, et al: Adaptive Mentalization-Based Integrative Treatment: A Guide for Teams to Develop Systems of Care. Oxford, UK, Oxford University Press, 2017

Blair RJ: The neurobiology of psychopathic traits in youths. Nat Rev Neurosci 14(11):786–799, 2013 24105343

Blair RJ, Colledge E, Murray L, et al: A selective impairment in the processing of sad and fearful expressions in children with psychopathic tendencies. J Abnorm Child Psychol 29(6):491–498, 2001 11761283

Blair RJ, White SF, Meffert H, et al: Disruptive behavior disorders: taking an RDoC(ish) approach. Curr Top Behav Neurosci 16:319–336, 2014 24048954

Buck KA: Understanding adolescent psychopathic traits from early risk and protective factors: relations among inhibitory control, maternal sensitivity, and attachment representation. J Adolesc 44:97–105, 2015 26255247

Center on the Developing Child: The science of neglect: the persistent absence of responsive care disrupts the developing brain. Working Paper No. 12. Cambridge, MA, Center on the Developing Child, Harvard University, 2012

Chabrol H, van Leeuwen N, Rodgers RF, et al: Relations between self-serving cognitive distortions, psychopathic traits, and antisocial behavior in a non-clinical sample of adolescents. Pers Individ Dif 51:887–892, 2011

Cicchetti D, Rogosch FA: Equifinality and multifinality in developmental psychopathology. Dev Psychopathol 8:597–600, 1996

Corriveau KH, Harris PL, Meins E, et al: Young children's trust in their mother's claims: longitudinal links with attachment security in infancy. Child Dev 80(3):750–761, 2009 19489901

Csibra G, Gergely G: Natural pedagogy as evolutionary adaptation. Philos Trans R Soc Lond B Biol Sci 366(1567):1149–1157, 2011 21357237

Dadds MR, Hawes DJ, Frost AD, et al: Learning to 'talk the talk': the relationship of psychopathic traits to deficits in empathy across childhood. J Child Psychol Psychiatry 50(5):599–606, 2009 19445007

Dadds MR, Allen JL, McGregor K, et al: Callous-unemotional traits in children and mechanisms of impaired eye contact during expressions of love: a treatment target? J Child Psychol Psychiatry 55(7):771–780, 2014 24117894

de Wied M, van Boxtel A, Matthys W, et al: Verbal, facial and autonomic responses to empathy-eliciting film clips by disruptive male adolescents with high versus low callous-unemotional traits. J Abnorm Child Psychol 40(2):211–223, 2012 21870040

Deligianni F, Senju A, Gergely G, et al: Automated gaze-contingent objects elicit orientation following in 8-month-old infants. Dev Psychol 47(6):1499–1503, 2011 21942669

Dodge KA, Pettit GS: A biopsychosocial model of the development of chronic conduct problems in adolescence. Dev Psychol 39(2):349–371, 2003 12661890

Edens JF, Skopp NA, Cahill MA: Psychopathic features moderate the relationship between harsh and inconsistent parental discipline and adolescent antisocial behavior. J Clin Child Adolesc Psychol 37(2):472–476, 2008 18470783

Egyed K, Király I, Gergely G: Communicating shared knowledge in infancy. Psychol Sci 24(7):1348–1353, 2013 23719664

Erskine HE, Ferrari AJ, Nelson P, et al: Epidemiological modelling of attention-deficit/hyperactivity disorder and conduct disorder for the Global Burden of Disease Study 2010. J Child Psychol Psychiatry 54(12):1263–1274, 2013 24117530

Fairchild G, Passamonti L, Hurford G, et al: Brain structure abnormalities in early onset and adolescent-onset conduct disorder. Am J Psychiatry 168(6):624–633, 2011 21454920

Fearon RP, Bakermans-Kranenburg MJ, van Ijzendoorn MH, et al: The significance of insecure attachment and disorganization in the development of children's externalizing behavior: a meta-analytic study. Child Dev 81(2):435–456, 2010 20438450

Fonagy P: Towards a developmental understanding of violence. Br J Psychiatry 183:190–192, 2003 12948988

Fonagy P: Early life trauma and the psychogenesis and prevention of violence. Ann N Y Acad Sci 1036:181–200, 2004 15817738

Fonagy P, Twemlow SW, Vernberg EM, et al: A cluster randomized controlled trial of child-focused psychiatric consultation and a school systems-focused intervention to reduce aggression. J Child Psychol Psychiatry 50(5):607–616, 2009 19207633

Fonagy P, Luyten P, Allison E: Epistemic petrification and the restoration of epistemic trust: a new conceptualization of borderline personality disorder and its psychosocial treatment. J Pers Disord 29(5):575–609, 2015 26393477

Fontaine NM, McCrory EJ, Boivin M, et al: Predictors and outcomes of joint trajectories of callous-unemotional traits and conduct problems in childhood. J Abnorm Psychol 120(3):730–742, 2011 21341879

Foulkes L, McCrory EJ, Neumann CS, et al: Inverted social reward: associations between psychopathic traits and self-report and experimental measures of social reward. PLoS One 9(8):e106000, 2014 25162519

Frick PJ, Ellis M: Callous-unemotional traits and subtypes of conduct disorder. Clin Child Fam Psychol Rev 2(3):149–168, 1999 11227072

Frick PJ, O'Brien BS, Wootton JM, et al: Psychopathy and conduct problems in children. J Abnorm Psychol 103(4):700–707, 1994 7822571

Frick PJ, Cornell AH, Barry CT, et al: Callous-unemotional traits and conduct problems in the prediction of conduct problem severity, aggression, and self-report of delinquency. J Abnorm Child Psychol 31(4):457–470, 2003 12831233

Frick PJ, Ray JV, Thornton LC, et al: Annual research review: a developmental psychopathology approach to understanding callous-unemotional traits in children and adolescents with serious conduct problems. J Child Psychol Psychiatry 55(6):532–548, 2014 24117854

Galica VL, Vannucci A, Flannery KM, et al: Social media use and conduct problems in emerging adults. Cyberpsychol Behav Soc Netw 20(7):448–452, 2017 28715261

Jaffee SR, Caspi A, Moffitt TE, et al: Nature X nurture: genetic vulnerabilities interact with physical maltreatment to promote conduct problems. Dev Psychopathol 17(1):67–84, 2005 15971760

Jones AP, Happé FG, Gilbert F, et al: Feeling, caring, knowing: different types of empathy deficit in boys with psychopathic tendencies and autism spectrum disorder. J Child Psychol Psychiatry 51(11):1188–1197, 2010 20633070

Kapur N: Paradoxical functional facilitation in brain-behaviour research. A critical review. Brain 119(Pt 5):1775–1790, 1996 8931597

Kim-Cohen J, Caspi A, Moffitt TE, et al: Prior juvenile diagnoses in adults with mental disorder: developmental follow-back of a prospective-longitudinal cohort. Arch Gen Psychiatry 60(7):709–717, 2003 12860775

Kochanska G, Kim S: Toward a new understanding of legacy of early attachments for future antisocial trajectories: evidence from two longitudinal studies. Dev Psychopathol 24(3):783–806, 2012 22781855

Kochanska G, Aksan N, Prisco TR, et al: Mother-child and father-child mutually responsive orientation in the first 2 years and children's outcomes at preschool age: mechanisms of influence. Child Dev 79(1):30–44, 2008 18269507

Kochanska G, Kim S, Boldt LJ, et al: Children's callous-unemotional traits moderate links between their positive relationships with parents at preschool age and externalizing behavior problems at early school age. J Child Psychol Psychiatry 54(11):1251–1260, 2013 23639120

Kochanska G, Boldt LJ, Kim S, et al: Developmental interplay between children's biobehavioral risk and the parenting environment from toddler to early school age: prediction of socialization outcomes in preadolescence. Dev Psychopathol 27(3):775–790, 2015 25154427

Koós O, Gergely G: A contingency-based approach to the etiology of 'disorganized' attachment: the 'flickering switch' hypothesis. Bull Menninger Clin 65(3):397–410, 2001 11531135

Kroneman LM, Hipwell AE, Loeber R, et al: Contextual risk factors as predictors of disruptive behavior disorder trajectories in girls: the moderating effect of callous-unemotional features. J Child Psychol Psychiatry 52(2):167–175, 2011 20735513

Kumsta R, Sonuga-Barke E, Rutter M: Adolescent callous-unemotional traits and conduct disorder in adoptees exposed to severe early deprivation. Br J Psychiatry 200(3):197–201, 2012 22116980

Lahey BB, McBurnett K, Loeber R: Are attention-deficit/hyperactivity disorder and oppositional defiant disorder developmental precursors to conduct disorder? in Handbook of Developmental Psychopathology. Edited by Sameroff A, Lewis M, Miller SM. New York, Plenum, 2000, pp 431–446

Latimer K, Wilson P, Kemp J, et al: Disruptive behaviour disorders: a systematic review of environmental antenatal and early years risk factors. Child Care Health Dev 38(5):611–628, 2012 22372737

Loeber R, Burke JD, Lahey BB: What are adolescent antecedents to antisocial personality disorder? Crim Behav Ment Health 12(1):24–36, 2002 12357255

Lösel F, Bender D: Resilience and protective factors, in Cambridge Studies in Criminology Early Prevention of Adult Antisocial Behaviour. Edited by Farrington DP, Coid J. Cambridge, UK, Cambridge University Press, 2003, pp 130–204

Marsh AA, Finger EC, Schechter JC, et al: Adolescents with psychopathic traits report reductions in physiological responses to fear. J Child Psychol Psychiatry 52(8):834–841, 2011 21155775

Matthys W, Vanderschuren LJ, Schutter DJ: The neurobiology of oppositional defiant disorder and conduct disorder: altered functioning in three mental domains. Dev Psychopathol 25(1):193–207, 2013 22800761

Maughan B, Rutter M: Antisocial children grown up, in Conduct Disorders in Childhood and Adolescence. Edited by Hill J, Maughan B. Cambridge, UK, Cambridge University Press, 2001, pp 507–552

McCabe KM, Hough R, Wood PA, et al: Childhood and adolescent onset conduct disorder: a test of the developmental taxonomy. J Abnorm Child Psychol 29(4):305–316, 2001 11523836

Moffitt TE, Caspi A: Childhood predictors differentiate life-course persistent and adolescence-limited antisocial pathways among males and females. Dev Psychopathol 13(2):355–375, 2001 11393651

Moffitt TE, Caspi A, Harrington H, et al: Males on the life-course-persistent and adolescence-limited antisocial pathways: follow-up at age 26 years. Dev Psychopathol 14(1):179–207, 2002 11893092

Murray J, Farrington DP: Risk factors for conduct disorder and delinquency: key findings from longitudinal studies. Can J Psychiatry 55(10):633–642, 2010 20964942

Ortiz J, Raine A: Heart rate level and antisocial behavior in children and adolescents: a meta-analysis. J Am Acad Child Adolesc Psychiatry 43(2):154–162, 2004 14726721

Panksepp J: Affective Neuroscience: The Foundations of Human and Animal Emotions. Oxford, UK, Oxford University Press, 1998

Pardini DA, Loeber R: Interpersonal callousness trajectories across adolescence: Early social influences and adult outcomes. Crim Justice Behav 35(2):173–196, 2008 21394215

Pardini DA, Lochman JE, Frick PJ: Callous/unemotional traits and social-cognitive processes in adjudicated youths. J Am Acad Child Adolesc Psychiatry 42(3):364–371, 2003 12595791

Pardini DA, Lochman JE, Powell N: The development of callous-unemotional traits and antisocial behavior in children: are there shared and/or unique predictors? J Clin Child Adolesc Psychol 36(3):319–333, 2007 17658977

Pasalich DS, Dadds MR, Hawes DJ, et al: Attachment and callous-unemotional traits in children with early onset conduct problems. J Child Psychol Psychiatry 53(8):838–845, 2012 22394435

Patton GC, Sawyer SM, Santelli JS, et al: Our future: a Lancet commission on adolescent health and wellbeing. Lancet 387:2423–2478, 2016 27174304

Pedersen CA: Biological aspects of social bonding and the roots of human violence. Ann N Y Acad Sci 1036:106–127, 2004 15817733

Ravens-Sieberer U, Wille N, Bettge S, et al: Psychische Gesundheit von Kindern und Jugendlichen in Deutschland. Ergebnisse aus der BELLA-Studie im Kinder- und Jugendgesundheitssurvey (KiGGS) [Mental health of children and adolescents in Germany. Results from the BELLA study within the German Health Interview and Examination Survey for Children and Adolescents (KiGGS)] [in German]. Bundesgesundheitsblatt Gesundheitsforschung Gesundheitsschutz 50(5–6):871–878, 2007 17514473

Ridenour TA, Cottler LB, Robins LN, et al: Test of the plausibility of adolescent substance use playing a causal role in developing adulthood antisocial behavior. J Abnorm Psychol 111(1):144–155, 2002 11866167

Rowe R, Maughan B, Moran P, et al: The role of callous and unemotional traits in the diagnosis of conduct disorder. J Child Psychol Psychiatry 51(6):688–695, 2010 20039995

Savage J: The association between attachment, parental bonds and physically aggressive and violent behavior: a comprehensive review. Aggress Violent Behav 19:164–178, 2014

Senju A, Csibra G: Gaze following in human infants depends on communicative signals. Curr Biol 18(9):668–671, 2008 18439827

Sharp C, Fonagy P, Goodyer I: Social Cognition and Developmental Psychopathology. Oxford, Oxford University Press, 2008

Sperber D, Clement F, Heintz C, et al: Epistemic vigilance. Mind Lang 25:359–393, 2010

Staebler K, Renneberg B, Stopsack M, et al: Facial emotional expression in reaction to social exclusion in borderline personality disorder. Psychol Med 41(9):1929–1938, 2011 21306661

Stevens D, Charman T, Blair RJ: Recognition of emotion in facial expressions and vocal tones in children with psychopathic tendencies. J Genet Psychol 162(2):201–211, 2001 11432605

Sylvers PD, Brennan PA, Lilienfeld SO: Psychopathic traits and preattentive threat processing in children: a novel test of the fearlessness hypothesis. Psychol Sci 22(10):1280–1287, 2011 21881061

Taubner S, White LO, Zimmermann J, et al: Attachment-related mentalization moderates the relationship between psychopathic traits and proactive aggression in adolescence. J Abnorm Child Psychol 41(6):929–938, 2013 23512713

Taubner S, Zimmermann L, Ramberg A, et al: Mentalization mediates the relationship between early maltreatment and potential for violence in adolescence. Psychopathology 49(4):236–246, 2016 27548462

Theule J, Germain SM, Cheung K, et al: Conduct disorder/oppositional defiant disorder and attachment: a meta-analysis. J Dev Life Course Criminol 2:232–255, 2016

Tomasello M: Origins of Human Communication. Cambridge, MA, MIT Press, 2008

Treffert DA: Savant syndrome: realities, myths and misconceptions. J Autism Dev Disord 44(3):564–571, 2014 23918440

Tremblay RE: Developmental origins of disruptive behaviour problems: the 'original sin' hypothesis, epigenetics and their consequences for prevention. J Child Psychol Psychiatry 51(4):341–367, 2010 20146751

Tremblay RE, Nagin DS, Séguin JR, et al: Physical aggression during early childhood: trajectories and predictors. Pediatrics 114(1):e43–e50, 2004 15231972

Twemlow SW, Fonagy P, Sacco FC, et al: Assessing adolescents who threaten homicide in schools. Clin Soc Work J 36:131–142, 2008

Viding E, McCrory EJ: Genetic and neurocognitive contributions to the development of psychopathy. Dev Psychopathol 24(3):969–983, 2012 22781866

Viding E, Price TS, Jaffee SR, et al: Genetics of callous-unemotional behavior in children. PLoS One 8(7):e65789, 2013 23874384

Wagner G, Zeiler M, Waldherr K, et al: Mental health problems in Austrian adolescents: a nationwide, two-stage epidemiological study applying DSM-5 criteria. Eur Child Adolesc Psychiatry 26(12):1483–1499, 2017 28540609

Waller R, Shaw DS, Neiderhiser JM, et al: Toward an understanding of the role of the environment in the development of early callous behavior. J Pers 85(1):90–103, 2017 26291075

Willoughby MT, Waschbusch DA, Moore GA, Propper CB: Using the ASEBA to screen for callous unemotional traits in early childhood: Factor structure, temporal stability, and utility. J Psychopathol Behav Assess 33(1):19–30, 2011 21483647

Wilson D, Sperber D: Meaning and Relevance. Cambridge, UK, Cambridge University Press, 2012

Wilson DS, Hayes SC, Biglan A, et al: Evolving the future: toward a science of intentional change. Behav Brain Sci 37(4):395–416, 2014 24826907

Woodworth M, Waschbusch D: Emotional processing in children with conduct problems and callous/unemotional traits. Child Care Health Dev 34(2):234–244, 2008 18028474

CHAPTER 19

BORDERLINE PERSONALITY DISORDER

Anthony Bateman, M.A., FRCPsych

Peter Fonagy, Ph.D., FBA, FMedSci, FAcSS

Chloe Campbell, Ph.D.

Borderline personality disorder (BPD) is the clinical disorder around which both the theory of mentalizing and the mentalization-based treatment (MBT) approach were initially elaborated (Bateman 1995; Fonagy 1991). As MBT has expanded, it has been adapted to treat a range of mental disorders, as described across other chapters of this book. However, the mentalizing profile associated with BPD has continued to hold a rich and paradigmatic source of interest in formulating mentalizing theory, as it manifests so acutely the social-cognitive distortions and interpersonal distress associated with psychopathology.

BPD is a severe condition with an estimated lifetime prevalence of up to 6% (Grant et al. 2008). Comorbidity is a very common feature of BPD: the disorder is often diagnosed alongside mood disorders, anxiety disorders, bipolar disorder, and schizotypal and narcissistic personality disorders. BPD may be particularly common in outpatient and forensic psychiatric populations, in which between one-quarter and one-third of individuals may be expected to meet criteria for the diagnosis.

The fifth edition of *Diagnostic and Statistical Manual of Mental Disorders* (DSM-5; American Psychiatric Association 2013) lists nine criteria for BPD, of which at least five must be present for the disorder to be diagnosed. These can be summarized as follows: a pattern of unstable, intense relationships; inappropriate, intense anger; frantic efforts to avoid abandonment; affective instability; impulsive, potentially self-damaging actions; recurrent self-injurious behavior and suicidality; chronic feelings of emptiness; transient, stress-related paranoid thoughts or severe dissociative symptoms; and identity disturbance (American Psychiatric Association 2013). The group of patients captured by the DSM-5 criteria for the diagnosis of BPD is wide, and there has been some dispute about the strength of the DSM-5 categorical approach to diagnosing BPD, to the extent that an alternative model for diagnosis of personality disorders is presented in Section III of the same edition of the manual (American Psychiatric Association 2013). According to this model, the diagnostic criteria for personality disorders are made up of three components. The first component is level of personality functioning: severity of impairment predicts whether the individual's presentation meets the general criteria for personality disorder, with more severe impairment predicting whether an individual can be diagnosed with more than one personality disorder, or one of the more typically severe forms of personality disorder. The four elements of personality function are *identity* and *self-direction* (which fall into the category of functioning in relation to the self), and *empathy* and *intimacy* (which fall into the category of interpersonal functioning). The second component consists of specific personality disorder diagnoses, of which there are six in the Section III model (as opposed to 10 in the existing model): antisocial personality disorder, avoidant personality disorder, borderline personality disorder, narcissistic personality disorder, obsessive-compulsive personality disorder, and schizotypal personality disorder. The final component is made up of a system of pathological personality traits, which are organized into five domains: negative affectivity, detachment, antagonism, disinhibition, and psychoticism.

At the heart of recent discourse on the conceptualization of personality disorder lies the following three-pronged, unresolved question: a) to what extent it can be understood as a single dimensional continuum, or b) whether it should be understood as being made up of discrete but overlapping diagnostic categories, or c) whether a hybrid model combining dimensional and categorical approaches is the most fitting. There is, however, increasing consensus that BPD consists of three related core features: emotion dysregulation, impulsivity, and social dysfunction. We will consider each of these features in terms of a mentalizing framework.

CORE FEATURES OF BPD

Before describing the core features of BPD, we wish to emphasize that the reality of living with BPD is that these features, while helpful from a clinical and theoretical perspective, are often not clearly delineated; they are interrelated, and one feature may end up triggering another. An example of this is the way in which emotion dysregulation can easily be the cause as well as the consequence of dysfunctional social relationships. Intense emotion almost invariably causes social dysfunction. When an individual with BPD behaves in an emotionally dysregulated way, it is likely to severely disrupt social (and particularly intimate) relationships. Whoever is with the person with BPD is quite likely to act in a way that causes the person's further emotional reaction, and a spiral of dysregulation might follow. Alternatively, the person's attempt to control his or her emotion dysregulation may entail impulsive behaviors such as self-harm.

Emotion Dysregulation

Emotion dysregulation is often apparent as intense, inappropriate anger. Affective instability and intensity of affect may underlie the frantic efforts to avoid abandonment that are a key characteristic of BPD, but may also drive many other symptoms of BPD (e.g., impulsive actions). For example, experimental studies have confirmed that patients with a diagnosis of BPD are less willing to experience distress in order to pursue goal-directed behavior (Gratz et al. 2006; Salsman and Linehan 2012), have significantly prolonged anger reactions (Jacob et al. 2008), are less able to inhibit their response to negative emotional stimuli (Domes et al. 2006; Gratz et al. 2010), show abnormalities in processing unpleasant emotional stimuli (Baer et al. 2012; Hazlett et al. 2007), and are more likely to behave impulsively when in a negative mood (Chapman et al. 2008), compared with people with no BPD features. Over any specific time period, they are likely to experience dramatic shifts in mood states (Reich et al. 2012; Santangelo et al. 2014) and increases in heart rate not associated with metabolic activity (Reisch et al. 2008; Trull et al. 2008). Compared with healthy control subjects, people with BPD experience sudden and large decreases in positive mood states (Ebner-Priemer et al. 2007; Houben et al. 2016). Studies of daily emotional dynamics show that the frequency with which people with BPD experience shifts between positive and negative moods is no different from that with which individuals without BPD experience such shifts, but the change in emotional intensity is larger in BPD patients than in controls.

People with BPD also report more complex emotions and experience greater problems in identifying specific emotions associated with higher levels of distress (Bornovalova et al. 2011; Ebner-Priemer et al. 2008; Preißler et al. 2010) than individuals with low levels of BPD features, although this may be an effect rather than the cause of emotional hyperreactivity (Domes et al. 2009).

Emotion dysregulation is a well-recognized core feature of BPD. From a clinical point of view, however, we need to explain emotion dysregulation from a mentalizing perspective. We contend that overwhelming emotional arousal causes significant mentalizing imbalances. In terms of the mentalizing dimensions (see Chapter 1, "Introduction"), this involves being temporarily restricted to the affective polarity of the cognitive–affective dimension, with thinking also characterized by an automatic and nonreflective form of mentalizing (on the automatic–controlled dimension). When someone is in a state of stress, it is natural for automatic mentalizing to dominate. Up to a point this is a normal fight/flight response to stress, which has the advantage of allowing a person to respond to physical danger immediately and without the need to reflect on his or her actions. However, in situations of social interpersonal stress, it is clearly important to be able to function in a more cognitive and reflective way, and inability to use the more controlled and conscious mentalizing skills can lead to real difficulties. For example, before someone acts on the desire to yell or scream, he or she might think about how it might frighten a child he or she is with, and considering the child's mental state has a calming, regulating effect. If it is hard for the individual concerned to access the sense of perspective that can help to regulate his or her heightened affect by appraising the context, it may also make him or her behave in a way that generates responses that escalate interpersonal stress and worsen social difficulties and dysfunctions. Returning to the example above, shouting or screaming would dysregulate the child, which may in turn further dysregulate the adult.

The nonmentalizing mode that may be most closely linked to emotion dysregulation is *psychic equivalence*. As described in Chapter 1, in this mode emotion is felt as overly real, and when sufficiently intense, it leaves no room for any doubt. This mode makes the experience of internal events (thoughts and feelings) seem concrete rather than subjective, as having the same weight and significance as a physical incident; this may be what makes the impact of emotional arousal so overwhelming. It is one thing to *feel* tired and unattractive first thing in the morning, but quite another to regard that feeling as proof that one *is* ugly and undesirable. When this emotional way of experiencing the world is extended to cognitions—that is, when both thoughts and feelings become "too real"—it leads to a state of mind that allows no alternative perspective. It makes the emotions themselves feel highly immediate and completely unquestionable; this experience can be powerful and overwhelming. When such points arise in therapy, the best strategy for the clinician is to avoid being drawn into a nonmentalizing discourse. We see dysregulated emotional thinking as triggering the concreteness of the psychic equivalence mode, which in turn makes it difficult for the individual to accept alternative perspectives that could help to contextualize and downregulate the intensity of the experience.

Impulsivity

Impulsivity—of which the most disquieting aspect is suicidality—is the second core feature of BPD. Three-quarters of BPD patients attempt suicide at least once (Black et al. 2004). Affective instability, particularly negative mood amplitude and the intensity of negative mood (Links et al. 2008), has been associated with an increased likelihood of impulsivity (Gratz et al. 2010). A diagnosis of major depressive disorder, substance use disorder, or posttraumatic stress disorder; the presence of self-harm; being sexually assaulted in adulthood; having had a caregiver who died by suicide; affective instability; and more severe dissociation have each been shown to increase suicidal behavior (Wedig et al. 2012, 2013). Suicide risk has been associated with poor social adjustment and the absence of supportive family, work, and social relationships (Soloff and Fabio 2008; Soloff et al. 2008; Wedig et al. 2013).

We understand impulsivity in terms of imbalance among the dimensions of mentalizing: it involves a heavy emphasis on the automatic pole of the automatic–controlled dimension. Impulsive behavior will result if there is insufficient reflection concerning the impact of the individual's actions on others, or on himself or herself. Any such reflection is most likely to be disconnected from reality: that is, it is likely to be *hypermentalizing* or *pseudomentalizing* (see Chapter 1, "Introduction," and Chapter 17, "Borderline Personality Pathology in Adolescence"). In this mode, if individuals with BPD have done something for which they have no explanation, they will develop a reason retrospectively, usually in terms of their "intentions" and "beliefs" and/or the intentions and beliefs of others around them. For example, if the context for a person's actions was an imagined slight because her partner did not respond immediately to a text message she sent him, the person's explanation will be marked by extravagant assumptions about what might have been going on. If the individual then discusses this event in therapy, she will entangle herself and the clinician in extended analyses but will offer little compelling evidence for any of her assertions. The person might urgently seek validation for her view, but even when this is provided, it is meaningless because the person is simultaneously aware that she made up her explanation; thus, confirming or elaborating it only increases her sense of emptiness and meaninglessness. In such a situation, the clinician would be most helpful by interrupting this nonmentalizing process—and the sooner the better. This style of functioning, when mentalizing becomes highly impaired, develops into the *pretend mode* of nonmentalizing (or *prementalizing*), in which there is an inadequate link between inner and outer reality; this can often result in impulsive behavior, as it is not tempered by a measured hold on external reality.

Impulsivity can also result from the *teleological stance*. The teleological mode of prementalizing involves a heavy emphasis on observable physical outcomes. In teleological mode, the individual cannot accept anything other than a physical action as a true expression of the other person's intentions. In the case of such a patient, his partner or parents might constantly assure him of their love and support, yet none of that feels real to him: it does not address the "hole" into which the patient "falls" at certain—especially lonely—times when he feels a terrible emptiness. For such a patient, what does seem to help are physical actions that make him feel real—for example, scratching himself a little too violently. In this mode, intentions can be accepted only if they are proven by actions, and are meaningless unless they produce physically observable outcomes; this can explain acts of self-harm, which demonstrate to the individual that he or she still has the power of self-agency, or acts of aggression toward others for similar reasons. The feeling that interpersonal affection can be real only if it is accompanied by physical behavior certainly explains some risky sexual behavior, but it also explains the need to create physical distraction that helps with the feeling that all verbal expressions of interpersonal affection are meaningless. The teleological stance is a state of nonmentalizing that is highly fixed on the exterior pole of the internal–external dimension of mentalizing and reflects the momentary loss of controlled mentalizing.

Social Dysfunction

Social dysfunction is typically seen as the third factor in the triad of core BPD symptom clusters. For example, patients with BPD experience greater social problem-solving difficulties compared with other clinical groups and report high levels of disturbances in romantic relationships. Difficulties in social problem-solving are likely to be directly connected to *dysfunctional attachment processes*. In one study of a sample of patients with BPD (Fonagy et al. 1996), which controlled for conditions that commonly co-occur with BPD, a particular association between BPD and preoccupied attachment was reported (75% of patients who met criteria for BPD fell into the rarely used adult attachment subgroup of "fearfully preoccupied with respect to trauma").

We, along with many others working in this area of clinical practice and research, have highlighted a characteristic pattern in BPD patients of fearful attachment (attachment anxiety and relational avoidance), painful intolerance of aloneness, a marked hypersensitivity to social situations, alertness to a hostile response from others, and greatly reduced positive memories of dyadic interactions (e.g., Gunderson and Lyons-Ruth 2008).

As mentalizing is at the heart of social cognition, it is clear that these social difficulties are more likely to arise in individuals whose mentalizing is poor and who find it difficult to moderate their automatic assumptions about others by using reflective thought. Numerous studies have reported that individuals with BPD appear to anxiously expect, readily perceive, and intensely react to social rejection. BPD patients score higher than either healthy controls or patients with anxiety disorders (including social phobia) or mood disorders on a questionnaire measuring rejection sensitivity (Downey and Feldman 1996). Compared with either of the other groups, they expect rejection more—and even perceive it when it is not present. The "cyberball" game, in which the experience of social rejection can be reliably induced under experimental conditions, shows similar results (Staebler et al. 2011). Participants engage in an online ball-tossing game with partners who access the game from elsewhere—players whom they believe to be co-participants but are in fact virtual players preprogrammed to play in a specific way. In the "inclusion" condition, all players receive the same number of ball tosses and the game is completely fair, whereas in the "exclusion" condition the virtual players stop tossing the ball to the participant and favor each other, thereby excluding the participant from the game. Individuals with BPD feel more rejected than healthy controls independent of the experimental conditions—that is, they feel rejected when they are excluded, but they also feel rejected when they are being included equally. During social rejection, individuals with BPD show altered processing in the frontolimbic regions: specifically, activity in the medial prefrontal cortex increases (Ruocco et al. 2010). Overall, the data from these studies suggest that individuals with BPD have difficulty in discriminating between social situations and tend to hypermentalize during social encounters (Domsalla et al. 2014).

Social dysfunction is inevitable if the individual places undue emphasis on mentalizing based on exterior cues as indicators of mental states. Difficulties in understanding and connecting with the individual's own thoughts and feelings can drive a constant and intense need for reassurance to protect against feelings of emptiness and meaninglessness. This can lead to the neediness and dependence on others that is a common aspect of the social dysfunction associated with BPD. The focus on exterior cues can create an attitude of hypervigilance, which, combined with what others might see as unreasonable demands for reassurance, can actually increase the likelihood of being rejected. The dependence on others is driven by hypersensitivity to others' moods and to what they say, the *chameleon effect* (the unconscious tendency to mimic others' behavior), and the attendant fear that the self will disappear. A rejection triggers panic that others' affirmations and reassurance will disappear. The threat that others represent to the sense of self is hard to overestimate: an impingement can feel existential. One way to meet this vulnerability may be through brittle and assertive actions that seek to force recognition of the individual's identity in interactions with others. Although this approach may be understandable, this kind of aggressive or dominating behavior will cause others to respond defensively, often leading to conflict and intense affect, which serve to further undermine the individual's mentalizing capacity.

MENTALIZING PROFILE OF BPD ACROSS THE FOUR DIMENSIONS OF SOCIAL COGNITION

We will briefly consider how the mentalizing strengths and weaknesses of a typical individual with BPD may be apparent across the four dimensions of social cognition discussed in Chapter 1—automatic versus controlled, self versus other, internal versus external, and cognitive versus affective.

Automatic Versus Controlled

Individuals with BPD often tend toward a form of mentalizing that is unhelpfully automatic or implicit. This mentalizing can appear simplistic; it is normally automatic, nonquestioning, and nonconscious; it is impossible for the individual with BPD to genuinely verbally explicate, because the underlying logic is intuitive, unreasoned, and nonverbal; and it is marked by an unwarranted certainty, which betrays its unreflective origin. Particularly when arousal increases, as is typical in the context of intense attachment relationships, people with BPD may readily switch to automatic mentalizing. As a consequence, they often show severe impairments in social cognition; for example, they may be overly distrustful (paranoid) or, the opposite, overly trustful (naive). Their thinking is impulsive: they make quick assumptions about others' thoughts and feelings, which are not reflected upon or tested. Because these individuals likely find it challenging to consider and reflect on the impact they are having on others around them, they can become embroiled in interpersonal conflicts. Furthermore, because of these individuals' lack of perspective taking, a degree of (unintended) cruelty can enter into their thinking and actions. In place of genuine reflectiveness, pseudomentalizing can occur. In addition, their mentalizing is frequently excessive, as it is not circumscribed by being tested against reality; this phenomenon has been described as *hypermentalizing*, and it may be particularly characteristic of adolescents with personality disorder (Sharp 2014; see also Chapter 17).

Self Versus Other

Patients with some borderline traits may show excessive concern about their own internal state (i.e., they hypermentalize in relation to the self). At the same time, these views of the self develop without reference to social reality (an awareness of how others perceive them). Failure to balance self-perception with sincere curiosity about how they are perceived by others can lead to exaggerations of the self-image in both positive and negative directions. A balanced, adaptive form of self-mentalizing is absent, and the reality of the individual's identity becomes lost in hypermentalized fantasy.

Internal Versus External

People with BPD tend to perform poorly on tasks that require them to understand the intentions of other people. However, they can be hypersensitive to facial expressions; in fact, in some studies of sensitivity to visual cues about emotional states, individuals with BPD outperform those without BPD. The heightened sensitivity to emotional experiences that is characteristic of BPD seems to be intrinsically related to increased sensitivity to external features of self and others as a source of knowledge about mental states, and perhaps links to BPD patients' tendency to be excessively affected by the emotional states of those around them. Excessive focus on the external may make an individual hypervigilant about what others feel or think, yet unable to make accurate assessments based on anything other than surface judgments.

This type of mentalizing impairment may become apparent only when the balance of internal and external cues used to establish the mental states of others is assessed. For example, an accurate depiction of how committed the individual's clinician is can come only from recognizing the level of motivation normally required for a clinician to attend regularly, when most likely receiving relatively low financial compensation and little explicitly expressed gratitude. However, if such evaluations of *internal* states are inaccessible to a person, then *external* indicators of attitudes feel crucial. Tiny indicators of a lack of commitment, such as the clinician arriving late for a session, can be seen as devastating evidence of betrayal. In MBT, mentalizing interventions often need to start by accepting the patient's subjective experience, which can often be overwhelming, rather than yielding to the temptation to review the evidence, which, in more balanced circumstances, would be accepted as evidence that the other person's internal state is different from what the patient, in his or her state of high emotional arousal, holds to be true.

Cognitive Versus Affective

Patients with borderline traits are often overwhelmed by automatic, feeling-driven mentalizing and lack the ability to balance this affective mentalizing with more reflective, cognitive modes of function. This is seen clinically as overwhelmingly dysregulated emotions that are inadequately balanced (or not balanced at all) by cognition, and these emotions come to dominate behavior, leading to catastrophizing.

By their nature, cognitions have doubt built into them. Being aware that a thought is just a thought enables someone to distinguish what he or she is thinking from what he or she knows to be actual. By contrast, emotions always feel real. If someone is in pain, it is hard to persuade the person that this sensation is a product of his or her imagination. While cognitions typically come with doubt, feelings have a built-in quality of bodily or physical reality—and normally cognitions and affect are not separate: they come as a package. This allows people to balance the immediate compelling quality of feeling states with the perspective given by cognition. However, for individuals with BPD, when an imbalance on the cognitive–affective dimension occurs, cognition is experienced as firmly located in the self, and emotions in individuals with BPD persist without the moderation of cognition. For example, if a person senses ("feels") that someone sees him or her as second-rate or inferior, and simply experiences this thought without reflecting on it, the thought will carry with it some of the inner conviction of physical pain—it will become something with which the person cannot argue.

To compound this problem, intense emotion can disrupt the process that normally helps to regulate it: that is, cognitive appraisal. Returning to the above example, if an individual's sense of being thought second-rate by a friend creates an intense emotional response, the individual is no longer capable of testing her assumptions against everything else she knows about the friend and their past experiences with each other. The absence of cognition can also lead to an oversensitivity to emotional cues and, in a social context, to overwhelming experiences of emotional contagion when one person's intense emotional experience triggers an emotional reaction in another, which, in turn, can become challenging to regulate. Thus, the person may respond to her friend's imagined slight by slighting (or even overtly insulting) him—something to which he understandably does not take kindly. In this situation, a person may lose the capacity for boundaries around the self and may more readily attribute his or her own mental states to others. The individual sees the friend's response as a clear indication of his vulnerable sense of self, and his modest attempt to protect himself as an equally clear indication of his untrustworthiness and unreliability; the individual ends up feeling let down by him and quite abandoned and isolated. Thus, despite the apparent emotionality shown by people with BPD in relation to others, emotional storms can lead to serious limitations in their capacity for genuine empathy, and they may show self-oriented distress, rather than genuine other-oriented empathy, when confronted with sadness or pain in others.

PUTTING THE DIMENSIONS INTO CLINICAL PRACTICE

A dimensional framework of mentalizing helps the clinician to formulate and focus on the specific failures in mentalizing that create problems for the person with BPD. Any reasonable referral letter should contain indicators of a patient's mentalizing vulnerabilities, and so the clinician will explore these areas more specifically during assessment of the patient (see Chapter 3, "Assessment of Mentalizing," for a discussion of the assessment of mentalizing).

Example Referral Letter

In the case of Sally, a number of pointers suggest her problems with self-mentalizing. She finds it difficult to be on her own for normal periods of time, she persists in asking for reassurance that she is loved, she constantly compares herself with previous girlfriends, and she has to go out to meet people with whom she flirts (and at times eventually engages in risky sexual behavior). In the past she was controlled by another man who dictated to her and was coercive and violent toward her.

All this information suggests that the clinician needs to assess Sally's ability to access reliable internal self-states. Sally is overly reliant on others' states of mind, leaving her vulnerable to exploitation. Positively, she has a more robust sense of herself as a mother, when she is with her son. Probing this area of function suggested that her relationship with him was "mechanical" to a large degree, with her son's physical needs cared for but his emotional needs unmet. Affectively, she describes mood fluctuations, which are unbalanced by cognitive processing and primarily addressed through changes in the external world: she finds men who "like" her and who will engage in sexual interaction. Teleologically, this gives her a stronger sense of her own feeling that she is lovable.

Finally, her relationships suggest that she has a fearful-avoidant attachment pattern characterized by attachment anxiety and relational avoidance and a painful intolerance of aloneness. This is likely to be activated early in treatment. Already, the referrer has remarked on Sally as a likeable person. More importantly, she may experience anxiety quickly in treatment, worrying whether the clinician likes her; she may ask for reassurance and confirmation that she is "doing the right thing" in the sessions. Her support from the session and experience of help from the clinician may be short-lived, and so she might increase her contact between sessions. All these behaviors, based on mentalizing vulnerabilities, are predictable using a dimensional approach to assessment, and so can be discussed with Sally before starting treatment.

CONCLUSION

Elsewhere, we have explored the idea that the features associated with BPD, along with the high level of comorbidity that is characteristic of the disorder, suggest that BPD may represent a general lack of psychological resilience, and be a core marker for the general psychopathology factor (see Chapter 4, "Mentalizing, Resilience, and Epistemic Trust," and Fonagy et al. 2017a, 2017b). We have also suggested that the vulnerabilities associated with BPD that make it so paradigmatic in relation to general psychopathology are related to impairments in epistemic trust and consequent impairments in the individual's ability to benefit from his or her social environment (see Chapters 1 and 4 and Fonagy et al. 2015). The quality of rigidity, or being "hard to reach," that clinicians have traditionally ascribed to patients with BPD is an outcome of the difficulties in social communication that arise from epistemic mistrust. Patients may, for all their apparent need for social contact and willingness to discuss their feelings, struggle to benefit from and build on constructive social relations in a sustainable manner because the social learning that this requires is not accessible to them. This has significant implications in terms of clinical practice, which is discussed more fully in Chapter 10, "Therapeutic Models." Here, we would like simply to emphasize that balanced mentalizing is the fundamental tool for social learning and benefiting from social communication. New learning about the social world and how to operate within it is achievable only if the social environment is accurately interpreted; being able to understand the mental states of others' actions and reactions—that is, adequate mentalizing—is critical to this. Furthermore, it is possible to reap the benefits of constructive social experiences only through the ongoing maintenance of improved relationships, emotion regulation, and good behavioral control; once again, improved mentalizing is essential for these. BPD is a condition that is often characterized by intense interpersonal distress and feelings of social isolation; helping individuals to develop more balanced mentalizing provides the fundamental social building blocks that make possible the construction of more benign and cooperative relationships with people in the wider social environment.

REFERENCES

American Psychiatric Association: Diagnostic and Statistical Manual of Mental Disorders, 5th Edition. Arlington, VA, American Psychiatric Association, 2013

Baer RA, Peters JR, Eisenlohr-Moul TA, et al: Emotion-related cognitive processes in borderline personality disorder: a review of the empirical literature. Clin Psychol Rev 32(5):359–369, 2012 22561966

Bateman AW: The treatment of borderline patients in a day hospital setting. Psychoanal Psychother 9:3–16, 1995

Black DW, Blum N, Pfohl B, et al: Suicidal behavior in borderline personality disorder: prevalence, risk factors, prediction, and prevention. J Pers Disord 18(3):226–239, 2004 15237043

Bornovalova MA, Matusiewicz A, Rojas E: Distress tolerance moderates the relationship between negative affect intensity with borderline personality disorder levels. Compr Psychiatry 52(6):744–753, 2011 21257162

Chapman AL, Leung DW, Lynch TR: Impulsivity and emotion dysregulation in borderline personality disorder. J Pers Disord 22(2):148–164, 2008 18419235

Domes G, Schulze L, Herpertz SC: Emotion recognition in borderline personality disorder—a review of the literature. J Pers Disord 23(1):6–19, 2009 19267658

Domes G, Winter B, Schnell K, et al: The influence of emotions on inhibitory functioning in borderline personality disorder. Psychol Med 36(8):1163–1172, 2006 16700964

Domsalla M, Koppe G, Niedtfeld I, et al: Cerebral processing of social rejection in patients with borderline personality disorder. Soc Cogn Affect Neurosci 9(11):1789–1797, 2014 24273076

Downey G, Feldman SI: Implications of rejection sensitivity for intimate relationships. J Pers Soc Psychol 70(6):1327–1343, 1996 8667172

Ebner-Priemer UW, Kuo J, Kleindienst N, et al: State affective instability in borderline personality disorder assessed by ambulatory monitoring. Psychol Med 37(7):961–970, 2007 17202005

Ebner-Priemer UW, Kuo J, Schlotz W, et al: Distress and affective dysregulation in patients with borderline personality disorder: a psychophysiological ambulatory monitoring study. J Nerv Ment Dis 196(4):314–320, 2008 18414126

Fonagy P: Thinking about thinking: some clinical and theoretical considerations in the treatment of a borderline patient. Int J Psychoanal 72(Pt 4):639–656, 1991 1797718

Fonagy P, Leigh T, Steele M, et al: The relation of attachment status, psychiatric classification, and response to psychotherapy. J Consult Clin Psychol 64(1):22–31, 1996 8907081

Fonagy P, Luyten P, Allison E: Epistemic petrification and the restoration of epistemic trust: a new conceptualization of borderline personality disorder and its psychosocial treatment. J Pers Disord 29(5):575–609, 2015 26393477

Fonagy P, Luyten P, Allison E, et al: What we have changed our minds about: Part 1. Borderline personality disorder as a limitation of resilience. Borderline Personal Disorder Emotion Dysregul 4:11, 2017a 28413687

Fonagy P, Luyten P, Allison E, et al: What we have changed our minds about: Part 2. Borderline personality disorder, epistemic trust and the developmental significance of social communication. Borderline Personal Disorder Emotion Dysregul 4:9, 2017b 28405338

Grant BF, Chou SP, Goldstein RB, et al: Prevalence, correlates, disability, and comorbidity of DSM-IV borderline personality disorder: results from the Wave 2 National Epidemiologic Survey on Alcohol and Related Conditions. J Clin Psychiatry 69(4):533–545, 2008 18426259

Gratz KL, Rosenthal MZ, Tull MT, et al: An experimental investigation of emotion dysregulation in borderline personality disorder. J Abnorm Psychol 115(4):850–855, 2006 17100543

Gratz KL, Breetz A, Tull MT: The moderating role of borderline personality in the relationships between deliberate self-harm and emotion-related factors. Pers Ment Health 4:96–107, 2010

Gunderson JG, Lyons-Ruth K: BPD's interpersonal hypersensitivity phenotype: a gene-environment-developmental model. J Pers Disord 22(1):22–41, 2008 18312121

Hazlett EA, Speiser LJ, Goodman M, et al: Exaggerated affect-modulated startle during unpleasant stimuli in borderline personality disorder. Biol Psychiatry 62(3):250–255, 2007 17258691

Houben M, Vansteelandt K, Claes L, et al: Emotional switching in borderline personality disorder: a daily life study. Pers Disord 7(1):50–60, 2016 26098377

Jacob GA, Guenzler C, Zimmermann S, et al: Time course of anger and other emotions in women with borderline personality disorder: a preliminary study. J Behav Ther Exp Psychiatry 39(3):391–402, 2008 18171575

Links PS, Eynan R, Heisel MJ, et al: Elements of affective instability associated with suicidal behaviour in patients with borderline personality disorder. Can J Psychiatry 53(2):112–116, 2008 18357929

Preißler S, Dziobek I, Ritter K, et al: Social cognition in borderline personality disorder: evidence for disturbed recognition of the emotions, thoughts, and intentions of others. Front Behav Neurosci 4:182, 2010 21151817

Reich DB, Zanarini MC, Fitzmaurice G: Affective lability in bipolar disorder and borderline personality disorder. Compr Psychiatry 53(3):230–237, 2012 21632042

Reisch T, Ebner-Priemer UW, Tschacher W, et al: Sequences of emotions in patients with borderline personality disorder. Acta Psychiatr Scand 118(1):42–48, 2008 18582346

Ruocco AC, Medaglia JD, Tinker JR, et al: Medial prefrontal cortex hyperactivation during social exclusion in borderline personality disorder. Psychiatry Res 181(3):233–236, 2010 20153143

Salsman NL, Linehan MM: An investigation of the relationships among negative affect, difficulties in emotion regulation, and features of borderline personality disorder. J Psychopathol Behav Assess 34:260–267, 2012

Santangelo P, Bohus M, Ebner-Priemer UW: Ecological momentary assessment in borderline personality disorder: a review of recent findings and methodological challenges. J Pers Disord 28(4):555–576, 2014 22984853

Sharp C: The social-cognitive basis of BPD: a theory of hypermentalizing, in Handbook of Borderline Personality Disorder in Children and Adolescents. Edited by Sharp C, Tackett JL. New York, Springer, 2014, pp 211–226

Soloff PH, Fabio A: Prospective predictors of suicide attempts in borderline personality disorder at one, two, and two-to-five year follow-up. J Pers Disord 22(2):123–134, 2008 18419233

Soloff PH, Feske U, Fabio A: Mediators of the relationship between childhood sexual abuse and suicidal behavior in borderline personality disorder. J Pers Disord 22(3):221–232, 2008 18540795

Staebler K, Renneberg B, Stopsack M, et al: Facial emotional expression in reaction to social exclusion in borderline personality disorder. Psychol Med 41(9):1929–1938, 2011 21306661

Trull TJ, Solhan MB, Tragesser SL, et al: Affective instability: measuring a core feature of borderline personality disorder with ecological momentary assessment. J Abnorm Psychol 117(3):647–661, 2008 18729616

Wedig MM, Silverman MH, Frankenburg FR, et al: Predictors of suicide attempts in patients with borderline personality disorder over 16 years of prospective follow-up. Psychol Med 42(11):2395–2404, 2012 22436619

Wedig MM, Frankenburg FR, Bradford Reich D, et al: Predictors of suicide threats in patients with borderline personality disorder over 16 years of prospective follow-up. Psychiatry Res 208(3):252–256, 2013 23747235

ANTISOCIAL PERSONALITY DISORDER IN COMMUNITY AND PRISON SETTINGS

Anthony Bateman, M.A., FRCPsych

Anna Motz, B.A., C.Foren.Psychol., DipClinPsych

Jessica Yakeley, M.B. B.Chir., MRCP, FRCPsych

In this chapter, we outline a mentalizing understanding of antisocial personality disorder (ASPD), summarize mentalization-based treatment for ASPD (MBT-ASPD), and argue that implementation of this clinical intervention in both community and prison contexts will be of benefit both to the individual and to society if treatment reduces reactive aggression toward others. MBT-ASPD currently targets male clients because of the high prevalence of ASPD in this group in society and prison populations.

ASPD AND COMMUNITY SETTINGS: GENERAL CONSIDERATIONS FOR TREATMENT

Within the general population, the prevalence of men with ASPD has been estimated at 1%–6% (Coid et al. 2006; Torgersen et al. 2001); the disorder is more common among individuals in mental health services, the judicial system, and prison settings. ASPD is associated with significant comorbidity, particularly substance dependence (Compton et al. 2005), anxiety, and depressive disorders (Lenzenweger et al. 2007), and also with physical health conditions (Byrne et al. 2013). Moreover, people with ASPD have an increased risk of early death, predominantly through reckless behavior and putting themselves in positions of danger but also due to higher rates of suicide (Black et al. 1996; Martin et al. 1985).

Despite the relatively high occurrence of ASPD within the community and the heavy burden placed on services due to comorbid mental health and physical illnesses, there remains a lack of treatment for those with ASPD in community settings within both health and criminal justice systems in the United Kingdom. This is in obvious contrast to the growth in the past decade of dedicated treatment services for individuals with borderline personality disorder (BPD). Although many individuals with ASPD tend to be treatment avoidant, others will present to their general medical practitioner/primary care physician or are referred to secondary mental health services with anxiety, depression, or complaints of physical ill-health. Yet, professionals often decline to provide treatment once an individual's history of violence and antisocial behavior is uncovered; this is perhaps due to the challenges associated with increased risk, substance misuse, treatment noncompliance, and the persistent beliefs of many clinicians that ASPD is untreatable. Difficulties in engaging antisocial individuals are frequently due to their reluctance to think of themselves as having a mental health disorder, as this is equated in their minds with weakness and associated with feelings of shame and humiliation. Their unwillingness to access and receive treatment adds to the likelihood that their personality disorder will remain untreated. In some cases, suicidality remains undetected, not only because of shame in acknowledging such feelings and failure to inform others, but also as a result of the focus by professionals on the risk posed by the individual with ASPD to others, rather than risk to the self.

MENTALIZING PROFILE OF ASPD

In a sense, it is self-evident that ASPD entails mentalizing difficulties and that a common path to violence is via momentary inhibition of the capacity to mentalize. However, it would be too simplistic to assert that individuals with ASPD have an outright mentalizing deficit. For example, evidence suggests that however paradoxically, better mentalizing ability in some areas may be linked with violence in individuals with certain mental disorders. Violent individuals with schizophrenia, for example, tend to outperform their nonviolent counterparts on complex theory-of-mind tasks. As with BPD, thinking in terms of mentalizing profiles and the subjective states they engender rather than thinking of "mentalizing" as a single entity is vital when working with ASPD.

From the point of view of implementing a mentalization-based therapy program for people with ASPD, the nature of their mentalizing deficits in terms of the dimensions of mentalizing need to be identified. To summarize our overall view: antisocial characteristics stabilize mentalizing by "rigidifying" otherwise unpredictable interpersonal relationships with the use of prementalizing modes of thinking. Individuals with ASPD show imbalances of mentalizing and, surprisingly, may even be better than normal at external rather than internal, cognitive rather than affective, and impulsive-intuitive (automatic) rather than reflective (controlled) forms of mentalizing.

Automatic Versus Controlled: Failure of Automatic Mentalizing

Controlled or explicit mentalizing, particularly when it is of a higher order, can be the apparent substance of psychological therapy. This is a significant clinical problem in the treatment of people with ASPD, who may be asked to undertake explicit mentalizing of both themselves and others: they do not attach any emotional salience to the understanding. Consequently, they overuse automatic mentalizing, which is rapid and reflexive. Their limited ability to resonate with others and reduced interest in what others think and feel result in a failure to recruit controlled mentalizing. This results in a failure of automatic mentalizing because their assumptions remain unquestioned and uninformed, and thus lack nuance.

Cognitive Versus Affective: Failure of Affective Mentalizing

The link between cognition and emotional experience in both the self and others is tenuous; individuals with ASPD may show considerable cognitive understanding of mental states but are not in touch with the affective core of human experience. Cognitions, because of their "disembodied" character, can readily be distorted in largely self-serving ways, so that they end up extensively distorting, rather than representing, reality—the person believes his own story despite evidence to the contrary. This makes the possibility of genuine compassion for themselves or empathy for others elusive, and some individuals may even feel excitement in response to, or enjoyment of, others' pain (Decety et al. 2009).

Clinical Illustration

In a group, one client became manifestly upset and indicated that he did not want to talk further about the problem he had been addressing. The clinician empathized with this and sensitively moved the group to another topic. However, another client questioned this change of topic, asking the clinician whether the group was "about talking to each other about difficult things." The clinician had to agree with this, and the second client then went on to interrogate the first client, who became increasingly upset. It was apparent that the questioning client gained pleasure from making the first client feel uncomfortable.

Self Versus Other: Failure to See Self in the Other

In the example above, the client is misusing his capacity to understand the cognitive and affective states of another in a self-serving way. Individuals with ASPD are relative experts at reading the inner states of others from a cognitive perspective, but are unable to identify empathically with these states and be compassionate toward them. This asymmetry facilitates pervasive disregard for the rights of others. It is this sense of partial recognition of the mind of the other that is critical in permitting antisocial behavior. Recognition of the other person as having a separate mind will inhibit violence; the loss of mentalizing makes it possible for the individual to use the other person to fulfill his own needs or to carry out a physical attack on him or her, as he or she becomes no more than a body or threatening presence. This mechanism can characterize assaults even on highly vulnerable targets, including young children, as they are seen solely as objects, or as malevolent creatures who intend to "wind them up"; in either account there is little sense of another subjective being with a mind.

Having limited capacity to resonate with others, people with ASPD feel that their explicit ideas about the other—however accurate these might be—lack meaning and therefore do not serve to regulate their own behavior. Experience of the other's reaction and feeling does not constrain them. Put simply, the person with ASPD does not care about others; he would rather engage with others only to satisfy his own aims. This excessive concentration on either the self or the other leads to one-sided relationships and distortions in social interaction. Inevitably, this will be reflected in how individuals present for treatment and interact with their clinicians, and it makes treatment "through" and "with" others particularly problematic. People with ASPD tend to "fix" at one pole of the self–other dimension, depending on context.

Internal Versus External: Failure to See the Inside From the Outside

Internal mentalizing is a focus on the individual's own or others' internal states—that is, thoughts, feelings, and desires. External mentalizing relies on external features, such as facial expressions and behavior. Individuals with ASPD may focus on themselves and their own internal states and become selective experts in getting others to do things for them to meet their requirements. However, in general, they do not reflect on their own internal states, making it difficult to ask them to explore their current experiences.

With regard to external mentalizing, people with ASPD have been shown to have a limited response to expressed facial or otherwise externally depicted emotion; this suggests that mechanisms for acquiring information about mental states quickly and easily are profoundly compromised in these individuals, perhaps increasing their use of automatic mentalizing. Individuals with ASPD show a particular inability to read facial expressions that convey affect. If an individual can mentalize someone else so that he or she "feels" what the other feels, it makes it harder to hurt the other person, as the individual is constrained by the other's feelings. Aggressive acts are possible if mentalizing is (temporarily) inhibited or decoupled.

ASPD AND THE PREMENTALIZING MODES

The significant characteristics of the mentalizing profile of people with ASPD all reflect a shift to nonmentalizing (or prementalizing) ways of operating. We assume that in some individuals—perhaps those who have experienced attachment-related trauma such as severe parental maltreatment or exposure to domestic violence—activation of the attachment system inhibits aspects of mentalizing.

In psychic equivalence, everything is "for real." Concrete thinking is a consequence of mentalizing that is excessively based on external cues and is implicit and nonreflective. There is a tendency to assume motives based merely on external appearance. This causes real social problems. The overemphasis on external indicators of internal states, unchecked by reflection, generates deeply disturbing expectations of other people's intentions.

Pretend mode allows the individual to undertake violence in a disconnected way, as if there is no psychological victim involved in a crime, or as if the victim's mind is so alien and different from the perpetrator's that no continuity between the two could be established. In the absence of an appropriate balance between mentalizing the self and the other, thoughts and feelings can become dissociated almost to the point of meaninglessness. Emotional capacities such as guilt, love of others, and fear of consequences normally help to restrain violent behavior, but the loss of mentalizing and stunted ability of some violent individuals to fully experience and resonate with such feelings prevent these inhibitory mechanisms from functioning.

The teleological mode tends to dominate motivation for actions in individuals with ASPD. In this mode, experience is felt to be valid only when its consequences are visibly and palpably apparent. The stereotypical depiction of a successful antisocial individual as wearing ostentatious jewelry or an expensive watch, driving a luxury car, and demonstrating loyalty through violent attacks on enemies (and, similarly, requiring others to demonstrate loyalty to him in a similar way) may be a fantasy of scriptwriters, but it is based on an appreciation of the massive value placed by antisocial individuals on appearance and "face" (Gilligan 2000). Retribution has to be physical and observable. The justice system has, by and large, adopted the same teleological stance; the logic of "justice being seen to be done" is acceptable to prisoners and prison guards in equal measure. Deviating from these simple principles and attempting to introduce psychological-mindedness into the system is disconcerting to all and often avoided. We discuss the attempts to create a more mentalizing environment in prisons later in this chapter.

ASPD AND THE ALIEN SELF

Individuals with ASPD need relationships, whether within a gang-like group or in a more personal context. These relationships tend to be hierarchical and rigidly organized. However, the controlled and often limited nature of interactions within such relationships should not lead to underestimating their intensity and significance; these relationships are often characterized by a strong sense of loyalty to and identification with the other. Such relationships can be of great importance to people with ASPD because they stabilize their sense of self for two reasons. First, they can affirm and validate the individual's state (and this sense of affirmation and validation is often a rare experience for individuals with ASPD, given that their behavior often serves to alienate others); second, social relationships often function as a place where the alien self can be externalized (see Chapter 1, "Introduction"). The imperative to externalize the alien self creates challenges for treatment—the rigidity with which relationships are conceptualized needs to be challenged by the clinician, but with great care, as such a challenge may arouse feelings of violence and aggression because any perceived changes in relationships unleash a need for the violent assertion of control as an automatic response; however, it also creates opportunities. For example, the MBT-ASPD program is organized around group work to harness these individuals' loyalty to others and to explore the bonds formed through identification with others with ASPD who have similar attitudes.

MBT-ASPD: GROUP TREATMENT

Group work is crucial for people with ASPD if disorganized behavior in their social and intimate lives is to be addressed. Many people with ASPD live within a subculture of barely restrained violence and implicit threats; in this regard they are more likely to be influenced by their peer group than by clinicians whom they see as unlikely to understand the sociocultural context and constant mental alertness about others' motives that is required if they are to survive in the community in which they live. People with ASPD may gain from sharing with others and from recognition that they are not alone in their struggle for autonomy and desire to have more constructive relationships.

A number of additional reasons suggest that group work may be beneficial. First, people with ASPD tend to seek relationships that are organized hierarchically. Group work stimulates a hierarchical process within a peer group, which can be harnessed in vivo by the clinicians working with the group to explore participants' sensitivity to hierarchy and authority and the mentalizing distortions that ensue. Second, participants are more likely to demonstrate overcontrol of their emotional states within well-structured, schematic attachment relationships, such as avoidance of interaction or anxious ambivalence when relating to members of the group, which becomes obvious in a group. Third, emotional capacities such as guilt and love toward others and fear for the self may restrain people from engaging in violent behavior, but the loss of mentalizing and attenuated ability of people with ASPD to experience such feelings prevent these inhibitory mechanisms from being mobilized. The absence of these social emotions, which normally structure behavior toward others, must be addressed in the group. Finally, if the reduction in ability to recognize others' emotions is more pervasive than being restricted to fear and sadness, then a focus in treatment on recognizing *all* emotions in the self and others is essential. Generating nuance and variability in the emotions that are expressed is necessary. In certain subcultures with a high prevalence of ASPD (e.g., in probation hostels), even when emotions are experienced, when these relate to vulnerability, loss, or sadness they are muted or denied, while anger, pride, and thirst for vengeance are socially accepted.

Group treatment, which is usually delivered by two clinicians, is described fully elsewhere (Bateman and Fonagy 2016; Bateman et al. 2013). A brief summary is given here (for a general discussion of mentalizing and group therapy, see Chapter 7, "Group Therapy for Adults and Adolescents").

Engagement

People with ASPD are naturally wary and distrusting, given their backgrounds and experience. They do not initially accept that others' motives might be benign. In view of this, the clinician first needs to develop a treatment plan that is relevant to the individual. In MBT-ASPD the clinician explores the client's values first by asking a number of questions about personal topics, such as:

1. *"Do other people think that something should be important to you, or do you think so? Is 'the something'—for example, less violence, loving relationships, employment—important to you?"* The client must consider a focus of treatment to be meaningful to him personally. It is not possible to engage people with ASPD in treatment if they feel that the focus is important to society and not to them.
2. *"Is it still important if nobody knows about it and if nobody would judge you?"* This ensures that the person is motivated by a wish to be different, rather than from external pressure.
3. *"Is it important to you although it might not play a role in your current life?"*

Exploration around these questions enables the clinician and client to address personally important concerns, as well as generate longer-term aims. In the end, the clinician and client consider how the client would like to be rather than how he is. Gradually, they build a focus for treatment and jointly identify goals. These goals should have a broader focus than preventing aggression or violence, which is seen as an end-product of, rather than the problem for, therapeutic work. Clients with ASPD complain that they are seen as "angry men" and sent to anger management classes, which merely serve to make them feel stereotyped and misunderstood.

Focus of Group Treatment

In MBT-ASPD, attention is paid equally to increasing mentalizing abilities that are underdeveloped and decreasing those that are overdeveloped. The core areas of focus include 1) affective understanding of self and others and 2) identification of relational patterns, and exploration of their desirable and undesirable consequences. Before joining a group focusing on interpersonal processes, clients undertake an introductory group program that offers psychoeducation about mentalizing and ASPD with the aim of developing personal reflection about emotional and relational difficulties. This program provides an introduction to mentalizing, helps clients understand attachment processes and mapping of relationship patterns, and addresses problems that are anticipated to be encountered in treatment.

INCREASING AFFECTIVE UNDERSTANDING OF SELF AND OTHERS

In the group work, clinicians are sensitive not only to the clients' compromised ability to express emotions but also to their consummate ability to avoid emotions. People with ASPD avoid recognizing self-affect states and so, to counter this tendency, the clinician persistently asks the client to describe his current subjective experience—this approach is distinct from asking the client how he feels. Most clients are unable to say how they feel but they can talk about their current experience—for example, whether they are comfortable or uncomfortable in the group, or are distant or involved. Validation of their experience is important with some exploration of the cause. Asking clients to identify these generic experiences in the group and exploring them is one of the first tasks of the group work. Only after they are comfortable can they begin to describe more specific feelings, such as concern, worry, or hurt, and give these feelings context from their life or from their experience in the group. Importantly, the clinician avoids evoking acute shame or embarrassment stimulated by interaction between members of the group.

The ability of an individual to identify how others feel and to be compassionate about it—that is, to be empathic—is an important part of mentalizing. Because of the problems people with ASPD have with "tuning in" to how others may be feeling (outlined earlier in this chapter), clinicians may need to ask a client directly what he thinks another participant feels, and inquire how he came to that conclusion. This is then checked out with the person in question—*"Is he right about how you feel?"* Different understanding from group participants of how someone feels can be explored. The aim is to continually build representations of affect states of self and others that are accurate and functional, increasing the cohesion of the interactions and interpersonal compassion.

IDENTIFICATION OF RELATIONAL PATTERNS: INCREASING CONSTRUCTIVE INTERACTION AND DECREASING DESTRUCTIVE INTERACTION

Each client who attends MBT-ASPD has been supported in the early phase of treatment to recognize his attachment patterns and identify how these are represented in his relationships. In particular, avoidant, overinvolved, controlling, and hierarchical patterns are considered. These are written down in the formulation jointly constructed with the client. On entry to the group, the client carries a "relational passport," which is part of the formulation (see Chapter 6, "Individual Therapy Techniques"), and hopefully has developed some level of personal mental representation of this pattern, since it has been discussed during the assessment phase. At his first group session, he is asked to present his problems and relationship style, with the aid of the clinicians. Sensitivity on the part of the clinicians is required to ensure that embarrassment and shame are not triggered for the participant. Commonly, one of the clinicians asks the current clients of the group to outline their own reasons for attending the group first, along with a description of their relational patterns. The aim is for all participants to begin to reflect on how they relate to others and for the clinicians to be attentive to the interactions in terms of the clients' relational patterns.

The clinician actively alights on relational interactions in the group, trying to identify constructive interactions as much as problematic interactions. Commonly, it is within destructive interactions that the alien self becomes apparent, with rigid, fixed interactions and schematic characterization of others. However, people with ASPD can be very supportive of one another, bonding through talk of being victimized by the police or criminal justice system, for example. This supportive process is also effected through activation of the alien self—externalization of blame to an external organization or system—so this needs to be differentiated from activation of the alien self in the context of intimacy. The externalization of problems to social systems and society creates a sense of shared difficulty, which increases group cohesion. This is important because harnessing shared experience creates a functioning group. So, first the clinician empathically validates the clients' sense of suffering at the hands of the system to maintain group cohesion, but eventually challenge is required because the rigid externalization to "the other" lacks self-and-other reflection, as pretend mode can become entrenched. Clients are therefore asked to explore their own contributions to their difficulties and regain some balance in self–other mentalizing.

More importantly, the clinician needs to move toward an understanding in the group that affective interaction between participants in the group is significant. Activation of each client's attachment strategies, identified at the beginning of treatment, becomes apparent. Exploration of interpersonal interactions in the group leads to an understanding of the processes that interfere with the generation of satisfying intimate relationships in clients' lives.

A particular finding from outcome research on the treatment of people with personality disorders is that their lives remain impaired (Bateman and Fonagy 2008). In the context of the poor social circumstances that are common in the lives of people with ASPD, everyday stressors and the social environment may easily undo the generation of positive change in therapy—hence the necessity to support such clients in the real world in which they live. In MBT for individuals with substance abuse problems (see Chapter 24, "Comorbid Substance Use Disorder and Personality Disorder"), this problem is addressed by having a social focus as an integrated part of treatment, with a social worker as a member of the professional team. This approach has not been specifically included in MBT-ASPD. However, current MBT-ASPD programs are implemented within probation services, which themselves have a designated task of supporting clients' rehousing and personal social development in terms of employment. Further integration of these services into the MBT-ASPD program is likely to bring benefits. To this end, some probation officers are trained to deliver the MBT program while simultaneously managing the client's risk to himself and others and supporting adaptation to life in the community after leaving prison.

MBT IN FORENSIC COMMUNITY SETTINGS

Delivering MBT programs to individuals within community probation services carries particular challenges. People with ASPD are often socially isolated and reluctant to leave their homes because of fears of acting on their impulses, especially in response to perceived threats from others, which activate intolerable emotions associated with vulnerability. This underscores the necessity of intervening proactively to engage and maintain clients in treatment, by, for example, telephoning clients after missed sessions or assessing them in settings that they find easier to travel to, such as their local probation office. Anxieties associated with being in crowded places or traveling on public transport can be addressed later in treatment.

Therapy may also be interrupted by frequent visits by the client to other health professionals, seeking treatment for physical complaints. Although these complaints may be strongly suspected to be psychosomatic in origin, they need to be taken seriously in therapy and the symptoms validated and given mental representation if they are psychosomatic in origin. At the same time, liaison with the client's general medical practitioner and other involved health services is required to promote the integration of MBT within the client's overall treatment plan and pathway.

Liaison with other professionals, especially those involved in the criminal justice system, is also essential regarding issues of risk; as noted earlier, these issues may comprise risk to the self and/or others. Here, the balance of maintaining the person's confidentiality and maintaining his trust and a positive therapeutic alliance versus disclosure of the perceived risk, and the possibility that the person will drop out of treatment, must be carefully considered. Thresholds for disclosure differ between health and criminal justice settings. These issues need to be clarified at the onset of treatment with the other professionals involved, and discussed with the clients/offenders, so that they understand the conditions under which their confidentiality may be breached. This clarification and openness between professionals and the client is an example of dealing with the "elephant in the room" and the subject of an affect focus. MBT promotes a therapeutic stance of transparency and openness; individuals with ASPD are often particularly sensitive to opaqueness in others, which they are apt to find persecutory, and it is therefore crucial that clinicians are candid in their communications and that the boundaries of therapy are agreed at the beginning of treatment. Negotiating boundaries may be particularly vexatious if the individual remains involved with a criminal subculture, including gang membership, which is increasingly common for younger offenders. Clients or offenders in group therapy may know others in the group from their past or present criminal associations or previous contacts in prison, and this may inhibit them from engaging in therapy and revealing details of their offending due to fears of retribution.

An important factor predicting positive outcomes of any therapy is the motivation of the person to engage in treatment. When such motivation is lacking, therapy is more likely to be ineffective. This poses a problem in working with individuals with ASPD, given their frequent antipathy toward treatment; the option of mandatory treatment, albeit being mandated through the courts or as a condition of their probation license, should be considered. Compulsory treatment may seem at odds with the ethos of MBT, which promotes flexibility of thinking and mutual respect within interpersonal relationships. However, almost all existing treatment programs for offenders within the criminal justice system, including those in community settings such as open prisons and probation, are mandatory. This arrangement may be therapeutically counterproductive for some individuals, but for others, who are equally suspicious and rejecting of treatment, exposure to a less structured and more flexible therapy such as MBT may unexpectedly engage their interest and trust in a new process. Engagement in treatment is also likely to be enhanced if others involved in the person's management, such as probation officers, have some understanding of the mentalizing model and how it differs from other more structured and offense-focused treatment programs.

MBT IN PRISON SETTINGS

Treatment for people with ASPD should ideally begin within prison settings and not be delayed until they are released into the community. Because of this, MBT-ASPD is now being offered within custodial settings, with the aim of making it continuous with treatment on release.

The application of MBT-ASPD to prison populations offers a unique opportunity for engaging clients in treatment, and a chance for even high-risk men facing long sentences to develop a new way of understanding how and why they have developed entrenched, destructive ways of relating to others. The groups offer the members effective psychological interventions that can both reduce the risk of reoffending on release and enhance the chances of early release, decreasing the likelihood of adjudications in custody.

Pragmatic Considerations for Implementation

When clinicians are considering whether to establish MBT groups within a prison, it is essential to bear certain pragmatic concerns in mind, including the need for senior management within the prison to be fully supportive of the group program, the need for training and supervision for staff, and the length of average stay for prisoners. Senior management support is essential to support the training, supervision, and time required for the psychological clinicians to run the groups, and such support also means that prison wing staff will ensure the prisoners attend the groups. The purpose of the group should be clear to the prison staff and senior managers, so that they understand its purpose and can respect and maintain the boundaries required for group attendance. All too often, if different subsystems within the prison service are not working together, group attendance in prisons is disrupted by alternative activities being organized that conflict with group time.

Other considerations include securing the ethical agreement required to film or audio record the sessions for supervision or research purposes, establishing the limits of confidentiality, setting ground rules for the disclosure of sensitive information that could place a prisoner at risk of harm from others (e.g., disclosing a sexual offense), determining how and where to record session notes, and establishing group ground rules (e.g., that violence will not be tolerated within the group, that members are expected to respect confidentiality). Furthermore, the emotional toll on the prisoners of attending this group should be acknowledged, as MBT is designed to engage them on an affective as well as a cognitive level and may leave them feeling moved by, or reflective about, disturbing experiences in their own early lives. It may be that prison wing staff will need to be informed if a group member is thought to require additional support and monitoring after a group.

One fundamental difference from a community-based setting is that prisoners live in very close proximity to one another. Clearly, any disruption or conflict within a group between prisoners who are housed together in the prison may create tension that could spill out on the accommodation wing, and this issue needs consideration. Resolution of conflict within the MBT group will thus be a priority; in most cases, skilled clinicians will be able to address conflicts within the group and not leave the group members feeling that they need to resolve issues outside the group. In some cases, however, confidentiality will need to be broken so that prison wing staff are alerted to the risk of some ongoing conflict between prisoners. The limits of confidentiality need to be clearly explained within the group from the outset. In addition, the clinicians should make clear the expectation that all group members attend reliably, especially in the shorter MBT-Introductory (MBT-I) groups (see Chapter 6), which last only 8–12 weeks.

Tips for Delivery of Treatment

The usual principles of MBT-ASPD apply within the prison setting, but here we emphasize aspects of delivery that may require special attention.

ENSURE CLINICIANS ARE TRAINED IN MBT AND SUPERVISION STRUCTURES ARE IN PLACE

Treatment in prisons poses particular challenges to the clinicians providing the treatment. Clinicians must have at least basic training in MBT and must demonstrate skill in adopting an MBT stance. Identifying suitable clinicians to run the groups is key: they must be consistent and reliable, and the same two clinicians must both be available each week. Furthermore, once identified, the clinicians need to establish a clear system of working together and being able to call on one another during groups 1) to monitor group members' arousal levels and 2) to check out and clarify themes, process, and points of confusion in the group. The clinicians' ability to model open dialogue and to acknowledge areas of confusion, or points during a session when the clinicians themselves are not able to mentalize, will be invaluable for group members. Regular supervision of clinicians is essential for ensuring the groups are adherent to the MBT-ASPD model.

MAINTAIN A NOT-KNOWING STANCE
AND EMPHASIZE ENGAGEMENT

The ongoing stance of curiosity, "not-knowing," and empathic interest may be difficult to maintain in the face of frightening or disturbing material that the prisoners will no doubt bring, but it is essential to hold on to this stance. The prisoners will often describe situations that are not familiar to the lives of the clinicians and allude to a value system that they have encoded, as well as some rote behavior that is alien to nonoffenders. Clinicians must remain curious about how these beliefs and feelings arise. Rather than assuming that they know what prisoners are feeling, clinicians must help them explore, while remaining curious, interested, and empathic as the prisoners begin to think about their own minds. As described earlier in this chapter, engagement is essential and particularly challenging for groups with ASPD.

GET MENTALIZING BACK ON TRACK
RATHER THAN JOINING WITH NONMENTALIZING

One risk is that clinicians will often join with nonmentalizing that inevitably occurs in the group in an attempt to explore or challenge it. Instead, they need to stop the ineffective mentalizing and then try to reflect with the prisoner on what was going on before he became aroused and unable to mentalize. This task may require techniques such as "stop and rewind" and "microslicing" of the nonmentalizing speech or description (Bateman and Fonagy 2016); these techniques bring the prisoner back to a lower level of arousal where he is able to reflect and to link thoughts and feelings, and can begin to gain a fuller understanding of his own mind and its emotional content.

TRACK THE PROCESS OF NONMENTALIZING
RATHER THAN ARGUING WITH THE CONTENT
OF NONMENTALIZING DESCRIPTIONS

One of the major challenges for clinicians will be the need to manage some prisoners' vehement descriptions of groups of people (e.g., women, prison staff, people from other cultures, sex offenders) using highly derogatory terms, with little room for questioning. This type of speech and attitude is a consequence of activation of the alien self, as described earlier. Managing it is often an emotional challenge to clinicians, who may worry about appearing to "collude" with views that run contrary to their own, or who may struggle with their own countertransference feelings about individuals who espouse unpleasant, frightening, or otherwise disturbing views and beliefs. In the face of this emotional onslaught, clinicians must remember to track the nonmentalizing process that is being demonstrated, rather than to get caught up in arguing with the prisoners about being "racist," "sexist," or "wrong." The clinicians must resist being drawn into arguments about the nonmentalizing content, as such arguments will not only antagonize and "lose" the prisoners, but also actually increase the nonmentalizing. Instead, clinicians should express interest, curiosity, and empathy with the underlying feelings once the nonmentalizing "rant" has been stopped. It is essential to the efficacy of the treatment that these beliefs and accompanying feelings be understood, deconstructed, and challenged, by use of an empathic and exploratory approach. Only this approach will allow the prisoners themselves to get to the point where they can challenge their own generalizations and identify the underlying feelings that led to them.

START WITH MENTALIZING THE SELF

This tip relates to a general principle with which clinicians, particularly those used to working in offense-specific models of treatment, may be unfamiliar: *to mentalize others requires the capacity to mentalize the self.* For example, it is simply not possible to jump from feeling furious with others to empathizing with them. The naive view of establishing empathy through cognitive challenges, in the absence of full identification and elaboration of the affective component of nonmentalizing, is enshrined in many offense-specific treatment programs. MBT clinicians are asked to be circumspect about this dynamic and are advised initially to focus more on mentalizing the self before exploring the understanding of others' mental states.

RETAIN HUMANITY, HUMOR, AND THE CAPACITY TO APOLOGIZE

Clinicians who are used to being in a clear authority role in relation to offender clients may be loath to apologize or to admit to "getting things wrong," and may even unconsciously equate this type of honesty with "losing control." MBT requires such authenticity, however. This approachwill prove invaluable in enabling the prisoners both to respect the clinicians and to recognize that everyone can misunderstand another's mental state, or inadvertently trigger anger, embarrassment, or fear in another person. A clinician who can acknowledge his own misunderstandings and the unintended impact they have on a prisoner will go much further in engaging the prisoner than someone attempting to retain authority at all times. Retaining a sense of humility and being able to acknowledge the clinician's own mentalizing lapses will be far more effective when working with individuals with ASPD who distrust authority figures.

Clinical Illustration

The Irish Prison Service began training psychologists in MBT with a view to rolling out an MBT program across the prison service in 2018, with specialist training and supervision provided by the Anna Freud National Centre for Children and Families (AFNCCF), London, beginning in 2016 with a pilot project with two sites. The experience of these clinicians has been a high level of engagement in the project by the prisoners, exploration of areas that were previously untouched in traditional offense-specific work, and reduced rates of adjudications for the men involved in the groups.

The clinicians have enjoyed the experience of using a new therapeutic model, in which neither traditional psychoanalytic methods nor strict cognitive-behavioral approaches are used; both approaches are integrated within an attachment-based model. Some of the challenges of the approach became evident in the pilot.

- First was the need to consider the impact of the close proximity of group members outside the groups, as the prisoners lived together on the wings. It was essential that group members agreed to respect the confidentiality condition of the MBT group, and not to take information gleaned about one another on to the wing.
- Second, the men were filmed for the purpose of supervision of the clinicians; this meant that their trust in the group clinicians needed to be developed fully, and it was essential that they not be inhibited by the presence of the cameras. For this purpose, the clinicians also needed to obtain ethical consent and draw up clear guidelines on how these recordings would be used and stored.

- Third, the limited resources in terms of clinicians' time meant that the groups were MBT-I groups rather than the longer-term and more intense MBT process groups. It also was not possible to offer individual sessions; and thus, the prisoners had to bring their most pressing issues to the group.

Despite these limitations, the engagement and quality of the groups was high. The clinicians are now all involved in the rollout, with a view to developing an MBT-ASPD center of excellence in Ireland, under the supervision of the AFNCCF, with a clear research plan to demonstrate outcomes.

CONCLUSION

MBT-ASPD is an innovative treatment that is being tested in a randomized controlled trial (ongoing at the time of writing) and is implemented in a range of settings. Treatment uses a mentalizing framework to understand ASPD and focus interventions. People with ASPD are more likely to respond to peer process than to a hierarchically structured intervention, so MBT-ASPD is organized as a group intervention. Effective implementation can occur only if the system around the person with ASPD supports the intervention; it is thus essential for the clinicians to work with the criminal justice system and the prison system. In custodial settings, the prison officers are trained in mentalizing skills; in probation services, the probation officers may themselves participate in the groups. Engagement of clients is supported by "experts by experience," who have participated in MBT treatment. In keeping with the mentalizing model, an individual with ASPD is more likely to experience a sense of being understood if his difficulties, and solutions to them, are presented to him by someone who shares his perspectives and experiences.

REFERENCES

Bateman A, Fonagy P: 8-year follow-up of patients treated for borderline personality disorder: mentalization-based treatment versus treatment as usual. Am J Psychiatry 165(5):631–638, 2008 18347003

Bateman A, Fonagy P: Mentalization-Based Treatment for Personality Disorders: A Practical Guide. Oxford, UK, Oxford University Press, 2016

Bateman A, Bolton R, Fonagy P: Antisocial personality disorder: a mentalizing framework. Focus 11:178–186, 2013

Black DW, Baumgard CH, Bell SE, et al: Death rates in 71 men with antisocial personality disorder. A comparison with general population mortality. Psychosomatics 37(2):131–136, 1996 8742541

Byrne SA, Cherniack MG, Petry NM: Antisocial personality disorder is associated with receipt of physical disability benefits in substance abuse treatment patients. Drug Alcohol Depend 132(1–2):373–377, 2013 23394688

Coid J, Yang M, Tyrer P, et al: Prevalence and correlates of personality disorder in Great Britain. Br J Psychiatry 188:423–431, 2006 16648528

Compton WM, Conway KP, Stinson FS, et al: Prevalence, correlates, and comorbidity of DSM-IV antisocial personality syndromes and alcohol and specific drug use disorders in the United States: results from the national epidemiologic survey on alcohol and related conditions. J Clin Psychiatry 66(6):677–685, 2005 15960559

Decety J, Michalska KJ, Akitsuki Y, et al: Atypical empathic responses in adolescents with aggressive conduct disorder: a functional MRI investigation. Biol Psychol 80(2):203–211, 2009 18940230

Gilligan J: Violence: Reflections on Our Deadliest Epidemic. London, Jessica Kingsley, 2000

Lenzenweger MF, Lane MC, Loranger AW, et al: DSM-IV personality disorders in the National Comorbidity Survey Replication. Biol Psychiatry 62(6):553–564, 2007 17217923

Martin RL, Cloninger CR, Guze SB, et al: Mortality in a follow-up of 500 psychiatric outpatients. I. Total mortality. Arch Gen Psychiatry 42(1):47–54, 1985 3966852

Torgersen S, Kringlen E, Cramer V: The prevalence of personality disorders in a community sample. Arch Gen Psychiatry 58(6):590–596, 2001 11386989

AVOIDANT AND NARCISSISTIC PERSONALITY DISORDERS

Sebastian Simonsen, Ph.D.

Sebastian Euler, M.D.

Both avoidant personality disorder (AvPD) and narcissistic personality disorder (NPD) are characterized by an insecure, predominantly avoidant attachment style that seriously impairs mentalizing capacity and consequently makes it difficult for patients with these disorders to maintain satisfying social lives. Individuals with either of the two disorders also have in common a vulnerability, in that their sense of self-worth is unstable and heavily influenced by how they believe they are viewed by others. Narcissism is often conceptualized as consisting of both grandiose and vulnerable features (Ronningstam 2005). Grandiose features are not common in AvPD, but vulnerable narcissism and AvPD share many characteristics, especially avoidance, shame proneness, and overuse of fantasy (Dickinson and Pincus 2003). In this chapter we view the symptomatology of the two disorders from a mentalizing perspective and provide some guidance in regard to taking a mentalization-based therapeutic stance.

AVOIDANT PERSONALITY DISORDER

Core Pathology

AvPD is common in outpatient settings (Zimmerman et al. 2005) and services specializing in the treatment of personality disorders (Karterud and Wilberg 2007; Simonsen et al. 2017). Despite being a common presentation, AvPD has existed quietly in the shadow of more prominent disorders such as borderline personality disorder (BPD) and social phobia. The unsatisfying status of research on psychopathology and treatment of AvPD has been pointed out in recent studies and reviews (Eikenaes et al. 2013; Lampe 2016). In addition, patients in the few randomized controlled trials that have been conducted do not seem representative of the more poorly functioning end of the AvPD spectrum (for a recent review, see Bateman et al. 2015). Mentalizing may provide a clinically useful framework for clinicians to use with patients with AvPD.

Individuals with AvPD are most often characterized by *hypermentalizing*—using thoughts and reflection as a way of distancing themselves from whatever emotions are evoked in situations (Bateman and Fonagy 2012). AvPD is thus also often considered a disorder of inhibition and viewed as being the opposite of BPD (Dimaggio et al. 2007a). Hypermentalizing may resemble mentalizing but tends to come across as an overly analytical, cognitive style that lacks authentic affectivity (see Chapter 1, "Introduction," for further discussion of hypermentalizing). In addition, when hypermentalizing, people tend to be focused only on a very particular, often self-serving perspective, which hinders the ability to shift perspective, for example, from self to other or from cognition to affect (Bateman and Fonagy 2015). This lack of openness is often an important obstacle to development in general and therapeutic progress in particular.

Attachment and Avoidance

Patients with AvPD often show high levels of both attachment anxiety and avoidance, consistent with a fearful attachment style (Eikenaes et al. 2016; Riggs et al. 2007). Hence, both the view of the self and that of others are quite consistently negatively biased. Thus, although everyone may sometimes feel that "hell is other people," the inner world of many patients with AvPD is even more painful and bewildered, with patients often reporting that they oscillate between hypermentalizing and avoiding emotions, which could be labeled *hypomentalizing*. Millon (1981) described the typical object representation of people with AvPD as being caught in the worst of both worlds, meaning that patients with AvPD are able neither to find ease within themselves nor to seek refuge and comfort in others. From this perspective, these patients in some ways seem harder to reach than patients who are more preoccupied, needy, and explicit about how they feel about others. On the basis of recent developments in mentalizing theory emphasizing the (re)establishment of epistemic trust (see Chapter 4, "Mentalizing, Resilience, and Epistemic Trust," and Chapter 10, "Therapeutic Models") as a core feature of the treatment of personality disorders, AvPD, like BPD, may be understood as a communication breakdown. Anxiety and fearful attachment are then a result of social signaling in the familial context inscribing specific mentalizing capacities that will be outlined in the following sections. Such a model with specific environmental causes for AvPD is in accordance with twin studies supporting qualitative differences between social anxiety disorder and AvPD (Torvik et al. 2016) and developmental models of psychopathology (Nolte et al. 2011).

From the beginning, the mentalizing literature in regard to BPD has focused especially on attachment and affiliation (Fonagy and Target 1997). However, the psychopathology of patients with AvPD necessitates greater awareness of the social-status system (Dimaggio et al. 2015; Liotti and Gilbert 2011). Patients with AvPD may fear separation, but in many cases—as with NPD—they may also be focused on issues of autonomy and relational power dynamics.

Impaired Mentalizing

There are few studies of mentalizing in patients with AvPD, and the results of those that exist are not consistent, probably because of measurement, sample, and contextual issues; for example, Arntz et al. (2009) reported that Cluster C patients outperformed both a nonclinical sample and patients with BPD on an advanced measure of explicit theory of mind. Within the theory of metacognition, important mind-reading characteristics of patients with AvPD have been described, with pronounced problems in the basic ability to monitor mental states (Semerari et al. 2014). While patients with BPD are often characterized by considerable affective instability and variance in mentalizing across situations, the basic failure in monitoring function in AvPD results in a more stable, but persistent, problem that affects most interpersonal areas, situations, and relationships. A mentalizing profile (Figure 21–1) can be described by using the four mentalizing dimensions (see Chapter 1, "Introduction," and Chapter 3, "Assessment of Mentalizing"). Mentalizing functioning in one dimension often affects mentalizing in other dimensions, and thus the dimensions cannot be completely separated. However, the dimensions do provide a useful structure for understanding psychopathology, including both AvPD and NPD, in terms of typical patterns of mentalizing.

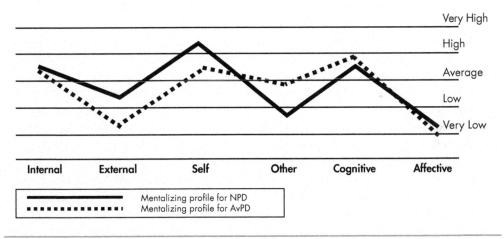

Figure 21–1. Mentalizing profiles for narcissistic personality disorder (NPD) and avoidant personality disorder (AvPD).

IMPLICIT–EXPLICIT DIMENSION

Moroni et al. (2016) found that patients with AvPD in particular are characterized by difficulties with monitoring mental states. These patients are often very uncertain or confused about their own feelings or thoughts about something. Shifting to the explicit mode is challenging, because many of these patients are then faced with a profoundly negative self-image without sufficient nuance; for example, *"I am worthless"* or *"I feel only shame about who I am."* From this perspective, it is completely understandable that patients shy away from an explicit mentalizing focus, even though this is, arguably, exactly what is needed. Therapists working with AvPD should be aware of this self-perpetuating cycle and strive to mentalize with the patient as to when and why explicit mentalizing becomes too painful.

SELF–OTHER DIMENSION

Patients with AvPD often have a fearful attachment style. Thus, mentally benign good object representations are fragile and insufficiently developed. They avoid others both behaviorally and mentally. The default mentalizing position of individuals with AvPD is the self rather than others (Dimaggio et al. 2007a, 2008a). This is somewhat confusing, as AvPD is also often comorbid with social phobia (40%–45%; Bögels et al. 2010; Friborg et al. 2013), which involves an exaggerated focus on how the individual is evaluated by others in social situations. However, AvPD patients have more severe metacognitive difficulties with both alexithymia and the capacity for decentration—that is, dealing with the fact that others have a different perspective from their own (Moroni et al. 2016; Nicolò et al. 2011). From an interpersonal perspective, social phobia and AvPD are probably not qualitatively different, as both positions are defined by a marked tendency toward social avoidance and nonassertiveness (Eikenaes et al. 2013; Wright et al. 2009). If there are qualitative differences, these are more likely to be found in how the self or the person mentally and behaviorally handles and regulates this interpersonal challenge (Marques et al. 2012).

COGNITIVE–AFFECTIVE DIMENSION

Patients with AvPD tend to be more cognitive than affective in their mentalizing stance. With regard to primary emotions, they have marked difficulties with accessing feelings of play and curiosity (Karterud et al. 2016). Anxiety and shame often dominate, but these emotions are also avoided, both internally, via hypomentalizing and hypermentalizing (e.g., intellectualization and rumination), and externally, by means of social withdrawal. In the most severe cases, mentalized affectivity is more or less absent. In support of this, Johansen et al. (2013) found that patients with AvPD had significantly lower levels of global affect consciousness and conceptual expressivity compared with patients with BPD. A functional magnetic resonance imaging (fMRI) study comparing AvPD patients with healthy controls found amygdala hyperreactivity in anticipation of an explicit emotion-regulation task (Denny et al. 2015). Thus, a common sequence, especially prior to social engagement, would be hypermentalizing leading to heightened amygdala responses, followed by avoidance and hypomentalizing. People with AvPD have great difficulty sharing their feelings with others, and even close relatives are often not fully aware of the pain experienced by these individuals (Carlson et al. 2013). In mentalizing terms, this may be viewed as gross communication problems, both with the congruency of affective mirroring and with the marking of emotions.

INTERNAL–EXTERNAL DIMENSION

An fMRI study found that during repeated viewings of negatively valent pictures (e.g., showing a car accident or an aggressive dog), AvPD patients exhibited less insula–ventral anterior cingulate functional connectivity than both healthy subjects and patients with BPD (Koenigsberg et al. 2014). This difference in connectivity would translate into problems with implicit habituation, especially with the process of making connections between internal bodily sensations and relevant external stimuli (interoceptive awareness). A similar dysfunction has been found in general social anxiety disorder (Klumpp et al. 2012). In terms of external mentalizing, Rosenthal et al. (2011) found that compared with control subjects without AvPD, patients with

AvPD were significantly more likely to misclassify fully expressed fear (when viewing morphed pictures). No other significant differences were found in speed or classification with regard to recognizing other emotions. Although emotional regulation was not assessed in this study, the finding may be explained as an implicit attentional strategy whereby patients with AvPD regulate arousal by diverting attention away from the source of discomfort, that is, by avoidance. With external mentalizing, the main problem may be not with recognition, but instead with expression or display. If emotions are not expressed verbally and, especially, nonverbally, others will find it harder to mentalize the person. This may make social interactions (including therapy) less helpful. In addition, mirroring and mimicry are involved in both learning and affiliation (Kavanagh and Winkielman 2016), which may thus be affected by blunted expressivity, especially in group settings (Kongerslev et al. 2015).

Nonmentalistic Modes and Mentalization-Based Treatment

Overall, the default setting for AvPD is internal mentalizing; affects, others, and external information are not sufficiently processed. The main mode is hypermentalizing: patients often focus on very specific aspects, which are then interpreted and considered in so many ways that the essence is lost, others are unable to follow the patient's thoughts, and the patient becomes exhausted. In many cases, the motive behind such a pattern is probably to avoid expected criticism from others and thus to achieve a sense of safety. When the fear of condemnation is so strong, it is almost impossible to retain the capacity for curiosity and mentalizing. Many patients with AvPD are virtually obsessed with being liked, in contrast to most nonavoidant individuals, who, when they do not feel authentically recognized for who they are, react with rejection or indifference. In therapy with AvPD patients, the exact opposite should be the aim, and balancing safety and curiosity is a continuous focus of attention in drawing patients away from the internal, fearful, hypermentalizing position about being liked or disliked in which they are trapped.

Across different therapy models, a common countertransference reaction toward patients with AvPD is a parental and supportive stance (Betan et al. 2005). This may be viewed as the underlying affect focus, whereby the therapist's probing of the patient's mind leads to an uncomfortable state that rather than being addressed directly, leads to reassuring and advice-giving interventions. In general, one helpful tool for countering avoidance in both patient and therapist is to introduce predefined tasks and exercises that trigger explicit mentalizing. A powerful example is the video task developed by David Clark (2001) for social phobia. In this task, patients are filmed while giving a 3-minute speech in a group and are then interviewed about what they believe they will see when they subsequently view the video. The exercise is a powerful way to make the patients' negative automatic thoughts explicit along with their thoughts on how and why their perception of themselves differs from other people's view of them.

Like individuals with BPD, many AvPD patients fear abandonment (Pedersen et al. 2015), but often they also have a sense of being controlled, criticized, and ridiculed, without being able to mentalize explicitly that this is what is going on inside them. Sometimes, this emotional theme may manifest as passive-aggressive behavior, but mostly it is manifest as a feeling in the therapist of not "being on the same wavelength" as the patient. The therapist needs to be aware that such reactions from the patient are not necessarily about discomfort with affiliation, but may just as well have been triggered by the patient's feeling that his or her autonomy is threatened.

Even when they have some emotional awareness, patients with AvPD are unlikely to disclose and display feelings and will therefore not be contained and shifted by relevant mentalizing from others. This poses a challenge for the therapist, who needs to both identify and mark emotions that are often only vaguely expressed. Dimaggio et al. (2015) point out that therapists working with these patients need to be especially aware of nonverbal cues of elicited emotions, and that such displays should be reinforced and enriched. This technique may of course easily be overdone or be perceived as being too direct or even confrontational by the patient, triggering exactly the withdrawal pattern that the therapist is trying to counteract.

From a mentalizing perspective, therapists treating patients with AvPD are particularly challenged in their ability to be open, curious, and playful. This may be highly challenging because the mental material brought forth by the patient, compared with ordinary standards, provides very little material to work with. It is important that therapists working with AvPD are able to discuss patients and receive regular supervision lest they end up colluding with the patient's avoidance or acting out feelings of boredom; above all, therapists need help in order to stay emotionally alive.

NARCISSISTIC PERSONALITY DISORDER

Core Pathology

NPD is defined as a concentration of the psychic interest on the self, combined with an overwhelming need for admiration (Moore and Fine 1968; Wink 1991), and is primarily characterized by difficulties with interpersonal relationships (American Psychiatric Association 2013). Patients usually seek psychotherapeutic help for social implications or when compensatory gratifications in interpersonal relationships fall away. Many patients do not genuinely suffer from their underlying structural psychopathology (Ronningstam 2005). Comorbid depression, addiction, and suicidal crises are common (Euler et al. 2015; Ronningstam 2010). From a developmental perspective, the self of a person with NPD is marked by feelings of inferiority, insufficiency, shame, anger, and envy as a result of neglect or a chronic lack of support from attachment figures (Bennett 2006; Lorenzini and Fonagy 2013). The regulating second-order representations are not well integrated to handle these negative self-states because interpersonal matching by the caregivers during infantile personality development will have been repeatedly noncontingent and contradictory (Blatt and Levy 2003; Fonagy et al. 2008; Kernberg 1985; Otway and Vignoles 2006).

The abovementioned characteristics lead to particular difficulties for the psychotherapeutic treatment of patients with NPD, including a high dropout rate and frequent aversive countertransference reactions (Ellison et al. 2013; Ronningstam 2017; Tanzilli et al. 2017). Because emotional dysregulation and interpersonal dysfunction are key features of both BPD and NPD, although the disorders are highly distinctive in their phenomenology, it is especially challenging when the two disorders co-occur (comorbidity is frequent, with a prevalence of up to 40%; Stinson et al. 2008) and their specific mentalizing deficits accumulate (Diamond et al. 2014).

As conventional psychological and diagnostic descriptions tend to overemphasize grandiose aspects of narcissism (Olssøn et al. 2016; Pincus and Lukowitsky 2010; Skodol et al. 2014), the phenotypic description of vulnerable and grandiose features of narcissism is widely accepted today (Cain et al. 2008; Gore and Widiger 2016; Levy 2012; Miller and Campbell 2008). In the current literature, the terminology of "vulnerable" versus "grandiose" has largely replaced the formerly used descriptions of "thin-skinned" versus "thick-skinned" (Rosenfeld 1987) or "covered" versus "uncovered" (Wink 1991), although the terms are not necessarily synonymous. A dimensional understanding of narcissism has broad clinical implications, because grandiosely and vulnerably narcissistic patients differ in terms of psychopathology, treatment utilization, and countertransference reactions (Ellison et al. 2013; Euler et al. 2018; Rosenfeld 1987). Intrapersonal fluctuations of both facets are frequent in narcissistic patients, even within the same psychotherapeutic session (Bateman 1998; Gore and Widiger 2016).

Attachment and Narcissism

As with other disorders, impaired mentalizing in NPD is conceptualized around attachment theory. The individual's dependency on the caregiver in early life has not been experienced as secure, which has led to an inability to tolerate interpersonal dependency in adulthood. Consequently, many narcissistic patients maintain a hypoactive attachment system by detaching from others (Britton 2004; Dimaggio et al. 2008b). In narcissistic pathology, especially in grandiose narcissism, the attachment behavior is avoidant, that is, dismissive (Diamond et al. 2014). Unrecognized attachment needs are accompanied by compulsive self-reliance and the denial of environmental threats (Bowlby 1969; Dickinson and Pincus 2003; Lorenzini and Fonagy 2013). Because of a negative self-image, attachment in vulnerable narcissism might be both avoidant and anxious. Primary fears of rejection and hypersensitivity to criticism lead to secondary avoidant attachment behavior (Otway and Vignoles 2006; Smolewska and Dion 2005). Vulnerable narcissists would then look for agreement and deny interpersonal differences between minds (Bateman 1998). However, the evidence is partly contradictory, with some findings of secure attachment in grandiose narcissism, and anxious, but not avoidant, attachment in narcissism in general (Dickinson and Pincus 2003; Kealy et al. 2015). These contradictions support the abovementioned point that both facets of narcissism go hand in hand in patients, and thus, activated attachment patterns may consist of both avoidant and anxious elements. In any case, most of the evidence indicates that attachment patterns in NPD are insecure, with predominantly anxious attachment in vulnerable narcissism and predominantly avoidant attachment in grandiose narcissism. Insecure attachment leads to high rates of dropout from therapy, because the patients do not form a secure bond with the therapist. Therapists' relational approach is perceived as a threat to narcissistic patients, especially when they do not feel entirely understood or are confronted with therapists' disagreement or challenging interpersonal processes—but also when exposed to sometimes overwhelming "therapeutic" sympathy. Patients try to avoid interpersonal relatedness, including feelings of dependency and need (Lorenzini and Fonagy 2013). Their distant, disdainful, and discrediting behavior may also lead to aversive reactions from therapists, for instance, by rejecting patients' boundary and corroborative needs (Bennett 2006; Luchner et al. 2008).

Impaired Mentalizing in NPD

IMPLICIT–EXPLICIT DIMENSION

Individuals with NPD feel easily threatened with respect to a potential loss of interpersonal control. The greater they perceive this threat to their self-agency, the more profoundly their distorted attachment system will be activated. In consequence, mentalizing switches to an automatic mode. Mentalizing is then marked by stereotypic patterns—that is, it becomes less dynamic and flexible (Luyten and Fonagy 2015; Ronningstam 2010).

SELF–OTHER AND COGNITIVE–AFFECTIVE DIMENSIONS

According to the framework of mentalizing, narcissistic individuals are generally characterized as being mainly focused on their own mental state (see Figure 21–1). They control what others do for them in order to achieve an inner psychic benefit, but they find it difficult to empathize with someone else's state of mind (Bateman et al. 2013). Deficits have been found in affective, but not cognitive, empathy (Ritter et al. 2011); this finding corresponds with reduced gray matter in the insula (Schulze et al. 2013). Furthermore, lower deactivation of the insula during empathy is associated with narcissism (Fan et al. 2011). Patients with NPD are able to describe others' thoughts and emotions from their own point of view but find this difficult when someone else's mental state differs from their own. They also have difficulty describing different facets of affects and the underlying interpersonal context, as well as sympathizing with others (Dimaggio et al. 2008b). The underdeveloped self–other distinction leads to emotional stress when patients with NPD are forced to mentalize others' state of mind. Furthermore, their self-centeredness makes it difficult for them to perceive when others are empathizing with them. The neurobiological underpinnings of self–other distinctive mentalizing with impaired functional perception of the other have been outlined previously (Mitchell et al. 2006; Mizen 2014).

INTERNAL–EXTERNAL DIMENSION

Narcissistic patients are primarily focused on the internal regulation of their sense of self-worth. They may also focus on the internal states of others in order to control others' behavior with regard to their own intentions.

Nonmentalistic Modes and Mentalization-Based Treatment

In mentalization-based treatment (MBT), grandiose and dismissive behavior is not understood as an intrapsychological pathology that projects into the relationship; instead, it is regarded as reflecting a relationally based need for secure attachment. This requires optimal responsiveness from the therapist (Bateman and Fonagy 2016; Bennett 2006). A secure base is considered a prerequisite for exploring mental states (i.e., as occurs in psychotherapy), with respect for the consequences of the caregiver's misattunement with the patient's needs during childhood. Distancing the patient through neutrality or a transference interpretation is seen as an iatrogenic default when the attachment is experienced as insecure. We consider these kinds of interventions to cause harm, rather than benefit, specifically during precarious patient–therapist interactions. These approaches may then be interpreted as an enactment of a countertransference reaction, for instance, with the therapist's purpose of detaching from the patient in order to protect himself or herself from the projection of the patient's alien self (see Chapter 1).

In MBT, therapists take the responsibility to hold and contain emerging arousal (e.g., flooding of negative affects) by considering that they themselves genuinely contribute to an activation of the narcissistic patient's insecure attachment system by their relational approach (Bateman and Fonagy 2016; Bennett 2006). Otherwise, the therapist may cause the patient to detach into self-centeredness (pretend mode) or to devalue, or even dismiss, the therapist (psychic equivalence mode). Promoting the narcissistic patient's reflection on his or her own and the other's state of mind requires making the patient feel understood (and "felt") in order to foster epistemic trust (Fonagy and Allison 2014; Fonagy et al. 2015); this is done by the use of ostensive cues (see Chapter 10), for example. The mentalizing therapist needs to be well attuned to the patient's affective needs to generate strong emotional and interactional experiences that differ from the patient's attachment history.

MENTALIZING SELF AND OTHER

Several challenges for therapeutic interventions arise from the impaired self–other dimension of mentalizing in NPD patients. It has been proposed that fostering mentalizing of others may seem too threatening before the individual has mentalized himself or herself in a self-attentive manner; hence, therapeutic work should initially focus on self-reflection (Dimaggio et al. 2008b). On the other hand, such an approach may support narcissistic self-centeredness (Dimaggio et al. 2007b). Furthermore, successful mentalizing of others may lead to improved mentalizing of the self through mutual interdependence: *"If she felt hurt, perhaps I had provoked her by a subtle display of hostility."* However, this mentalizing is counterproductive if self-knowledge is used to apply stronger control to others. In this respect, affective mentalizing of the self is a prerequisite for social behavior (Bateman et al. 2013). Consequently, in MBT it is recommended that the therapist constantly monitor the self–other dynamics of the patient's mentalizing and intervene carefully by means of contrary moves (see Chapter 6, "Individual Therapy Techniques") in favor of a more integrated and equilibrated view of self and others. However, this is a challenging endeavor, as the patient's self-centeredness is also reflected in the patient–therapist interaction. Narcissistic patients often bring up self-centered, nonmentalistic "stories" in psychotherapy sessions, commonly engaging in lengthy narratives, as if the therapist were not present (pretend mode), or lacking any critical distance from their narrative (psychic equivalence mode). Furthermore, NPD patients tend to defend their own knowledge—even when they assume that it is incorrect—whenever they feel threatened by someone else challenging their assumptions or remembering things differently from their own perspective (psychic equivalence mode) (Fonagy and Allison 2014). Therapists must bear in mind that narcissistic patients may display an "allergic reaction" to others' thoughts or opinions (Britton 2004). They may feel that their own state of mind is being eliminated if they perceive an attack on their integrity.

SUPPORTIVE AND EMPATHIC VALIDATION

Overly self-elevating narratives and behavior indicate a reduced capability to mentalize in insecure attachment situations. Thus, the narcissistic patient's need for gratification requires supportive and empathic validation, particularly in the early stages of treatment (for an illustration, see the clinical example of an admission interview later in this chapter). At the same time, the therapist needs to tolerate feelings of insufficiency and devaluation in his or her countertransference. Empathic validation requires the therapist to find *something* to validate in the narrative; for example, that the patient has done well in his or her endeavor to support others. It is helpful to validate with a gentle and sometimes slightly questioning—but nonironic—tone in order to achieve *marked mirroring*. This helps the patient draw a line between self and other. When the patient does not feel safe enough, the projective identification of the alien self will not be challenged but will be maintained and contained as part of the *collaborative stance*.

NOT-KNOWING STANCE

The therapist promotes the patient's sense of security by adopting a sympathetic, respectful, honest, unprejudiced stance. He or she must be ready to adopt a not-knowing stance and *follow* the conversation instead of leading the process. The therapist must also sometimes show humility. As some patients may perceive a not-knowing stance as malignant, because it is not seen as sufficiently acknowledging their special significance and properly understanding them, all interventions must be highly responsive and finely tuned, that is, *contingent*. If the therapist's interventions fail in this regard and cause ruptures, the therapist takes responsibility for this.

When challenging the patient, the therapist should describe his or her perspective as an uncertain possibility resulting from a subjective perception, while maintaining an openness to alternative views.

AFFECT FOCUS

During affect focus, the therapist must be particularly aware of the danger of the patient pseudomentalizing by constantly checking the authenticity of his or her *mentalized affectivity*. Otherwise, the presence of pseudomentalizing or hypermentalizing with a self-serving (i.e., self- and cognitive-focused) perspective risks an extended therapeutic discourse in pretend mode. According to the four dimensions of mentalizing, the therapist will attempt a *contrary move* when the affective or self pole is underrepresented. In doing so, the therapist helps the patient to engage in full mentalizing whenever possible. Describing affects and accepting that thinking and acting are permanently influenced by emotions through affect elaboration and affect focus are hallmarks of MBT. If feelings of insufficiency, shame, fear, or insecurity are permitted by the narcissistic patient during treatment, it is important to observe whether the patient has sufficient capacity for mentalizing in the therapeutic situation. These feelings may be perceived in psychic equivalence mode, leading to a sudden breakdown of mentalizing. The therapist consistently accepts a shared responsibility for helping the patient overcome the affects that the therapist evokes. A narcissistic patient only gradually comes to command the second-order representation necessary for dealing with negative affective states in psychic equivalence mode.

MENTALIZING THE RELATIONSHIP

Eventually, the narcissistic patient will be able to mentalize the relationship with the therapist, but only once he or she has sufficiently mentalized himself or herself through affect elaboration and affect focus. To develop the other dimension, the patient must have a certain mentalizing capacity. A premature focus on mentalizing the relationship places the patient at risk of falling into pretend mode with a cognitive self-reflection that disregards the therapist's mind and relational dimensions. Hence, the therapy must be well structured, following the interventional hierarchy and trajectories of MBT (discussed in Chapter 6).

Clinical Example: Admission Interview in a Multicomponent Day Hospital for Personality Disorders

The patient is a 24-year-old male with NPD and comorbid cannabis and heavy internet abuse. Assessment interviews, diagnosis, and provision of a treatment plan were conducted before the interview by the psychologist in the outpatient unit. After being received by the staff, the patient is sent to the recreation room and told that the therapist will pass by during the course of the morning.

Attending: Patient (P), nurse (N), therapist (T)

The patient is welcomed, and everybody takes a seat.

P *(in a loud voice):* Is it normal procedure that the therapist does not come on time? Shouldn't she apologize for being late?

T: I am sorry, Mr. R, for your wait. I just got the call that we now have time for the intake interview. So I hurried and came straight here from another ward.

P: That is unbelievable. I came here this morning, and since then, nobody has told me a thing about the procedure. No one cares. I am in a room, waiting. After several hours, someone came in and told me to go downstairs for the interview. No one was there. So I waited even longer. That is so unprofessional. Finally, the therapist arrives, and she's not even willing to apologize.

N: I am really sorry for that. You are right, the planning wasn't ideal. Unfortunately. Sorry again.

P: Yeah, whatever.

N: Would it be okay to proceed with the treatment plan?

P: Mm.

N reads the treatment plan out loud and explains each point in detail. P vigorously interrupts N.

P: I already know all that. They told me at the outpatient unit. Can't we skip it?

N: Okay, good to know. I'll try to keep it brief.

N continues with the regulations (general hospital rules, agreements about use of drugs and the personal computer)

P: Why do I have to sign the online access agreement? I'm not even a computer gamer!

T: The psychologist at the outpatient unit informed us that you might have problems with that stuff.

P: So what? It's just not true. Cannabis yes, hospital rules, yes, but online access? I told her there was a time I played computer games, from age 10 to 15. Then I quit. I completely lost interest. I knew from the beginning this woman was incompetent.

T: Okay, let's see.

P: I can sign it. That is not the problem.

T: I suggest that I check again whether this particular agreement is necessary and let you know as soon as possible.

P: Whatever!

Meanwhile, the chief resident (CR) opens the door.

CR: Hello, everybody. Is it a good time to introduce myself?

T *(shaking her head)*: Sorry. Not right now, we are in the middle of something.

CR leaves the room. All attendants sign the agreements. N leaves the room.

P *(furious)*: Couldn't you shake your head a little more *(shakes his head vigorously)*? What would he think? Why didn't you just tell him to leave?

T: I'm sorry. That might make you feel embarrassed.

P *(expressing contempt)*: I'm not embarrassed! This place is a joke. It's exactly like the other place [*psychiatric hospital where he had been a few months earlier*]. I left after 6 hours. This is ridiculous!

T: Mm. I see. The thing is, I don't know why you left the other hospital. Could you explain it to me?

P: The treatment was unprofessional, as it is here. I felt isolated, and I was disappointed. I went there for help, but no one helped me. I was all alone in my room. You can't leave someone with depression alone in their room. And here, it's the same. No one cares.

T: Yes, I understand. Now I can better understand why you are so upset. Could you tell me more about yourself and what you are struggling with in life?

P: I have had depressive episodes for the past 6 years. That's why I go to therapy. Besides, I struggle with a sleep disorder. During these episodes I become more irritable, less tolerant, and I try to avoid people. Also, I have issues with others, like with my brother. I want to tell him something, but he just doesn't get it. Then he tells me to leave him alone and goes away. I don't understand that.

T: Do you have any idea why?

P: I don't know. People don't get me.

T: I see. But that would probably make me feel angry.

P: Yes, it does.

T: Is this issue one of the reasons why you are here?

P: Hm. I don't know why I'm here, actually.

T: I see you're really struggling with these issues, and I'm sorry we had a rough start. Thank you for sharing some of your burden with me. We will have time to talk about this. May I tell you how the next days are organized now? After that, the chief resident will come back to welcome you. Okay?

P agrees and seems calmer and less agitated.

The insecure boundary situation triggers the patient's anxious attachment pattern, leading to open entitlement rage and dismissive behavior toward the staff. Initially, the patient has no mentalizing capacity at all. He is in a teleological mode (being late means being totally unprofessional and ridiculous; preparing an online gaming agreement confirms the incompetence of the psychologist in the outpatient unit; the therapist's shaking her head gives the chief resident a signal about "something" about the patient). The therapist's submissive and open-minded stance helps "cool down" the patient's attachment system, and even enables the patient to point to certain aspects of his personal history and to name some affects he perceived earlier. In this description, vulnerable narcissistic features become obvious. The therapist decides not to enter too deeply into these issues due to the precarious attachment situation when the patient answers in pretend mode (*"I don't know"*). Because of the patient's limited mentalizing capacity at this point, the therapist simply shows empathic validation after the patient has calmed down and feels more comfortable. She then does a contrary move toward the organizational structure of the following days. The main issue of the admission interview, from the therapist's point of view, is to create an ambience of epistemic trust and safety, to foster the patient's capacity to mentalize during the upcoming psychotherapeutic process.

CONCLUSION

The purpose of this chapter is to provide some compelling reasons why the mentalizing framework and consequently MBT might be promising in the treatment of AvPD and NPD. However, as of the time of this writing, no well-controlled treatment studies of MBT have been done for either AvPD or NPD. Much work is needed before MBT can be used with more confidence of efficacy, including such trials and further studies of neurobiology and social cognition. Research on both disorders has previously been primarily psychopathological and cross-sectional in nature, so, little is known about dynamic, developmental, and therapeutic processes over time. Studies with multiple time-point measurements would likely be of great value in identifying the most important contextual factors and mechanisms of change, including in particular shifts in mentalizing and affect consciousness. However, from our point of view, until this work has been done, practicing MBT in the treatment of patients with AvPD and NPD is an auspicious approach.

REFERENCES

American Psychiatric Association: Diagnostic and Statistical Manual of Mental Disorders, 5th Edition. Arlington, VA, American Psychiatric Association, 2013

Arntz A, Bernstein D, Oorschot M, et al: Theory of mind in borderline and cluster-C personality disorder. J Nerv Ment Dis 197(11):801–807, 2009 19996717

Bateman A, Fonagy P: Borderline personality disorder and mood disorders: mentalizing as a framework for integrated treatment. J Clin Psychol 71(8):792–804, 2015 26190067

Bateman A, Fonagy P: Mentalization-Based Treatment for Personality Disorders: A Practical Guide. Oxford, UK, Oxford University Press, 2016

Bateman A, Bolton R, Fonagy P: Antisocial personality disorder: a mentalizing framework. Focus 11:178–186, 2013

Bateman AW: Thick- and thin-skinned organisations and enactment in borderline and narcissistic disorders. Int J Psychoanal 79(Pt 1):13–25, 1998 9587805

Bateman AW, Fonagy P: Handbook of Mentalizing in Mental Health Practice. Washington, DC, American Psychiatric Publishing, 2012

Bateman AW, Gunderson J, Mulder R: Treatment of personality disorder. Lancet 385(9969):735–743, 2015 25706219

Bennett CS: Attachment theory and research applied to the conceptualization and treatment of pathological narcissism. Clin Soc Work J 34:45–60, 2006

Betan E, Heim AK, Zittel Conklin C, et al: Countertransference phenomena and personality pathology in clinical practice: an empirical investigation. Am J Psychiatry 162(5):890–898, 2005 15863790

Blatt SJ, Levy KN: Attachment theory, psychoanalysis, personality development, and psychopathology. Psychoanalytic Inquiry 23:102–150, 2003

Bögels SM, Alden L, Beidel DC, et al: Social anxiety disorder: questions and answers for the DSM-V. Depress Anxiety 27(2):168–189, 2010 20143427

Bowlby J: Attachment and Loss, Vol 1: Attachment. London, Hogarth Press and Institute of Psycho-Analysis, 1969

Britton R: Narcissistic disorders in clinical practice. J Anal Psychol 49(4):477–490; discussion 491–473, 2004 15317528

Cain NM, Pincus AL, Ansell EB: Narcissism at the crossroads: phenotypic description of pathological narcissism across clinical theory, social/personality psychology, and psychiatric diagnosis. Clin Psychol Rev 28(4):638–656, 2008 18029072

Carlson EN, Vazire S, Oltmanns TF: Self-other knowledge asymmetries in personality pathology. J Pers 81(2):155–170, 2013 22583054

Clark DM: A cognitive perspective on social phobia, in International Handbook of Social Anxiety: Concepts, Research and Interventions Relating to the Self and Shyness. Edited by Crozier WR, Alden LE. Chichester, UK, Wiley, 2001, pp 405–430

Denny BT, Fan J, Liu X, et al: Elevated amygdala activity during reappraisal anticipation predicts anxiety in avoidant personality disorder. J Affect Disord 172:1–7, 2015 25451388

Diamond D, Levy KN, Clarkin JF, et al: Attachment and mentalization in female patients with comorbid narcissistic and borderline personality disorder. Pers Disord 5(4):428–433, 2014 25314231

Dickinson KA, Pincus AL: Interpersonal analysis of grandiose and vulnerable narcissism. J Pers Disord 17(3):188–207, 2003 12839099

Dimaggio G, Procacci M, Nicolo G, et al: Poor metacognition in narcissistic and avoidant personality disorders: four psychotherapy patients analysed using the Metacognition Assessment Scale. Clin Psychol Psychother 14:386–401, 2007a

Dimaggio G, Semerari A, Carcione A, et al: Psychotherapy of Personality Disorders: Metacognition, States of Mind and Interpersonal Cycles. Hove, UK, Routledge, 2007b

Dimaggio G, Lysaker PH, Carcione A, et al: Know yourself and you shall know the other... to a certain extent: multiple paths of influence of self-reflection on mindreading. Conscious Cogn 17(3):778–789, 2008a 18394921

Dimaggio G, Nicolò G, Fiore D, et al: States of minds in narcissistic personality disorder: three psychotherapies analyzed using the grid of problematic states. Psychother Res 18(4):466–480, 2008b 18815998

Dimaggio G, Montano A, Popolo R, et al: Metacognitive Interpersonal Therapy for Personality Disorders: A Treatment Manual. Hove, UK, Routledge, 2015

Eikenaes I, Hummelen B, Abrahamsen G, et al: Personality functioning in patients with avoidant personality disorder and social phobia. J Pers Disord 27(6):746–763, 2013 23786266

Eikenaes I, Pedersen G, Wilberg T: Attachment styles in patients with avoidant personality disorder compared with social phobia. Psychol Psychother 89(3):245–260, 2016 26332087

Ellison WD, Levy KN, Cain NM, et al: The impact of pathological narcissism on psychotherapy utilization, initial symptom severity, and early treatment symptom change: a naturalistic investigation. J Pers Assess 95(3):291–300, 2013 23186259

Euler S, Sollberger D, Bader K, et al: Persönlichkeitsstörungen und Sucht: Systematische Literaturübersicht zu Epidemiologie, Verlauf und Behandlung [A Systematic Review of Personality Disorders and Addiction: Epidemiology, Course and Treatment] [In German]. Fortschr Neurol Psychiatr 83(10):544–554, 2015 26588717

Euler S, Stöbi D, Sowislo J, et al: Grandiose and vulnerable narcissism in borderline personality disorder. Psychopathology 51(2):110–121, 2018 29466803

Fan Y, Wonneberger C, Enzi B, et al: The narcissistic self and its psychological and neural correlates: an exploratory fMRI study. Psychol Med 41(8):1641–1650, 2011 21144117

Fonagy P, Allison E: The role of mentalizing and epistemic trust in the therapeutic relationship. Psychotherapy (Chic) 51(3):372–380, 2014 24773092

Fonagy P, Target M: Attachment and reflective function: their role in self-organization. Dev Psychopathol 9(4):679–700, 1997 9449001

Fonagy P, Gergely G, Target M: Psychoanalytic constructs and attachment theory and research, in Handbook of Attachment: Theory, Research, and Clinical Applications, 2nd Edition. Edited by Cassidy J, Shaver PR. New York, Guilford, 2008, pp 783–810

Fonagy P, Luyten P, Allison E: Epistemic petrification and the restoration of epistemic trust: a new conceptualization of borderline personality disorder and its psychosocial treatment. J Pers Disord 29(5):575–609, 2015 26393477

Friborg O, Martinussen M, Kaiser S, et al: Comorbidity of personality disorders in anxiety disorders: a meta-analysis of 30 years of research. J Affect Disord 145(2):143–155, 2013 22999891

Gore WL, Widiger TA: Fluctuation between grandiose and vulnerable narcissism. Pers Disord 7(4):363–371, 2016 26986960

Johansen MS, Normann-Eide E, Normann-Eide T, et al: Emotional dysfunction in avoidant compared to borderline personality disorder: a study of affect consciousness. Scand J Psychol 54(6):515–521, 2013 24107113

Karterud S, Wilberg T: From general day hospital treatment to specialized treatment programmes. Int Rev Psychiatry 19(1):39–49, 2007 17365157

Karterud S, Pedersen G, Johansen M, et al: Primary emotional traits in patients with personality disorders. Pers Ment Health 10(4):261–273, 2016 27257161

Kavanagh LC, Winkielman P: The functionality of spontaneous mimicry and its influences on affiliation: an implicit socialization account. Front Psychol 7:458, 2016 27064398

Kealy D, Ogrodniczuk JS, Joyce AS, et al: Narcissism and relational representations among psychiatric outpatients. J Pers Disord 29(3):393–407, 2015 23398104

Kernberg OF: Borderline Conditions and Pathological Narcissism. New York, Jason Aronson, 1985

Klumpp H, Angstadt M, Phan KL: Insula reactivity and connectivity to anterior cingulate cortex when processing threat in generalized social anxiety disorder. Biol Psychol 89(1):273–276, 2012 22027088

Koenigsberg HW, Denny BT, Fan J, et al: The neural correlates of anomalous habituation to negative emotional pictures in borderline and avoidant personality disorder patients. Am J Psychiatry 171(1):82–90, 2014 24275960

Kongerslev M, Simonsen S, Bo S: The quest for tailored treatments: a meta-discussion of six social cognitive therapies. J Clin Psychol 71(2):188–198, 2015 25557904

Lampe L: Avoidant personality disorder as a social anxiety phenotype: risk factors, associations and treatment. Curr Opin Psychiatry 29(1):64–69, 2016 26651009

Levy KN: Subtypes, dimensions, levels, and mental states in narcissism and narcissistic personality disorder. J Clin Psychol 68(8):886–897, 2012 22740389

Liotti G, Gilbert P: Mentalizing, motivation, and social mentalities: theoretical considerations and implications for psychotherapy. Psychol Psychother 84(1):9–25, discussion 98–110, 2011 22903828

Lorenzini N, Fonagy P: Attachment and personality disorders: a short review. Focus 11:155–166, 2013

Luchner AF, Mirsalimi H, Moser CJ, et al: Maintaining boundaries in psychotherapy: covert narcissistic personality characteristics and psychotherapists. Psychotherapy (Chic) 45(1):1–14, 2008 22122361

Luyten P, Fonagy P: The neurobiology of mentalizing. Pers Disord 6(4):366–379, 2015 26436580

Marques L, Porter E, Keshaviah A, et al: Avoidant personality disorder in individuals with generalized social anxiety disorder: what does it add? J Anxiety Disord 26(6):665–672, 2012 22705954

Miller JD, Campbell WK: Comparing clinical and social-personality conceptualizations of narcissism. J Pers 76(3):449–476, 2008 18399956

Millon T: Disorders of Personality: DSM-III, Axis II. New York, Wiley, 1981

Mitchell JP, Mason MF, Macrae CN, et al: Thinking about others: the neural substrates of social cognition, in Social Neuroscience: People Thinking About Thinking People. Edited by Cacioppo JT, Visser PS, Pickett CL. Cambridge, MA, MIT Press, 2006, pp 63–82

Mizen R: On the capacity to suffer one's self. J Anal Psychol 59(3):314–332, 2014 24919626

Moore BE, Fine BD: A Glossary of Psychoanalytic Terms and Concepts, 2nd Edition. New York, American Psychoanalytic Association, 1968

Moroni F, Procacci M, Pellecchia G, et al: Mindreading dysfunction in avoidant personality disorder compared with other personality disorders. J Nerv Ment Dis 204(10):752–757, 2016 27227557

Nicolò G, Semerari A, Lysaker PH, et al: Alexithymia in personality disorders: correlations with symptoms and interpersonal functioning. Psychiatry Res 190(1):37–42, 2011 20800288

Nolte T, Guiney J, Fonagy P, et al: Interpersonal stress regulation and the development of anxiety disorders: an attachment-based developmental framework. Front Behav Neurosci 5:55, 2011 21960962

Olssøn I, Svindseth MF, Dahl AA: Is there an association between the level of grandiose narcissism severity of psychopathology? Nord J Psychiatry 70(2):121–127, 2016 26212624

Otway LJ, Vignoles VL: Narcissism and childhood recollections: a quantitative test of psychoanalytic predictions. Pers Soc Psychol Bull 32(1):104–116, 2006 16317192

Pedersen G, Eikenæs I, Urnes Ø, et al: Experiences in Close Relationships – Psychometric properties among patients with personality disorders. Pers Ment Health 9(3):208–219, 2015 26033784

Pincus AL, Lukowitsky MR: Pathological narcissism and narcissistic personality disorder. Annu Rev Clin Psychol 6:421–446, 2010 20001728

Riggs SA, Paulson A, Tunnell E, et al: Attachment, personality, and psychopathology among adult inpatients: self-reported romantic attachment style versus Adult Attachment Interview states of mind. Dev Psychopathol 19(1):263–291, 2007 17241494

Ritter K, Dziobek I, Preissler S, et al: Lack of empathy in patients with narcissistic personality disorder. Psychiatry Res 187(1–2):241–247, 2011 21055831

Ronningstam E: Narcissistic personality disorder: a review, in Personality Disorders. Edited by Maj M, Akiskal HS, Mezzich J, Okasha A. Chichester, UK, Wiley, 2005, pp 277–327

Ronningstam E: Narcissistic personality disorder: a current review. Curr Psychiatry Rep 12(1):68–75, 2010 20425313

Ronningstam E: Intersect between self-esteem and emotion regulation in narcissistic personality disorder—implications for alliance building and treatment. Borderline Personal Disorder Emotion Dysregul 4:3, 2017 28191317

Rosenfeld H: Destructive narcissism and the death instinct, in Impasse and Interpretation. London, Tavistock Publications, 1987, pp 105–132

Rosenthal MZ, Kim K, Herr NR, et al: Speed and accuracy of facial expression classification in avoidant personality disorder: a preliminary study. Pers Disord 2(4):327–334, 2011 22448805

Schulze L, Dziobek I, Vater A, et al: Gray matter abnormalities in patients with narcissistic personality disorder. J Psychiatr Res 47(10):1363–1369, 2013 23777939

Semerari A, Colle L, Pellecchia G, et al: Metacognitive dysfunctions in personality disorders: correlations with disorder severity and personality styles. J Pers Disord 28(6):751–766, 2014 24689762

Simonsen S, Heinskou T, Sørensen P, et al: Personality disorders: patient characteristics and level of outpatient treatment service. Nord J Psychiatry 71(5):325–331, 2017 28635555

Skodol AE, Bender DS, Morey LC: Narcissistic personality disorder in DSM-5. Pers Disord 5(4):422–427, 2014 23834518

Smolewska K, Dion KL: Narcissism and adult attachment: a multivariate approach. Self Ident 4:59–68, 2005

Stinson FS, Dawson DA, Goldstein RB, et al: Prevalence, correlates, disability, and comorbidity of DSM-IV narcissistic personality disorder: results from the wave 2 national epidemiologic survey on alcohol and related conditions. J Clin Psychiatry 69(7):1033–1045, 2008 18557663

Tanzilli A, Muzi L, Ronningstam E, et al: Countertransference when working with narcissistic personality disorder: an empirical investigation. Psychotherapy (Chic) 54(2):184–194, 2017 28581327

Torvik FA, Welander-Vatn A, Ystrom E, et al: Longitudinal associations between social anxiety disorder and avoidant personality disorder: a twin study. J Abnorm Psychol 125(1):114–124, 2016 26569037

Wink P: Two faces of narcissism. J Pers Soc Psychol 61(4):590–597, 1991 1960651

Wright AG, Pincus AL, Conroy DE, et al: Integrating methods to optimize circumplex description and comparison of groups. J Pers Assess 91(4):311–322, 2009 20017060

Zimmerman M, Rothschild L, Chelminski I: The prevalence of DSM-IV personality disorders in psychiatric outpatients. Am J Psychiatry 162(10):1911–1918, 2005 16199838

CHAPTER 22

EATING DISORDERS

Paul Robinson, M.D., FRCP, FRCPsych

Finn Skårderud, M.D., Ph.D.

Few symptoms create stronger reactions in therapists than those of eating disorders, particularly anorexia nervosa—and few require more forbearance and self-questioning. Eating disorders are challenging for mental health practitioners in both clinical and intellectual terms. Severe eating disorders may last for decades, cause patients to retreat from normal social and family activity, and destroy and break up families. Anorexia nervosa has the highest standardized mortality rate of all psychiatric disorders. Eating disorders most often start during adolescence, which is a critical phase for many people, during which changes occur to both their physiology and their identity. In addition, adolescence is a period when the brain is still immature. The psychological consequences of impaired somatic health result in an increase in symptoms. In this chapter, we propose that the model of mentalizing is highly relevant to furthering both the understanding of eating disorders and clinical practice. Not least, we assert that severely impaired mentalizing in patients tends to compromise the therapist's mentalizing, with the consequent risk of enactments, ineffective treatment, or iatrogenic effects.

Let us start with an example. A young person—apparently with everything to look forward to—starves herself to near death. When told how dangerous the situation is, she rejects feeding and has to be forced, apparently preferring to die rather than accept nutrition. For most people, this behavior is very hard to understand. The task of the therapist is to work toward an understanding of the patient's thinking and moti-

---

We are grateful to Patrick Luyten, Ph.D., Alex Bogaardt, M.Sc., Ajay Clare, B.M., B.S., M.Sc., and Sofia Sacchetti, M.Sc., who contributed to the research illustrated in Table 22–1.

vation. This is not an easy task, and some therapists can only manage to accept the patient's thinking, without understanding it. This can be enough to allow the therapist to work with the patient. Without such an acceptance, staff who work with patients with eating disorders can have very destructive feelings about the patients, which can lead to the patients being criticized and rejected by staff. Such strong feelings also occur with patients who engage in self-injurious behavior and/or substance misuse, who regularly find themselves devalued in hospital emergency departments as "time wasters," not worthy of medical care. Implementing the model of mentalizing in eating disorders, therefore, includes both the thoughts and the feelings that staff have about the patient, as well as, of course, how the patient thinks and feels about himself or herself and others.

All psychiatric disorders involve varied impairments in mentalizing. Treatment innovation is guided by an understanding of the processes underpinning psychopathology. This treatment innovation can then, in turn, be subject to empirical investigation. In other words, treatment should be tailored to the disorder (Fonagy and Bateman 2006; Kazdin 2004). As a basis for our clinical approach, we first describe the psychopathology of severe eating disorders, using the language of the mentalizing model. We understand these disorders as manifestations of an underlying self-disorder. This underlying disorder should be the central focus of psychotherapy. Mentalization-based treatment for eating disorders (MBT-ED) of course aims to reduce symptoms, but it also aims to enhance the psychological and social competences that are involved in understanding the individual's own and other people's minds. The essence of MBT is its systematic attentiveness to achieving such understanding and, through that, improved affect regulation.

The role for MBT-ED, a therapy that explicitly teaches about and addresses problems with mentalizing, has not been established. In the absence of a clear evidence base, it is reasonable to think of MBT-ED as an intervention for patients who have been treated with less elaborate therapies, such as specialist supportive clinical management for eating disorders (SSCM-ED; Robinson et al. 2014, 2016) and extended cognitive-behavioral therapy for eating disorders (CBT-E) (Fairburn et al. 2009)—and remain unwell. For patients with a combination of an eating disorder and borderline personality disorder (BPD) who do not respond adequately to initial therapy, MBT-ED could also be regarded as a rational choice. This patient group was the subject of a randomized controlled trial (Robinson et al. 2016). The results were not definitive, and the attrition rate was high, but there was some evidence that MBT-ED was superior to a control treatment. We regard MBT-ED as a treatment for eating disorders that is yet to be supported by an evidence base. We present here the theory and practice relevant to the application of MBT in the field of eating disorders.

EATING DISORDERS AS SELF-DISORDERS

In this section, we describe the theoretical basis for the proposal that mentalizing is disturbed in eating disorders. This will contribute to the rationale for the use of a treatment model with the specific aim of enhancing mentalizing—that is, MBT-ED.

From observation, sound evidence supports the categorization of eating disorders as disorders of emotional and somatic regulation (e.g., Guarda 2008; Skårderud and Fonagy 2012). Such a categorization opens up the possibility of integrating different explanatory and descriptive models in medicine and psychology. Advances in neuro-biology and developmental psychology, theories of affect, research on infant development, trauma research, new concepts of personality development, and current concepts in psychoanalysis have all contributed to conjectures concerning a new and distinct conceptual entity: that of *self-regulation in general and of affect regulation in particular*. The tradition around mentalizing is a prominent example of this general intellectual trend, with an emphasis on how insecure attachment can contribute to impairment of regulation. (For a review of studies on eating disorders and attachment measured by the Adult Attachment Interview [AAI], see Zachrisson and Skårderud 2010.) In general, the prevalence of secure attachment classifications is low across all diagnostic subgroups.

Persons with eating disorders may attempt to drown out their anguished feelings by frantic self-stimulatory activities. Such activities could be seen as a common denominator to behaviors such as starvation, bingeing, vomiting, and hyperactivity. The symptoms can be seen as misguided attempts to organize emotions and other internal states more meaningfully. The absence of reliable internal self-regulation may cause the patient with an eating disorder to feel inadequate, ineffective, and out of control.

The psychiatrist and psychoanalyst Hilde Bruch (1904–1984) developed new perspectives for understanding and conceptualizing the psychopathology of eating disorders (Bruch 1970, 1973, 1988; Skårderud 2009). Bruch regarded the psychopathology of primary anorexia as *a deficient sense of self*, involving a wide range of deficits in conceptual developments, body image and awareness, and individuation (Taylor et al. 1997). Bruch (1962) suggested that patients with anorexia find it difficult to accurately perceive or interpret stimuli arising in their bodies, such as hunger and satiety, as well as the physiological signs of malnutrition, such as fatigue and weakness. She observed that patients with anorexia experience their emotions in a bewildering way. In addition, she described how patients were often unable to describe their emotions, with disconnections between the physiological, subjective feeling components of emotion, and language. For Bruch, the person with anorexia is therefore *one who does not know*, because he or she is a *person who has not learned to distinguish*. The relationship between experience and category has not been established in a valid manner. Bodily experiences are "miscategorized." When patients do not know *what* they feel and need, they are close to experiencing loss of their own reality. Anorexia nervosa becomes a struggle for a reality and a sense of identity.

To sum up, Bruch's clinical and theoretical descriptions of eating disorders anticipated later models of impaired mentalizing, not least by stressing how such compromised competences affect both the individual's own mental states—*minding one's own mind*—and the individual's own somatic sensations—*minding one's own body*.

The term *embodied mentalizing* (see Chapter 2, "Contemporary Neuroscientific Research") is now used to emphasize the corporeal aspects of the mentalizing process. With eating disorders, there is an unduly negative focus on the exterior, combined with an impaired awareness of the individual's bodily sensations. This *concretization* is one of the major challenges of clinical work with severe eating disorders. The body of the person with an eating disorder is emotionally and cognitively experienced more via the weight scales than by *feeling* his or her own *lived body* (Merleau-Ponty 1962). Pollatos et al. (2008) describe reduced perception of bodily signals in anorexia nervosa such that in eating disorders the person's body may at the same time be experienced as *too real* and *too unreal.*

EATING DISORDERS AND PSYCHIC MODES OF REALITY

Prementalistic modes of reality are described in more detail in Chapter 1, "Introduction."

Psychic Equivalence and Pretend Mode

Psychic equivalence as a construct means equating the internal world with the external world (Fonagy et al. 2002). Eating disorders most often start during adolescence. For many young people, adolescence is a critical phase characterized by both physiological changes and changes in identity. Attempts to modify the body—for example, through controlling the appetite—may represent an effort to maintain inner control and cohesion. There is psychic equivalence between the experience of body shape and its concrete parameters: to be thinner is felt to be superior and therefore *is* superior. Mental states, which are unable to achieve representation as ideas or feelings, come to be represented in the bodily domain:

> Physical attributes such as weight come to reflect states such as internal well-being, control, sense of self-worth, and so on, far beyond the normal tendency for this to happen in adolescence. (Fonagy et al. 2002, p. 405)

Skårderud (2007a) gives numerous examples of psychic equivalence based on transcripts from research interviews and therapy sessions with adults with anorexia nervosa. Sensorimotor experiences and bodily qualities and sensations, such as hunger, size, weight, and shape, are physical entities that function as sources of metaphors for nonphysical phenomena. In psychic equivalence, bodily metaphors do not function mainly as *representations* capable of containing an experience, but as *presentations*, which are experienced as concrete facts in the here and now and are difficult to negotiate with. In this mode, "as if" turns into "is." Psychic equivalence is *too real, here and now.* The psychic pain for the patient is that he or she is trapped in this harsh corporeality here and now and does not satisfactorily mentalize how his or her body functions as a metaphorical source for emotional life, and vice versa.

The alexithymic patient may lack words for his or her inner life, while the patient in pretend mode has words, but they are "not yet his or her own." The described outer-directedness, with the patient trying to interpret and satisfy other persons' needs (Buhl 2002; Skårderud 2007b), may also lead to *hypermentalizing,* an exaggerated but emotionally meaningless interest in thoughts and feelings. The combination of pseudomentalizing and hypermentalizing may contribute to confusion in the therapeutic relationship.

Teleological Mode

In this mode, there is a focus on understanding actions in terms of their physical, as opposed to mental, outcomes: *"I don't believe it unless I see it."* Few clinical conditions illustrate this concept better than eating disorders. In the world of psychiatric disorders, eating disorders represent a special case, insofar as the therapist can identify an initial active wish for change in the histories of patients: they want to change themselves in terms of self-esteem and social acceptance, and they seek to achieve these changes *physically,* by modifying their bodies. The patients' solution is to lose weight, because in the personal psyche (and also, to a degree that should not be underestimated, in the cultural context) losing weight teleologically represents mastery and self-control. A general feeling of distrust is expressed as distrust about something specific (e.g., weighing scales or the number of calories or grams in food). The patient with an eating disorder might also be a person who engages in self-injurious behavior, in which internal pain is concretized as and regulated by physical pain.

The feelings of distrust experienced by a person with an eating disorder may also be expressed as distrust of other people, including health personnel and helpers. The patient's fear of not being in psychological control can lead to controlling behavior, such a checking, double-checking, and controlling behavior toward the therapist. In group therapy, patients may define each other by their weight, body shape, and their reports about dieting, restriction, bingeing, purging, physical activity, and so on. Insecure identity generates a patient's tendency to compare himself or herself with others in terms of their concrete achievements and bodily qualities.

RESEARCH INDICATING IMPAIRED MENTALIZING IN EATING DISORDERS

Emotional Theory of Mind

Theory of mind (ToM) refers to the way individuals can be aware of other people's thoughts. For example, if an individual sees someone on a bus take a ticket from the driver and place it in a pocket, he or she will know that the person will probably look in that pocket if an inspector later asks to see the ticket. The observer is able to do this because he or she can surmise what is in the person's mind about the whereabouts of the ticket. Emotional theory of mind (eToM) extends this capacity to feelings. For example, if the inspector asks for the ticket and the person cannot find it, the observer will understand that the person is likely to be feeling perplexed and anxious. There is evidence of poor eToM in some patients with eating disorders. Oldershaw et al. (2010), using the Level of Emotional Awareness Scale, found that patients who were currently underweight because of anorexia nervosa had poorer eToM than control subjects or patients who had recovered from anorexia nervosa. Recovered patients performed poorly on some eToM tasks, suggesting either that a problem was present before the onset of the eating disorder or that the difficulty was a result ("scar") of having had the condition.

Reflective Functioning

Reflective functioning (RF) attempts to measure the capacity of an individual to think about his or her own and others' mental states. Fonagy et al. (1996) reported significantly lower scores on the Reflective Self-Function Scale on AAI transcripts in a small group of inpatients with eating disorders, and Pedersen et al. (2015), using the AAI, found that the RF of patients with bulimia nervosa did not differ statistically from that of control subjects. However, the distribution of scores did differ, with some high and some low values, suggesting that there may be atypical patients with abnormal values. Müller et al. (2006), using a modification of the AAI in 24 inpatients (16 with eating disorders and the remainder with depression), found "questionable or low" RF in the entire patient group. Rothschild-Yakar et al. (2010), using the Reflective Functioning Scale, found significantly lower RF scores in a group of 34 adolescents with binge–purge anorexia nervosa. Lastly, our own data (Table 22–1) showed abnormal scores in a group of patients with bulimia nervosa; notably, the effect sizes are large. The group contained a high proportion of patients with BPD; the influence of BPD on the RF of patients in this group remains to be determined.

TABLE 22–1.　**Results from unpublished data of different measures of mentalizing in patients with bulimia nervosa (BN) with features of borderline personality disorder, compared with healthy control subjects (HC)**

Group	Measure	Mean	SD	n	P	Effect size[a]
BN	ORI mother	5.55	1.08	53	<0.001	0.42 (M)
HC	ORI mother	6.19	0.82	87		
BN	ORI father	5.9	0.91	53	<0.001	0.45 (M)
HC	ORI father	6.31	0.91	87		
BN	ORI self	5.38	1.04	53	<0.001	1.08 (L)
HC	ORI self	6.44	0.92	87		
BN	RFQ-c	2.56	2.53	53	<0.001	1.46 (L)
HC	RFQ-c	7.9	4.76	51		
BN	RFQ-u	8.9	4.47	53	<0.001	1.90 (L)
HC	RFQ-u	1.9	2.88	51		
BN	RMET	26.09	3.88	53	<0.01	0.62 (M)
HC	RMET	28.27	3.19	51		

Note.　ORI=Object Relations Inventory; RFQ-c=Reflective Functioning Questionnaire—Certainty scale; RFQ-u=Reflective Function Questionnaire—Uncertainty scale; RMET=Reading the Mind in the Eyes Test.
[a]L=large; M=moderate.

Object Relations

The capacity of an individual to make emotionally satisfying relationships with family members, friends, partners, and therapists, among others, can be used as a proxy for mentalizing ability. Blatt and Auerbach (2003) developed the Object Relations Inventory (ORI), in which subjects are invited to provide descriptions of their parents and themselves. These descriptions are rated by trained observers according to the maturity and complexity of the descriptions. This measure was used in a study by Rothschild-Yakar et al. (2013) of inpatient adolescents with anorexia nervosa. The study found that the patients had significantly lower levels of mentalizing and symbolization and had more malevolent working models of their parents in comparison with control participants without eating disorders. In unpublished findings from the

NOURISHED study (Robinson et al. 2016), the ORI was used with adult patients with bulimia nervosa and symptoms of BPD. Patients with bulimia had significantly lower scores than control subjects when describing their mothers, their fathers, and themselves. Effect sizes were moderate to large (see Table 22–1).

Emotion Recognition and Expression

Patients with eating disorders have problems with both reading other people's expressions and making their own expressions. Harrison et al. (2010) found that patients with anorexia nervosa had poor emotion recognition in both the acutely ill and the recovered state, suggesting that this deficit may be long-lasting. Participants in this study showed increased latency of response when presented with angry faces. Lang et al. (2016) found that patients with anorexia nervosa had reduced expression of positive emotions. In a review of this area, Oldershaw et al. (2011) reported deficits in emotional expression in anorexia nervosa.

The Reading the Mind in the Eyes Test (RMET)[1] was introduced by Baron-Cohen et al. (2001). Harrison et al. (2010) found that scores on this test were significantly lower in a group of patients with anorexia nervosa who were acutely ill. In the NOURISHED study, Robinson et al. (2016), using the same test on patients with bulimia nervosa and borderline features, found significantly poorer performance in the patients compared with healthy control subjects; the effect size was moderate (Table 22–1).

Social Cognition

Further evidence suggesting the relevance of a mentalizing approach to eating disorders comes from research in social cognition. A mentalizing approach, based on the notion that people understand actions in others and in themselves by imagining that thoughts and feelings underpin these actions, seems relevant to eating disorders because beliefs, desires, and needs are the common currency of social interchange and are nested in all family environments. Mentalizing—like language—emerges in a form that is specific to a culture, and is learned in the context of attachment relationships. It is assumed that both genetics and early family environments play a role in making mentalizing less robust in some individuals than others. Disturbance in the family and in attachment relationships undermines the full development of this capacity (Fonagy et al. 2002), leading to significant challenges in handling social pressures and emotionally loaded social situations (Skårderud and Fonagy 2012). As suggested at the beginning of this chapter, eating disorder symptoms may be best understood as attempted solutions to underlying problems of social (self-)regulation.

The bulk of studies with adults with eating disorders have confirmed anomalies in social cognition (Oldershaw et al. 2010, 2011). A range of studies has pointed to difficulties with self-regulation in eating disorders. There are indications that eating disorders are associated with problems of self-regulation, manifested in individuals as the following: difficulties in identifying and describing their own emotions (Beadle et al. 2013; Bydlowski et al. 2005); impairment in mentalizing others' emotional experience (Harrison et al. 2009; Taube-Schiff et al. 2015); problems with attention and ex-

---

[1] Available at: https://www.autismresearchcentre.com/arc_tests; see the "Eyes Test (Adult)."

ecutive function (Gillberg et al. 2010); and reduced self-agency (Caglar-Nazali et al. 2014). Taking these difficulties together suggests that symptoms of eating disorder may be linked to challenges in self-regulation. Phenomenological accounts of eating disorder provide rich evidence for quite exceptional capacities for self-discipline and self-regulation in the physical domain, sometimes intercurrent with dramatic failures of this capacity (binge eating). The mentalizing model of eating disorders would suggest that dramatic attempts at controlling eating behavior might be the consequence of failed attempts at regulation of a social self.

Are these difficulties in attachment and mentalizing the consequence (or at least the correlate) of eating problems, or are they a genuine cause? Developmental psychopathology studies point to a potential causal relationship. Two reviews of the association of eating disorder with attachment in young people (Jewell et al. 2016; Zachrisson and Skårderud 2010) identified 14 studies in which attachment insecurity correlated with eating disorder in childhood and adolescence. The early roots matter less than adolescent relationships based on interpersonal competence. Attachment insecurity in infancy appears to be a weak predictor of eating pathology, whereas preadolescent attachment insecurity does predict eating disorder a year later rather well. Attachment to peers predicts eating pathology in midadolescence better than attachment to parents, again highlighting the importance of social adjustment and competence. Similarly, difficulties with emotion recognition in adolescence predict eating disorders, particularly anorexia nervosa. Mentalizing difficulties are also directly associated with eating pathology. It is something of an open question whether mentalizing problems persist following recovery (discussed later in this chapter), but developmentally, they do seem to precede the eating disorder.

The systematic review and meta-analysis of "systems for social processes" in eating disorders by Caglar-Nazali et al. (2014) identified more than 150 studies that measured constructs such as attachment, social communication, perception and understanding of self and others, and social dominance in people with eating disorder. They reported 11 meta-analyses with varying effect sizes that highlight a broad range of social, cognitive, and relational problems associated with the diagnosis, which point to the vulnerability of the social self of individuals with eating disorder. In terms of child–parent relationships, the authors provided strong evidence for attachment insecurity and indications of low parental care, and more limited indications for parental overprotection. While the reported effect size for impaired facial emotion recognition in individuals with eating disorder was modest (Cohen's $d=0.40$), those for impairment in facial communication and facial avoidance were higher ($d=2.1$ and 0.52, respectively). The meta-analyses confirm a significant reduction in self-agency, negative self-evaluation, poor understanding of mental states, and alexithymia, and increased sensitivity to social dominance. In other words, there is strong evidence for a broad range of social-cognitive problems associated with eating disorder, but the evidence is strongest when capacities are evaluated in social contexts.

That this limitation may represent a developmental vulnerability to social and cultural pressures is supported by findings such as those reported by McAdams and Krawczyk (2011), who demonstrated that even patients who had recovered from anorexia show reduced activation of the mentalizing network when a task calls for making social attributions. Both recovered individuals with a diagnosis of anorexia nervosa and patients with bulimia nervosa show reduced temporoparietal activation when asked to make judgments of social causation (McAdams and Krawczyk 2013). A task that required participants to read and respond to social adjectives presented in three different conditions showed that self-reflection was associated with more limited dorsal anterior cingulate and precuneus activation. Brain regions that serve as substrates for ToM and mentalizing and enable understanding of others as well as the individual's own self appear to be less active, pointing to problems of self-agency, self-knowledge, and self-awareness in both participants with bulimia nervosa and those with anorexia nervosa (McAdams and Krawczyk 2013).

The enhancement of mentalizing is important, not simply because of the close links between mental-state understanding of others and self-regulation, but because mentalizing improves the individual's capacity to negotiate the social world. Mentalizing enables connection to others. The extent to which individuals with eating disorder, particularly anorexia, can feel isolated is often seriously underestimated. Yet, making a connection with others is critical to ensure adaptation to a constantly changing (internal as well as external) world.

CLINICAL STRUCTURES IN MBT-ED

General Points

MBT has much in common with other approaches to psychotherapy. Careful behavioral and cognitive analysis will be familiar to CBT therapists, while attention to the therapist–patient relationship is a key part of psychoanalytically informed therapies. The defining characteristic of MBT is probably the clear objective in the mind of the therapist to enhance mentalizing. Although there is increasing evidence that patients with eating disorders have problems in mentalizing, it is not known to what extent these problems precede the development of the eating disorder (suggesting that eating disorders might be developmental disorders with roots in childhood), or whether the mentalizing difficulties are secondary to symptoms of eating disorder. It is probable that frequent binge eating and vomiting, as well as maintaining a very low body weight, can interfere with cognition and impair mentalizing, in the same way that drug and alcohol abuse can make accurate mentalizing difficult. The MBT-ED therapist must therefore be prepared to facilitate improvements in mentalizing as well as directly addressing physical risk, mental health risk, and symptoms of eating disorder. This is a major undertaking, and therapist training and experience (discussed later in this chapter) must reach acceptable standards of competence. The theory and practice of MBT-ED have been described at length in Robinson et al. (2019).

The overall structure of MBT-ED has not yet been decided. However, MBT-ED is *always* a combination of treatment models, to strengthen therapeutic alliances and prevent dropout. MBT-ED is a long-term program, structured as a combination of the following:

- Individual therapy.
- Group therapy.
- Group psychoeducation.
- Active use of written case formulations.
- Medical management.

In addition to the traditional MBT format (Bateman and Fonagy 2004, 2006, 2016), regular physical assessment is required for patients with eating disorders. An agreement between a medical doctor and the clinicians running the treatment program about how to divide responsibility is a precondition for participation. Sometimes, family crises or important issues in the patient's family or couple relationships may lead to a limited number of family or couple therapy sessions being included in the program. Other forms of crisis (e.g., suicide attempts or increased frequency of self-harm) may also lead to intensified therapeutic contact for a limited time. All therapy sessions should be recorded for training, supervision, and model development.

Individual Therapy

Individual therapy is preferred by most patients, who often describe the group (see below) as very challenging and find the individual context safer. In contrast, some patients feel that the group is a safer place (in a negative sense) because it is possible to hide in the group, by means of silence, unfruitful courtesy, withdrawal, or passivity; for these patients, individual therapy is experienced as more demanding because there are only two people in the room.

In individual therapy sessions, we base the work on MBT principles in general (described in Chapter 6, "Individual Therapy Techniques") and those more specifically developed for eating disorders, as outlined below. In the treatment model, we practice openness between the different treatment contexts—for example, the individual therapist is informed about the patient's ways of functioning in the group. In this way, the individual sessions are also an opportunity to work with the patient on how to use the group optimally.

Group Therapy

Many patients find the group sessions the most challenging part of the MBT-ED program. This makes sense in terms of some of the psychological traits frequently observed in patients with eating disorders, such as outer-directedness with an obsessive preoccupation with others' ideas about them and their bodies. Hence, the group treatment context inevitably activates the core pathology of eating disorders as self-disorders. Thus, while groups are very useful, they are challenging to run. Some moderate modifications in therapeutic stance from the MBT model for patients with BPD (Bateman and Fonagy 2004, 2006, 2016) are described for psychoeducational groups, discussed below.

Psychoeducational Groups

The psychoeducational groups, known as *introductory MBT group therapy* (MBT-I-ED), orient the patient to the treatment model and facilitate understanding of the clinical process (see Chapter 6 for more information on MBT-I). There are five to eight of these sessions, and the topics of each session are set and presented by the therapist. The psychoeducational groups are about mentalizing, with emphasis on communication, misunderstandings, difficulties in reading other people, and difficulties in knowing oneself. In each session, the therapist presents the topic briefly, using simple language, and then asks the participants to contribute their own examples. For a proposed list of topics, see Box 22–1.

BOX 22–1. **Psychoeducational groups: proposed themes**

- Mentalizing.
- The therapeutic model.
- The why and how of group therapy.
- Nutrition and somatic aspects of eating disorders.
- Emotions.
- Attachment.
- Personality traits and eating disorders.
- Embodied culture.

In these groups, we try to establish and maintain a playful atmosphere that is not too "hot" or emotionally intense. The emphasis is on a pedagogical stance (Csibra and Gergely 2006), with the therapist taking an active role in both sharing ideas and involving all participants. A concrete challenge for the therapist is to make these group sessions different enough from the weekly group therapy, with the latter intentionally dealing more with personally challenging material (i.e., being "hotter"). It is our experience that the patients are generally very supportive of this format.

In the NOURISHED study (Robinson et al. 2016), five sessions of MBT-I-ED preceded the main part of therapy, in which weekly individual and group sessions were provided for 12 months. There was a high dropout rate in the study, so conclusions are difficult to reach, but therapists reported that by 12 months, patients were often just starting to "get" MBT-ED. On this basis, it may be advisable to follow the lead of the MBT treatment program for BPD (Bateman and Fonagy 2009) and offer 18 months of MBT-ED, with the first 3 months consisting of psychoeducational MBT-I-ED.

TRAINING FOR MBT-ED

There is no formalized set of training standards for MBT-ED, although such standards do exist for MBT. We propose the following standards for MBT-ED therapists:

1. A mental health background (e.g., mental health nursing, clinical or counseling psychology, medical psychiatry).
2. At least 6 months' experience in treating patients with eating disorders in a specialist unit.
3. Attendance at a general training program in MBT.
4. Participation in either group (as co-therapist to a qualified MBT therapist) or individual MBT for at least 6 months with regular supervision and provision of therapy recordings.

There is no doubt that experience as an MBT-ED therapist under supervision gradually improves practice, and this improvement can continue for years.

WORKING IN A TEAM

Patients with complex needs usually require input from more than one professional. This may not be the case for some individuals with less severe eating disorders, but a patient with an eating disorder complicated by self-harm, substance misuse, chronicity (>5 years), serious medical problems, severe depression, or other serious comorbidities will need consultation with a range of specialist professionals. The expertise of professionals working in a team with the patient varies with the individual patient but usually includes medical, nursing, psychology and dietetic professionals, one of whom could be the MBT-ED therapist. Good communication between team members, a common written or computer record that is accessible to everyone in the team, and a system for raising concerns about risk are essential. Communication with the patient's primary care physician (in the United Kingdom, the general practitioner) should also occur regularly, although in most services this physician will not have access to all medical records. In England, some patients with high levels of need will be subject to the Care Programme Approach, which dictates the frequency of meetings and defines the role of each professional as well as the patient and his or her carers (National Institute for Health and Care Excellence 2017).

FORMULATION

The formulation should focus on the patient's current problems in light of his or her individual history and current situation, sketch the dynamic and other factors that seem to explain the clinical picture, and predict the likely impact of the foregoing factors on the process and outcome of therapy (Eells 2010; Perry et al. 1987); for further discussion of the formulation, see Chapter 6, "Individual Therapy Techniques"; Chapter 15, "Children"; and Chapter 17, "Borderline Personality Pathology in Adolescence." The formulation should also outline a mentalizing profile of the patient and the attachment strategies that are commonly activated, and clarify how these might become apparent in different contexts of therapy. The aim is for the formulation to capture these contexts—within both individual and group therapy—and indicate that cooperation between the therapists is necessary. The purpose is to paint a more holistic picture of the individual and his or her problems, to present hypotheses and propose a plan for treatment, and, not least, to set out the anticipated obstacles and challenges in therapy. Other aspects of the case formulation could include the individual's

- Beliefs about himself or herself.
- Beliefs about others.
- Bodily experiences.
- Relational difficulties.
- Strengths in mentalizing.

Guidelines for how to use therapy should also be presented.

The formulation is generated by the therapist and edited by the patient so that it becomes a jointly constructed document that is placed in the patient's records. The timing of when the formulation is generated varies, but usually it is begun after the first few sessions. The general idea of a formulation is that it encapsulates the problems presented by the patient and indicates what might be done in therapy to address them. It is important to describe the patient's mentalizing in the past and in the present, and how that capacity might be improved. Individuals with eating disorders can find mentalizing very difficult, because of the distracting nature of their symptoms. The degree to which this aspect of the disorder impedes the patient's mentalizing and the effect this may have on the symptoms themselves, and on interpersonal relationships, need to be included in the formulation.

It is recognized that the formulation may be written when only a few sessions have taken place, and many aspects of the patient's history, including relationships with family members and romantic/sexual relationships, may not yet have been touched on in therapy. The formulation can, of course, only contain information that has arisen in the sessions. A possible approach to the task of constructing the formulation is outlined in Box 22–2.

BOX 22–2. **Essential components of the formulation**

- Description of current problems.
- How difficulties with mentalizing can lead to symptoms.
- How mentalizing has been effective in the past and currently.
- How symptoms (both eating disorder symptoms and other issues such as substance misuse) can lead to difficulties with mentalizing.
- How mentalizing forms part of current relationships.
- Present and past attachment patterns, and vulnerabilities in relationships.
- Mentalizing and attachment in the therapeutic relationship.
- Planned approach to identified problems during individual and group therapy.

ACTION/CRISIS PLAN

A joint action/crisis plan is a document containing the patient's and therapist's treatment preferences for the management of symptoms and possible future crises (Moran et al. 2010). The plan is created with the aim of being "one step ahead" of future challenges and obstacles.

In MBT-ED the plan consists of two parts:

- How to deal with symptoms, such as weight restoration, excessive exercise, nutrition, bingeing and purging, and use of laxatives.
- How to deal with acute crises, such as suicidal thoughts and self-harm.

These two aims, addressing matters that can threaten both health and life, are approached within a mentalizing context. Behaviors that may endanger health are examined not only in physical terms but also in their accompanying mental nexus; that is, thoughts about physical harm, body image, and mortality are explored along with the intrapsychic and social processes that may determine these behaviors. In this way, exploring mentalizing becomes central to the therapist's approach to the potentially life-threatening behaviors that may accompany eating disorders.

Clinical Example

Sarah is 22 years old and has an 8-year history of anorexia nervosa with episodic bingeing and purging behavior. She has not been able to attend university for the past 2 years. She was hospitalized five times last year because of her physical state. She does not want to involve her family in therapy.

The following excerpts are from an action plan that was developed together with Sarah. All members of the treatment team have agreed upon this plan. The plan is reviewed and revised every 3 months.

MAIN SYMPTOMS TO WORK WITH IN THERAPY

Restrictive eating combined with episodes of bingeing and purging.

What Sarah Needs to Do

- Remember to eat regular meals according to her nutrition plan to prevent bingeing and purging.
- Try to make plans for the time immediately after meals (e.g., contacting her friends by e-mail or telephone).
- Eat together with her boyfriend when possible.

What Sarah and the Therapists Should Do

- Work with discrete episodes of bingeing and purging and explore the emotional and relational contexts of these episodes.
- Identify thoughts and feelings that precede episodes of bingeing and purging and changes in diet, and hence develop a mentalizing theory that applies to her eating-related symptoms.

WEIGHT RESTORATION

Sarah needs to restore her physical health, and this includes weight gain to normal weight.

What Sarah Needs to Do

- Stop weighing herself many times daily. She knows that this confuses her.
- Try to accept that her body needs better nutrition.
- Be honest about what she has been drinking before weighing herself.

What Sarah and the Therapists Should Do

- Sarah and the therapists have agreed that Sarah should gain approximately 0.5 kg (or 1 lb) every second week until she reaches normal weight.
- Track the changes in Sarah's thoughts and emotions related to changes in weight (and to lack of weight change) that relate to the mentalizing theory developed above.

- Conduct weekly weight checks in Sarah's individual sessions to make her feel safer about not gaining weight too quickly.
- If Sarah gains weight faster, reduce the nutrition plan.
- Relate rapid weight gain to the mentalizing theory above.
- Work with Sarah's body image distortion and how it fluctuates with emotional and relational contexts. Elaborate when she feels more comfortable in her own body.
- Track changes in Sarah's body image alongside thoughts and feelings about her body and other aspects of her life. Further develop the mentalizing theory.
- Track Sarah's feelings about her therapist (and others in her life) and how the latter may be responding to changes or lack of changes in bingeing and purging symptoms and weight.
- Modify the agreed formulation to incorporate these developments.

DEALING WITH SELF-HARM

Sarah engages in self-injurious behavior and has suicidal thoughts. Known triggers for acts of self-injury are feelings of rejection, difficulties in relation to others, and strong feelings of self-contempt in the wake of overeating.

What Sarah Needs to Do

- Try to delay her behavior by
  - Playing loud music, watching a movie, or surfing the internet.
  - Sending an SMS (text) or calling her boyfriend or close friends.
  - Writing down her thoughts and feelings in her diary.
  - Writing an e-mail to her therapist. It helps Sarah to know that someone else knows about her difficult feelings.
- Think about the consequences of self-injury (e.g., feelings of shame afterward and the scars).
- If Sarah is starting to cut herself, contact the service. Sarah has been given the phone numbers for daytime and for evenings and nights.

What Sarah and the Therapists Should Do

- Identify thoughts and feelings that precede and accompany urges to engage in self-injurious behavior.
- Relate these thoughts and feelings to fluctuations or other changes in relationships with significant others in Sarah's life.
- Relate these thoughts and feelings to changes in the therapeutic relationship and thoughts about the therapist.

CONCLUSION

This chapter has provided evidence in favor of the suggestion that eating disorders can be regarded as disorders of the self, with roots in disturbed attachment and symptoms that represent frantic attempts to escape the anxieties that ensue as a result of chronic insecurity. We propose that this model of eating disorders is a useful framework for therapy and fits with the insecure attachment patterns we see in our patients. The mentalizing model can be used in any therapy and, we contend, forms a part of many successful approaches to treatment in which patients are encouraged to understand themselves better and to become more aware of the thoughts and feelings produced in their interactions with other people, including the therapist and their family. Indeed, a mentalizing service, in which these processes are incorporated into relationships between team members and with the patient and family, seems to us to improve the chances that it will be effective. For example, take the situation in which a patient confides in one team member but asks that the information be kept from the other members of the team. A systemic approach will allow the team member to predict the splitting and disruption of treatment that could occur, while the mentalizing model can, in addition, allow the mental states of the patient, the family, and the therapist and other team members to be taken into account, with clear benefits for the functioning of the therapeutic process.

This approach can be introduced whatever the therapeutic model—whether cognitive-behavioral or psychodynamic, inpatient, day-patient (partial hospitalization), or outpatient. Although the evidence base for MBT-ED is at present inadequate, we propose that MBT-ED could well be a reasonable therapeutic model for patients who have failed to respond to therapy, or who present with severe and enduring eating disorders or with a combination of an eating disorder and emotional dysregulation or borderline symptoms.

REFERENCES

Baron-Cohen S, Wheelwright S, Hill J, et al: The "Reading the Mind in the Eyes" Test revised version: a study with normal adults, and adults with Asperger syndrome or high-functioning autism. J Child Psychol Psychiatry 42(2):241–251, 2001 11280420

Bateman A, Fonagy P: Psychotherapy for Borderline Personality Disorder: Mentalization-Based Treatment. Oxford, UK, Oxford University Press, 2004

Bateman A, Fonagy P: Mentalizing and borderline personality disorder, in Handbook of Mentalization-Based Treatment. Edited by Allen JG, Fonagy P. Chichester, UK, Wiley, 2006, pp 185–200

Bateman A, Fonagy P: Randomized controlled trial of outpatient mentalization-based treatment versus structured clinical management for borderline personality disorder. Am J Psychiatry 166(12):1355–1364, 2009 19833787

Bateman A, Fonagy P: Mentalization-Based Treatment for Personality Disorders: A Practical Guide. Oxford, UK, Oxford University Press, 2016

Beadle JN, Paradiso S, Salerno A, et al: Alexithymia, emotional empathy, and self-regulation in anorexia nervosa. Ann Clin Psychiatry 25(2):107–120, 2013 23638441

Blatt SJ, Auerbach JS: Psychodynamic measures of therapeutic change. Psychoanal Inq 23:268–307, 2003

Bruch H: Perceptual and conceptual disturbances in anorexia nervosa. Psychosom Med 24:187–194, 1962 13873828

Bruch H: Psychotherapy in primary anorexia nervosa. J Nerv Ment Dis 150(1):51–67, 1970 5416686

Bruch H: Eating Disorders: Obesity, Anorexia Nervosa, and the Person Within. New York, Basic Books, 1973

Bruch H: Conversations With Anorexics. London, Jason Aronson, 1988

Buhl C: Eating disorders as manifestations of developmental disorders: language and the capacity for abstract thinking in psychotherapy of eating disorders. Eur Eat Disord Rev 10:138–145, 2002

Bydlowski S, Corcos M, Jeammet P, et al: Emotion-processing deficits in eating disorders. Int J Eat Disord 37(4):321–329, 2005 15856501

Caglar-Nazali HP, Corfield F, Cardi V, et al: A systematic review and meta-analysis of "Systems for Social Processes" in eating disorders. Neurosci Biobehav Rev 42:55–92, 2014 24333650

Csibra G, Gergely G: Social learning and social cognition: the case for pedagogy, in Processes of Change in Brain and Cognitive Development Attention and Performance XXI. Edited by Johnson MH, Munakata Y. Oxford, UK, Oxford University Press, 2006, pp 249–274

Eells TD: Handbook of Psychotherapy Case Formulation, 2nd Edition. New York, Guilford, 2010

Fairburn CG, Cooper Z, Doll HA, et al: Transdiagnostic cognitive-behavioral therapy for patients with eating disorders: a two-site trial with 60-week follow-up. Am J Psychiatry 166(3):311–319, 2009 19074978

Fonagy P, Bateman AW: Mechanisms of change in mentalization-based treatment of BPD. J Clin Psychol 62(4):411–430, 2006 16470710

Fonagy P, Leigh T, Steele M, et al: The relation of attachment status, psychiatric classification, and response to psychotherapy. J Consult Clin Psychol 64(1):22–31, 1996 8907081

Fonagy P, Gergely G, Jurist E, et al: Affect Regulation, Mentalization, and the Development of the Self. New York, Other Press, 2002

Gillberg IC, Billstedt E, Wentz E, et al: Attention, executive functions, and mentalizing in anorexia nervosa eighteen years after onset of eating disorder. J Clin Exp Neuropsychol 32(4):358–365, 2010 19856232

Guarda AS: Treatment of anorexia nervosa: insights and obstacles. Physiol Behav 94(1):113–120, 2008 18155737

Harrison A, Sullivan S, Tchanturia K, et al: Emotion recognition and regulation in anorexia nervosa. Clin Psychol Psychother 16(4):348–356, 2009 19517577

Harrison A, Tchanturia K, Treasure J: Attentional bias, emotion recognition, and emotion regulation in anorexia: state or trait? Biol Psychiatry 68(8):755–761, 2010 20591417

Jewell T, Collyer H, Gardner T, et al: Attachment and mentalization and their association with child and adolescent eating pathology: a systematic review. Int J Eat Disord 49(4):354–373, 2016 26691270

Kazdin AE: Psychotherapy for children and adolescents, in Bergin and Garfield's Handbook of Psychotherapy and Behavior Change, 5th Edition. Edited by Lambert M. New York, Wiley, 2004, pp 543–589

Lang K, Roberts M, Harrison A, et al: Central coherence in eating disorders: a synthesis of studies using the Rey Osterrieth Complex Figure Test. PLoS One 11(11):e0165467, 2016 27806073

McAdams CJ, Krawczyk DC: Impaired neural processing of social attribution in anorexia nervosa. Psychiatry Res 194(1):54–63, 2011 21872451

McAdams CJ, Krawczyk DC: Neural responses during social and self-knowledge tasks in bulimia nervosa. Front Psychiatry 4:103, 2013 24065928

Merleau-Ponty M: Phenomenology of Perception. Translated by Smith C. London, Routledge & Kegan Paul, 1962

Moran P, Borschmann R, Flach C, et al: The effectiveness of joint crisis plans for people with borderline personality disorder: protocol for an exploratory randomised controlled trial. Trials 11:18, 2010 20178572

Müller C, Kaufhold J, Overbeck G, et al: The importance of reflective functioning to the diagnosis of psychic structure. Psychol Psychother 79(Pt 4):485–494, 2006 17312866

National Institute for Health and Care Excellence: Eating Disorders: Recognition and Treatment. NICE Guideline NG69. 2017. Available at: https://www.nice.org.uk/guidance/ng69. Accessed June 12, 2018.

Oldershaw A, Hambrook D, Tchanturia K, et al: Emotional theory of mind and emotional awareness in recovered anorexia nervosa patients. Psychosom Med 72(1):73–79, 2010 19995886

Oldershaw A, Hambrook D, Stahl D, et al: The socio-emotional processing stream in Anorexia Nervosa. Neurosci Biobehav Rev 35(3):970–988, 2011 21070808

Pedersen SH, Poulsen S, Lunn S: Eating disorders and mentalization: high reflective functioning in patients with bulimia nervosa. J Am Psychoanal Assoc 63(4):671–694, 2015 26316406

Perry S, Cooper AM, Michels R: The psychodynamic formulation: its purpose, structure, and clinical application. Am J Psychiatry 144(5):543–550, 1987 3578562

Pollatos O, Kurz AL, Albrecht J, et al: Reduced perception of bodily signals in anorexia nervosa. Eat Behav 9(4):381–388, 2008 18928900

Robinson P, Barrett B, Bateman A, et al: Study Protocol for a randomized controlled trial of mentalization based therapy against specialist supportive clinical management in patients with both eating disorders and symptoms of borderline personality disorder. BMC Psychiatry 14:51, 2014 24555511

Robinson P, Hellier J, Barrett B, et al: The NOURISHED randomised controlled trial comparing mentalisation-based treatment for eating disorders (MBT-ED) with specialist supportive clinical management (SSCM-ED) for patients with eating disorders and symptoms of borderline personality disorder. Trials 17(1):549, 2016 27855714

Robinson PH, Skårderud F, Sommerfeldt B: Hunger: Mentalization-Based Treatments for Eating Disorders. Cham, Switzerland, Springer, 2019

Rothschild-Yakar L, Levy-Shiff R, Fridman-Balaban R, et al: Mentalization and relationships with parents as predictors of eating disordered behavior. J Nerv Ment Dis 198(7):501–507, 2010 20611053

Rothschild-Yakar L, Waniel A, Stein D: Mentalizing in self vs. parent representations and working models of parents as risk and protective factors from distress and eating disorders. J Nerv Ment Dis 201(6):510–518, 2013 23686159

Skårderud F: Eating one's words, part I: 'Concretised metaphors' and reflective function in anorexia nervosa—an interview study. Eur Eat Disord Rev 15(3):163–174, 2007a 17676686

Skårderud F: Eating one's words: Part III. Mentalisation-based psychotherapy for anorexia nervosa—an outline for a treatment and training manual. Eur Eat Disord Rev 15(5):323–339, 2007b 17701977

Skårderud F: Bruch revisited and revised. Eur Eat Disord Rev 17(2):83–88, 2009 19241426

Skårderud F, Fonagy P: Eating disorders, in Handbook of Mentalizing in Mental Health Practice. Edited by Bateman AW, Fonagy P. Washington, DC, American Psychiatric Publishing, 2012, pp 347–384

Taube-Schiff M, Van Exan J, Tanaka R, et al: Attachment style and emotional eating in bariatric surgery candidates: the mediating role of difficulties in emotion regulation. Eat Behav 18:36–40, 2015 25875114

Taylor GJ, Bagby RM, Parker JDA: Disorders of Affect Regulation. Alexithymia in Medical and Psychiatric Illness. Cambridge, UK, Cambridge University Press, 1997

Zachrisson HD, Skårderud F: Feelings of insecurity: review of attachment and eating disorders. Eur Eat Disord Rev 18(2):97–106, 2010 20148392

CHAPTER 23

DEPRESSION

Patrick Luyten, Ph.D.

Alessandra Lemma, M.A., M.Phil., D.Clin.Psych.

Mary Target, M.Sc., Ph.D.

Depression is among the most prevalent disorders worldwide. Population-based studies suggest a lifetime prevalence for unipolar depression of approximately 15%, with rates of up to 25% in women (Alonso et al. 2004; Blazer et al. 1994; Kessler et al. 2003; Thornicroft et al. 2017). Mood disorders are the chief cause of suicide and suicide attempts (Bernal et al. 2007). In the 2013 Global Burden of Disease study (Global Burden of Disease Study 2013 Collaborators 2015), major depressive disorder was the second leading cause of years lived with disability worldwide, and the first to fourth leading cause in different regions of the world. Moreover, by the year 2020 depression is expected to be the second most serious disorder with respect to global disease burden (Murray and Lopez 1996). Depression is also associated with serious economic costs (Donohue and Pincus 2007), particularly because most patients with depression either do not seek treatment or receive inadequate treatment (Thornicroft et al. 2017).

Studies have shown that current pharmaceutical and psychotherapeutic treatments have limited effects for a considerable subgroup of individuals with depression, with only about 50% of patients responding to such treatments (Cuijpers et al. 2010; Luyten and Blatt 2007; Luyten et al. 2006); more recent trials in more clinically representative samples have found even lower remission rates (Driessen et al. 2013). As we discuss in more detail later in this chapter, prevention of relapse is one of the main aims of the mentalization-based approach to depression. This is a particularly important aim in the treatment of patients with chronic and treatment-resistant depression, who are at high risk of relapse even after successful treatment (Fonagy et al. 2015b; Town et al. 2017). We believe that fostering the mentalizing capacities of individuals vulnerable to depression enables them to cope better with the stresses of life when faced with adversity, thereby decreasing the likelihood of relapse; moreover, this approach may also reduce the probability of the intergenerational transmission of depression.

In this chapter, we first explain the rationale for applying the concept of mentalizing to depression. We then present a discussion of the basic assumptions of the mentalization-based approach to depression. Next, we discuss the relationship between mood and mentalizing, and the roles that individual differences in attachment history play in specific mentalizing impairments. Finally, we outline the role of mentalizing in current treatments for depression, including dynamic interpersonal therapy, a brief psychodynamic treatment for depression that incorporates an explicit mentalizing focus (Lemma et al. 2011a).

THE CASE FOR A MENTALIZATION-BASED APPROACH

Interpersonal problems in people with depression are well documented (McFarquhar et al. 2018). A focus on mentalizing may therefore be particularly apt in the treatment of these individuals. More specifically, depression has been associated with so-called dysfunctional interpersonal transactional cycles (Kiesler 1983), implying that the individual's interpersonal style leads to exactly those behaviors and reactions in others that the individual fears and attempts to avoid, and that this in turn confirms his or her negative expectations about others and the self. Hence, it has been shown not only that depressed mood influences relationships negatively but also that individuals who are vulnerable to depression actively select and evoke maladaptive interpersonal environments, leading to much conflict and ambivalence in relationships and potentially to social exclusion and isolation (Luyten and Blatt 2012). This view of the interpersonal nature of depression is further reinforced by findings that interpersonal factors play an important role in explaining the outcome of current evidence-based treatments for depression (Blatt et al. 2010; McFarquhar et al. 2018).

Consistent with the key role of interpersonal difficulties in depression, studies have quite consistently reported impairments in mentalizing, based on a wide variety of tasks, in patients with both unipolar and bipolar disorder (Billeke et al. 2013; Bistricky et al. 2011; Weightman et al. 2014). Importantly, these deficits have been found to predict relapse in major depression and have been demonstrated in euthymic patients, even when basic cognitive dysfunctions associated with depressed mood were controlled for. This finding clearly suggests that mentalizing impairments continue to exist outside depressive episodes and thus may be involved in the onset and recurrence of mood disorders. Furthermore, most of these studies found that the duration and severity of depression negatively influenced mentalizing capacities.

Mentalizing in depressed patients may of course be context dependent—for example, it may be particularly pronounced with regard to experiences of loss, separation, or failure, rather than reflecting a general impairment in social cognition—and may also be heavily influenced by current mood, particularly in severely depressed patients or patients with strong mood reactivity to either positive or negative events. Hence, whereas depressed patients are often prone to hypomentalizing, they may also show hypersensitivity to mental states and may be highly attuned to the mental states of others (Montag et al. 2010). Similarly, depressed patients may show hypermentalizing (i.e., excessive speculation about the mental states of the self and/or others), as discussed in more detail later in this chapter (see also Luyten and Blatt 2012).

A final and important reason why the mentalizing approach may be relevant for the conceptualization and treatment of depression is that depression shows high comorbidity with other disorders that are characterized by marked mentalizing deficits as well as interpersonal problems and pathology of the self, most notably borderline personality disorder. Hence, many depressed patients present with borderline features, and vice versa, which has important implications for treatment (Luyten and Fonagy 2014).

DEPRESSION AND MENTALIZING: THEORETICAL PERSPECTIVES

Basic Assumption of the Mentalizing Approach

The basic assumption of the mentalizing approach to depression is that depressive symptoms reflect responses to threats to attachment relations, and thus threats to the self, because of (impending) separation, rejection, or loss; (impending) failure experiences; or a combination of both. It is further assumed that these responses result in impaired and/or distorted mentalizing with regard to both the individual's own and other people's motivations and desires (Lemma et al. 2011a).

Moreover, depressed mood leads to further increases in arousal and stress levels, resulting in further impairments and distortions in mentalizing, which in turn lead to a loss of resilience in the face of stress and to a vicious cycle of increasing depressed mood (Figure 23–1). In the following sections, we review the evidence for these assumptions.

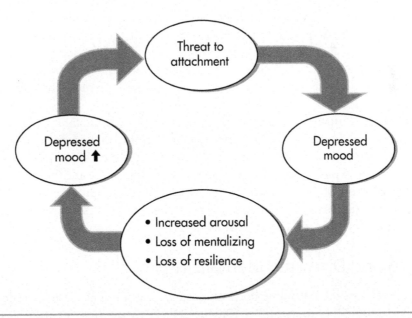

FIGURE 23–1. Relationship between threats to attachments, mood, and mentalizing.

Attachment, Stress Regulation, Reward, and Depression

Insecure attachment has been related to vulnerability to depression in children, adolescents, and adults (Grunebaum et al. 2010; Lee and Hankin 2009). It has also been shown to play a central role in explaining impairments in three central domains of functioning of depressed patients: 1) problems with stress and emotion regulation, 2) a decreased capacity for enjoyment related to a decreased sensitivity to reward, and 3) mentalizing problems (Luyten and Fonagy 2018).

The central role of attachment experiences in the causation of depression is further emphasized by findings of the important role of early adversity and disruptive attachment experiences (in particular, abuse and neglect) in the etiology of depression, with profound effects on the developing stress, reward, and mentalizing systems (Luyten and Fonagy 2018). Insecure attachment has been shown to mediate the relationship between early adversity and vulnerability to depression in later life through impaired affect regulation, stress responsivity, and social problem-solving skills (Bifulco et al. 2006; Styron and Janoff-Bulman 1997).

Several studies have lent strong support to the notion that there are intimate ties between attachment experiences, stress regulation, sensitivity to reward, and mentalizing in depression. Research in this area suggests that the attachment system is an evolutionarily developed system that is closely associated with the brain systems that reward affiliative behavior and regulate stress, and that it has stress-attenuating features that reinforce the interpersonal regulation of stress, increase trust in others, and reinforce the capacity for metacognition and mentalizing (Luyten and Fonagy 2018).

Further support for these assumptions comes from research showing that the ability to continue to mentalize, even under considerable stress, leads to so-called *broaden-and-build* (Fredrickson 2001) cycles of attachment security, which reinforce feelings of secure attachment, personal agency, and affect regulation ("build"), leading to individuals being drawn into different and more adaptive environments ("broaden") (Mikulincer and Shaver 2007). Indeed, studies on resilience have shown that positive attachment experiences are related to resilience in part through *relationship recruiting*—that is, the capacity of resilient individuals to become attached to caring others (Hauser et al. 2006). Hence, high levels of mentalizing and the associated use of security-based attachment strategies when faced with stress can explain the effect of relationship recruiting on resilience in the face of stress.

In contrast, insecure attachment strategies (discussed in detail later in this chapter) have been shown to limit the ability to "broaden and build" in the face of stress. Moreover, they have been shown to inhibit other behavioral systems that are involved in resilience, such as exploration, affiliation, and caregiving (Insel and Young 2001; Mikulincer and Shaver 2007; Neumann 2008). These findings might explain the key role of interpersonal distress and problems in depression, as well as the high rates of intergenerational transmission of depression.

Impaired and Distorted Mentalizing

Clinical experience and a growing body of research suggest that disturbed mood impairs individuals' ability to mentalize (Billeke et al. 2013; Bistricky et al. 2011; Luyten and Fonagy 2018; Weightman et al. 2014). Moreover, when depressed individuals attempt to mentalize, mentalizing is likely to be distorted, as expressed in the reemergence—either temporarily or more chronically—of modes of thinking that antedate full mentalizing (Lemma et al. 2011a).

Impairments and distortions of mentalizing due to depressed mood are most likely to be encountered in severely depressed patients. From a mentalizing perspective, when working with these patients, discussions of etiological issues (e.g., trauma, dysfunctional attitudes) that presume a capacity for insight and reflectiveness are contraindicated in the early stages of treatment. Such discussions may be counterproductive because they are likely to exceed the depressed patient's ability to mentalize effectively about these issues. Early introduction of these topics can create a vicious cycle of increasing self-criticism, rumination, helplessness, and suicidal thoughts, which also tends to make the therapist feel helpless and superfluous.

The recovery of mentalizing is typically the first therapeutic task at hand in moderately and severely depressed patients. The therapist's mentalizing stance and use of basic mentalizing techniques (see Chapter 6, "Individual Therapy Techniques") can be quite effective in this regard. The use of contrary moves, and a general inquisitive, not-knowing stance rooted in a supportive and empathic attitude on the part of the therapist that attempts to clarify and validate the patient's subjective mental states, typically provide an important counterweight to nonmentalizing states of mind. Empathic challenge and a focus on affect in the here and now are other mentalizing techniques that are helpful in this phase of the treatment, particularly as the patient is often unaware of affective states besides those related to depressed mood. For instance, although the patient may exclaim that everything is meaningless and that he or she feels completely depressed, there might be a smile on his or her face when talking about what happened earlier in the day. Marking such "islands of happiness" may play an important role in challenging psychic equivalence and teleological thinking. Similarly, a focus on affect may counterbalance feelings of emptiness and meaninglessness in patients in pretend mode.

These techniques thus also counter the second negative influence of depressed mood on mentalizing, as depressed mood is likely to be associated not only with reduced mentalizing but also with the reemergence of distorted modes of mentalizing. Foremost among these nonmentalizing modes in depression is the *psychic equivalence mode*, in which inner and outer reality are equated. The sometimes extreme accounts of inner pain and devastation, chronic fatigue, and physical pain in depressed patients are linked to psychic equivalence, where mental states may be experienced as physical conditions. A state of hyperembodiment ensues, in which subjective experiences are experienced as too real: a sense of rejection can generate acute mental and physical pain.

Consistent with our view that depressive symptoms reflect responses to threats to attachment relations and thus threats to the self, rumination and self-criticism often also have interpersonal functions—not only as a cry for attention and help but also as an attempt to regulate internal mental states in the presence of another. These interpersonal functions, particularly attempts to coregulate arousal and stress in the context of a relationship with an attachment figure, can be a primary target for interventions aimed at fostering mentalizing, as they mean that the patient is open to interpersonal communication, however distorted that communication may be at the time.

In this regard, it is important to note that *depressive realism* is relatively well documented in individuals with mood problems, meaning that their perceptions, including perceptions of the self and others, sometimes may be more accurate than those of nondepressed individuals (Moore and Fresco 2007; Yeh and Liu 2007). Hence, deficits in mentalizing may be context- or relationship-specific, so that depressed individuals may primarily show mentalizing impairments with regard to themes of loss, separation, or failure; with regard to specific attachment figures (e.g., mother or partner); and/or only with increasing levels of arousal or stress. In line with this assumption, studies have shown that depressed patients' accounts of their attachment history are not necessarily distorted, but rather appear to reflect the adverse circumstances in which many of them grew up (Hardt and Rutter 2004). Yet this depressive realism is not invariably "realistic" in the sense of adaptive, because it is often accompanied by psychic equivalence: grim reality is unquestioned or even insisted on—"*that's just how it [always] is*"—and the possibility of alternatives is ruled out.

Hypomentalizing is also often surprisingly accompanied by *extreme pretend mode* or *hypermentalizing accounts* in which the relation to reality is severed. Clinicians may be led astray by what seem to be elaborate, differentiated, and largely accurate narratives involving the self and others that moderately depressed patients often provide during assessment. These reports may—on first impression—seem to be based on genuine mentalizing. Yet, on closer listening, several features may distinguish such pretend-mode accounts from genuinely high levels of mentalizing, including 1) they are often overly detailed, long, and repetitive, permeated by depressive themes such as guilt and shame; 2) they often have a self-serving function (e.g., to prompt attention, compassion, or guilt in others, a hidden coercion); 3) they are either overly cognitive, out of touch with the underlying affective core of the experiences ("*she is too narcissistically fragile, I just ignore her*"), or affectively overwhelmed ("*I don't know, I am too disgusting to think about*"); 4) the total absence of feelings of self-worth, self-liking, and perceived control (excessive depressive realism); and 5) the inability to switch perspectives (e.g., from a focus on the self to what could have motivated others in a specific situation: "*I really have no idea; probably because she hates me*"). Genuine mentalizing should thus not be confused with hypermentalizing or with rumination.

A third nonmentalizing mode that can be typically observed in depressed individuals is the *teleological mode* or stance, in which desires and feelings are equated with observable behavior and/or material causes. Many depressed patients can feel loved only if their partner, or any other significant other, physically expresses his or her love (e.g., by being present, buying gifts, staying at home with the patient rather than going out with friends). This stance may lead to often frantic attempts to induce attachment figures, including the therapist, to show that they care about, like, and/or love the patient. Hence, patients may demand longer or more sessions and, in more extreme cases, demand to be touched, caressed, or hugged by the therapist, which may lead to boundary violations. Alternatively, many depressed patients are desperately looking for "objective proof" of their illness.

TREATMENT IMPLICATIONS

General Principles

The therapist's basic mentalizing stance and use of mentalizing interventions may help patients recover their capacity for mentalizing. Together, these typically result in the patient realizing that thoughts and feelings are *mental states* that can be reflected on, however painful or anxiety-provoking they are. Such reflection, however, may be particularly challenging in severely depressed and/or treatment-resistant patients (Luyten et al. 2012) and in patients with severe personality disorder (Luyten and Fonagy 2014) (see Box 23–1). In these patients, any attempt at mentalizing, particularly early in treatment, may be short-circuited (e.g., *"What is the point of this, it's all meaningless"*), and there is always the danger of acting out aggressive urges (e.g., self-harm, suicidal gestures) and alien-self parts (see Chapter 1, "Introduction").

BOX 23–1. Key features distinguishing depressed patients with marked personality problems

- Difference in depressive experiences: greater affective instability, greater painfulness of depressive feelings, more feelings of emptiness, abandonment, self-criticism, and shame.

- More profound mentalizing impairments in terms of both intensity and content.

- More profound attachment disruptions (i.e., attachment disorganization).

- Profound epistemic distrust/hypervigilance.

Fostering a more mentalizing stance in these patients therefore typically takes considerable persistence, patience, and skill, particularly as the therapist might be overwhelmed by the unmentalized alien-self states of depressed patients and may start feeling helpless and useless as well. Alternatively, the therapist may begin to feel like an intrusive perpetrator who revictimizes the patient by insisting on the need to reflect on what is happening in the here and now of the session. Judicious use of mentalizing these transference experiences is often needed in these instances, and therapists need to make sure that they validate the patient's experience and recognize their own contribution to it (see Chapter 6). Depressed patients with marked personality problems revert more readily to nonmentalizing modes, a shift that when combined with a propensity to externalize alien-self parts and also epistemic hypervigilance, makes these patients unsuitable for brief focused treatments that presume a capacity for reflective functioning and epistemic trust, and a capacity to form a working alliance—which is largely absent. In these patients there is first and foremost a need to foster the *process* of mentalizing. Interventions early in treatment should be primarily focused on recovering the patients' capacity for mentalizing, rather than focusing on the dynamics underlying depression, as such interventions may far exceed patients' mentalizing capacities at that time.

Basic containing interventions are also important in this context. Although merely being there—being with the patient, listening carefully, and recognizing his or her suffering—may not fully contain depressive experiences, it at least provides a holding function. The therapist's acceptance of the intensity of the patient's negative emotional states and inability to change them may, paradoxically, empower the patient to recognize that his or her usually unbearable feelings are mental as opposed to physical states—that these feelings are a subjective rather than concrete reality, and something that can be engaged with mentally (as the therapist is doing) rather than something from which the patient dissociates.

A particular clinical issue in treating depressed people in this context is the high prevalence of suicidal thoughts experienced by these patients. Many hypotheses have been advanced to explain these thoughts, ranging from feelings of helplessness and hopelessness to more complex explanations involving anger turned toward the self, fantasies about killing hated parts of the self, and omnipotent fantasies about reunion with lost loved ones. At the level of mentalizing, what seems to happen is that the un-

derlying emotions and fantasies are experienced as "too real" and concretely excruci-
ating. This agonizing experience leads patients to images or acts of suicide in a last
attempt to silence inner pain, and perhaps at the same time to obliterate what is felt
to be the cause—often the image of someone else's thoughts, also experienced as in-
trusively too real, and possible to get rid of only through violence (Fonagy and Target
1995). It is the abnormal experience of internal states in the self and other, particularly
in the psychic equivalence and teleological modes, but also the dissociation linked to
pretend-mode functioning, that increases suicidal ideation and the risk of suicide attempts. For example, shame, a common emotional experience that is enhanced in depression, feels literally self-annihilating when experienced in psychic equivalence.

Process and Content Focus

While the mentalizing approach to depression primarily focuses on the process of
mentalizing itself, there is no process without content, that is, the mental states (feelings, wishes, desires, and attitudes) that are typically organized around typical patterns of relating to the self and others. A focus on content (and particularly on typical
recurring attachment patterns that are implicated in depression, as discussed below)
requires relatively solid reflective capacities. Hence, as treatment advances, there is
typically a gradual shift from process to content. This dual focus in the treatment of
depression enables the therapist to tailor treatment and titrate it to the patient's level
of mentalizing. When arousal increases, as characteristically occurs in the context of
the discussion of a recurring pattern of relation to self and others, mentalizing may
become impaired or temporarily lost; in this scenario, a focus on the process of mentalizing is then indicated. Such a focus also helps to foster the capacity for mentalizing
even in high-arousal contexts, which in turn helps the patient to recognize these typical patterns of relating to self and others more readily outside of the treatment situation—an essential condition for change.

The dual focus on process and content is a key feature of *dynamic interpersonal therapy*, an integrative psychodynamic treatment that incorporates supportive, expressive, and directive techniques with an explicit focus on mentalizing, given the often
pervasive impairments in mentalizing of depressed patients (Lemma et al. 2011a).
From a mentalizing perspective, we believe that any effective treatment contains pro-
cess- and content-related interventions (Luyten et al. 2013a).

Tailoring Treatment: Attachment Deactivating and Hyperactivating Strategies

A focus on the content of the dynamics involved in the onset and perpetuation of depressed mood in relation to mentalizing is particularly important given the heterogeneous nature of depression. A "one size fits all" approach to the treatment of depression
is unlikely to be effective. To help clinicians match their interventions to specific patients, a focus on the role of differences in attachment history in relation to mentalizing
in depression is particularly helpful (Table 23–1; Figures 23–2 and 23–3).

As noted, substantial evidence indicates that vulnerability to depression is associated with 1) attachment anxiety and attachment avoidance and 2) the use of hyperactivating and deactivating attachment strategies, respectively (Mikulincer and Shaver

TABLE 23–1.	Attachment hyperactivating and deactivating dimensions in depression	
	Attachment hyperactivating	**Attachment deactivating**
Associated personality dimensions	Dependency/sociotropy	Self-criticism/autonomy
Experiential mode	Affective, figurative, visual	Logical; focused on overt behavior, clear cause-effect relationships
Cognitive style	Simultaneous processing, synthesis of discrete elements into cohesive total	Manifest form, analytic, detailed
Interpersonal relatedness	Seeking relatedness, harmony, and fusion; more field-dependent	Influenced by internal disposition instead of social environment; more field-independent
Stress regulation strategies (defensive style)	Recruit the support of others	Isolation, noninterpersonal regulation
Typical mentalizing profile	Hypersensitivity to mental states of others; affect-driven hypermentalizing accounts concerning love, rejection, enmeshment with attachment figures	Cognitive hypermentalizing; disconnection from emotions; often derogation of mental life as such

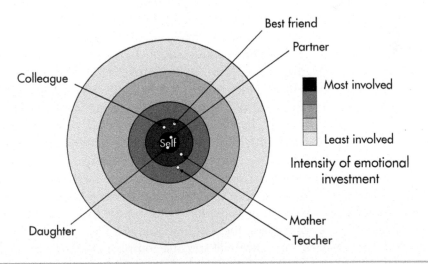

FIGURE 23–2. Hierarchy of relationships associated with high attachment anxiety in dependent/sociotropic depressed individuals.

2007). Attachment hyperactivating strategies, which are typically used by anxious attached individuals (i.e., those with a preoccupied attachment style), are aimed at finding and keeping protection, leading to frantic efforts to find support and reassurance, often expressed in demanding, clinging behavior. Attachment deactivating strategies,

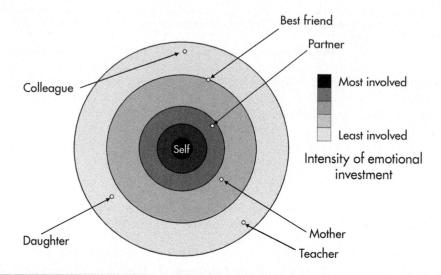

FIGURE 23–3. Hierarchy of relationships associated with attachment avoidance in self-critical/autonomous depressed individuals.

which are typically observed in avoidant individuals (i.e., those with fearful-avoidant and, in particular, dismissive attachment styles), involve denial of attachment needs and assertion of independence and strength in an attempt to avoid or reduce stress.

ATTACHMENT DEACTIVATING STRATEGIES

Depressed individuals who primarily use attachment deactivating strategies in response to threats to attachment relationships tend to defensively inhibit mentalizing, which would link thoughts and feelings, by using cognitive hypermentalizing, a pattern of overactivity, or a combination of both. Activity and work enable the depressed individual to avoid reflecting on his or her past or current life, which would be too painful and threatening. In these individuals, mentalizing is defensively inhibited because of underlying feelings of sadness, emptiness, or rage that are developmentally linked to attachment experiences. In addition, this deactivating strategy often serves to push back feelings of failure or worthlessness, with the activity proving to the individual that he or she is "good" or "achieving important things in life."

These individuals also often seem to be disconnected from their emotions and their bodies, an observation congruent with findings that attachment avoidance is associated with a dissociation between subjective and bodily stress. This finding links to the alexithymic-like features of some of these individuals and the high comorbidity between mood disturbances and functional somatic complaints among these patients (Luyten et al. 2013b). Attachment deactivating strategies are often associated with a derogation of mental life as such and with a dominance of the teleological mode, leading to an idealization of action and prioritization of "objective" knowledge. These patients may also show gross "mind-blindness" to the internal states of others, and sometimes also to their own mental states. For instance, they may be either unaware of the fact that others do not like them or, alternatively, exaggerate dislike by others.

However, in some patients, this mind-blindness may alternate with a kind of cognitive mentalizing involving highly detailed, typically self-centered narratives, particularly when they are asked to talk about their situation. Such accounts may be difficult to distinguish from genuine mentalizing, but the tightly woven, egocentric texture of such accounts, combined with their rather fixed "objectivity," which actually seems decoupled from reality, may indicate pseudomentalizing in pretend-mode functioning. Furthermore, under increasing stress, mentalizing typically breaks down, leading to the reemergence of strong feelings of dependency, helplessness, and hopelessness, sometimes with anger or panic. Much easier to identify as failures of mentalizing are the highly dismissive accounts in which some avoidant individuals almost completely deny the problematic nature of their behavior and relationships, for example, denigrating everyone else as weak or stupid, or the highly idealizing accounts in which some patients minimize painful experiences or exaggerate positive aspects of their attachment history or current relationships, usually without being able to give any concrete examples or making implausible claims. For example: *"It was good for me to go to boarding school from age 4, and I finally had to overrule my wife to send our kids at 8, which was probably too late. It upsets her when they cry, but that's just a reflex."*

The first task in working with these patients is to foster a mentalizing stance before addressing underlying psychological issues, thus focusing on mentalizing as a process and a capacity, with the history and underlying dynamics giving material for mentalizing that is salient to the patient rather than being elaborated for its own sake.

ATTACHMENT HYPERACTIVATING STRATEGIES

Individuals who primarily use attachment hyperactivating strategies in response to threats to attachment relationships often show a paradoxical pattern of hypersensitivity to the mental states of others yet simultaneous defensive inhibition of mentalizing, because they are easily overwhelmed by emotions related to attachment threats in the present and past (e.g., related to memories of abuse or neglect). They are easily overwhelmed by fear of rejection and abandonment and by fears about their own aggression and rage. Hence, in contrast to those who primarily use attachment deactivating strategies, these individuals readily decouple mentalizing and are subsequently typically slow to start mentalizing again. Particularly when under acute stress, or when severely depressed, they can be completely overwhelmed by negative emotions, which can lead to total inhibition of the capacity to reflect. Moreover, attempts at genuine mentalizing are also often short-circuited because of hypersensitivity to the mental states of others, including the therapist (Blatt 2004). Hence, early in treatment, these patients will often try very hard to please the therapist and to say "what the therapist wants to hear" while in fact trying not to hear much themselves in case they become more overwhelmed. They may be vulnerable to emotional contagion, confusing their own mental states with those of others; this is particularly likely to happen in patients with comorbid borderline features (Fonagy and Luyten 2009).

A preoccupation with negative emotion and perceived threats to attachment relationships is expressed not only in hypersensitivity to rejection, separation, and loss, but also in a bias toward interpreting the behavior of others in terms of rejection. For instance, when the therapist looks at the time, the patient believes that he or she is bored; when the therapist gives the dates of a future holiday break, the patient feels completely rejected and thinks the therapist would like to get rid of him or her and is perhaps taking a break only from him or her, rather than an actual holiday. This bias can be very difficult to correct.

A teleological stance, in which actions speak but words are distrusted, is also expressed in a strong need to be reassured, liked, and cared for, which may lead to demands for the (constant) availability of attachment figures, including the therapist—no holiday breaks, extra session time, e-mail or phone contact as needed—and other "objective proofs" of acceptance and care. This pattern may be accompanied by hypermentalizing as expressed in detailed, repetitive, or confusing accounts and fantasies about perfect or rejected love, or by attachment narratives that betray a continuing enmeshment with attachment figures (e.g., mother, father, partner, and, increasingly, therapist) that can be further exacerbated by self–other confusion. Particularly in higher-functioning patients (e.g., those with histrionic or hysterical features), such accounts may be quite elaborate and dominated by endless possible scenarios about past, present, or future relationships, in which the self is generally the victim of the bad intentions or indifference of others.

MENTALIZING IN VIVO

Particularly in the early stages of treatment, while therapists inevitably activate the patients' attachment system in order to engage them in treatment, there is a constant risk of the decoupling of mentalizing (as with patients who predominantly use deactivating strategies, as described earlier), particularly if interventions are aimed at clarifying links between symptoms and interpersonal conflict and ambivalence. In lower-functioning patients, such interventions may lead to a rapid decoupling of mentalizing, with ensuing rage, and thus may be a threat to the therapeutic alliance. In higher-functioning patients, these interventions may lead to denial, rage that threatens to "bite the hand that feeds it," decoupling of mentalizing, and sometimes disengagement from treatment.

What is in MBT called *mentalizing the relationship* (see Chapter 6) may counteract this tendency, as it provides an "online" and in-vivo experience that communicates to the patient that his or her feelings are understandable but, at the same time, come with a high intrapersonal and interpersonal cost (Lemma et al. 2011a).

Addressing the Patient's Interpersonal Functioning

Patients who present as depressed invariably also present with difficulties and distress about their relationships, leading to problems with responding in an open and flexible way to their (changing) social environment. This has also been described as *epistemic petrification*: patients no longer trust others (or themselves) as a reliable source of knowledge about themselves, others, and interpersonal relationships (Fonagy et al. 2015a). Rather, they impose a set of expectations that have been well honed in other relationship contexts, and they are not responsive to any new social information that could modify those expectations. To put this another way: regardless of his or her current experience, the patient applies social schemata that are too rigid and poorly fit the actual interpersonal situation, and this generates relational tension that further contributes to his or her preexisting difficulties. For instance, particular patterns of social interaction are created that persistently devalue the relationships that an individual may form. Reactions can be provoked in others that generate criticism, disappointment, betrayal, or rebuff. These in turn generate a loss of trust in others and confidence in the self, reducing the chance of better social experiences that could correct the preexisting expectations. As described in Chapter 4 ("Mentalizing, Resilience, and Epistemic Trust") and Chapter 10 ("Therapeutic Models"), a consistent mentalizing stance on the part of the therapist may reactivate the capacity for epistemic trust in the patient, as it is typically associated with an experience of feeling validated—that is, recognized as an agentive human being.

CONCLUSION

From a mentalizing perspective, the presenting symptoms of depression can be reformulated as responses to interpersonal difficulties or perceived threats to attachments and hence also to the self. These perceived threats can both result from and cause difficulties in mentalizing—that is, in thinking clearly and realistically not only about the external world but also about the internal world of the individual's own thoughts, feelings, and experiences with others. The therapist reframes the patient's symptoms of depression as manifestations of a relational disturbance that the patient cannot understand, or understands in a maladaptive way, attributing unlikely or unhelpful motivations to himself or herself and others. Change occurs because the individual gradually feels able to abandon the constraining set of expectations, a process that is facilitated by an increased capacity for mentalizing. This in turn serves to reduce interpersonal tensions and facilitates the recovery of personal capacities that improve coping and resilience.

Evidence is mounting for the effectiveness of a mentalizing approach in treating major depressive disorder (Bressi et al. 2017; Jakobsen et al. 2014; Lemma and Fonagy 2013; Lemma et al. 2011b) and in addressing depression and related features in patients with borderline personality disorder (Bateman and Fonagy 2008; Rossouw and Fonagy 2012). More research is needed to further investigate the efficacy of mentalizing approaches to depression and the purported mechanisms of change. In the meantime, however, a mentalizing approach to depression appears to be a welcome addition to the established treatment approaches.

REFERENCES

Alonso J, Angermeyer MC, Bernert S, et al; ESEMeD/MHEDEA 2000 Investigators, European Study of the Epidemiology of Mental Disorders (ESEMeD) Project: Prevalence of mental disorders in Europe: results from the European Study of the Epidemiology of Mental Disorders (ESEMeD) project. Acta Psychiatr Scand Suppl 109(420):21–27, 2004 15128384

Bateman A, Fonagy P: 8-year follow-up of patients treated for borderline personality disorder: mentalization-based treatment versus treatment as usual. Am J Psychiatry 165(5):631–638, 2008 18347003

Bernal M, Haro JM, Bernert S, et al; ESEMED/MHEDEA Investigators: Risk factors for suicidality in Europe: results from the ESEMED study. J Affect Disord 101(1–3):27–34, 2007 17074395

Bifulco A, Kwon J, Jacobs C, et al: Adult attachment style as mediator between childhood neglect/abuse and adult depression and anxiety. Soc Psychiatry Psychiatr Epidemiol 41(10):796–805, 2006 16871369

Billeke P, Boardman S, Doraiswamy PM: Social cognition in major depressive disorder: a new paradigm? Transl Neurosci 4:437–447, 2013

Bistricky SL, Ingram RE, Atchley RA: Facial affect processing and depression susceptibility: cognitive biases and cognitive neuroscience. Psychol Bull 137(6):998–1028, 2011 21895353

Blatt SJ: Experiences of Depression: Theoretical, Clinical and Research Perspectives. Washington, DC, American Psychological Association, 2004

Blatt SJ, Zuroff DC, Hawley LL, et al: Predictors of sustained therapeutic change. Psychother Res 20(1):37–54, 2010 19757328

Blazer DG, Kessler RC, McGonagle KA, et al: The prevalence and distribution of major depression in a national community sample: the National Comorbidity Survey. Am J Psychiatry 151(7):979–986, 1994 8010383

Bressi C, Fronza S, Minacapelli E, et al: Short-term psychodynamic psychotherapy with mentalization-based techniques in major depressive disorder patients: relationship among alexithymia, reflective functioning, and outcome variables—a pilot study. Psychol Psychother 90(3):299–313, 2017 27801544

Cuijpers P, van Straten A, Bohlmeijer E, et al: The effects of psychotherapy for adult depression are overestimated: a meta-analysis of study quality and effect size. Psychol Med 40(2):211–223, 2010 19490745

Donohue JM, Pincus HA: Reducing the societal burden of depression: a review of economic costs, quality of care and effects of treatment. Pharmacoeconomics 25(1):7–24, 2007 17192115

Driessen E, Van HL, Don FJ, et al: The efficacy of cognitive-behavioral therapy and psychodynamic therapy in the outpatient treatment of major depression: a randomized clinical trial. Am J Psychiatry 170(9):1041–1050, 2013 24030613

Fonagy P, Luyten P: A developmental, mentalization-based approach to the understanding and treatment of borderline personality disorder. Dev Psychopathol 21(4):1355–1381, 2009 19825272

Fonagy P, Target M: Understanding the violent patient: the use of the body and the role of the father. Int J Psychoanal 76(Pt 3):487–501, 1995 7558608

Fonagy P, Luyten P, Allison E: Epistemic petrification and the restoration of epistemic trust: a new conceptualization of borderline personality disorder and its psychosocial treatment. J Pers Disord 29(5):575–609, 2015a 26393477

Fonagy P, Rost F, Carlyle JA, et al: Pragmatic randomized controlled trial of long-term psychoanalytic psychotherapy for treatment-resistant depression: the Tavistock Adult Depression Study (TADS). World Psychiatry 14(3):312–321, 2015b 26407787

Fredrickson BL: The role of positive emotions in positive psychology. The broaden-and-build theory of positive emotions. Am Psychol 56(3):218–226, 2001 11315248

Global Burden of Disease Study 2013 Collaborators: Global, regional, and national incidence, prevalence, and years lived with disability for 301 acute and chronic diseases and injuries in 188 countries, 1990–2013: a systematic analysis for the Global Burden of Disease Study 2013. Lancet 386(9995):743–800, 2015 26063472

Grunebaum MF, Galfalvy HC, Mortenson LY, et al: Attachment and social adjustment: relationships to suicide attempt and major depressive episode in a prospective study. J Affect Disord 123(1–3):123–130, 2010 19819021

Hardt J, Rutter M: Validity of adult retrospective reports of adverse childhood experiences: review of the evidence. J Child Psychol Psychiatry 45(2):260–273, 2004 14982240

Hauser ST, Allen JP, Golden E: Out of the Woods: Tales of Resilient Teens. Cambridge, MA, Harvard University Press, 2006

Insel TR, Young LJ: The neurobiology of attachment. Nat Rev Neurosci 2(2):129–136, 2001 11252992

Jakobsen JC, Gluud C, Kongerslev M, et al: Third-wave cognitive therapy versus mentalisation-based treatment for major depressive disorder: a randomised clinical trial. BMJ Open 4(8):e004903, 2014 25138802

Kessler RC, Berglund P, Demler O, et al; National Comorbidity Survey Replication: The epidemiology of major depressive disorder: results from the National Comorbidity Survey Replication (NCS-R). JAMA 289(23):3095–3105, 2003 12813115

Kiesler DJ: The 1982 interpersonal circle: a taxonomy for complementarity in human transactions. Psychol Rev 90:185–214, 1983

Lee A, Hankin BL: Insecure attachment, dysfunctional attitudes, and low self-esteem predicting prospective symptoms of depression and anxiety during adolescence. J Clin Child Adolesc Psychol 38(2):219–231, 2009 19283600

Lemma A, Fonagy P: Feasibility study of a psychodynamic online group intervention for depression. Psychoanal Psychol 30:367–380, 2013

Lemma A, Target M, Fonagy P: Brief Dynamic Interpersonal Therapy: A Clinician's Guide. Oxford, Oxford University Press, 2011a

Lemma A, Target M, Fonagy P: The development of a brief psychodynamic intervention (dynamic interpersonal therapy) and its application to depression: a pilot study. Psychiatry 74(1):41–48, 2011b 21463169

Luyten P, Blatt SJ: Looking back towards the future: is it time to change the DSM approach to psychiatric disorders? The case of depression. Psychiatry 70(2):85–99, 2007 17661536

Luyten P, Blatt SJ: Psychodynamic treatment of depression. Psychiatr Clin North Am 35(1):111–129, 2012 22370494

Luyten P, Fonagy P: Psychodynamic treatment for borderline personality disorder and mood disorders: a mentalizing perspective, in Borderline Personality Disorder and Mood Disorders: Controversies and Consensus. Edited by Choi-Kain L, Gunderson J. New York, Springer, 2014, pp 223–251

Luyten P, Fonagy P: The stress-reward-mentalizing model of depression: an integrative developmental cascade approach to child and adolescent depressive disorder based on the research domain criteria (RDoC) approach. Clin Psychol Rev 64:87–98, 2018 29107398

Luyten P, Blatt SJ, Van Houdenhove B, et al: Depression research and treatment: are we skating to where the puck is going to be? Clin Psychol Rev 26(8):985–999, 2006 16473443

Luyten P, Fonagy P, Lemma A, et al: Depression, in Handbook of Mentalizing in Mental Health Practice. Edited by Bateman A, Fonagy P. Washington, DC, American Psychiatric Association, 2012, pp 385–417

Luyten P, Blatt SJ, Fonagy P: Impairments in self structures in depression and suicide in psychodynamic and cognitive behavioral approaches: implications for clinical practice and research. Int J Cogn Ther 6:265–279, 2013a

Luyten P, Van Houdenhove B, Lemma A, et al: Vulnerability for functional somatic disorders: a contemporary psychodynamic approach. J Psychother Integration 23:250–262, 2013b

McFarquhar T, Luyten P, Fonagy P: Changes in interpersonal problems in the psychotherapeutic treatment of depression as measured by the Inventory of Interpersonal Problems: a systematic review and meta-analysis. J Affect Disord 226:108–123, 2018 28968563

Mikulincer M, Shaver PR: Attachment in Adulthood: Structure, Dynamics, and Change. New York, Guilford, 2007

Montag C, Ehrlich A, Neuhaus K, et al: Theory of mind impairments in euthymic bipolar patients. J Affect Disord 123(1–3):264–269, 2010 19748680

Moore MT, Fresco DM: Depressive realism and attributional style: implications for individuals at risk for depression. Behav Ther 38(2):144–154, 2007 17499081

Murray CJL, Lopez AD: The Global Burden of Disease: A Comprehensive Assessment of Mortality and Disability From Diseases, Injuries, and Risk Factors in 1990 and Projected to 2020. Cambridge, MA, Harvard University Press, 1996

Neumann ID: Brain oxytocin: a key regulator of emotional and social behaviours in both females and males. J Neuroendocrinol 20(6):858–865, 2008 18601710

Rossouw TI, Fonagy P: Mentalization-based treatment for self-harm in adolescents: a randomized controlled trial. J Am Acad Child Adolesc Psychiatry 51(12):1304.e3–1313.e3, 2012 23200287

Styron T, Janoff-Bulman R: Childhood attachment and abuse: long-term effects on adult attachment, depression, and conflict resolution. Child Abuse Negl 21(10):1015–1023, 1997 9330802

Thornicroft G, Chatterji S, Evans-Lacko S, et al: Undertreatment of people with major depressive disorder in 21 countries. Br J Psychiatry 210(2):119–124, 2017 27908899

Town JM, Abbass A, Stride C, et al: A randomised controlled trial of Intensive Short-Term Dynamic Psychotherapy for treatment resistant depression: the Halifax Depression Study. J Affect Disord 214:15–25, 2017 28266318

Weightman MJ, Air TM, Baune BT: A review of the role of social cognition in major depressive disorder. Front Psychiatry 5:179, 2014 25566100

Yeh ZT, Liu SI: Depressive realism: evidence from false interpersonal perception. Psychiatry Clin Neurosci 61(2):135–141, 2007 17362430

COMORBID SUBSTANCE USE DISORDER AND PERSONALITY DISORDER

Nina Arefjord, Cand.Psychol.

Katharina Morken, Cand.Psychol., Ph.D.

Kari Lossius, Cand.Psychol.

In modern treatment of substance use disorder (SUD), it remains a challenge to offer effective outpatient treatment for patients with SUD and severe personality disorders (PDs). Outpatient programs need to be comprehensive and intensive, and treatment must be effective in terms of reducing the use of inpatient crisis admittance. Patients with comorbid PD and SUD often show problems with regular attendance in outpatient programs. These difficulties are due not only to the SUD and the patients' varying motivation and lack of endurance, but also to their difficulties in coping with their feelings and interpersonal problems. SUD therapists are in need of useful tools to be able to offer effective outpatient treatment to these patients. There is a need for therapy programs with a good structure, theoretical consistency, and continuity. In this chapter, we describe how mentalization-based treatment for substance use disorder (MBT-SUD) can be implemented for SUD, why this model and its theoretical foundation make sense, and how it broadens our understanding of SUD patients with severe PDs (Morken et al. 2014, 2017a, 2017b).

COMORBIDITY BETWEEN PERSONALITY DISORDER AND SUBSTANCE USE DISORDER

Many studies have demonstrated the frequent comorbidity between PD and SUD (Fenton et al. 2012; Hasin and Kilcoyne 2012; Trull et al. 2010; Verheul 2001). One review found that the comorbidity of PD among SUD patients ranged from 25% to 75% (Cacciola et al. 2001). The most prevalent PDs in clinical SUD populations are antisocial PD (ASPD), at 23%–28%, and borderline PD (BPD), at 7%–18% (Fridell and Hesse 2005; Verheul 2001).

Cluster B personality traits (i.e., antisocial, borderline, histrionic, and narcissistic) have been found to be independent risk factors both for developing SUD and for the persistence of SUD (Cohen et al. 2007; Fenton et al. 2012; Walter et al. 2009); however, in the course of a 10-year study, remission of SUD in BPD patients was also common (Zanarini et al. 2011).

The risk for treatment attrition is higher among patients with PD and SUD than with SUD alone, and comorbidity has been found to negatively influence outcome for SUD patients (Ball et al. 2006; Brorson et al. 2013; Vaglum 2005). Cluster B traits have been found to be a barrier to forming a therapeutic alliance with SUD patients and also to provoke more distance in helpers, which explains why countertransference processes (described later in this chapter) could influence the treatment negatively (Olesek et al. 2016; Thylstrup and Hesse 2008).

COMPROMISED MENTALIZING AND EMOTIONAL DYSREGULATION

"Without mentalizing there can be no robust sense of self, no constructive social interaction, no mutuality in relationships, and no sense of personal security" (Bateman and Fonagy 2016, p. 3). This sentence characterizes the core problem for many patients with BPD and comorbid SUD: an unstable sense of self and poor self–other mentalizing, specifically, being unable to identify and mentalize their own internal states. Substances are then used to stabilize the collapse in self-states. Emotional dysregulation is characterized by strong emotions, which undermine the capacity to think clearly. Mentalizing failures are characterized by being unable to express feelings in an appropriate way. Substance use can be considered as one of several self-soothing strategies used by patients who struggle with personality problems (Phillips et al. 2012). As one patient expressed it: *"I intoxicate myself to be able to bear my intense/strong feelings, and at the moment that is my only coping strategy."*

The dysregulation is partly caused by insecure attachment patterns characterized by mistrust of others and a belief that other people cannot be of any help (Bateman and Fonagy 2016; Fonagy and Bateman 2016); the mistrust may jeopardize commitment to and compliance with treatment. Substance use undermines mentalizing capacities further, aggravating the patient's condition.

ATTACHMENT, SUBSTANCE USE, AND NEUROBIOLOGY

Substance dependency and attachment share a common neurobiology (Insel 2003; Phillips et al. 2012). Many patients with BPD and SUD are traumatized, with concentration problems, thought disorder, and disabling flashbacks. Of 228 female patients with substance use, 50% reported emotional abuse, 42% reported physical abuse, and

42% reported sexual abuse (Haller and Miles 2004). SUD patients who had polydrug use had the highest prevalence of PDs. The women who had been exposed to sexual abuse had a doubled risk for ASPD. Emotional and physical abuse was connected to increased risk for BPD. Painful attachment experiences increase negative emotions; negative emotionality and impulsivity are among the underlying personality traits that are considered to explain the comorbidity between SUD and BPD (James and Taylor 2007; Karterud et al. 2017).

Below follows a clinical example from our MBT-SUD program. This patient demonstrates how vulnerable she is in relationships and how compromised she is by her negative emotions, which in turn lead to impulsive drinking as a strategy to cope.

> A patient with prolonged traumatic childhood experiences of being in the middle of her parents' bitter conflicts was exploring what could be behind her teacher's behavior and intentions. She had been drinking heavily after a difficult meeting with the teacher. The patient was naming different emotions: feeling excluded and jealous, with a fixed view that her teacher preferred other students to her. The patient was in both a psychic equivalence and a hypermentalizing mode. She had fragmented explanations of how she understood her teacher's behavior, but these were not contextualized or grounded in reality. She summarized her understanding of herself as: *"I must be a monster, having these feelings."*

NEUROBIOLOGY OF SUBSTANCE USE DISORDER

Every substance has slightly different effects on the brain, but all addictive drugs, including alcohol, opioids, and cocaine, produce a pleasurable surge of the neurotransmitter dopamine in the basal ganglia region of the brain. This area is part of the reward system and controls the ability to learn on the basis of reward. Some drugs (i.e., cocaine and morphine) influence the nucleus accumbens directly and can interfere with and hijack the reward system, with the result that the individual prefers substances instead of social interaction. These same circuits control the ability to derive pleasure from ordinary rewards such as food, sex, and social interaction, and when they are disrupted by substance use, the rest of life can feel less and less enjoyable to the user when he or she is not using substances. It seems likely that these pathways and the genes underlying them evolved not for drug abuse but for mediating the motivational aspects of social interaction, including pair bonding, maternal attachment to infants, and, presumably, infant attachment to the mother (Insel 2003; Phillips et al. 2012). Healthy adults are usually able to control their impulses when necessary because these impulses are balanced by the judgment and decision-making circuits of the prefrontal cortex. These prefrontal circuits are disrupted in SUD and in PD. This explains why SUD is said to involve compromised self-control. It is not a complete loss of autonomy—substance-dependent individuals are still accountable for their actions, but they are much less able to override the powerful drive to seek relief from withdrawal provided by alcohol or drugs (U.S. Department of Health and Human Services Office of the Surgeon General 2016). Two factors found in both SUD and PD—decreased ability to take pleasure or reward from social interaction, and compromised self-control—can partly explain why SUD complicates the treatment course of PDs and why, when comorbid PD occurs in people presenting primarily with SUD, both disorders need to be treated.

DUAL-TRACK TREATMENT FOR COMORBID SUBSTANCE USE DISORDER AND PERSONALITY DISORDER

A review of psychotherapies for comorbid BPD and SUD found 10 controlled studies of BPD/SUD patients (Lee et al. 2015). The authors concluded that although the evidence base for treatment of co-occurring BPD and SUD needs to be expanded with more research, there is some preliminary evidence of benefit from dialectical behavior therapy and dynamic deconstructive psychotherapy. Many studies have claimed the need for targeted treatments for this group of patients (Ravndal et al. 2005; van den Bosch and Verheul 2007). MBT trials have had successful outcomes with BPD patients, but MBT has not been tried for patients in whom SUD is the main disorder. Morken et al. (2017a) summarize various randomized controlled trials and naturalistic cohort studies in which MBT has shown promising outcomes with BPD; and the strength of MBT has been demonstrated when the severity of PD is taken into consideration (Bales et al. 2012, 2015; Bateman and Fonagy 2001, 2009; Jørgensen et al. 2014; Kvarstein et al. 2015; Rossouw and Fonagy 2012).

THE BERGEN MBT-SUD MODEL: CLINICAL EXPERIENCE

The Bergen Clinics MBT-SUD program in Norway adheres to the MBT model described by Bateman and Fonagy (2004, 2012, 2016) but extends the treatment period up to 3 years and integrates a social worker as part of the MBT team. MBT-SUD is a dual-track treatment that pays simultaneous attention to both addictive and personality problems and aims to focus on the patients' mentalizing processes around the psychological functions underlying their substance use. We have found in our clinical practice that patients' use of substances and alcohol frequently links with their psychological needs and a lack of more beneficial strategies to cope with those needs.

> A patient is talking about her excessive intake of benzodiazepines. When she elaborates on the last intake, the psychological pattern appears; she is struggling with self-imposed isolation and her coping mechanism is to use benzodiazepines.

Addiction-specific strategies in MBT-SUD include addressing the patient's coping mechanism in the sessions while identifying and exploring the underlying psychological pattern in a way that is meaningful to the patient.

In MBT-SUD the substance abuse is addressed directly by working toward abstinence, and indirectly by targeting emotional dysregulation and impulsivity and increasing self-regulation. The core mentalizing problem for these patients is their unstable sense of self, and an important therapeutic task is to increase and stabilize their ability to identify, know, and regulate their own self-states. However, reducing or stopping substance use means that the individual will become more aware of negative emotions and be thrown into dysregulating emotions without functional soothing strategies. The aim of treatment is for emotions to be eventually mastered by reflections on thoughts, affects, and interpersonal contact. This change is a demanding process and motivation is vital. Motivational interviewing is generally recommended in the initial phase to increase the therapeutic alliance and motivational process (Bateman and Fonagy 2004). A further focus is on interpersonal interactions in which mentalizing failure occurs and is followed by substance use. Risky substance use should be stabilized before the patient can fully benefit from MBT combination treatment. If the substance craving is too strong, the patient should initially be offered stabilizing treatment. Feelings of shame and defeat due to continual relapses may lead to risky behavior such as overdoses. The intake of substances must be continually addressed, especially at the start of treatment (Box 24–1).

BOX 24–1. Specific strategies in MBT-SUD

1. Consider the use of alcohol and drugs as a kind of "thermometer" that measures the patient's emotional mental state.

2. Monitor substance use by (a) awareness of and (b) addressing the intake of substances from the beginning of therapy.

3. Use motivational interviewing techniques at the beginning of treatment and if the patient has not been in SUD treatment previously.

4. Monitor whether reduction of SUD is replaced by an increase in eating disorder behavior.

5. Explore the mental function of SUD by using the interventions of the "mentalizing process trajectory" (Bateman and Fonagy 2016); this is a central component of MBT-SUD.

6. Be aware of feelings of shame and possible acting out—the "here and now" focus is vital.

7. Include a social worker on the MBT team to assist with social issues.

8. Address group attendance continually to maintain motivation, using motivational interventions. Phoning the patient after failed attendance is usually valued by the patient.

9. Increase reflection (in both patients and therapist) on how to understand nonattendance. Explore with a not-knowing stance; do not automatically assume that the reason for nonattendance is substance use.

The Bergen Clinics Foundation (BCF) was inspired by MBT and theories about personality development and decided to implement a pilot project for female patients. The BCF has a policy of gender-responsive programs that consider the needs of women in all aspects of program design and delivery, including location, staff, program development, program contents, and materials (Morken et al. 2014, 2017a, 2017b). The project was advertised within the clinic but also received referrals from mental health clinics, asking for participants who were "difficult to treat" and had a tentative diagnosis of BPD and SUD. Eighteen patients were included in the project. Four patients left the treatment. Inclusion criteria were being female and having a diagnosis of SUD together with a PD with clinically significant borderline traits according to the Structural Clinical Interview for DSM-IV Axis II Personality Disorders (SCID-II; First et al. 1997). Patients in the project were assessed by a standardized battery of interviews, and general function, symptoms, interpersonal function, and substance use were carefully monitored over time. A full diagnosis of BPD was not necessary in order to be accepted for treatment. Exclusion criteria were a diagnosis of schizophrenia and use of substitute opiate medication (Morken et al. 2017a). All patients had dependent SUD when they were included in the project, with the most commonly used substances being alcohol, cannabis, amphetamine, heroin, γ-hydroxybutyric acid (GHB), buprenorphine (Subutex), and benzodiazepines. The primary outcome measured was reduction of SUD and PD. Thirteen patients were interviewed at a follow-up 2 years after completing treatment; two patients had dependent SUD, and 11 had full remission.

The patients' core personality problems were an unstable sense of self and problems knowing their own internal states, leading to emotional dysregulation and mentalizing failures characterized especially by compromised self–other mentalizing. The consequences of these problems were frequent interpersonal misunderstandings, interactional problems, and escape into intoxication. Based on these findings, secondary treatment outcomes were social function, symptoms, and interpersonal functioning. The patients showed positive change in all measures after an average of 21 months in MBT-SUD treatment following the guidelines and manuals of MBT (Bateman and Fonagy 2004, 2006; Karterud and Bateman 2010, 2011; Morken et al. 2017a).

All therapists went through extensive MBT training. The team had weekly internal supervision in addition to an external supervisor once a month. All sessions were videotaped. Supervision was considered vital for managing MBT-SUD group therapy and avoiding destructive group processes. It took longer for the patients to commit to group therapy compared with individual therapy. Gradually, most patients became attached to the group, but PD/SUD patients' attendance had to be monitored and addressed continually to maintain their motivation for group treatment (see Box 24–1). The main motivational interventions used in MBT-SUD are demonstrating support, reassurance, and empathy in addition to exploring the patients' mind while the therapist models reflectivity (Bateman and Fonagy 2016).

An MBT-informed social worker is an integral part of the team (Box 24–1). The social worker assists patients with crucial issues of daily living, helping them to negotiate affairs of finances, housing, social welfare rights, the judicial system, and child protection agencies. The social worker position strengthens the patient's alliance with the treatment program through offering practical assistance, and home visits are made when necessary. The social worker contributes to the concerted effort to increase the patients' motivation to try psychotherapy and to control their substance use when many important issues in their lives are in a mess or unsolved. His or her work allows the therapists to concentrate on their share of the task—that is, to do psychotherapeutic work according to the guidelines of MBT. The importance of this last point can hardly be emphasized enough. As Bateman and Fonagy (2016) note

> MBT recommends that early in therapy the patient's social context is stabilized. Change will be impossible if housing, financial, employment, probation and other stressors are dominant. (p. 34)

The authors recommend an active focus on these issues by the clinician, and we found that the extent of social issues experienced by our patients is best assisted by a social worker.

RISK FACTORS FOR DROPOUT FROM TREATMENT

MBT emphasizes the need for awareness of two important risk factors in treatment if they are not properly addressed during therapy: a mental state of *pseudomentalizing* in the patient and *countertransference* in the therapist. MBT-SUD therapists need to continuously monitor themselves not to overestimate their patients' mentalizing capacity. The theory of mentalizing has contributed to understanding rigid and distorted patterns of thoughts in terms of theories of human development. As outlined in more detail in Chapter 1 ("Introduction"), pretend mode, psychic equivalence, and teleological thinking describe children's understanding of the mental world before the age of 4–5 years. These pre-mentalistic ways of thinking can also influence adults. Pretend mode, seen often as pseudomentalizing in clinical interaction, is characterized by emotions and thoughts that are not connected but isolated like different and fragmented experiences. The patient does not "own" his or her own emotions and cannot contain them or give them meaningful expression through language (Bateman and Fonagy 2004, 2016).

Pseudomentalizing mental states occur frequently in SUD treatment. However, it can be difficult to become aware of them in the session, especially if the clinician is not "listening" for them. This has been noted as an important clinical phenomenon through rating of numerous videotaped sessions of MBT-SUD. Patients might be overwhelmed by feelings within the session, and if there is no real mentalizing in the session, risky substance use might be the result to enable the patient to cope with painful feelings. The therapist might have been "fooled" by the patient's pseudomentalizing and believed that the patient was in contact with (rather than dysregulated by) emotions because the patient was describing his or her feelings. However, in pseudomentalizing these descriptions are not rooted in reality with clear links to mental representations. They are "floating" without a representational tether, and so are unbound and lack context. This can lead to sudden uncontrolled dysregulation. In SUD treatment, the use of alcohol and drugs is an indicator of the patient's emotional mode. This is why monitoring and focusing on, and constantly being aware of, the intake of substances, and the mental functions associated with the substance abuse, are central components of MBT-SUD. Addressing the intake of substances from the beginning avoids "elephants in the room"—that is, important topics being ignored. For example, the therapist needs to monitor whether a reduction of SUD is replaced by an increase in an eating disorder, which is a common but unrecognized side effect of treatment for BPD/SUD patients (see Box 24–1). The patient in the following clinical example had been treated for an eating disorder but had then replaced binge eating with the use of alcohol.

> The patient explored her last encounter with her mother. The patient talked fast and described feeling sad, desperate, and unhappy. The therapist believed the patient was able to mentalize the emotions during the session, but later the patient got excessively drunk and exposed herself to risky situations. When exploring her actions in the next session and aiming to mentalize the affects, the patient described feeling "empty" after the previous session and only being able to fill herself with alcohol, having no other self-soothing strategies available.

If the clinician is not closely monitoring the patient's mentalizing state, the clinician is in danger of talking to the patient as if she had the capacity to mentalize in the moment. But the patient is in danger of acting out by intoxicating herself:

> Patient: I drank half a bottle of vodka on Thursday. I felt desperate and had to drink.
> Therapist: It sounds like you felt you had no other options to calm down at the moment, but I am still surprised that you drank so heavily. What do you make of it?
> Patient: After having sex I didn't want to have, I felt devastated, and I didn't know what to do except drink and drink; I was not able to talk about it with anybody.

The goal is for the patient to gradually develop a language for emotions that substances have formerly been used to control and suppress (Bateman and Fonagy 2004, 2012, 2016).

SUBSTANCE USE DISORDER AND SHAME

Regular attendance in the group is a challenge when a patient is not able to gain control of his or her substance use. If the patient denies his or her level of substance intake, this is an important issue to address. Patients usually feel relieved of their shame following "hidden" substance use when they are able to mentalize it in the group. But it is vital that the clinician is aware that shame and guilt are "negative" or uncomfortable emotions. Shame involves a negative evaluation of the entire self vis-à-vis social and moral standards; guilt focuses on specific behaviors (not the self) that are inconsistent with such standards. Shame and guilt lead to different "action tendencies" (Lindsay-Hartz 2016): guilt is apt to motivate reparations, while shame is apt to motivate efforts to disappear (nonattendance) or attack, and the therapist needs to skillfully address the shame while closely monitoring the patient's mental state. MBT is tailored to address and focus on the mentalizing processes and the losses of mentalizing both within and outside the sessions. In MBT the therapist is reminded about his or her responsibility to monitor the patient's emotional activation and that the capacity to mentalize can fluctuate within a session. The therapist's self-reflection and the ability to maintain his or her own mentalizing in the session is highlighted by the model, and this strengthens the safety of MBT-SUD treatment.

COUNTERTRANSFERENCE: FEELING WITHIN THE CLINICIAN

Substance use is prone to evoke moral feelings in treatment, and treatment systems that use confrontation as a main method of treatment for SUD patients continue to be used. This approach can be risky for BPD/SUD patients because of their neurobiological vulnerability and emotional dysregulation when under psychological stress. Treatment of patients with comorbid BPD and SUD has been described as difficult because of high dropout rates and relational problems that make the process of establishing a therapeutic alliance challenging (Karterud et al. 2009; Vaglum 2005). Given the emotional challenges clinicians face when working with patients with BPD and SUD, team supervision is vital. The therapist is vulnerable to many sorts of feelings, such as care, fear, anger, rejection, and anxiety. We consider that providing a safe environment for the MBT-SUD team to discuss these countertransference issues is important. Our clinical experience can perhaps be best explained by the words of Bateman and Fonagy (2016, p. 192):

> Yet, whatever definition is used, a core persists, namely, that "countertransference" refers to feelings in the clinician and links to his/her self-awareness, which in turn relies on his/her affective pole of mentalizing....As clinicians, we need to be mindful of the fact that our mental states might unduly color our understanding of the patient's mental states and that we tend to equate our own mental states with those of the patient without adequate foundation. The clinician has to "quarantine" his/her feelings. These feelings are defined as those experiences, both affective and cognitive, that the clinician has in sessions and which he/she thinks might help to further develop an understanding of mental processes relevant to the problems of the patient or those in treatment itself.

Our clinicians have found MBT's understanding of the feelings within the clinician, and the weekly team supervision, to be most valuable for reminding them of the importance of being self-aware and not acting on these feelings by, for example, either rejecting or being overly protective of the patient. The not-knowing stance is valuable to see our clinical practice from different perspectives, and being part of a team with a coherent model and theory is experienced as important to prevent both dropout by patients and burnout for the therapists.

> Patient: In this therapy you are talking to us patients in a different way than in my other therapies. I got insecure and just talked and talked when the therapist was mainly nodding and…hmm…here I almost always know what you are thinking about our conversation, I learn from it.

FORMING AN ALLIANCE THROUGH PSYCHOEDUCATION, CRISIS PLANNING, AND MENTALIZING CASE FORMULATION

MBT is collaborative in style. Collaboration is achieved through specific strategies and attitudes such as psychoeducation, mentalizing crisis planning, development of a mentalizing case formulation, combination group and individual therapy, and video-based team supervision. These interventions and strategies are ideal for consistent treatment of BPD/SUD patients and help prevent dropout from treatment. In the pilot project of MBT-SUD, the psychoeducational sessions were experienced as an important component to prepare the patients for treatment, increase knowledge, and contribute to a shared understanding between patients and clinicians about how the patients' actual mental problems could be understood. The psychoeducational component was experienced as meaningful and an important component of the treatment:

> Patient: "Mentalizing": I didn't know its meaning. Psychoeducation contributed a lot.
>   I could better see the unifying theme between my problems.

Psychoeducational groups last 1.5 hours with a break in the middle. SUD is linked to each of the major topics addressed. The patients are asked to reflect on different ways of understanding excessive substance use linked to mental health and mentalizing. They are encouraged to introduce examples from their own life of times when they used substances to regulate difficult emotions:

> Patient: My ex called to say I couldn't have the children; he is taking them on a trip.
>   I couldn't believe him; how could he just decide this? I couldn't think, I just blanked out and drank until I passed out.

Crisis plans are an important preventive intervention for patients prone to acting out during crisis. The process of the clinician writing the crisis plan together with the patient engages the patient in reflecting about the mental processes that trigger crises for him or her:

> In the process of working out Liv's crisis plan, the most important precursor to Liv's dissociating and using drugs was discovered through exploration of which mental state she was in before she used benzodiazepines. Initially, Liv had had no idea: *"It just happened."* In fact, she does not want be in contact with her father due to a very disturbing relationship, but he continues to phone her. When the phone rings, Liv sits immobilized and goes into a state of dissociation, and then numbs herself with benzodiazepines.

Liv's crisis plan:
What is useful: To put on music and to look at photos of my daughter.
What is not useful: Taking pills to escape.

The system—what is useful: When I call Linda [the social worker], she should just listen to me. If she is not available, I can talk to some of the milieu therapists at the female unit.
The system—what is not useful: To tell me that I should not bother about my father.

The most important thing is that the patient is involved in the development of his or her crisis plan and that the therapist helps the patient reflect about the mental precursors of crises (Bateman and Fonagy 2004).

Another important part of the early phase of treatment is the development of a mentalizing case formulation, which focuses on problematic intersubjective self-regulation. Our experience is that clinicians need training in formulating these mental connections and summarizing them in a language that the patient can understand and relate to. Many SUD patients are sensitive toward the use of professional language and might interpret it as the clinician feeling superior. This phenomenon has mostly appeared in group therapy: *"The therapists are just wanting to show their cleverness using a language that I do not understand, and this new patient in the group is just showing off that he is an academic too, and that he is superior to us."*

If the clinician succeeds with the formulation, he or she is rewarded: *"The formulation I received from you was fantastic. It was like I had written it myself. I read it several times. You have really understood what it is all about. This comprises what I think myself, and I like it in writing."* In this case the patient was doing well outside therapy; however, when given such a positive response, the clinician should be aware that the patient might simply be agreeing, for example, to avoid conflict or to gain the clinician's favor, and it becomes an agreement based in pseudomentalizing. If this is the case, the formulation will not increase the patient's motivation or embed epistemic trust in his or her relationship with the clinician. The patient's use of pseudomentalizing will become apparent through monitoring closely whether the patient's formulated treatment aims actually are associated with improvements. The addiction-specific strategies are summarized in Box 24–1.

In a 2-year follow-up study after completing treatment, the patients in the MBT-SUD pilot project described what were, in many cases, the major mental changes that had occurred during the treatment (Morken et al. 2017b). The patients first achieved self-regulating competencies, which then influenced and increased their interpersonal competencies and gave them a sense of having an agentive self. Reduced impulsivity and increased ability to think though mind states in the moment increased the patients' ability to tolerate negative feelings and to control and resist substance use and other self-destructive behaviors. The ability to self-regulate increased interpersonal mentalizing, by which the patients were able, as they described it, "to see themselves from the outside." This mentalizing capacity was influenced by a more stable sense of self. Drugs or alcohol were no longer necessary to stabilize frequent collapses of internal states, which had previously caused unbearable mental pain. Core personality problems—namely, continuously unstable self-states, mistrust of others' intentions, difficulty in understanding others, and emotional dysregulation—all improved. More stable self-states influenced the patients' agentive self and understanding of others. Self-agency was a result of this new mode of experiencing their own mind and was important for their ability to reduce or cease substance use (Morken et al. 2017b).

CONCLUSION

In this chapter we have highlighted how MBT has added necessary and useful theory, knowledge, and competencies to the treatment of patients with BPD and comorbid SUD. After completion of the pilot project with female patients, the BCF is now offering an MBT program to both male and female patients with severe PDs and SUD. The treatment program adheres to the MBT model (Bateman and Fonagy 2004, 2012, 2016) but includes addiction-specific strategies and adaptations. MBT groups with male BPD/SUD patients are now also part of the MBT-SUD program. Our clinical experience is that the model is as suitable for male as for female patients; however, no formal qualitative or quantitative studies have been carried out so far. Occasionally, the groups contain patients with ASPD as well as BPD. So far, our experience is that the diagnosis in itself does not predict the patient's adjustment to the group, and the group dynamic tolerates mixed PDs. We would prefer to have separate groups for patients with ASPD/SUD and those with BPD/SUD, but so far our population of individuals with comorbid ASPD/SUD who are motivated to take up this treatment is not big enough to make a dedicated ASPD/SUD group viable.

We suggest that without the MBT model, the therapists would have had less opportunity to focus on the patients' self-reflection and understanding of their interpersonal and emotional problems associated with their drug abuse. Why is this the case? The BPD/SUD patients' vulnerability in treatment has already been described. The patients' and therapists' needs are met through the collaborative style, and the therapist is not alone, given the requirement to attend supervision. MBT is a structured treatment offering both a theoretical model to understand interpersonal problems and a clinical model to act as a framework to address therapeutic challenges that might occur throughout the course of therapy. MBT includes manual-based interventions that increase the clinician's ability to explore, cope with, and understand the patient's attachment and emotional problems, motivational difficulties, and interpersonal conflicts as they appear in treatment. Early in the therapeutic process, the goal is to stimulate the patient's active participation in the therapy. The inclusion in the program of an ambulant social worker, mentalizing crisis plans, mentalizing case formulations, and psychoeducational groups helps ensure that these aims are met. Well-structured weekly video supervision and cooperation between the individual and group therapists enables motivational difficulties and interpersonal conflicts to be better handled and understood as they appear in individual and group therapy. On the basis of frequent supervision and videotaping sessions, we believe that the MBT-SUD conducted in BCF has adhered to the MBT model and that the patients' mentalizing capacities improved as a result of treatment.

Both the quantitative results measured after the completion of treatment and the patients' own reports at 2-year follow-up suggest that their mental changes involved new ways of perceiving emotions, thinking about mind states, and self-reflecting in interpersonal encounters, and that there was an improvement in their ability to explore others' intentions in interpersonal encounters (Morken et al. 2017a, 2017b). These general aims became the means to achieve the primary goals of increased substance use control/remission and better social functioning. Of course, we do not know whether these changes will last over the long term. The patients had severe psychological and substance use problems and had been in numerous inpatient treatments for both their mental health and their SUD. Self-harm, suicide attempts and overdoses, violent episodes, and severe childhood trauma characterized the patients' histories. The dual-track treatment of MBT-SUD that is the combination of MBT with addiction-specific strategies renders the therapist more able to meet the patient's interpersonal vulnerability by being informed and aware of the patient's attachment insecurity and recognizing that the patient–therapist relationship is an attachment relationship. The relationship needs to be mentalized, and affects associated with the patient–therapist interaction need to be carefully defined and marked by the therapist in terms of their interaction with substance use. We can interpret patients' reports after treatment to mean that the concept of mentalizing and the tailoring of interventions helped them to understand misunderstandings by recapturing the mind states that led to such misapprehensions (Bateman and Fonagy 2016). This is valuable knowledge for clinicians too. Organizing an MBT team, and including staff from other units during monthly supervision, has increased the BCF's staff's knowledge about PDs and about patient and therapist vulnerabilities when delivering complex therapy. This can only be to the benefit of many clients of BCF.

> Patient: Do you know how much effort it takes to come back to normal life after being a drug addict? I did lose many years of my life, and I still feel very lost sometimes. I think human beings are too complicated, myself included. I think and feel so much, it makes me dizzy sometimes, trying to mentalize myself, the group, and my family, it is too much for me…[*with a smile*]

REFERENCES

Bales D, van Beek N, Smits M, et al: Treatment outcome of 18-month, day hospital mentalization-based treatment (MBT) in patients with severe borderline personality disorder in the Netherlands. J Pers Disord 26(4):568–582, 2012 22867507

Bales DL, Timman R, Andrea H, et al: Effectiveness of day hospital mentalization-based treatment for patients with severe borderline personality disorder: a matched control study. Clin Psychol Psychother 22(5):409–417, 2015 25060747

Ball SA, Carroll KM, Canning-Ball M, et al: Reasons for dropout from drug abuse treatment: symptoms, personality, and motivation. Addict Behav 31(2):320–330, 2006 15964152

Bateman A, Fonagy P: Treatment of borderline personality disorder with psychoanalytically oriented partial hospitalization: an 18-month follow-up. Am J Psychiatry 158(1):36–42, 2001 11136631

Bateman A, Fonagy P: Psychotherapy for Borderline Personality Disorder: Mentalization-Based Treatment. Oxford, UK, Oxford University Press, 2004

Bateman A, Fonagy P: Mentalization-Based Treatment for Borderline Personality Disorder: A Practical Guide. Oxford, UK, Oxford University Press, 2006

Bateman A, Fonagy P: Randomized controlled trial of outpatient mentalization-based treatment versus structured clinical management for borderline personality disorder. Am J Psychiatry 166(12):1355–1364, 2009 19833787

Bateman A, Fonagy P: Mentalization-Based Treatment for Personality Disorders: A Practical Guide. Oxford, UK, Oxford University Press, 2016

Bateman AW, Fonagy P: Handbook of Mentalizing in Mental Health Practice. Washington, DC, American Psychiatric Publishing, 2012

Brorson HH, Ajo Arnevik E, Rand-Hendriksen K, et al: Drop-out from addiction treatment: a systematic review of risk factors. Clin Psychol Rev 33(8):1010–1024, 2013 24029221

Cacciola JS, Alterman AI, McKay JR, et al: Psychiatric comorbidity in patients with substance use disorders: do not forget Axis II disorders. Psychiatr Ann 31:321–331, 2001

Cohen P, Chen H, Crawford TN, et al: Personality disorders in early adolescence and the development of later substance use disorders in the general population. Drug Alcohol Depend 88(Suppl 1):S71–S84, 2007 17227697

Fenton MC, Keyes K, Geier T, et al: Psychiatric comorbidity and the persistence of drug use disorders in the United States. Addiction 107(3):599–609, 2012 21883607

First MB, Gibbon M, Spitzer RL, et al: User's Guide for the Structured Clinical Interview for DSM-IV Axis II Personality Disorders: SCID-II. Washington, DC, American Psychiatric Press, 1997

Fonagy P, Bateman AW: Adversity, attachment, and mentalizing. Compr Psychiatry 64:59–66, 2016 26654293

Fridell M, Hesse M: Personality Disorders in Substance Abusers (NAD Publ No 47). Helsinki, Sweden, Nordic Council for Alcohol and Drug Research, 2005

Haller DL, Miles DR: Personality disturbances in drug-dependent women: relationship to childhood abuse. Am J Drug Alcohol Abuse 30(2):269–286, 2004 15230076

Hasin D, Kilcoyne B: Comorbidity of psychiatric and substance use disorders in the United States: current issues and findings from the NESARC. Curr Opin Psychiatry 25(3):165–171, 2012 22449770

Insel TR: Is social attachment an addictive disorder? Physiol Behav 79(3):351–357, 2003 12954430

James LM, Taylor J: Impulsivity and negative emotionality associated with substance use problems and Cluster B personality in college students. Addict Behav 32(4):714–727, 2007 16842928

Jørgensen CR, Bøye R, Andersen D, et al: Eighteen months post-treatment naturalistic follow-up study of mentalization-based therapy and supportive group treatment of borderline personality disorder: clinical outcomes and functioning. Nordic Psychol 66:254–273, 2014

Karterud S, Arefjord N, Andresen NE, et al: Substance use disorders among personality disordered patients admitted for day hospital treatment. Implications for service developments. Nord J Psychiatry 63(1):57–63, 2009 19172500

Karterud S, Bateman A: Manual for Mentaliseringsbasert Terapi (MBT) og MBT Vurderingsskala: Versjon Individualterapi [Manual for Mentalization-Based Therapy (MBT) and MBT Rating Scale: Individual Therapy Version]. Oslo, Norway, Gyldendal Akademisk, 2010

Karterud S, Bateman A: Manual for Mentaliseringsbasert Psykoedukativ Gruppeterapi (MBT-I) [Manual for Mentalization-Based Psychoedical Group Therapy (MBT-I)]. Oslo, Norway, Gyldendal Akademisk, 2011

Karterud S, Wilberg T, Urnes Ø: Personlighetspsykiatri, 2nd Edition. Oslo, Gyldendal Akademisk, 2017

Kvarstein EH, Pedersen G, Urnes Ø, et al: Changing from a traditional psychodynamic treatment programme to mentalization-based treatment for patients with borderline personality disorder—does it make a difference? Psychol Psychother 88(1):71–86, 2015 25045028

Lee NK, Cameron J, Jenner L: A systematic review of interventions for co-occurring substance use and borderline personality disorders. Drug Alcohol Rev 34(6):663–672, 2015 25919396

Lindsay-Hartz J: Contrasting experiences of shame and guilt. Am Behav Sci 27:689–704, 2016

Morken K, Karterud S, Arefjord N: Transforming disorganized attachment through mentalization-based treatment. J Contemp Psychother 44:117–126, 2014

Morken KTE, Binder P-E, Molde H, et al: Mentalization-based treatment for female patients with comorbid personality disorder and substance use disorder: a pilot study. Scandinavian Psychologist 4:e16, 2017a

Morken KTE, Binder P-E, Arefjord N, et al: Juggling thoughts and feelings: how do female patients with borderline symptomology and substance use disorder experience change in mentalization-based treatment? Psychother Res 17:1–16, 2017b

Olesek KL, Outcalt J, Dimaggio G, et al: Cluster B personality disorder traits as a predictor of therapeutic alliance over time in residential treatment for substance use disorders. J Nerv Ment Dis 204(10):736–740, 2016 27356120

Phillips B, Kahn U, Bateman A: Drug addiction, in Handbook of Mentalizing in Mental Health Practice. Edited by Bateman A, Fonagy P. Washington, DC, American Psychiatric Publishing, 2012

Ravndal E, Vaglum P, Lauritzen G: Completion of long-term inpatient treatment of drug abusers: a prospective study from 13 different units. Eur Addict Res 11(4):180–185, 2005 16110224

Rossouw TI, Fonagy P: Mentalization-based treatment for self-harm in adolescents: a randomized controlled trial. J Am Acad Child Adolesc Psychiatry 51(12):1304.e3–1313.e3, 2012 23200287

Thylstrup B, Hesse M: Substance abusers' personality disorders and staff members' emotional reactions. BMC Psychiatry 8:21, 2008 18402658

Trull TJ, Jahng S, Tomko RL, et al: Revised NESARC personality disorder diagnoses: gender, prevalence, and comorbidity with substance dependence disorders. J Pers Disord 24(4):412–426, 2010 20695803

U.S. Department of Health and Human Services Office of the Surgeon General: Facing Addiction in America: The Surgeon General's Report on Alcohol, Drugs, and Health. Washington, DC, U.S. Department of Health and Human Services, 2016

Vaglum P: Personality disorders and the course and outcome of substance abuse: a selective review of the 1984 to 2004 literature, in Personality Disorders:Current Research and Treatments. Edited by Reich J. New York, Routledge, 2005, pp 105–126

van den Bosch LM, Verheul R: Patients with addiction and personality disorder: treatment outcomes and clinical implications. Curr Opin Psychiatry 20(1):67–71, 2007 17143086

Verheul R: Co-morbidity of personality disorders in individuals with substance use disorders. Eur Psychiatry 16(5):274–282, 2001 11514129

Walter M, Gunderson JG, Zanarini MC, et al: New onsets of substance use disorders in borderline personality disorder over 7 years of follow-ups: findings from the Collaborative Longitudinal Personality Disorders Study. Addiction 104(1):97–103, 2009 19133893

Zanarini MC, Frankenburg FR, Weingeroff JL, et al: The course of substance use disorders in patients with borderline personality disorder and Axis II comparison subjects: a 10-year follow-up study. Addiction 106(2):342–348, 2011 21083831

CHAPTER 25

PSYCHOSIS

Martin Debbané, Ph.D.

Anthony Bateman, M.A., FRCPsych

Schizophrenia spectrum and other psychotic disorders (as defined in the DSM-5; American Psychiatric Association 2013) arguably represent the most challenging mental health conditions to treat. Because psychosis deeply alters the person's experience of being an agentive self in the world, life after the diagnosis rarely fully catches up to preonset levels of functioning. This pessimistic depiction of psychosis is not intended to undermine the important progress made in the past century to help affected individuals cope with the debilitating effects of the positive, negative, and disorganized symptoms that characterize psychosis. The advances in psychopharmacology have significantly contributed to modulation of the debilitating effects of hallucinations, delusions, negative symptoms, disorganized cognition, and the inherent thwarted sense of self the condition can cause in a person's life. Investment in quality psychotherapeutic and psychosocial treatments, which work best when the patient's family is engaged and/or the wider social context is addressed, can effectively sustain a significant degree of reinsertion into an active social role and contribute to increased fulfilment for individuals with psychosis. Some psychotherapeutic models of intervention have also shown promising effects (de Jong et al. 2016; Garrett 2016). Notwithstanding these important strides in treating psychosis, when examined from the perspective of quality of life, satisfaction with interpersonal relationships, and socioprofessional autonomy, the combined therapeutic effects of all these interventions pale in comparison to the lifelong loss of function and psychological suffering that the majority of individuals experience after receiving their first diagno-

The authors would like to thank George Salaminios, M.Phil., for his helpful comments on this chapter.

sis (Carbon and Correll 2014). For most mental health workers, the experience is of effectively treating the "fever," but too often remaining powerless at getting to the heart of the disease.

Although positive symptoms of psychosis, such as hallucinations and delusional beliefs, can be controlled, the residual condition for most individuals still dramatically perturbs social cognition to the point where self-confidence, trust in others, interpersonal relationships, and professional endeavors cannot be embraced in any constructive and consistent fashion, meaning that the prognosis is often bleak during adult life. Over the past three decades, experts in the field have begun to more closely examine the premorbid, prodromal, and early phases of the disease to gain further information about the emerging illness (McGlashan et al. 2010; McGorry 2000). The lessons learned from this research provide tremendous insight into the pathophysiological and clinical processes of emerging psychosis. Most importantly, perhaps, a contemporary approach to psychosis has become resolutely developmental; this approach distinguishes between genetic risk, distal risk, proximal risk, and maintenance/relapse factors (Debbané 2015).

It is well known that genetics play a role in the development of psychosis, whose degree of heritability is second only to that of autism spectrum disorder (Hilker et al. 2018). Most experts assume a multifactorial polygenic threshold model (Lenzenweger 2010), in which epigenetic interactions and social learning during infancy, childhood, adolescence, and early adulthood influence the expression of the disease (Debbané and Barrantes-Vidal 2015). Genetic programming will have an impact on early neurodevelopment and might also have an effect on adolescent brain maturation (Lamblin et al. 2017). Years before the onset of the illness, distal risk factors, which include prenatal and perinatal stress factors, as well as attachment trauma, constitute a set of strong but nonspecific factors potentiating the risk for psychotic psychopathology in later life (Brent and Fonagy 2014). During adolescence, atypical maturation trajectories of cortical brain areas devoted to social cognition, and more specifically to mentalizing, appear to predict onset in those at clinical high risk for psychosis (Cannon et al. 2015). Finally, proximal risk factors of interpersonal stress within attachment relationships with family members, romantic partners, and peers often precede the onset of the first psychotic break (Day et al. 1987; Tessner et al. 2011).

Considering the evidence gathered from prospective studies, it appears that attachment and mentalizing are confirmed as relevant to the study of psychosis, and potentially to its treatment, all along the continuum of psychosis (Brent 2009). However, evidence suggests that attachment and mentalizing may not represent etiological, causal, necessary factors in the development of psychosis. Still, as argued elsewhere (Debbané et al. 2016b), attachment and mentalizing may represent key protective factors that can 1) attenuate the clinical course of emerging psychosis in those at increased risk and 2) sustain recovery in affected individuals. In other words, a mentalization-based approach to psychosis seeks to enhance protective mechanisms in the early part of the disease, and to strengthen the "nonpsychotic" part of the personality (Bion 1957) in affected individuals, to promote partial or complete recovery.

In the first section of this chapter, we discuss evidence linking attachment and mentalizing to the trajectories of psychosis along its continuum of expression. In the second section, we describe neuroscientific studies pointing to the pathways associated with psychotic psychopathology; importantly, these pathways are also sensitive to attachment adversity and may thus represent the neurobiological grounds upon which both genetic and environmental vulnerabilities have an impact on risk for psychosis. This section will underline how developmental interactions of risk factors hinder the development of mentalizing, especially processes dedicated to mentalizing the self. In the third section of the chapter, we present the clinical rationale for using a mentalization-informed approach for psychotherapy, and in the fourth section, we discuss preventive treatment for affected individuals as indicated.

ATTACHMENT ALONG THE PSYCHOSIS CONTINUUM

Mentalizing function is fostered within the context of early attachment relationships, although genetic factors are also known to exert a moderate influence on psychological processes of mental-state understanding (Warrier et al. 2018). Multiple interactional pathways during development may lead to compromised mentalizing in the context of risk for psychosis.

Attachment disturbances are very common in the developmental history of individuals with psychosis. The evidence for the association between attachment disturbances, mentalizing, and psychosis comes from three stands of research along the continuum of severity for psychosis. Starting with the most severe forms of the disorder, studies have found that individuals with first-episode psychosis (FEP) (MacBeth et al. 2011), similar to those with chronic psychosis (Mickelson et al. 1997), report very high rates of insecure attachment. Insecure attachment, especially avoidant attachment, in these groups is associated with the severity of both positive and negative symptoms (Gumley et al. 2014). Other studies have reported modest but significant associations between positive symptoms and attachment anxiety/preoccupation (Berry et al. 2007b; Gumley et al. 2014). These results have been questioned on the grounds of the unlikeliness that patterns of behavior acquired in childhood play an important role in understanding the nature of a pathology that manifests itself in adulthood (Fisher et al. 2011).

Although attachment may not be etiologically linked to psychosis, it certainly appears to play an important role in response to treatment. Avoidant attachment is known to reduce help-seeking behaviors, undermine the therapeutic alliance, and increase service disengagement (Debbané et al. 2016b). By contrast, attachment security acts as a protective factor, because it favors help-seeking behaviors and treatment engagement, as well as a stronger therapeutic alliance, among individuals with established schizophrenia (Berry et al. 2007b).

Further evidence can be found in the preclinical phases of psychosis, among individuals diagnosed with prodromal syndromes, and even in nonclinical samples of individuals reporting above-average expression of schizotypy, a personality trait that provides a personality basis for increased vulnerability to the development of psychotic disorders (Debbané et al. 2015; Lenzenweger 2010), in a way similar to the relationship between impulsivity and antisocial disorders. Among individuals reporting subthreshold psychotic symptoms consistent with the contemporary clinical high-risk criteria (CHR; Schultze-Lutter et al. 2015), 80% of young adults with CHR show evidence of insecure attachment (Gajwani et al. 2013). It appears that the clinical outcomes for these young people relate to their level of fearful and dismissing/avoidant attachment styles at baseline (Quijada et al. 2015). Studies in nonclinical samples have reported significant relationships between attachment avoidance and positive schizotypy expression (delusion and hallucination-like manifestations). Furthermore, both attachment avoidance and attachment anxiety correlate with expressions of negative schizotypy—that is, interindividual differences in social withdrawal, flat affect, and social anxiety traits (Berry et al. 2007a; Sheinbaum et al. 2013, 2014).

The fact that attachment relates to expressions of psychosis all along its developmental continuum attests to the profound influence that disturbances in attachment may have. In addition to the evocative empirical and clinical accounts of this influence (Berry et al. 2007b; Liotti 2004), contemporary neuroscience research is starting to uncover the neurobiological pathways on which attachment disturbances may promote the grounds for the onset of psychosis.

NEUROBIOLOGICAL PATHWAYS CONTRIBUTING TO EMERGING PSYCHOSIS ALONG THE PSYCHOSIS CONTINUUM

Evidence supports the existence of at least five key neural systems (i.e., hypothalamic-pituitary-adrenal stress-response system, dopaminergic system, oxytocin system, inflammation, and oxidative stress) through which attachment may play a role in the development of mentalizing functions, in parallel to increasing resilience to psychosis proneness (Debbané et al. 2016b). These five systems and their links to attachment and mentalizing are reviewed in the following sections.

Hypothalamic-Pituitary-Adrenal Stress-Response System

Research in animals has identified the hypothalamic-pituitary-adrenal (HPA) stress-response system as a key contributor to the neurobiology of attachment. Disturbances of the early care environment have been linked with long-term HPA axis system dysfunction and chronically elevated corticosterone levels (Sullivan 2012). A longitudinal study observed increased cortisol levels among at-risk individuals who transitioned to clinical psychosis (Walker et al. 2010). In samples of patients with schizophrenia, increases in glucocorticoid levels also point to a possible link between early life stress and psychosis (Mondelli et al. 2010). Atypicalities in cerebral function and structure attributable to early life stress critically have an impact on cognitive processes associated with psychosis, namely, higher-order social-cognitive processes (Arnsten and Rubia 2012). Brent and Fonagy (2014) argue that adverse caregiving environments that generate chronic elevations of corticosterone in the brain may fundamentally affect its integrity and, more precisely, render early acquired self-referential processing systems vulnerable. During middle childhood, these vulnerabilities may underpin premorbid difficulties such as subtle alterations in the capacity to differentiate between self and nonself cues (Brent et al. 2014b). Furthermore, dysfunction of the HPA axis sustained by trauma and insecure attachment brings the psychosis-prone individual closer to the clinical threshold, whereas supportive early social experiences associated with maternal care appear to promote the modulation of HPA-axis-based threat reactivity, thus fostering flexibility and resilience in the face of novel stress-inducing social situations (Gunnar and Quevedo 2007). The HPA axis thus represents one possible biological path toward increased psychosis proneness; importantly, this system interacts with the other biological pathways leading to psychosis.

Dopaminergic and Oxytocinergic Systems

Four decades of research encompassing biological, neuroimaging, and genetic methodologies have provided evidence for the role of the dopaminergic system in the development and maintenance of psychosis-spectrum illnesses (Howes and Kapur 2009). Some of the candidate genes for schizophrenia can be directly connected to dopaminergic pathways. As has been observed in animal studies, early life adversity within the caregiving environment chronically affects the dopaminergic system by increasing the rates of dopamine synthesis and release in response to acute stress (Strathearn 2011). Furthermore, chronic exposure to stress has been shown to decrease tonic activity in the midbrain, which is normally responsible for regulating dopamine levels in the nucleus accumbens (Phillips et al. 2006). Therefore, the dopaminergic system is not connected to genetic vulnerability in isolation; rather, it meaningfully relates to interpersonal stress in attachment relationships.

In another significant interaction with the HPA axis, the hypothalamic oxytocin-release system modulates stress responses and rejection-related ideas, allowing individuals to relate to others constructively. Indeed, a number of nonclinical studies have reported that central oxytocin administration modulates social cognition and social behavior (Shamay-Tsoory and Abu-Akel 2016), sometimes in paradoxical ways (Debbané 2018). The oxytocinergic system further links to dopamine regulation. Oxytocin and arginine vasopressin are neuropeptide hormones/neurotransmitters synthesized primarily in the paraventricular and supraoptic nuclei of the hypothalamus and stored in the pituitary. These systems influence social behaviors that are important for the developmental acquisition of social cognition. Adverse experiences within early attachment relationships may exert a prolonged impact on the development and function of the oxytocinergic system (Feldman et al. 2016).

With regard to the early mother–infant relationship, it has been argued that attachment insecurity may have an impact on dopaminergic functioning because it is associated with decreased levels of available oxytocin (Brent et al. 2014a). Dysregulation of striatal dopamine, however, could be additionally affected by depletion of available oxytocin and overactivation of the HPA axis system, both of which have been associated with a dysfunctional early care environment. For example, oxytocin has been shown to have a modulatory effect on excessive mesolimbic dopamine in rodents receiving psychostimulants, leading to a number of studies evaluating oxytocin's intrinsic antipsychotic properties (Rich and Caldwell 2015). Additionally, overactivation of the HPA axis has been associated with elevated dopamine synthesis and alterations of striatal dopamine receptors (Walker and Diforio 1997). Taking the evidence from these studies together, we suggest that early neurobiological alterations of the attachment system could potentiate a premorbid susceptibility to striatal dopamine dysregulation and therefore increase the risk of psychosis during later adolescent/early adult development.

Neuroinflammation, Oxidative Stress, and Psychosis

Chronic inflammation in the brain (neuroinflammation) occurs as a manifestation of the immune system's breakdown in defending against infections or injuries. Neuroinflammation leads to disruptions in the blood–brain barrier through increased microglial activation and inflammatory cytokine release, causing alterations in brain function (Kirkpatrick and Miller 2013). A number of studies have reported evidence of inflammation along the continuum of psychosis. In a sample of youths and young adults at clinical high risk for psychosis, individuals who eventually converted to clinical psychosis showed higher plasma levels of proinflammatory cytokines at baseline evaluations (Cannon et al. 2015). Importantly, plasma levels of proinflammatory cytokines were strongly predictive of atypically elevated gray matter reduction in the prefrontal cortex. In patients with FEP, neuroinflammatory abnormalities can be observed, independent of neuroleptic use (Martínez-Gras et al. 2012). Furthermore, preliminary reports of correlational evidence link clinical status to higher cytokine concentrations in blood (Miller et al. 2011). From the developmental perspective, well-known distal risk factors for schizophrenia, such as preterm labor, maternal gestational diabetes, and preeclampsia, but also maternal depression and anxiety, which have often been associated with insecure attachment (Kirkpatrick and Miller 2013), may be mediated through the neuroinflammatory response. As exemplified by Buka et al. (2001), maternal concentrations of cytokines during pregnancy increase the offspring's risk for psychosis.

Oxidative stress due to aberrant reduction–oxidation (redox) control (Bitanihirwe and Woo 2011) represents yet another pathway through which early stress can increase psychosis proneness (Do et al. 2015). Do et al. (2009) showed that genetically based disruptions in antioxidant control (i.e., reductions in glutathione) interact with pro-oxidative environmental risk factors (including childhood and adolescent attachment adversity and stress) during critical periods of neurodevelopment. These interactions can significantly disrupt the processes of neural connectivity and synchronization, particularly in relation to prefrontal areas associated with self-referential and sociocognitive processing (Brent et al. 2014a). In this line of research, Aydin et al. (2015) examined the impact of caregiver attachment style and expressed emotion on schizophrenia participants' oxidative-stress parameters. Results showed that reduced and oxidized forms of glutathione (glutathione and glutathione disulfide, respectively), plasma lipid peroxidation, and urine malondialdehyde levels of patients with schizophrenia were higher than those measured in the control group of healthy individuals. Importantly, the caregivers' emotional overinvolvement and anxious-ambivalent attachment style were found to best predict the participants' oxidative stress levels (Aydin et al. 2015). As with the other neurobiological pathways associated with psychosis, contemporary neuroscience research is slowly unveiling the complex matrix of associations among neurobiological maturation, interpersonal relationships, and the potential perturbations in sense of self and self-in-relation-to-others-and-the-world central to the phenomenology of psychotic states.

The five neurobiological pathways reviewed above—HPA stress-response system, dopaminergic system, oxytocin system, neuroinflammation, and oxidative stress—are not exclusive to psychosis; indeed, similar pathways may lead to different psychopathological outcomes (Tiwari and Gonzalez 2018). What may be more specific to psychosis is how risk along these pathways occurs in the context of *trait abnormalities*, which in the field of schizophrenia research are conceptualized as genetically based characteristics of the information processing functions, in which sensory processing functions (e.g., habituation and gating responses to incoming stimuli) play a prominent role (Adams et al. 2013). Importantly, as is outlined in the next section, sensory processing lies at the root of higher social-cognitive development and thus is key to mentalizing (see Chapter 2, "Contemporary Neuroscientific Research").

A MENTALIZATION-INFORMED APPROACH ALONG THE PSYCHOSIS CONTINUUM

Even at the start of the 21st century, when philosophers and Buddhists enthusiastically engage in research with brain imaging techniques, it remains difficult to bridge the gap between the neurosciences and subjective experience, let alone clinical practice. The following discussion will ingloriously prove this point, yet the aim of this section is to engage the reader to attend to the possible directions that both the neuroscience and the psychotherapy of psychosis may take in a sort of cross-fertilizing joint venture.

The brain is often thought of as a part of the body that is somehow different because one cannot "feel" it as being a part of one's body. Yet, physical sensations are a constitutive part of what we experience as "real," and this sense of certainty about sensory experience is specifically conferred by the brain to sustain, among other things, a sense of self-continuity. Phenomenologically, psychosis is defined not by symptoms of hallucinations, but primarily by a disturbance in the sense of self, which can be expressed in a number of different forms of psychotic subjectivity, as charted by instruments such as the Examination of Anomalous Self-Experience (Parnas et al. 2005) and the German approach to basic symptoms (Schultze-Lutter et al. 2016). Important to the discussion around sensory experience and the sense of reality is the ubiquity and consistency of bodily cues, which constantly provide signals of the individual's position in space (Rudrauf et al. 2017) and firmly ground his or her basic sense of continuity as a unitary, continuous being. In addition, the sense of self-agency, and, more importantly, the capacity for self-regulation established in the context of embodied engagements with caregivers during infancy (through multiple initiations and interactions, which gradually foster control and regulatory capacity over bodily signals) are essential in establishing a minimal self (Fotopoulou and Tsakiris 2017). When such processes go awry in early development, as in autism spectrum disorder or other neurodevelopmental conditions, the development of interpersonal selfhood is significantly affected (Hobson 1990). It is probable that manifestations such as auto-stimulating and repetitive stereotypical behaviors emerge from the need to regain control over bodily signals that challenge the maintenance of self-continuity. Therefore, dysfunctions within the sensory and self-monitoring processes necessarily alert the individual to attend to and manage the states of vulnerability that are threatening the basis of self-integrity. Accordingly, in the domain of schizophrenia research, sensory and cognitive self-monitoring disturbances have been conceptualized as processes leading to psychotic symptoms, perhaps as a way of managing the associated disturbance in the sense of self.

Within this framework, a mentalization-based approach provides a legitimate starting point to address the central problem of psychosis—that of alterations in the sense of self. The construct of mentalizing assumes an interactive integration between systems sustaining low-level embodied experience and systems sustaining imaginative processes, which need to interact to foster the individual's understanding of self, self-in-relation-to-others, and others-in-relation-to-self. As Debbané et al. (2016b) have proposed, many types of dysregulation may arise in the interactive integration between the sensory and cognitive systems, or from the inability of one system to influence the other. Mental states arising from these impairments may translate to aberrant *embodied mentalizing,* in which too little or too much weight is given either to prior beliefs (as in persecutory delusions) or to sensory-affective evidence (as in hallucinatory phenomena), leading to heightened, rigid states of certainty decoupled from shared reality with others (see also Chapter 2).

In this context, the process of psychotherapeutic work focused on mentalizing would consist of fostering embodied mentalizing—that is, the capacity to flexibly employ bodily cues to understand the individual's own feelings in relation to self and others, within and beyond the therapeutic relationship. The process by which embodied mentalizing can be generated and generalized in the context of treatment for psychosis requires examination, but the rationale for this approach is to support mentalizing function as a mechanism of resilience. A number of clinical research projects are under way in Spain, the United States, and Switzerland, and a clinical trial in the Netherlands has recently been described (Debbané et al. 2016a; Lana et al. 2015; Weijers et al. 2016, 2018). The format of mentalization-based treatment (MBT) for psychosis follows the usual arrangement of MBT and typically includes a group approach to sustain mentalizing in interpersonal relationships, combined with individual therapy and/or family therapy when possible. The detail of the intervention remains to be defined, especially with regard to specific techniques that would sustain the recovery of embodied mentalizing. However, a number of issues have become clear from clinical experience.

Patients liable to psychotic symptoms tend to overregulate emotional expression, meaning that outwardly, MBT group sessions may be quiet, with limited interaction between participants. However, this lack of overtly expressed emotion gives a false impression of a lack of stress in the participants. Research has shown that patients susceptible to psychosis are actually more emotionally reactive to stress than nonpatients, while at the same time they often show flattened affective expression (Cohen et al. 2015). This can make it very difficult for the clinician to gauge the stress levels of the patient. The clinician needs to keep in mind the basic tenets of the relationship between attachment and mentalizing and social interaction: patients meet in the group, and the interaction between them inevitably activates their attachment processes, which in turn will increase their mentalizing difficulties. This results in problems in managing social interaction effectively. The natural self-protective response is withdrawal and attachment avoidance. Indeed, for new patients, joining the group initially requires preparation in individual sessions. Thus, the quiet that may be a feature of group sessions is actually a symptom of high arousal, as patients attempt to manage the internal threat to the stability of their sense of self. Related to this, social evaluation is one of the key interpersonal features increasing anxiety and provoking potentially psychotic cognitions and perceptions in patients. Furthermore, studies have demonstrated the different ways in which individuals with psychosis deal with uncertainty, ranging from concreteness to hyperreflexivity (Freeman et al. 2002; Jones and Fernyhough 2007). In this psychological context, it is unsurprising that patients with psychosis approach mental states and others' minds with an extremely high degree of vigilance. They avoid interpersonal conflict and do not express clear self-autonomy or let other patients know if they feel anxious or threatened. Avoidant attachment strategies are dominant. The clinician must therefore be sensitive to the idiosyncratic signs of emotional disturbance of each patient, which often involve subtle bodily expressions, such as slowing of speech, increased incoherence, or lack of eye contact.

Attachment avoidance implies that bonds to the therapist or the group are not easily established and generally remain fragile. Even if a patient has attended several months of group therapy, he or she may find it easy to drop out of therapy, seemingly forgetting about the other group members and the therapists. Keeping patients in therapy, especially after they have missed a few sessions, requires that they experience a sense that they are still represented in the minds of the clinicians and the other patients in the group. Tools that are tailored to the special needs of psychotic patients include smartphone apps (Firth and Torous 2015), regular telephone calls, or house visits after missed sessions to revitalize their connectedness with therapy.

Clinicians find mentalizing the relationship between the patient and clinician problematic. Although this is a common finding in MBT (see Chapter 6, "Individual Therapy Techniques")—perhaps especially with patients who engage in avoidant strategies—the clinician may be concerned that a focus on relationships will provoke excessive stress and increase the patient's withdrawal, rather than addressing it. For this reason, mentalizing the relationship is approached with caution, and clinicians often address this problem from a third-person perspective, through the use of materials in which interacting minds can be visually represented—for example, a drawing of two minds that are interacting with each other. Mentalizing the relationship is still a necessary ingredient of therapy to increase the patient's resilience to social interaction, which is so troublesome for people with psychotic symptoms.

Dropout from therapy may be preceded by an increase in psychotic symptoms, which, if present during interactions in the group, can lead to self-protective withdrawal of the patient from the group. In addition to this anxious avoidance, the patient may feel ashamed about how he or she behaved; returning to the group embodies that shame, leading to further instability. In this context, psychoeducation about mentalizing in relation to symptoms appears essential to prepare patients for the possibility of rupture–repair processes in group therapy. Similar to self-harming behaviors in individuals with borderline personality disorder, psychotic symptoms may be formulated as states that when acute, can lead the individual to withdraw from treatment, and as such represent an obstacle to treatment. In this situation, individual sessions to restabilize mentalizing may be necessary if the patient is to return to the group.

PREVENTION AND PROTECTION

MBT may be relevant not only to fully developed forms of psychotic disorders but also during the developmental phases of these disorders. As mentioned earlier, impairments in mentalizing may not constitute a necessary condition to develop schizophrenia; there is, however, reason to believe that mentalizing may represent a protective factor mitigating the risk—as well as the clinical impact—of psychotic thought processes. Beyond clinical descriptions of resilience afforded by robust mentalizing skills in psychotic disorders (Debbané et al. 2016b), some recent empirical evidence supports a protective role of mentalizing along the developmental continuum of psychosis. A longitudinal study in nonclinical adolescents reporting auditory verbal hallucinations (AVHs) observed that participants with good baseline theory-of-mind skills were less likely to develop secondary delusional beliefs linked to their AVHs (Bartels-Velthuis et al. 2011). In parallel to these findings, a recent study in late-stage schizophrenia patients demonstrated that theory-of-mind skills mitigate the negative influences of persistent delusions on social functioning (Phalen et al. 2017). Focusing less on the other-oriented dimension of mentalizing and more on the self-oriented mechanisms, an interesting project involving adults aimed to compare the differences in psychological functioning among nonclinical voice-hearers, adults diagnosed with a psychotic disorder who reported positive symptoms, and nonhallucinating healthy control subjects (Peters et al. 2016). The comparisons were performed on a range of interview and self-report measures of features including mood and anxiety, satisfaction and well-being, perceived stress, core schemas, and mindfulness. Interestingly, mindfulness was the only measure distinguishing the voice-hearers among both the control subjects and the psychotic patients. In other words, nonpsychotic voice-hearers were found to report greater mindfulness in comparison to the other two groups. This result indicates that mindfulness, which conceptually overlaps with mentalizing about the self, may represent a factor that protects voice-hearing individuals from the psychopathological effects of AVHs.

The evidence presented here originates from studies employing conceptual "cousins" to the concept of mentalizing: mindfulness and theory of mind. Studies using measures of mentalizing in combination with other measures are needed to elucidate the general and specific associations between these higher-order processes and psychotic expression. Nevertheless, the current evidence does point to a protective effect of mentalizing along the psychosis continuum, motivating innovations for indicated preventive treatment informed by a mentalization-based approach to psychosis.

REFERENCES

Adams RA, Stephan KE, Brown HR, et al: The computational anatomy of psychosis. Front Psychiatry 4:47, 2013 23750138

American Psychiatric Association: Diagnostic and Statistical Manual of Mental Disorders, 5th Edition. Arlington, VA, American Psychiatric Association, 2013

Arnsten AF, Rubia K: Neurobiological circuits regulating attention, cognitive control, motivation, and emotion: disruptions in neurodevelopmental psychiatric disorders. J Am Acad Child Adolesc Psychiatry 51(4):356–367, 2012 22449642

Aydin M, Kuscu MK, Eker B, et al: Effect of caregivers' expressed emotion and attachment patterns on the oxidative stress level in schizophrenic patients. Bull Clin Psychopharmacol 25:S177, 2015

Bartels-Velthuis AA, Blijd-Hoogewys EM, van Os J: Better theory-of-mind skills in children hearing voices mitigate the risk of secondary delusion formation. Acta Psychiatr Scand 124(3):193–197, 2011 21426312

Berry K, Band R, Corcoran R, et al: Attachment styles, earlier interpersonal relationships and schizotypy in a non-clinical sample. Psychol Psychother 80(Pt 4):563–576, 2007a 17535544

Berry K, Barrowclough C, Wearden A: A review of the role of adult attachment style in psychosis: unexplored issues and questions for further research. Clin Psychol Rev 27(4):458–475, 2007b 17258365

Bion WR: Differentiation of the psychotic from the non-psychotic personalities. Int J Psychoanal 38(3–4):266–275, 1957 13438602

Bitanihirwe BK, Woo TU: Oxidative stress in schizophrenia: an integrated approach. Neurosci Biobehav Rev 35(3):878–893, 2011 20974172

Brent B: Mentalization-based psychodynamic psychotherapy for psychosis. J Clin Psychol 65(8):803–814, 2009 19572277

Brent B, Fonagy P: A mentalization-based treatment approach to disturbances of social understanding in schizophrenia, in Social Cognition and Metacognition in Schizophrenia. Edited by Lysaker PH, Dimaggio G, Brüne M. London, Academic Press, 2014, pp 245–257

Brent BK, Holt DJ, Keshavan MS, et al: Mentalization-based treatment for psychosis: linking an attachment-based model to the psychotherapy for impaired mental state understanding in people with psychotic disorders. Isr J Psychiatry Relat Sci 51(1):17–24, 2014a 24858631

Brent BK, Seidman LJ, Thermenos HW, et al: Self-disturbances as a possible premorbid indicator of schizophrenia risk: a neurodevelopmental perspective. Schizophr Res 152(1):73–80, 2014b 23932148

Buka SL, Tsuang MT, Torrey EF, et al: Maternal cytokine levels during pregnancy and adult psychosis. Brain Behav Immun 15(4):411–420, 2001 11782107

Cannon TD, Chung Y, He G, et al; North American Prodrome Longitudinal Study Consortium: Progressive reduction in cortical thickness as psychosis develops: a multisite longitudinal neuroimaging study of youth at elevated clinical risk. Biol Psychiatry 77(2):147–157, 2015 25034946

Carbon M, Correll CU: Clinical predictors of therapeutic response to antipsychotics in schizophrenia. Dialogues Clin Neurosci 16(4):505–524, 2014 25733955

Cohen AS, Mohr C, Ettinger U, et al: Schizotypy as an organizing framework for social and affective sciences. Schizophr Bull 41(Suppl 2):S427–S435, 2015 25810057

Day R, Nielsen JA, Korten A, et al: Stressful life events preceding the acute onset of schizophrenia: a cross-national study from the World Health Organization. Cult Med Psychiatry 11(2):123–205, 1987 3595169

de Jong S, van Donkersgoed R, Pijnenborg GH, et al: Metacognitive Reflection and Insight Therapy (MERIT) with a patient with severe symptoms of disorganization. J Clin Psychol 72(2):164–174, 2016 26636663

Debbané M: Schizotypy: a developmental perspective, in Schizotypy: New Dimensions. Edited by Mason O, Claridge G. Hove, UK, Routledge, 2015, pp 83–98

Debbané M: Treating borderline personality disorder with oxytocin: an enthusiastic note of caution. Commentary to Servan et al. The effect of oxytocin in borderline personality disorder. Encephale 44(1):83–84, 2018 29402386

Debbané M, Barrantes-Vidal N: Schizotypy from a developmental perspective. Schizophr Bull 41(Suppl 2):S386–S395, 2015 25548385

Debbané M, Eliez S, Badoud D, et al: Developing psychosis and its risk states through the lens of schizotypy. Schizophr Bull 41(Suppl 2):S396–S407, 2015 25548386

Debbané M, Benmiloud J, Salaminios G, et al: Mentalization-based treatment in clinical high-risk for psychosis: a rationale and clinical illustration. J Contemp Psychother 46:217–225, 2016a

Debbané M, Salaminios G, Luyten P, et al: Attachment, neurobiology, and mentalizing along the psychosis continuum. Front Hum Neurosci 10:406, 2016b 27597820

Do KQ, Cabungcal JH, Frank A, et al: Redox dysregulation, neurodevelopment, and schizophrenia. Curr Opin Neurobiol 19(2):220–230, 2009 19481443

Do KQ, Cuenod M, Hensch TK: Targeting oxidative stress and aberrant critical period plasticity in the developmental trajectory to schizophrenia. Schizophr Bull 41(4):835–846, 2015 26032508

Feldman R, Monakhov M, Pratt M, et al: Oxytocin pathway genes: evolutionary ancient system impacting on human affiliation, sociality, and psychopathology. Biol Psychiatry 79(3):174–184, 2016 26392129

Firth J, Torous J: Smartphone apps for schizophrenia: a systematic review. JMIR Mhealth Uhealth 3(4):e102, 2015 26546039

Fisher HL, Craig TK, Fearon P, et al: Reliability and comparability of psychosis patients' retrospective reports of childhood abuse. Schizophr Bull 37(3):546–553, 2011 19776204

Fotopoulou A, Tsakiris M: Mentalizing homeostasis: the social origins of interoceptive inference. Neuro-psychoanalysis 19:3–28, 2017

Freeman D, Garety PA, Kuipers E, et al: A cognitive model of persecutory delusions. Br J Clin Psychol 41(Pt 4):331–347, 2002 12437789

Gajwani R, Patterson P, Birchwood M: Attachment: developmental pathways to affective dysregulation in young people at ultra-high risk of developing psychosis. Br J Clin Psychol 52(4):424–437, 2013 24117914

Garrett M: Introduction: Psychotherapy for Psychosis. Am J Psychother 70(1):1–4, 2016 27052603

Gumley AI, Taylor HE, Schwannauer M, et al: A systematic review of attachment and psychosis: measurement, construct validity and outcomes. Acta Psychiatr Scand 129(4):257–274, 2014 23834647

Gunnar M, Quevedo K: The neurobiology of stress and development. Annu Rev Psychol 58:145–173, 2007 16903808

Hilker R, Helenius D, Fagerlund B, et al: Heritability of schizophrenia and schizophrenia spectrum based on the nationwide Danish Twin Register. Biol Psychiatry 83(6):492–498, 2018 28987712

Hobson RP: On the origins of self and the case of autism. Dev Psychopathol 2:163–181, 1990

Howes OD, Kapur S: The dopamine hypothesis of schizophrenia: version III—the final common pathway. Schizophr Bull 35(3):549–562, 2009 19325164

Jones SR, Fernyhough C: A new look at the neural diathesis—stress model of schizophrenia: the primacy of social-evaluative and uncontrollable situations. Schizophr Bull 33(5):1171–1177, 2007 17105966

Kirkpatrick B, Miller BJ: Inflammation and schizophrenia. Schizophr Bull 39(6):1174–1179, 2013 24072812

Lamblin M, Murawski C, Whittle S, et al: Social connectedness, mental health and the adolescent brain. Neurosci Biobehav Rev 80:57–68, 2017 28506925

Lana F, Marcos S, Mollà L, et al: Mentalization based group psychotherapy for psychosis: a pilot study to assess safety, acceptance and subjective efficacy. International Journal of Psychology and Psychoanalysis 1(2):007, 2015

Lenzenweger MF: Schizotypy and Schizophrenia: The View from Experimental Psychology. New York, Guilford, 2010

Liotti G: Trauma, dissociation, and disorganized attachment: three strands of a single braid. Psychotherapy 41:472–486, 2004

MacBeth A, Gumley A, Schwannauer M, et al: Attachment states of mind, mentalization, and their correlates in a first-episode psychosis sample. Psychol Psychother 84(1):42–57, discussion 98–110, 2011 22903830

Martínez-Gras I, García-Sánchez F, Guaza C, et al: Altered immune function in unaffected first-degree biological relatives of schizophrenia patients. Psychiatry Res 200(2–3):1022–1025, 2012 22766011

McGlashan TH, Walsh BC, Woods SW: The Psychosis-Risk Prodrome: Handbook for Diagnosis and Follow-Up. New York, Oxford University Press, 2010

McGorry PD: The nature of schizophrenia: signposts to prevention. Aust N Z J Psychiatry 34(Suppl):S14–S21, 2000 11129299

Mickelson KD, Kessler RC, Shaver PR: Adult attachment in a nationally representative sample. J Pers Soc Psychol 73(5):1092–1106, 1997 9364763

Miller BJ, Buckley P, Seabolt W, et al: Meta-analysis of cytokine alterations in schizophrenia: clinical status and antipsychotic effects. Biol Psychiatry 70(7):663–671, 2011 21641581

Mondelli V, Dazzan P, Hepgul N, et al: Abnormal cortisol levels during the day and cortisol awakening response in first-episode psychosis: the role of stress and of antipsychotic treatment. Schizophr Res 116(2–3):234–242, 2010 19751968

Parnas J, Møller P, Kircher T, et al: EASE: Examination of Anomalous Self-Experience. Psychopathology 38(5):236–258, 2005 16179811

Peters E, Ward T, Jackson M, et al: Clinical, socio-demographic and psychological characteristics in individuals with persistent psychotic experiences with and without a "need for care." World Psychiatry 15(1):41–52, 2016 26833608

Phalen PL, Dimaggio G, Popolo R, et al: Aspects of Theory of Mind that attenuate the relationship between persecutory delusions and social functioning in schizophrenia spectrum disorders. J Behav Ther Exp Psychiatry 56:65–70, 2017 27432819

Phillips LJ, McGorry PD, Garner B, et al: Stress, the hippocampus and the hypothalamic-pituitary-adrenal axis: implications for the development of psychotic disorders. Aust N Z J Psychiatry 40(9):725–741, 2006 16911747

Quijada Y, Kwapil TR, Tizón J, et al: Impact of attachment style on the 1-year outcome of persons with an at-risk mental state for psychosis. Psychiatry Res 228(3):849–856, 2015 26032461

Rich ME, Caldwell HK: A role for oxytocin in the etiology and treatment of schizophrenia. Front Endocrinol (Lausanne) 6:90, 2015 26089815

Rudrauf D, Bennequin D, Granic I, et al: A mathematical model of embodied consciousness. J Theor Biol 428:106–131, 2017 28554611

Schultze-Lutter F, Michel C, Schmidt SJ, et al: EPA guidance on the early detection of clinical high risk states of psychoses. Eur Psychiatry 30(3):405–416, 2015 25735810

Schultze-Lutter F, Debbané M, Theodoridou A, et al: Revisiting the basic symptom concept: toward translating risk symptoms for psychosis into neurobiological targets. Front Psychiatry 7:9, 2016 26858660

Shamay-Tsoory SG, Abu-Akel A: The social salience hypothesis of oxytocin. Biol Psychiatry 79(3):194–202, 2016 26321019

Sheinbaum T, Bedoya E, Ros-Morente A, et al: Association between attachment prototypes and schizotypy dimensions in two independent non-clinical samples of Spanish and American young adults. Psychiatry Res 210(2):408–413, 2013 24011849

Sheinbaum T, Kwapil TR, Barrantes-Vidal N: Fearful attachment mediates the association of childhood trauma with schizotypy and psychotic-like experiences. Psychiatry Res 220(1–2):691–693, 2014 25095756

Strathearn L: Maternal neglect: oxytocin, dopamine and the neurobiology of attachment. J Neuroendocrinol 23(11):1054–1065, 2011 21951160

Sullivan RM: The neurobiology of attachment to nurturing and abusive caregivers. Hastings Law J 63(6):1553–1570, 2012 24049190

Tessner KD, Mittal V, Walker EF: Longitudinal study of stressful life events and daily stressors among adolescents at high risk for psychotic disorders. Schizophr Bull 37(2):432–441, 2011 19734244

Tiwari A, Gonzalez A: Biological alterations affecting risk of adult psychopathology following childhood trauma: A review of sex differences. Clin Psychol Rev 66:69–79, 2018 29433843

Walker EF, Diforio D: Schizophrenia: a neural diathesis-stress model. Psychol Rev 104(4):667–685, 1997 9337628

Walker EF, Brennan PA, Esterberg M, et al: Longitudinal changes in cortisol secretion and conversion to psychosis in at-risk youth. J Abnorm Psychol 119(2):401–408, 2010 20455612

Warrier V, Grasby KL, Uzefovsky F, et al: Genome-wide meta-analysis of cognitive empathy: heritability, and correlates with sex, neuropsychiatric conditions and cognition. Mol Psychiatry 23(6):1402–1409, 2018 28584286

Weijers J, Ten Kate C, Eurelings-Bontekoe E, et al: Mentalization-based treatment for psychotic disorder: protocol of a randomized controlled trial. BMC Psychiatry 16:191, 2016 27278250

Weijers J, Fonagy P, Eurelings-Bontekoe E, et al: Mentalizing impairment as a mediator between reported childhood abuse and outcome in nonaffective psychotic disorder. Psychiatry Res 259:463–469, 2018 29145104

Index

Page numbers printed in **boldface** *type refer to tables or figures.*
Specific mentalization-based treatments are abbreviated in subentries.